THE PRESCHOOL
CHILD

WILEY SERIES IN CHILD AND ADOLESCENT MENTAL HEALTH

Joseph D. Noshpitz, Editor

THE PRESCHOOL CHILD

ASSESSMENT, DIAGNOSIS, AND TREATMENT

PAUL V. TRAD

Child Outpatient Department
Cornell University Medical Center
Westchester Division

WILEY

A Wiley-Interscience Publication

JOHN WILEY & SONS

New York   Chichester   Brisbane   Toronto   Singapore

DSM-III-R material is reprinted with permission
from *The Diagnostic and Statistical Manual
of Mental Disorders, Third Edition, Revised,*
Copyright 1987 American Psychiatric Association.

Library of Congress Cataloging-in-Publication Data

Trad, Paul V.
    The preschool child : assessment, diagnosis, and treatment / Paul
V. Trad.
        p.   cm.—(Wiley series in child and adolescent mental
health)
    Bibliography: p.
    ISBN 0-471-61757-1
    1. Child psychopathology.   2. Preschool children—Mental health.
I. Title.   II. Series.
    [DNLM: 1. Child, Preschool.   2. Mental Disorders—diagnosis.
3. Mental Disorders—in infancy & childhood. WS 350 T763p]
RJ499.T73   1989
618.92'89—dc19
DNLM/DLC
for Library of Congress   88-20731
                                                                              CIP

Printed and bound by Quinn - Woodbine, Inc.

Series Preface

This series is intended to serve a number of functions. It includes works on child development; it presents material on child advocacy; it publishes contributions to child psychiatry; and it gives expression to cogent views on child rearing and child management. The mental health of parents and their interaction with their children is a major theme of the series, and emphasis is placed on the child as individual, as family member, and as a part of the larger social surround.

Child development is regarded as the basic science of child mental health, and within that framework research works are included in this series. The many ethical and legal dimensions of the way society relates to its children are the central theme of the child advocacy publications, as well as a primarily demographic approach that highlights the role and status of children within society. The child psychiatry publications span studies that concern the diagnosis, description, therapeutics, rehabilitation, and prevention of the emotional disorders of childhood. And the views of thoughtful and creative contributors to the handling of children under many different circumstances (retardation, acute and chronic illness, hospitalization, handicap, disturbed social conditions, etc.) find expression within the framework of child rearing and child management.

Family studies with a central child mental health perspective are included in the series, and explorations into the nature of parenthood and the parenting process are emphasized. This includes books about divorce, the single parent, the absent parent, parents with physical and emotional illnesses, and other conditions that significantly affect the parent-child relationship.

Finally, the series examines the impact of larger social forces, such as war, famine, migration, and economic failure, on the adaptation of children and families. In the largest sense, the series is devoted to books that illuminate the special needs, status, and history of children and their families, within all perspectives that bear on their collective mental health.

JOSEPH D. NOSHPITZ

Children's Hospital Medical Center and
The George Washington University
Washington, D.C.

Preface

The Preschool Child: Assessment, Diagnosis, and Treatment represents an integrated approach to deciphering the developmental phenomena that occur in children of preschool age. Previously, this population has not garnered the attention it truly deserves because most analyses either have focused on toddlerhood as a footnote to the period of infancy or have concentrated on young school-age children who have a full repertoire of verbal abilities. While both of these age groups offer compelling insights for the developmental clinician, the preschool period is equally worthy of scrutiny.

During this period from approximately 2 to 6 years of age, young children grapple with perceptions of emerging selfhood, acquire sophisticated linguistic skills, and begin a challenging journey away from the protective orbit of the family for the first time. No longer infants, but not yet independent youngsters, preschoolers are poised in a delicate chronological domain that motivates them to rapidly acquire sufficient developmental capacities to master the tasks posed by an exciting and occasionally forbidding external world. Moreover, their evolving fascination with the seemingly endless variety of the external world is paralleled by dramatic alterations in internal, psychological reality. It is during this period that a distinctive personality emerges, as the preschooler displays a full range of affective and cognitive dimensions. This book, then, elaborates on the myriad absorbing developmental changes that occur in these young children and explains how development can either proceed adaptively or become impaired during this most fascinating era of growth.

In elaborating on the themes that emerge during the preschool years, I selected a format that would highlight the most seminal developmental events of this period. I analyzed each of these events from the perspective of a clinician or practitioner who actually interacts with preschoolers on a daily basis. By integrating theoretical and practical approaches in this fashion, I divided the book into five fundamental sections. These include Developmental Perspective, Assessment, Clinical Syndromes, Specific Risk Factors During the Preschool Years, and Management. Numerous case histories are interspersed in the text to provide readers with an accessible interpretation of such developmental problems as borderline personality traits; developmental learning disorders; abuse; separation and conduct disorders; gender identity disorders; affective problems; and behavioral impairments that have a physiologic component such as enuresis and eating and sleeping disorders. In each instance, the reader is provided with the most recent interpretations of the etiology of the disorder, with insights for arriving at an accurate differential diagnosis and effective treatment strategies. It is my hope that all health-care professionals who work with the preschool population will benefit from exposure to this book and will experience a renewed sense of exhilaration from reading about this fascinating and compelling developmental period.

I owe special thanks and deep gratitude to Paulina F. Kernberg, M.D., Director of the Child and Adolescent Division, Department of Psychiatry, Cornell Medical College-Westchester Division, Eduardo Greenblatt, Ph.D., Jo Rosenberg, M.S.W., Stelle Schecter, M.S.W., and Marisa Horowitz, who have motivated me to explore the psychiatric challenges posed by the preschool population and have consistently demonstrated enthusiastic support for my academic efforts. I am also grateful to Lynn Yanuck, Director of the White Plains Day Care Center, and Martha Brogan, coordinator of Prime Time, for enabling me and the trainees rotating in our department to spend numerous happy hours meeting with preschoolers and their parents.

Stan Shaffer, Sara Lee Chazan, Ph.D., Henri Schwartz, M.D., and Walter Kass, Ph.D. contributed their invaluable critical skills to this work. I extend my deepest thanks to them. Sharon Yamamoto, Stephanie Hill, James Wtorkowski, and Vernon Bruette are also thanked for assistance in preparing the manuscript. I am especially thankful for the support and friendship of Richard H. White of Seattle, Washington, who has always encouraged my research and cheered me on. Finally, I wish to thank Wendy Luftig, whose qualities of dedication and good humor make me believe that all worthwhile pursuits are capable of being realized.

I would like to dedicate this book to my parents, George and Blanche Trad.

Paul V. Trad, M.D.
Cornell University Medical Center
White Plains, New York

Contents

PART V
MANAGEMENT

Introduction

ORGANIZATION OF THE BOOK

The nature of the therapeutic alliance between the preschool child and the therapist is indeed unique and serves as a pivotal model from which the child can learn adaptive behavior. Nevertheless, weaving the threads of this alliance into an integrated pattern can be problematic at times. Because the child projects overtones of unconscious attitudes toward the caregiver onto the therapist, both child and therapist are taxed when forging such a relationship.

During the evolution of this relationship, the child reenacts feelings associated with the loss of the ideal parent. Relinquishment of this omnipotent, beneficent, or disorganizing image usually occurs during the process of separating and individuating, and preschoolers in treatment can be expected to have accomplished this sometimes precarious developmental achievement. From the child's perspective, the therapist will be competing with an invisible, albeit ever-present, rival—the original introjected model of the parent. As a result, it becomes the therapist's task to empathically prove to the child that an adult can behave in a manner that differs from the child's unconsciously introjected experiences. The therapist must also be aware of the fact that the preschool child will be refocusing on the original model of the ideal parent each time the child experiences the therapeutic relationship as a threat to the existence of this internal model.

By continually helping the child to make this contrast—between the introjected ideal parent's behavior and the behaviors of the real therapist—the therapist helps the child exercise reality-testing skills. Progress is made toward adaptive behavior when the child candidly shares feelings and thoughts without fearing the side effects of resurrecting memories of a lost object. This seminal point in treatment will be reached when the child has resolved unconscious conflict aroused by either interaction with or loss of the caregiver to the extent that it is possible to establish new models for personal relationships without superimposing onto them the affective residue of previous experiences. The child has, in other words, overcome developmental impediments so that each encounter is viewed as a fresh and bold opportunity to master the nuances of a new relationship.

But this process can be arduous for preschoolers who are struggling to overcome the aftermath of imperfect developmental phenomena. During therapy with such young children, the past will eventually become identical to the present, as both therapist and child strive to maintain equilibrium in a psychological jungle that, for the child, is tangled with distortions from previous developmental traumas and terror at the new obstacles that await.

Another characteristic that is emblematic of caregivers who are engaged in an adaptive relationship with their children is *previewing*. Previewing is best described as the caregiver's proclivity to gradually introduce the child to imminent developmental achievements and then, just as gradually, to assist the child in returning to his or her current developmental status. As one illustration, a caregiver who is aware that an infant has begun to display inchoate crawling motions might slowly exercise the infant's legs in a pattern that simulates crawling, and when the infant begins to display signs of boredom or exhaustion, the caregiver will taper off the activity. Essentially, previewing serves two functions that promote adaptive development. First, previewing exercises provide the child with a flavor of accomplishments to come and allow him to revel in ever-increasing mastery over the environment. Second, by previewing development for the child, the caregiver conveys the message that she is present as a supportive partner for the child, thus consolidating the attachment bond between the pair. For these reasons, previewing behaviors exhibited by the caregiver tend to motivate and propel the child in the direction of adaptive development.

Even for children whose previous developmental history has not been troubled, however, the preschool years represent an especially vulnerable stage. This pivotal period is a time in the developmental chart when notions of *good* (nurturing) and *bad* (depriving) are detached and differentiated from one another. Prior to this age, these concepts were aspects of a unified, interconnected, and interdependent system. Just as during infancy children perceive of themselves as being one, integrated with their caregivers as a unit, so too are their notions of good and bad inextricably linked. But with toddlerhood and separation—both physical and psychological—from the exclusive orbit of their caregivers, preschoolers must begin coping with the differentiation of such concepts as good and bad and with the developmental sequelae accompanying these achievements.

Gradually, then, preschoolers come to realize that their emotional experiences are not necessarily identical to the emotional experiences of their caregivers, so that when they feel "good" it is possible for their caregivers to feel "bad" and vice versa. Even when both children and caregivers feel good simultaneously, moreover, during the preschool years children experience the new realization that they can control their "good" feelings. The growing ability to contrast this splitting of "good" and "bad" emerges because preschool children are now capable of maintaining internal representations and comparing present experiences with previous expectations. By virtue of this comparative process, "good" and "bad" become differentiated and separately identified.

Psychopathology during the preschool years derives from a form of stultified development that prevents the child from engaging in this process of comparison and differentiation. "Good" and "bad" are not distinguished as being separate, nor are the nurturing and depriving aspects of the caregiver perceived as being different, or separate, from aspects of the child's internal representations. This occurs if the caregiver is not nurturing, so that the child's experience is primarily one of deprivation. In contrast, children who experience a nurturing environment can *actively defy* episodes of deprivation, because they will recognize the presence of such episodes by comparing them with nurturing episodes. They will engage in protesting behavior, manifested by cries and irritability, when their interactions with caregivers are not sufficiently gratifying. Children whose environment is permeated with deprivation, however, will not be equipped to defy their caregivers.

It is important to remember that prior to the preschool years infants—whether in a nurturing or depriving ambience—empathically experience the mood fluctuations of their caregivers in a global fashion as if they were their own mood fluctuations. With the advent of toddlerhood, adaptive preschoolers begin to use defiance as a method for differentiating both the good and bad aspects of the caregiver's mood. This defiance often provokes caregivers to abandon a depriving stance and return to a nurturing attitude. But if a caregiver has created a maladaptive atmosphere for a child, one permeated by deprivation, the child mistakenly perceives that good and bad, as embodied in the child's behavior, are not experienced differently by the caregiver. Such children are not motivated to begin modifying their behavior or exhibiting defiance to evoke a particular response by the caregiver.

These specific abilities—to differentiate and to regulate—enable preschoolers to contrast and evaluate maternal response in a dynamic fashion. When the dyad is adaptive, this period marks the time when preschoolers can independently assess how their caregivers respond to their positive or negative feelings. After a time, infants begin to exert internal control over these feelings, displaying positive affects when they wish to elicit a positive response and negative affects when they wish to evoke change. By engaging in this form of experimentation, preschoolers begin to confirm that what they feel is different from what the caregiver feels. Moreover, by attributing meaning to the caregiver's responses, children learn how to differentiate their own intentions from those being communicated by the caregiver.

Thus, the phenomenon of differentiation is the emblematic developmental milestone of the preschool years, and differentiation in a multitude of formats typifies children's behaviors during this period. Not only do they learn to differentiate their own behaviors, but they also acquire the skill to differentiate their caregivers' behaviors and distinguish between the caregivers' intentions and their own. These rapid and dramatic changes in perceptions can occur only if the environment—particularly the environment created by the caregiver—is one geared to promote an infant's cognitive and affective maturation. When children are not provided with full reign to experiment flexibly with their emerging capabilities of differentiation, it is probable that psychopathology will develop.

The following chapters are devoted to an in-depth assessment of the developmental phenomena of this fascinating and challenging preschool period and to a discussion of how adaptation can be so thwarted during this period that psychopathology erupts.

In striving to provide a coherent description of children's developmental processes between the ages of 2 and 6 years, this book discusses both the historic and current views that shape diagnostic and treatment approaches in this young population. Pertinent case history material is interspersed throughout the text to provide readers with vivid illustrations of how psychopathology is manifested in children of this age.

This book is divided into five basic sections. Part One, "The Developmental Perspective," examines normative development through the interpretation of a single case study. In this section, the reader is provided with discussions of affective and cognitive development, the emergence of adaptive levels of aggression, beliefs about locus of control, and the evolution of play behaviors. Each of these areas is dissected individually and is subsequently compared to and interwoven with the discussion of the case study. Thus, the reader is encouraged to delve into the discrete features of each individual developmental process, as well as to conceptualize the overall tapestry of adaptive functioning.

Part Two, "Assessment," contains a systematic discussion of the nosological and epidemiological implications of various symptoms and symptom clusters. This section also contains a detailed description of guidelines for performing examinations of the mental status of young children. Specific strategies are analyzed for reliably eliciting and judging each of the behavioral nuances that can occur during interactions with preschool children. In addition, one chapter is devoted to examining the effect of each of the neuroendocrine agents during normative and dysfunctional emotional states. Detailed analysis is centered around the similar and dissimilar endocrinologic profiles that characterize each disorder.

Comparison analysis—both between normal and abnormal development and between the symptoms of various psychiatric disturbances—is the theme of Part Three, "Clinical Syndromes." Here, the attempt is made to integrate the symptoms of myriad disorders found in young children. This section represents one of the first attempts to catalog the symptoms of all of these psychiatric disturbances within one coherent scheme. It also offers the reader systematic guidelines for achieving differential diagnoses, since the critical aspects of overlap between normative development, symptoms, and syndromes are systematically discussed.

Certain special risk situations—such as parental psychopathology, separation reaction due to nursery attendance, divorce or death of a caregiver, and child abuse and neglect—which are known to be etiologic triggers to psychopathology—are discussed in Part Four, "Specific Risk Factors During the Preschool Years." In contrast to earlier discussion of specific disorders, the emphasis with these situational risk factors is on predicting the various types of scenarios that might emerge when these variables are present.

The fifth and final section of the book, "Management," develops treatment strategies and contains a comprehensive and original scheme for devising an appropriate protocol based on assessment of the individual case. Therapies are described and evaluated for each of the disorders cataloged.

Part I

The Developmental Perspective

CHAPTER ONE

A Developmental Analysis

Alain: Case Study of Aggressive Behavior

Alain is a $3\frac{1}{2}$-year-old white boy, the only child of two middle-income parents, both of whom work. Alain was born out of wedlock while his mother still lived with her parents. During the first year of his life, he lived with his mother and grandparents in their home. When he was 14 months old, Alain's mother married his natural father, and the new family moved into an apartment in the same community. For the next 2 years, Alain's father went to work each day while his mother stayed home and cared for her son.

During this time both parents report that Alain was a happy, energetic boy, engaging in numerous games and fantasies with his mother. He especially liked being read to by his mother and was very proficient with his hands, spending a considerable time each day playing with small toys and building with construction sets. Whenever Alain's mother needed a babysitter, one of his maternal grandparents would come over and watch after him. In general, Alain was exposed to relatively few people from outside the family circle, since his parents rarely entertained at home, preferring to go outside the home for their entertainment.

When Alain was 3 years, 6 months of age, his mother started working full time. Since his grandparents did not want the responsibility of full-time care, Alain was enrolled in a neighborhood day-care facility. He exhibited a relatively high level of stress for the first 2 weeks of being left at the pre-school each day. He would cry inconsolably for 1 or 2 hours and occasionally throw a temper tantrum, flinging the toys around him and refusing to be comforted by his teachers. However, Alain began to settle down during the third week at the day-care facility and continued to do well until, in the middle of the fifth week, he became involved in a fight with another, slightly older boy. Alain received a black eye and a slightly cut lip, but he managed to inflict some minor physical injuries on the other child as well.

His mother was very upset by the incident, but his teacher reassured her that such incidents occur occasionally and that there was no cause for undue alarm in light of Alain's good overall progress in adapting to the pre-school setting. However, following this incident, Alain became involved in conflict with his peers on an almost daily basis. These episodes were largely confined to the area of the room where the smaller games, toys, and construction sets were located. Alain was virtually always the instigator in the disruptive episodes.

Few of the incidents were as violent as the first one, but their frequency eventually led the teacher to agree with Alain's mother that it might be advisable to obtain an evaluation of his behavior.

INTRODUCTION

Rather than presenting specific developmental milestones this chapter will characterize normal development through the developmental analysis of the case of Alain, a child who, despite his difficult behavior, was not considered dysfunctional. If there is one need that generates a constant drive in the human organism it is the need for control. Whether they are reflected in dominance over the environment or over personal responses, manifestations of control are inevitably preferred to the inability to exert control. It can be said that the characteristic ways in which the individual attempts to control both self and the environment comprise the fundamental components of personality. In nonpathologic individuals, the objective of control by the ego is to reduce anxiety by achieving a maximum level of impulse expression while maintaining an acceptable margin of safety in interactions with the environment. For children, frustration arising from the inability to control all situations at all times causes a continuous but varying state of arousal.

When the ego fails too drastically in its attempts at control, the individual commonly reacts with behaviors indicative of *under-* or *overcontrol*. Those who become overcontrolled restrict their impulses and feelings, become unresponsive, inhibit their actions, and delay gratification. In children, this extreme self-suppression can lead to bouts of impulsive, aggressive behavior when the child's control falters in the face of overwhelming frustration. Undercontrol is characterized by the immediate expression of impulses and feelings, a high level of distractibility, hostile aggression, and lack of socialization. While both of these dysregulations of ego control are associated with aggressive outbursts and disordered behavior, Alain's symptomatology suggests the possibility of an undercontrolled coping style, since he is very active and freely expresses emotions.

When assessing the pathogenicity of Alain's behavior, it is essential to determine whether or not he is engaging in a truly damaging style of aggression. Parens (1979) has made a useful distinction regarding aggressive behavior, breaking it up into two subtypes. The first, nondestructive aggression, is merely directed at mastering certain challenges during the course of development. The second, hostile or destructive aggression, is directed at eliminating a social or physical structure that is perceived with intensely negative feeling as being extremely thwarting.

Whether Alain's behavior is of the hostile, pathologic type can be determined by assessing a number of factors known to be related to this type of aggression. Hostile aggression resulting from strong, threatening feelings of not being in control is accompanied by certain deficits in cognition, emotion, motivation, and self-esteem. Thus, evaluation of these parameters provides a good indication of the nature and intensity of aggression in a child. Furthermore, children who are repeatedly exposed to uncontrollable situations commonly develop an external locus of control and may even display signs of learned helplessness. Analysis of these factors, all of which are associated with feelings of uncontrollability that can foster aggression, will assist the clinician in evaluating the type and severity of Alain's aggressive behavior.

Play activities, both alone and with parents and peers, provide the richest and most immediate source of diagnostic information in the clinical setting. For children from 2 to 6 years of age, who lack the verbal skills to communicate their internal state, play behavior represents the primary means of expressing thoughts and feelings about the world. Furthermore, because play occurs in a make-believe situation, it provides a safe arena in which children can feel free to release emotions they might otherwise repress for fear of retribution. In this setting they are also free to demonstrate capabilities that are positive in nature, such as empathic understanding. Empathy has special significance for assessing aggressive behavior, since the ability to comprehend the feelings of others is a major inhibitor of aggressive actions.

COGNITION AND ITS RELATION TO AGGRESSIVE BEHAVIOR

Cognitive Stages and Their Implications

The greater a child's ability to form an internal representation of the world and of its cause and effect relationships, the greater his or her ability to achieve mastery and avoid high levels of frustration that can lead to feelings of uncontrollability and hostile aggression. Cognitive ability, however, develops in stages. As in all other areas of development, the child must move from undifferentiated, unregulated patterns of thought to more sophisticated systems of symbol encoding. Alain, who is $3\frac{1}{2}$ years old, would be expected to function cognitively at the level of Piaget's preoperational subperiod. Deficits in this level of functioning may indicate that Alain is vulnerable not only to aggressive behavior, but to depression as well (Trad, 1986, 1987).

The task posing the most formidable challenge to the development of cognition is that of making the distinction between which elements of perception emanate from inside and which emanate from outside the child. This distinction is most difficult to make for the child who is engaging in preoperational thinking, but it will become easier as the discriminative process becomes more sophisticated.

Preoperational thinking begins soon after decentering, when children become able to perceive of objects as being separate from themselves (Piaget, 1929, 1948). This realization gives rise to the development of signifiers, for example, pointing or an audible noise, that allow children to refer to things outside of themselves. However, their ability to manufacture symbols during this period is far in advance of their ability to understand the symbols in a socially integrated way.

Therefore, children form assumptive philosophies regarding the nature of people and the physical world (Elkind, 1976). During this period, animism (the projection of lifelike properties onto inanimate objects) and magical thinking (the attribution of cause-effect occurrences to a child's own powers) are at their height. A good deal of egocentric thought is also generated as a result of the gap between concept formation and social testing. (That is, children are likely to evolve numerous spurious causal theories and make false assumptions about the properties of objects based strictly on their own limited experiences. For example, clouds are assumed to be alive because, like children, they move.)

Later, at approximately age 6, children start to engage in Piaget's second level of cognition, concrete operations. The ability to conserve develops, allowing them to evaluate the relative permanencies in the properties of objects even when they change appearance. (For example, upon seeing liquid poured from a short, wide glass into a tall, narrow one a child will understand that the volume of the liquid remains constant. This is in contrast to the assumption that the amount of liquid changed, which would be made by a child engaging in preoperational thinking.) Ultimately, around puberty, normal children achieve Piaget's level of formal operations, in which reality is assessed in a mature fashion. In children of this age, constant comparisons are made and tested between what is real and what is imaginary, what is possible and what is not.

Stages of Emotional Development

Keeping pace with the developing child's cognitive advancement is the evolution of emotional sophistication. Lane and Schwartz (1987) have devised a system for describing the stages of emotional development that combines the work of Piaget with that of Werner and Kaplan (1963), who have exhaustively explored the ways in which symbols are formed to provide a mental representation of reality.

Combining Werner and Kaplan's observations regarding the development of symbols with Piaget's theory of cognitive development, Lane and Schwartz have mapped out five levels of structural transformation that occur during the development of emotional awareness. The first level is sensorimotor reflexive. In this earliest phase, the involuntary motor phenomena that accompany emotion become activated. These motor manifestations include such events as autonomic and neuroendocrine changes as well as autonomic facial expressions. During the second stage of emotional awareness, the sensorimotor enactive level, emotion is experienced as a conscious feeling state.

The third level of structural transformation occurs during Piaget's preoperational subperiod, the level of cognition that one might expect Alain to be in if his development has proceeded normally. At this stage of emotional development, emotion is transformed from a somatic experience to a psychological one. Significantly, for the first time it becomes possible to express emotion at will.

The fourth level of emotional awareness is analogous to concrete operational thinking. The child can perceive blends of feelings at this stage as emotional experience broadens. The fifth and highest level is analogous to the cognitive stage of formal operations, in that emotional appreciation of the feelings of others (e.g., empathy) becomes feasible as the individual is increasingly able to integrate different feelings and form blends of diverse emotions. Lane and Schwartz have observed that this cognitive-developmental scheme for the growth of emotional awareness provides the clinician with a clue as to whether emotion is experienced as being primarily somatic, somatopsychic (i.e., as an action tendency), or psychological. Thus, a means is provided for gauging the child's level of emotional development. This outline provides the clinician with a useful tool because the domains of cognition and emotion are different, and although they reach sophistication via the same internal dynamics, they may evolve at different rates.

With regard to Lane and Schwartz's scheme, Alain's emotional development appears to be proceeding in step with his cognitive evolution. His repetitive expressions of aggression demonstrate a volitional use of emotion. However, he does not seem able to perceive blends of emotions to any significant degree, since his interpretation of others' behaviors seems limited to perceiving only what others want from him. Alain is only beginning to be socially interactive, and so he may fail to understand the feelings of his peers in the same way as he does those of his parents. Nevertheless, it has been shown that children even younger than Alain have developed some empathic ability. Zahn-Waxler and Radke-Yarrow (1982), using highly contextualized perspective-taking measures, have demonstrated that very young children (18 to 24 months) are capable of offering comfort to distressed friends and family members and switching strategies if the first attempt at comfort fails. Therefore, Alain's play during nonaggressive periods was examined and, indeed, he did express empathic understanding toward his favorite playmates on several occasions.

Since empathy provides a major source of inner control against aggressive actions, it will be important to monitor Alain's empathic displays over time to assess the degree of his prosocial development. The fact that his aggressive behavior currently outdistances the inhibitions induced by empathic comprehension might be explained in part by his barely developed empathic system and by the observed fact that empathy more frequently emerges when ego needs are satisfied (Strayer, 1980). Alain, because of his discontent at being left in the day-care facility, is in the process of readjusting his ego demands and so may not yet feel inclined to inhibit his aggressive urges.

It may also be that, to some degree, Alain's repeated outbursts reflect his experimentation with the volitional expression of feelings. If this is the case, some of these outbursts may be attributable to the desire to "fire for effect," to see what this new behavioral mode elicits from the environment.

Mediational Role of the Caregiver

When discussing the development of the cognitive and emotional systems, it is vital to emphasize that the nature of the child's relationship with the caregiver plays a pivotal role in determining the degree of sophistication attained in both domains—and, hence, the degree to which aggressive behavior is incorporated in a nonpathologic fashion. The development of the child's ability to form symbols and use them to construct an inward, mental representation of the world outside signals not only the development of cognition and emotion, but also the beginning of separation from the caregiver. The attachment behaviors that then evolve over the course of interaction with the caregiver can be viewed as the external manifestations of an internal working model of the self. Therefore, if these behaviors become disorganized or dysregulated due to maternal overintrusiveness, overprotectiveness, or ambivalence, the child will experience difficulty in gaining mastery over the environment because he or she will be using an unstable internal working representation of the self based on the inconsistent interactions arising from an insecure attachment bond.

With respect to cognition, the importance of the attachment bond stems from the fact that *the process of separating from the mother forms the basis for self-object differentiation.* If an infant is overly afraid to separate, due to either a highly reactive temperament or maternal ambivalence that curtails the development of security, the infant will have difficulty in making other, later differentiations between self and outside objects.

There are three identifiable types of attachment between infant and caregiver (Ainsworth & Wittig, 1969). The *securely attached* infant is at least risk for developing pathological behavior, including hostile aggression. Such an infant is characterized by a wide range of emotional expressions and by an eagerness to reunite with the mother after brief separations. The *avoidant infant,* in contrast, shows little distress at the mother's departure and displays minimal desire to reunite with her when she returns. The third type of attachment bond, termed *resistant,* is characterized by either a great deal of distress or marked passivity during separations from the mother. The latter two types of attachment are indicative of children who are having difficulty in establishing object constancy with regard to the mother. Since the mother provides the template or touchstone for all objects, cognitive confusion is likely to emerge as these children attempt to apply the same anxious feelings and inconsistent rules that have developed in their attitude toward the mother to other objects in the environment. The success of their efforts at mastery is thereby blunted, and resultant feelings of rage and frustration may give rise to dysregulated aggressive behavior.

In addition to inaugurating the formation of the attachment bond, the loss of egocentrism upon gaining the ability to form mental representations also initiates the process of *separation-individuation*, as described by Mahler, Pine, and Bergman (1975). The beginning of the loss of egocentrism coincides with Mahler and co-workers' "differentiation subphase" of separation and individuation from the mother, which occurs at approximately 5 to 10 months of age. While an irritable mood typically accompanies this difficult time, the negative, fearful feelings of the differentiation subphase are somewhat offset when, at approximately 12 months of age, the "practicing subphase" begins to emerge. This period is characterized by the infant's further exploration of the environment and increased efforts to distance himself or herself from the caregiver. In the normally developing child, pleasurable feelings from exploratory efforts tend to counteract any negative feelings that arise when the child is not in the presence of the caregiver.

At approximately 16 months of age, following the practicing subphase, the "rapprochement subphase" begins. In terms of the genesis of aggressive behavior, this may be the most crucial stage in the child's development. During this period, the infant begins to display extreme separation reactions such as temper tantrums. While the particular behaviors depend on the interactions between the mother and infant, infants during this time show ambivalence about being with the caregiver, a tendency to change mood rapidly, and a certain free-floating dissatisfaction.

Children become highly activated during the rapprochement subphase because, in addition to the struggle to establish a consistent identity in the face of a growing awareness of separateness, they must also face three fears simultaneously: fear of object loss (i.e., the caregiver), fear of losing the object's love, and castration anxiety (Mahler et al., 1975). Pertinent to Alain's case, McDevitt (1985) has posited that there is an increased risk for inward-directed hostile aggressive behavior during this time. The ongoing process of identification merges with early superego formation to redirect aggressive impulses in toward the unconscious, where some may become encoded as fantasies while others may be acted upon. Hostile actions are directed not outward but toward the self, in accordance with the dictates of the undeveloped superego.

Since Alain is currently enmeshed in the phallic-Oedipal years, he also has the potential for outward-directed aggression, in terms of psychoanalytic theory (Cohen, Marans, Dahl, Marans, & Lewis, 1987). During this time, the child is trying to modulate aggressive urges stemming from sexual feelings about the opposite-sex parent and jealousy of the same-sex parent. Because psychoanalytic theory is concerned with the development of subjective experiences, viewing Alain's behavior in these terms may prove enlightening (Dare, 1985).

In psychoanalytic terminology, the years from age 3 to age 6 are characterized as the stage of initiative versus guilt. Sours (1980) has pointed out that there are many changes in ego functioning and even in instinctual functioning during this age period. These include (1) a shift from dependency toward adult object relationships; (2) the transition from suckling to eating; (3) progression from wetting and soiling to bladder and bowel control; (4) progression from irresponsibility in body management to responsibility; (5) growth from egocentricity to companionship; and (6) transitions from body concentration to the toy world and from play to work, as well as changes in the structure and function of dreams and fantasies.

Since Alain is just entering this period of development, he is likely experiencing a burst of energy and curiosity. Not only is he actively trying to win his mother's favor over his father, but he also sees himself as having a social role for the first time. He is no longer a baby, and he strives to act the part. However, he is still experiencing the pressure of instinctual drives that cannot be immediately gratified in reality. Therefore, he must refuse to believe that he is small and unable to partake of the pleasures available to adults (Cohen et al., 1987).

The need to repress the realization of the relative powerlessness of this period is crucial to survival because efforts powered by the great energy of youth at meeting the challenge to become an adult are inevitably met with frustration and denial. During this time, defeat and humiliation are ubiquitous.

It is through autonomy that Alain can combat his sense of shame and powerlessness, and it is through play that he can suspend disbelief and learn to experiment with a safe level of autonomous functioning. Thus, oppositional behavior is a common occurrence during this period, as the child strives to find an acceptable level of autonomous functioning. Since Alain is entering this phase and has not yet evolved elaborate play behaviors, it is reasonable to expect that his strivings for autonomy will be somewhat primitive and violent. Therefore, the relative pathogenicity of his behavior should be examined through this tempered lens.

The instinctual and ego changes Alain is experiencing basically characterize the fourth and final stage of separation-individuation, which Mahler and co-workers termed "consolidation of individuality and the beginnings of emotional object constancy"—a time in which the internal representation of the caregiver (i.e., love object) becomes integrated and consolidated (Mahler et al., 1975, p. 109). Again, as was true for aberrant attachment bonds, pathological processes within the separation-individuation scheme are predominantly brought about by caregivers who are neglectful; inhibit any expression of aggression; or are overly interfering, intrusive, anxious, or controlling during this developmental stage.

Since so much of cognitive development hinges on the ability to make self-object discriminations, and since this ability in turn centers around infant-caregiver interaction, it might be advantageous to pause for a moment to assess the level of Alain's risk for developing psychopathological behavior by evaluating observations of his interaction with his mother. At age $3\frac{1}{2}$, Alain appears well adjusted to short-term absences of his mother. Upon her departure, he quickly becomes engaged in play activities, and he exhibits happiness upon her return. However, Alain does not respond so favorably to the longer absences of his mother after she leaves him at the day-care facility. The teacher reports that he cries and is "fussy" for some time after his mother departs each day. Also of concern is the fact that Alain is reported to be very active during day-care activities. The possibility of hyperactivity must be considered, since the accompanying inability to control impulses can predispose a child to aggressive behavior.

There is minimal evidence of disturbed interaction between Alain and his mother. Not only did his mother care for him full time for the first 3 years of his life, but her manner of engaging with him demonstrates a balanced blend of respect, playfulness, and discipline, and he gives every indication of having reached a positive, viable internal representation of her and of his relationship with her. However, at this juncture the clinician must also consider the possibility of a precocious ego organization. If his mother did in fact display ambivalence toward him during the first year of his life (a possibility, since she may have experienced ambivalent feelings as a result of giving birth out of wedlock), Alain may have reacted during the rapprochement subphase by forming a precocious overidentification with the love object, an action that results in pseudo self-sufficiency. This process gives rise to a self-concept that is ill-equipped to deal with life situations (McDevitt, 1985). As a result, children with precocious personality organizations are vulnerable to pathological outcomes and the inappropriate use of behavioral manifestations such as aggression (Trad, 1986).

Another possibility, although one that seems less likely in Alain's case, is that a child can react to fruitless attempts to achieve a constant, dependable vision of the caregiver by practicing learned helplessness. This condition was first described by Seligman and Maier (1967). According to these researchers, after repeated trials in which an organism's response is unsuccessful, the organism will fail to respond even to painful stimuli because it has "learned" that its behavior is ineffectual.

While play analysis will assist in determining the probabilities of precocious organization and learned helplessness, it is reasonable to speculate now that Alain's high activity level, along with the high level of individual attention to which he is accustomed as an only child, may combine to frustrate his expectations of environmental control in the new school environment, thus giving rise to aggressive acts. Without benefit of play analysis, however, it is not possible to diagnose whether his activity level is truly hyperactive or he is merely at the high end of the activity dimension of temperament. Play analysis will also assist in determining Alain's status with respect to the other major variables of temperament—threshold, intensity, and distractibility (Thomas, Chess, Birch, Hertzog, & Horn, 1963).

Mechanisms of Cognitive Inhibition of Aggression

Language. Just as insecure attachments to the caregiver can lead to the dysregulated expression of behaviors such as aggression due to the infant's inability to form a coherent scheme of self–object discrimination, secure attachment to the caregiver can result in the evolution of cognitive mechanisms for controlling hostile aggressive urges and mobilizing nondestructive aggressive acts. Parens (1979) has emphasized that nondestructive aggression is vital in motivating the individual to strive for self-assertive behavior and autonomy.

Language is one element of normative cognitive development that fosters the construction of limits on the type and intensity of aggressive, self-assertive acts. White (1965) has pointed out that the expression of first-available responses to a stimulus (i.e., rapid responses dependent upon thinking patterns similar to those of an animal in the same circumstances) can be inhibited by the process of encoding these initial urges in language. In this way, further cognitive processing can proceed. It is possible that, rather than becoming immersed in an attempt to achieve a cognitive interpretation of the stimulus, some aggressive children fail to perform the initial step of encoding the response in language. These children tend to rely instead on associative processing, a type of learning based on conventional associations between stimulus and response (e.g., running away from a rapidly approaching dog without considering which dog it might be). Since Alain's attachment to his mother is a good one, it is hardly surprising that he demonstrates good linguistic encoding. Thus, it seems doubtful that his aggressive behavior derives from a failure to first encode his responses in language.

Empathy.   Another aspect of cognitive development that results in inhibition of aggressive urges is the comprehension of intentionality. This is a very important developmental milestone, since the failure to differentiate the internal processes of others, and hence their intentions, from one's own intentions can quickly result in pathological behavior. Without this discriminative ability, children can only interpret the behavior of others, and the results of those behaviors, in terms of external physical events—a process that can quickly lead to problems. For instance, abused children might feel responsible for and/or match violence that is inflicted upon them if they confuse their own intentions with those of their abusers. However, as children gradually come to understand the reasons for their own intentions, they will begin to comprehend the motives of others.

Again, the ability to understand and attribute the intentions of others is closely related to the success with which children can form mental representations of themselves and others, including, first and foremost, their caregivers. This is important because an accurate understanding of intention fosters the development of empathy. Many investigators (e.g., Staub, 1971) have found that the capacity to empathize with the recipient of an aggressive action (i.e., to understand when an action is intended to harm and to vicariously feel the results of that intention) is a major internal inhibitor of aggressive behavior. Alain's observed empathic acts, although infrequent, suggest that he is developing normally along these lines.

THE ROLE OF PLAY IN THE GENESIS AND DIAGNOSIS OF AGGRESSIVE BEHAVIOR

Play situations provide the first means by which a child can generate and coordinate distinctions between appearance and reality (Flavell, Green, & Flavell, 1986). Therefore, failure to master play situations can limit the child's ability to make these distinctions across the board, in play and nonplay circumstances alike. Using diagnostic measures of the healthy child at play, the clinician can make comparisons between age-adjusted normal behaviors and the actual behavior of the child. Ultimately, play behaviors can be used to diagnose emotional and/or cognitive deficits.

When searching for the various developmental functions that can be facilitated by pretend situations, it is most logical to look at the *motivations* that propel children into the realm of play. Fundamentally, play serves to promote the processes of assimilation and accommodation, the means by which children come to understand the world (Piaget, 1962). According to Piaget, children initially use play as a means of mastering sensorimotor skills. Following this, play acquires symbolic meanings, and ultimately culminates in shared games. The broad functions of play can then be described as achieving organization of language, object functionality, person constancy, and reduction of maladaptive egocentric behavior.

In general, descriptions of these functions fall within two contexts, the psychoanalytic and cognitive-developmental interpretations. Within the psychoanalytic perspective, Levin and Turgeon (1957) have described play as a means by which children can release emotions that they dare not express otherwise. Freud (1909, 1922) believed that the symbolic nature of play results from unmet, infantile fantasies. Conflict, anxiety, tension, and guilt associated with these desires can be mastered via make-believe situations. In a play environment that is controllable and nonthreatening, children are periodically able to act out frustrations and obstacles that they have thus far been forced to accept in real life (Freud, 1962). Additionally, through play, children can retrospectively master traumatic events.

Cognitive-developmental explanations of the function of play center around the child's burgeoning ability to make appearance–reality and self–object distinctions. For example, role playing is crucial to the development of the child's sense of self (Cottrell, 1969; Denzin, 1977; Stone, 1965). Developing infants perceive their caregivers' reactions in order to make judgments about their own internal state.

In the cognitive sense, pretend play provides the child with an infinite number of new interpretations of events within a limitless choice of contexts (Baldwin, 1911). Singer (1979) has noted that play provides an opportunity for children to reduce unintelligible experiences into more manageable models, allowing them to then apply the newly learned information to any new stimuli that might be encountered. Singer has also observed that play provides children with an immediate coping mechanism, one in which they can act out and rehearse behaviors that have not yet been fully mastered. All of these purposes are served by pretend play, the means by which children can experiment with the differences between appearance and reality. This process appears to be one that is directed more at the consolidation of old information than at the acquisition of new material (Piaget, 1962, in Fein, 1981).

Many investigators have tried to uncover the developmental milestones that delineate the developmental progression to adequate appearance–reality discrimination. Flavell, Green, and Flavell (1986) have pointed out that during the process of pretending, the initially egocentric thought processes of the child quickly acquire elements of perspective taking and dual coding, the ability to recognize the same object in different contexts (e.g., the father is an employee and also a father).

Pretend play appears at roughly age 12 months and grows increasingly complex up to the age of 5 or 6 years. The earliest pretend acts of children are directed toward the self, displaying the presence of egocentricity. Occurring at approximately 1 year of age, these acts are little more than simulations of their own activities (e.g., drinking and sleeping) (Fenson & Ramsay, 1980). It is not until the second year of life that symbolic play appears, since this mode of cognition is not possible until the advent of representational thought (Ungerer, Zelazo, Kearsley, & O'Leary, 1981).

Smilansky (1968) has defined four categories of play that are thought to develop in a predetermined sequence, the first of which, functional play, describes the egocentric, sensorimotor pretend acts of 1-year-olds. The second category, constructive play, involves the organization and/ or use of objects in order to achieve a goal. Next to develop is dramatic play, in which pretend, as-if situations are concocted in order to fulfill the personal wishes and needs of the child. Finally, the-games-with-rules stage develops. This category represents the child's recognition and acceptance of predetermined, conscious rules in an organized situation.

Focusing on the fact that a child's play activities evolve over time and proceed through different levels of development, Parten (1932) and Parten and Newhall (1943) have pointed out that the function of play also changes in such a way as to accommodate the child's evolving cognitive and emotional needs. Likewise, the social style in which the child plays also changes. Fein (1979) has observed that children's play is usually solitary in nature up to age 3. After this time, dramatic play begins to develop until, by 5 years of age, the child has mastered sensorimotor play sequences and is beginning to be able to integrate knowledge concerning reciprocal roles, complex plots, and a vast array of objects and meanings into coherent themes.

As play activities increase and intensify, the child develops flexibility, being able to move from play to reality with great agility. This process facilitates the development of dual encoding ability, as emotions are fully invested in play, yet the existence of reality is not denied. At some point the child will begin to transfer dual-encoded knowledge from play situations to real situations, hoping to master other dual-encoded information. As an example, a boy might dress in a skirt outside of peer play and observe the reactions of his parents to discover whether he is treated differently or their attitudes toward him remain essentially the same.

The point at which dual-encoded knowledge is experimentally transferred to other situations may take place at Level 2 of a scheme of structured play levels put forth by McCune-Nicolich (1981). This investigator has postulated that the first step, Level 1, involves the meaningful use of sensorimotor actions for purposes other than achieving their original objective. The child functioning at Level 2 begins to show an awareness of these meanings by using them playfully. However, functioning at this level is limited due to the fact that all schemes are still associated with the child's own sensorimotor actions. Level 3 describes the onset of symbolic play with a clear decentration of meanings. At Level 4, the various schemes become arranged into sequences (e.g., the child drinks, then gives a drink to a doll; or the scheme for drinking and for going to bed could be applied to the doll in sequence). At the last level, Level 5, games may be constructed mentally prior to performance instead of being elicited by others.

In sum, play provides a rich diagnostic and therapeutic context in which the child, while expressing unconscious thoughts and processes, allows the observer to analyze them in order to diagnose the child's area of conflict. The clinician, taking note of the developmental level and mental status of the child through observation of play, can thus identify psychopathological behaviors or risk factors for the child's development.

ASSESSMENT OF ALAIN'S PLAY BEHAVIORS: INTERACTIONS BETWEEN COGNITIVE DEVELOPMENT AND AGGRESSION

As noted previously, the degree to which children are able to form internal representations of the world has a direct bearing on their ability to achieve mastery and thereby avoid high levels of frustration that can result in hostile, aggressive behavior. This ability depends on their degree of success in making appearance-reality discriminations, a task that is initially facilitated by secure interaction with responsive caregivers and later reinforced by play activities such as role playing.

If Alain is developing normally, he should be well into Piaget's preoperational stage of thinking. Judging from his play activities, this appears to be the case. He shows a good ability to distinguish between events that occur inside and outside of himself in that he frequently uses signifiers to refer to outside objects, although he might not know their purpose. Alain also displays the assumptive philosophy of animism that is characteristic of children of this age.

In terms of aggressive behavior, Alain is in a volatile period since, according to Lane and Schwartz's (1987) scheme of emotional development, all emotions at this stage are making the transition from a somatic to a psychological experience. This is the first time the child is able to express emotion volitionally. Therefore, the likelihood of mistakes (e.g., inappropriate behavior) is high during this early emotional learning phase. Any interpretation of Alain's aggressive behavior regarding risk for later psychopathology should be somewhat conservative since it must take into account the volatility and trial-and-error nature of emotional expression that accompanies this phase of development.

In terms of overall play behavior, Alain appears to be exhibiting intermediate to advanced behavior for a child of his age. While he is not entirely devoid of egocentric thinking, and he still prefers to play alone (which is normal for a child of his age), he is well into Smilansky's (1968) stage of dramatic play, which is the last stage of play to occur before the final stage of games with rules. His relatively advanced level of play may be partially attributable to the numerous times his mother read fairy tales to him.

Alain's apparent low risk for potentially disordered behavior in terms of his level of cognitive development is supported by his use of language and a pronounced ability to display empathy. As mentioned, both of these talents are related to the child's ability to inhibit aggressive urges. Thus, given the relationship between poor cognitive development and aggressive behavior, Alain appears to be at very low risk for dysregulated use of this behavior—at least once he passes out of the initially volatile trial-and-error period of emotional expression.

RELATION OF LOCUS OF CONTROL BELIEFS TO AGGRESSIVE BEHAVIOR

Origins of Attributional Style

The vicissitudes of cognitive development and their relation to the development and expression of aggression have already been discussed. However, there is one more avenue of investigation that may prove fruitful in assessing Alain's risk for inappropriate aggression and other dysregulated behaviors: locus of control (LOC).

The objective of the developing ego is to maximize expression of impulse while maintaining a tolerable level of anxiety by engaging in safe-enough interactions with the environment. The degree to which the ego is successful in achieving this objective gives rise to an internal assumption about control. That is, the individual comes to feel that he or she has either an *internal* or an *external* LOC. Those who believe that the events in their lives occur mostly as a result of their own efforts have an internal LOC, while those who believe that events are relatively unrelated to their actions feel their LOC to be external.

Beliefs about control may be realistic or unrealistic. Those who strongly believe that they are in control run the risk of taking responsibility for outcomes that in fact happened independently of their actions. Individuals who perceive that most control comes from the environment may fail to appreciate the degree to which an outcome actually did depend on their efforts.

Over the long run, individuals will develop an *attributional style* in which their efforts are seen as being either important or unimportant to the outcome of events. This attributional style, reflecting their beliefs about their own degree of control over the environment, has been found to be a facet of personality that persists over time and applies to a wide range of phenomena (Hegland & Galejs, 1983; Galejs & Hegland, 1982).

Not surprisingly, different evaluations of a person's degree of control over the environment have been found to be associated with distinct coping styles. In general, those with an external LOC exhibit less effective coping styles than those who feel they are in control of events (Parkes, 1984). Developmentally, the subjective experience of control is rooted in the infant's first experiences of discrepancy, contingency, and expectancy. These interrelated lines of development have strong affective components that serve to reinforce the infant's early experience of control. Once the infant has developed the cognitive capacity to discriminate among stimuli with different degrees of appeal and to perceive cause–effect relationships, the infant may establish the first traces of perceptions about control.

Children may well develop beliefs about their degree of control over the environment by preschool age, since the primary focus of contingency is the caregiver, with whom interactions exist in abundance by this age. Theoretically, the caregiver is the most responsive element in the infant's environment. By displaying a response such as a smile, the infant can elicit a similar response in the caregiver, a process that generates positive affect in the infant.

Thus, by preschool, children usually have an attributional style that is well enough developed to influence many of their interactions with significant persons. Because the competence with which young children interact with others at a very young age has been shown to predict many types of competence later in childhood, attitudes about locus of control, which reflect the success of early interactions, may be an important indication of a child's future level of adaptation (Arend, Gove, & Sroufe, 1979).

Control and Aggression

Brehm (1966), Rothbaum (1980), and others have developed a theory describing the relationship between feelings of lack of control and aggressive behavior. This theory is called *reactance theory*, and it suggests that when a person's control of a specific behavior is threatened, the individual will increase efforts to engage in that particular behavior and may employ hostile aggressive behaviors to do so. In effect, this so-called reactance is the opposite of helpless behavior.

Rothbaum (1980), in attempting to account for the fact that different individuals perceive different levels of uncontrollability, has hypothesized that perceptions of relatively low levels of uncontrollability (i.e., feelings not reflecting a lack of control) lead to reactance behavior. In contrast, high levels of perceived uncontrollability lead to learned helplessness.

This hypothesis has been tested experimentally by Roth and Kubal (1975) and Tennen and Eller (1977), who conducted experiments in which adult subjects were first exposed to a series of unsolvable problems and then given a task that was solvable. They found that subjects who were exposed to a smaller number of unsolvable tasks demonstrated increased persistence in solving the latter task, while subjects exposed to a greater number of unsolvable trials showed less persistence (i.e., they showed helplessness). Significantly, the investigators also found that the higher degrees of uncontrollability that led to decreased persistence were associated with feelings of helplessness and powerlessness. Rothbaum further observed that the perception of *lack* of control might change in some cases to a perception of *loss* of control, which might then produce a change in feeling from apathy to anger.

ANALYSIS OF ALAIN'S AGGRESSIVE BEHAVIOR: LOCUS OF CONTROL

In light of the fact that Alain's potential risk for dysregulated aggressive behavior should be evaluated conservatively due to his stage of emotional development, and because he appears to be more than adequately advanced in terms of overall cognitive and empathic ability, the roots of his frequent aggressive behavior should be sought elsewhere, if possible.

It appears in this case that the problematic hostile aggression can be explained in terms of reactance theory. While Alain appears to be developing a healthy attributional style, displaying little of the negative affect that usually accompanies a sense of external locus of control, he may nevertheless experience feelings of anger when thwarted in his attempts to play with his favorite kinds of toys. These feelings, in combination with his anxiety over being left by his mother in a strange place, his inexperience in expressing emotion volitionally, and his somewhat pampered history as an only child, could well lead to aggressive acts.

However, it seems unlikely that these localized acts of aggression will result in lasting pathology. Alain is progressing admirably in his cognitive and emotional development. Furthermore, Feshbach and Feshbach (1969) have noted that peers evaluate aggression serving socially motivated purposes more positively than aggression purely in the service of the self. Thus, Alain's aggressive actions on his own behalf are likely to be unreinforced, paving the way to eventual extinction of this behavior. It seems likely that with more teacher supervision and more experience in expressing emotions while interacting with his peers, Alain will gradually relinquish the tendency to express his aggressive urges in so volatile a manner.

Part II

Assessment

CHAPTER TWO

Multiaxial Approach to Diagnosing Childhood Psychiatric Conditions

Steven: A Housewrecker

Steven is a 3-year, 7-month-old boy who lives with his older brother in a foster home. He was born of a full-term pregnancy. His mother, a single parent, abused alcohol and marijuana during the pregnancy. Steven reportedly reached developmental milestones within normal limits, and his medical history is remarkable only for mild scoliosis. Steven was removed from her care after it was found that he was being neglected by his mother and her most current boyfriend. When he was 14 months old, Steven was placed in foster care. A year later, Steven's foster parents brought him in for psychiatric assessment.

Steven's foster mother described him as a "housewrecker." She reported that he was destructive to property (ripped the mattress and inserted objects into the air conditioner), that he hoarded food under the bed, and that he lied about these activities. In addition, Steven's foster parents and his preschool teacher described him as "hyperactive and aggressive."

MENTAL STATUS EXAMINATION

In psychiatric assessments, many phenomena are difficult to describe in a manner devoid of personal, internal formulations. Thus, Jaspers (1963) developed a technique for accurately describing nonobjective occurrences; this technique is called *phenomenology,* and it is similar in format to listings in the revised edition of the *Diagnostic and Statistical Manual of Mental Disorders* (DSM-III-R) (American Psychiatric Association, 1987).

When noting the occurrence of psychopathological phenomena, observers need to differentiate clearly among those they observe directly, those that are derived from patient history, and those that are described by the patient. In recording, the clinician uses *sign* to denote his own observations and *symptom* to denote a patient's verbal indications. The psychiatric interview is the vehicle for collecting signs and symptoms, and these combine to constitute the mental status examination, which is used as a diagnostic tool.

Because children are not static beings (they are continuously growing and changing), it is important to view their signs and symptoms within a total developmental, environmental, and social context when making a diagnosis. Age-related susceptibility to different stressors, and comparison of patient data to epidemiologic findings also demand attention. Finally, a differential diagnosis must be performed before a course of treatment is formulated.

A multiaxial evaluation requires assessment of each case on several *axes,* or different types of information. There is a limited number of axes—5 in the DSM-III-R multiaxial classification—ensuring maximal clinical utility. Axes I, II, and III make up the official diagnostic assessment.

Use of the DSM-III-R multiaxial system ensures that attention is given to certain types of disorders, to aspects of the environment, and to areas of functioning that might be overlooked if the focus were on assessing a single presenting problem.

Each person is evaluated on each of the following axes:

Axis I Clinical Syndromes and V Codes
Axis II Developmental Disorders and Personality Disorders
Axis III Physical Disorders and Conditions
Axis IV Severity of Psychosocial Stressors
Axis V Global Assessment of Functioning

MULTIAXIAL ASSESSMENTS

Axes I and II: Mental Disorders and V Codes

Axes I and II make up the entire classification of mental disorders plus V Codes. The Axis I—Axis II distinction highlights the need to consider disorders involving the development of cognitive, social, and motor skills when evaluating children. (See Tables 2–1 and 2–2.)

Developmental disorders and personality disorders, listed on Axis II, usually present during childhood or adolescence and continue throughout adult life without either becoming more profound or going into remission. Axis I disorders are not usually characterized by these histories. It is not uncommon for disorders to occur on both Axis I and Axis II.

In some cases there may not be a disorder on Axis I or Axis II. What should be regarded is Axis I: No diagnosis or condition on Axis I; or conditions not attributable to a mental disorder. Axis II: No diagnosis on Axis II.

When more than one diagnosis is given, the one that initiated initial evaluation or clinical admission is regarded as the principal diagnosis, whether it is on Axis I or II. If the principal diagnosis is on Axis II, the clinician should note "principal diagnosis."

If there are disorders on both Axis I and Axis II, the principal diagnosis is assumed to be on Axis I unless the Axis II diagnosis is followed by the qualifying phrase "principal diagnosis." To describe the current condition, multiple diagnoses should be made on both Axis I and II as indicated.

When multiple diagnoses are made on either Axis I or Axis II, they are listed within each axis in order of focus of attention or treatment. Multiple diagnoses of specific developmental disorders are common within Axis II.

Specific personality traits or the habitual use of particular defense mechanisms can be indicated on Axis II, both when no personality disorder exists and to supplement a personality disorder diagnosis when personality traits are noted.

In some instances when there is not enough information to make a firm diagnosis, the clinician may wish to write "provisional" after the diagnosis to indicate that a significant diagnostic uncertainty exists.

Table 2–1. *Axis I Disorders Usually First Evident in Infancy, Childhood, or Adolescence*

Disorder	Age of Onset
Adjustment Disorder	May be at any age.
Autistic Disorder	Usually during infancy or during childhood (before 36 months).
Pica	Usually between 12 and 24 months, although it may begin earlier.
Avoidant Disorder of Childhood or Adolescence	At or after $2\frac{1}{2}$ years.
Rumination Disorder of Infancy	Usually between 3 and 12 months; may be later in children with Mental Retardation.
Functional Encopresis	Primary Functional Encopresis by age 4; Secondary between 4 and 8 years.
Functional Enuresis	Primary Functional Enuresis begins by age 5; Secondary between 5 and 8 years.
Gender Identity Disorder of Childhood	Majority of boys with this disorder begin to develop it before the 4th birthday. With females, onset is early, but exaggerated insistence on male activities and attire not apparent until late childhood or adolescence. Onset usually by 4 in males; onset also early in females, but characteristics not clearly apparent until late childhood or adolescence.
Multiple Personality Disorder	Almost invariably in childhood.
Psychogenic Fugue	Age variable.

Table 2–1.   Axis I Disorders Usually First Evident in Infancy, Childhood, or Adolescence (Continued)

Disorder	Age of Onset
Psychogenic Amnesia	Usually in adolescence.
Depersonalization Disorder	Usually in adolescence.
Mental Retardation	Before age 18 years.
Reactive Attachment Disorder of Infancy or Early Childhood	Before age 5.
Stuttering	Usually between 2 and 7 years (peak onset around age 5).
Cluttering	Usually after age 7.
Elective Mutism	Usually before age 5.
Major Depressive Episode	Usually in late 20s; may also be at any age, even infancy.
Dysthymia	Usually in childhood, adolescence, or early adult life.
Attention-Deficit Hyperactivity Disorder	Before age 7.
Conduct Disorder	Usually prepubertal, particularly of Solitary Aggressive Type.
Oppositional Defiant Disorder	Usually in early childhood (typical onset at age 8).
Stereotypy/Habit Disorder	Usually in childhood; may intensify in adolescence.
Chronic Motor or Vocal Tic Disorder	Before age 21.
Transient Tic Disorder	Before age 21.
Tourette Syndrome	Before age 21.
Separation Anxiety Disorder	Before age 18.
Overanxious Disorder	Information not available.
Schizophrenia	Usually during adolescence or early adulthood; may begin in middle or late adulthood.
Schizophreniform Disorder	Usually during adolescence or early adulthood; may begin in middle or late adulthood.
Identity Disorder	Late adolescence, young adulthood, or middle age.
Manic Episode	Early 20s.
Cyclothymia	Usually in adolescence or early adult life.
Anorexia Nervosa	Usually in adolescence; can range from prepuberty to early 30s (rare).

(continued)

Disorder	Age of Onset
Bulimia Nervosa	Usually in adolescence or early adult life.
Body Dysmorphic Disorder	Usually from adolescence through third decade.
Conversion Disorder	Usually in adolescence or early adulthood; may first appear in middle age or later.
Hypochondrias	Usually between ages 20 and 30; may begin at any age.
Somatization Disorder	Teen years.
Somatization Pain Disorder	May be at any age.
Transsexualism	Usually by late adolescence or early adulthood; may begin later.
Gender Identity Disorder of Adolescence or Adulthood, Nontranssexual Type (GIDAANT)	After puberty.
Dyssomnias	May be at any age (all dyssomnias).
Insomnia Disorders	
Insomnia Related to Another Mental Disorder.	
Insomnia Related to a Known Organic Factor.	
Primary Insomnia.	
Hypersomnia Disorders	
Hypersomnia Related to Another Mental Disorder.	
Hypersomnia Related to a Known Organic Factor.	
Primary Hypersomnia.	
Sleep-Wake Schedule Disorder	
Parasomnias	
Dream Anxiety Disorder	Usually before age 20.
Sleep Terror Disorder	Usually between 4 and 12 years.
Sleep Walking Disorder	Usually between 6 and 12 years.
Paraphilias:	
Exhibitionism	Usually before age 18.
Fetishism	Usually by adolescence; fetish may have been endowed with special significance in childhood.
Frotteurism	Usually by adolescence.
Pedophilia	Usually in adolescence; may begin at middle age.
Sexual Masochism	Likely in childhood.
Sexual Sadism	Likely in childhood.

Table 2-1. Axis I Disorders Usually First Evident in Infancy, Childhood, or Adolescence (Continued)

Disorder	Age of Onset
Transvestite Fetishism	Begins with cross-dressing in childhood or early adolescence.
Voyeurism	Usually before age 15.
Sexual Dysfunction	Usually in early adulthood.
Impulse control disorders not elsewhere classified:	
Intermittent Explosive Disorder	May be at any age.
Kleptomania	May be as early as childhood.
Pyromania	Usually in childhood.
Trichotillomania	Usually in childhood.
Pathological Gambling	Usually during adolescence in males; later in females.

Other Axis I diagnostic categories that are often appropriate for children and adolescents are the following:

Organic Mental Syndromes, e.g., Intoxication, Organic Hallucinosis
Organic Mental, e.g., Psychoactive Substance Use Disorders

Table 2-2. Axis II Disorders Usually First Evident in Infancy, Childhood, or Adolescence

Disorder	Age of Onset
I. Developmental Disorders	
Developmental Arithmetic Disorder	Usually by 8 years, and not after 10 years.
Developmental Expressive Writing Disorder	Usually by age 7 in severe cases; onset by age 10 if less severe.
Developmental Reading Disorder	Usually by 7 years (around 6 years when severe, 9 years when less severe).
Developmental Articulation Disorder	At 3 years if severe; onset at 6 years if less severe.
Developmental Expressive Language Disorder	Before 3 years if severe; may be until early adolescence if less severe.
Developmental Receptive Language Disorder	Usually before age 4 (2 years when severe, up to age 7 or older when mild).
Developmental Coordination Disorder	Usually when child first attempts such tasks as running, holding knife or fork, and/or buttoning clothes.

(continued)

35

Table 2–2. Axis II Disorders Usually First Evident in Infancy, Childhood, or Adolescence

Disorder	Age of Onset
II. V Codes.* Academic Problem	Age 18 or younger.
Borderline Intellectual Functioning	
Childhood or Adolescent Antisocial Behavior	
Malingering	
Noncompliance with Medical Treatment	
Occupational Problem	
Parent-Child Problem	
Other Interpersonal Problem	
Other Specified Family Circumstances	
Phase of Life Problem or Other Life Circumstance Problem	
Uncomplicated Bereavement	
III. Personality Disorders.** Antisocial Personality Disorder	Personality disorder categories may be applied to children or adolescents in those instances in which the particular traits appear to be stable. However, one exception to this rule is antisocial personality disorder. The diagnosis of conduct disorder should be made if the person is under 18 years of age.
Schizoid Personality Disorder	
Borderline Personality Disorder	
Paranoid Personality Disorder	
Schizotypal Personality Disorder	
Histrionic Personality Disorder	
Narcissistic Personality Disorder	
Obsessive Compulsive Personality Disorder	
Passive Aggressive Personality Disorder	
Avoidant Personality Disorder	

*V codes are conditions that are the focus of treatment or attention, and are not attributable to any mental disorder.
**Personality Traits* are "enduring patterns of perceiving, relating to, and thinking about the environment and oneself, and are exhibited in a wide range of important social and personal contexts." (DSM-III-R, p. 335).

"When personality traits are inflexible and maladaptive and cause either significant functional impairment or subjective distress then they constitute *personality disorders*." (DSM-III-R, p. 335).

Axis III: Physical Disorders or Conditions

On Axis III, the clinician can note any current physical disorder or condition that might be relevant to understanding or managing a case. In some instances the physical condition is etiologically significant, while in others it is not, but is still relevant to overall case management. In some cases the clinician may elect to note significant associated physical findings such as *soft neurologic signs*. Multiple diagnoses are permitted.

Axis IV: Severity of Psychosocial Stressors

Axis IV: The Severity of Psychosocial Stressors Scale is a scale used to code the overall severity of a psychosocial stressor or multiple psychosocial stressors that presented in the year preceding the current evaluation and that may have played a role in any of the following:

1. Development of a new mental disorder.
2. Recurrence of a prior mental disorder.
3. Exacerbation of an already existing mental disorder.

Although stressors often play a causative role in disorders, they might also be a consequence of a person's psychopathology.

Rating the Severity of the Stressor. Rating the severity of the stressor is based on the clinician's estimate of the stress that an *average* person, in similar circumstances and with similar sociocultural values, would endure as a result of a particular psychosocial stressor or stressors. This judgment entails considering (a) how much change is caused in the person's life by the stressor; (b) to what degree the occurrence is wanted and is under the person's control; and (c) what the number of stressors is.

Specific psychosocial stressors are then further specified as either *predominantly acute events* (duration of less than 6 months) or *predominantly enduring circumstances* (duration of more than 6 months).

Axis V: Global Assessment of Functioning

Axis V permits the clinician to present an overall judgment of a person's psychological, social, and occupational functioning using the Global Assessment of Functioning Scale, which assesses mental health or illness.

Ratings on the GAF Scale need to be made for two time periods:

1. Current—the level of functioning at the time of the evaluation.
2. Past year—the highest level of functioning that lasted for at least a few months during the past year. For children and adolescents, this should include at least a month during the school year.

Ratings of current functioning generally reveal the current need for treatment. Ratings of highest level of functioning during the past year often have prognostic significance, since a person usually returns to his or her prior level of functioning after an illness.

The following case provides an example of how the mental status examination can be used to diagnose disorders in preschool children.

During the mental status examination, Steven, a neatly dressed child, showed no evidence of postural abnormalities, nor did he display any difficulty with either gross or fine motor movements. Steven's affect was constricted; however, he generally expressed anger mixed with apprehension. Steven's social skills were age appropriate; at the start of the interview he appeared quite shy, but after a warm-up period, he was able to interact with the interviewer. Steven's thought content revealed a concern with mess and disorganization. Transient psychotic symptoms were not noted. Steven was able to indicate what toys he desired, he requested help from the therapist, and he cooperated in cleaning up at the end of the session. Steven denied the presence of hallucinations or delusions and showed no signs of either suicidal or homicidal ideation. He was noted to have a low frustration tolerance (throwing temper tantrums twice during the initial assessment interview), which interfered with his judgment. Steven's attention span was also limited by his impulsivity; he would not remain with a task consistently for an extended time period. Steven's intellectual functioning was noted to be in the low to average range as depicted by results on the Stanford-Binet Intelligence Test. His memory for the immediate, recent, and remote past was intact. Overall self-esteem was low.

These results, coupled with reports from Steven's foster parents, point to a diagnosis of conduct disorder, undifferentiated type. Although oppositional defiant disorder also includes some of the criteria necessary for a diagnosis of conduct disorder, it does not include violation of the basic rights of others and age-appropriate norms. Steven has reportedly stolen food, lied about hoarding food, and destroyed the property of others (ripped the mattress) for almost 1 year; thus, he meets the criteria for conduct disorder.

Steven also displays the features of attention deficit hyperactivity disorder, a common associated diagnosis. He is described as hyperactive and was found in the interview to be impulsive. Furthermore, it was noted that his self-esteem is low and his attention span is limited. A diagnosis of pervasive developmental disorder is inappropriate because Steven's social skills were found to be age-appropriate before he developed these behaviors.

Thus, Steven was diagnosed as meeting the criteria for conduct disorder and attention deficit hyperactivity disorder in Axis I; no diagnosis was addressed on Axis II (developmental or personality disorder) or

Axis III (physical disorder). The severity of Steven's psychosocial stressors (Axis IV) was considered to range from severe to extreme. The global assessment of Steven's functioning (Axis V) was considered to be poor over all. It was recommended that he begin weekly individual therapy and that he enter family therapy with his brother and their foster parents.

CHAPTER THREE

Familial Considerations for Assessment

Lisa: A Troubled Child of Troubled Parents

Lisa is a 5-year-old girl who has lived with her mother since her parents separated 8 months ago. Her parents were married, after a 3-year cohabitation, when Lisa's mother learned she was pregnant. Lisa's mother stated that her relationship with Lisa's father probably would have ended earlier if she had not become pregnant. Both of Lisa's parents are alcoholics, and their marriage included daily drinking. The father would sometimes destroy property during drinking binges. When Lisa was 2 years old, her mother attempted suicide by taking alcohol and Valium. Lisa was the only other person at home, and she saw her mother unconscious.

After this suicide attempt, Lisa's mother joined Alcoholics Anonymous, and she has not had a drink of alcohol in the ensuing 3 years. Lisa's father, however, did not alter his drinking behavior. Following Lisa's maternal grandfather's death (due, according to Lisa's mother, to his alcoholism), her father attempted suicide by taking alcohol and Valium. He did not suffer severe physical consequences, but Lisa and her mother did move out of the household at that time. After their departure, Lisa did not see her father until more than 2 weeks later, after her mother made formal visitation arrangements. A few months after the separation, Lisa's father went, uninvited, to the apartment where Lisa and her mother were living. Her mother would not let him in. The father pounded on the door and was verbally abusive. Lisa tried to let her father in, saying that her father needed to see her or else he would always feel sad. Lisa's mother prevented her from letting him in and told Lisa that the father had physically abused her in the past. Another time, Lisa's father tried to visit Lisa while her mother was at work. After being refused admission to the apartment by the babysitter, he tried to climb into Lisa's bedroom window.

Lisa's mother has noticed that since these two incidents Lisa has become hostile and oppositional toward her and her boyfriend of 18 months, to whom Lisa had previously been friendly. Lisa has also started to throw tantrums when left with a babysitter recently, even though she is accustomed to her mother's going out and she knows the babysitters. Another change her mother has noticed is that Lisa has become more aggressive toward her peers and is less willing to share. Although her nursery school teacher noted excellent social and academic school adjustment, Lisa's mother felt that Lisa should be evaluated regarding her recent regressive behavior trends. She was concerned that Lisa might have suffered as a result of the parents' relationship and behavior.

During the interview, Lisa displayed no evidence of attentional difficulties or psychoses. Her attitude was nondefensive and playful, and she drew during most of the interview. Although her drawing seemed obsessive, her pictures were not unusual for a girl of her age. Her intelligence was assessed as above average. Other elements of the mental status examination were judged as developmentally appropriate. It appears that Lisa's recent tantrums, aggressiveness with peers, and separation difficulties are isolated responses to stress. Lisa may also feel—as expressed by her verbalization that if her father did not see her he would always feel sad—that she is in some way responsible for her father's problems.

Lisa's responses to the stressors of her parents' separation and her maternal grandfather's death are mixed; they include sadness, aggression, and other feelings and point to a diagnosis of adjustment disorder with mixed emotional features. Her reactions to current stressors are maladaptive in that they interfere with her relationships in school and at home; therefore, the impairment is more pervasive than a V Code would imply. Assessment did not indicate that Lisa manifests any personality disorder traits either related to or in addition to her maladaptive adjustment behaviors. Physical assessment was also performed, and the possibility that Lisa's reaction could be in response to psychological factors affecting physical condition was ruled out. Recommendation was made for her to have weekly sessions for 3 months, with separate weekly sessions for her mother. It was also proposed that Lisa's father be seen at least once, to derive information for a complete picture.

INTRODUCTION

Psychiatrically disturbed preschool-age children such as Lisa have been the focus of mounting concern, not only in terms of diagnosis but with regard to treatment as well. Diagnosis of these children is especially complex, and it is often subject to various, sometimes mutually exclusive, interpretations. This is because there are many problems in this population that stand in the way of defining a symptomatic picture clearly enough to construct an effective treatment strategy.

First, children are inadequate to the task of fully and clearly delineating their feelings, and when diagnosticians rely on parents or teachers, there is a danger that the severity of the disturbance will be underestimated (Weissman et al., 1986). There is also a danger that the clinician may tend to blame the parent for the child's problem or may *underestimate* the value of the parent's information and *overvalue* the information derived during the assessment interview. A careful clinician must beware of such biases if the patient is to receive appropriate attention. In addition, it is necessary to take into account the developmental changes associated with normal maturation.

Perceiving the developmental context is crucial for a number of reasons, aside from the obvious need for information regarding normative behaviors at a given age. Knowing the age-appropriate range of normal behaviors also provides a means of assessing the degree to which a given disturbance has interfered with normal development. In this way it is possible to assess the severity of the disturbance. Also, the various phases of development carry with them different challenges and vulnerabilities that must be taken into account. Finally, it is necessary to understand the dynamics underlying normal development in order to assess and, if possible, correct the mechanism(s) responsible for aberrant development (Cox & Rutter, 1985).

An understanding of the progressive stages of development provides a sense of what events occur during which time periods in the course of normative development. An example is the Piagetian system of cognitive development in which a child moves in a stepwise progression away from egocentric thinking to contextual, concrete thinking. One manifestation of this process may be the finding in the study of preschool children by Kashani and Carlson (1987) that the number of somatic complaints in association with depression decreased with increasing age. Therefore, a child of 9 or 10 who is depressed and who also expresses somatic complaints may suffer from a lag or deficit in cognition. In fact, the delay in cognitive development may play a major role in the etiology of the depression (Trad, 1986, 1987).

Since a child's behavior is embedded in the overall context of maturation and development, emotional problems must be viewed as exaggerations or deficiencies of behavior patterns seen in every child (Plenk & Hinchey, 1985). Thus, symptoms in children cannot be viewed as a set of adjectives that may combine to describe a discrete psychological state. Rather, they are better viewed as existing, to one degree or another, along the entire behavioral continuum available to every child. Thus, testing for childhood psychopathology is largely, although not solely, a matter of assessing the behavior in question in terms of intensity, frequency, and duration.

In order to make these evaluations, the opportunity to interview both the child and the parents—and, if necessary, concerned individuals outside the family—is crucial. Behavior observation skills are required, as is the ability to rule out conditions that might be producing the same symptoms.

These skills and their attendant knowledge are necessary because of the heterogeneity of the childhood psychiatric population, which includes autistic children; those who are hyperactive, impulsive, and aggressive; children who have problems in habit training; others who are fearful and withdrawn; and still others who are mentally retarded or otherwise biologically impaired (Rescorla, 1986).

While assessing the psychological condition of these children demands considerable knowledge and expertise, there is good reason to believe that this expenditure of time and energy on the part of the clinician is justified. Numerous studies have indicated that preschool children with these behavioral problems are at risk for developing later psychopathology (Campbell, Endman, & Bernfield, 1977; Cantwell & Baker, 1980; Kohn & Rosman, 1972). An estimate of just how much greater the risk might be for these children than for others has emerged

from a study by Lerner, Inui, Trupin, and Douglas (1985), who prospectively studied 174 children aged 3 to 5 years prior to kindergarten entry.
These investigators found that aggressive children, children who are
withdrawn or hyperactive-distractible, and those with speech and language problems are at least twice as likely to develop specific psychiatric
disorders as children without these disabilities.

This introductory chapter to the clinical diagnosis section presents
an overview of the tools and perspective needed when diagnosing psychiatric conditions of childhood, including a description of proper interviewing techniques and a brief exposure to psychiatric tests. To the
same end, the relative specificity, or lack thereof, of certain key symptoms such as hallucinations and delusions also will be discussed.

FAMILY EVALUATION

Family Structure

While there are few proven direct correlations between family background and the development of specific psychopathologies in children,
there is little doubt that family variables are associated with risk for
developing many childhood psychopathologies. The clinician who is
alert to possible risk factors within a child's family will have valuable
information in addition to that gathered from interviews and testing.

One risk factor known to be associated with an increased risk for
childhood disorders is disordered parental marital status (i.e., separated, divorced, or remarried). One of the most thorough studies performed to date regarding this issue was undertaken by Brady, Bray, and
Zeeb (1986). These investigators studied 703 children in a clinic setting,
looking for interactions between family type and age and sex of child.

Using the 93-item Conners Parent Questionnaire, Brady and colleagues found that children from separated families displayed the most
severe problems over all, exhibiting more immature behavior, sleep disturbances, tension, and hyperactive behavior than those from intact
families. Interestingly, children from remarried families showed consistently more conduct problems and hyperactive behavior than children
from either divorced or separated families. In general, boys demonstrated more poor-conduct behaviors, hyperactive behavior, bowel
problems, and sibling rivalry than did girls, although girls tended to
show a higher level of sleep disturbances than the boys. Brady and colleagues pointed out that these sex differences have also been noted by
many other researchers.

Thus, in terms of general family background, it may be useful when
assessing a given child to know that boys in general tend to have more

difficulty adjusting to a disordered family life. Furthermore, the psycho-pathology of a child from a separated or remarried family may tend to be more severe than that of a child from an intact or divorced home, or perhaps, the etiology of the problem is more likely to be embedded in the home context of a child whose parent is separated or remarried.

Role of Parental Mediation

Maternal Depression. In attempting to narrow the focus of work such as that of Brady and co-workers, Fergusson, Horwood, and Shannon (1984) have examined the interrelationships between the effects of stressful life events on the mother and on the child. Using a cohort of 1,265 children who were examined at birth, 4 months, and annually up to 5 years of age, these investigators studied the role of maternal mood in the observed correlation between stressful life events and behavior problems in children.

Data were collected via structured interviews with the mothers and ongoing maternal diaries of their children's behavior, supplemented by information from hospital records and the records of general practitioners. Fergusson and co-workers found that, after excluding a range of the possible family and social characteristics (e.g., family type, family size, maternal educational level, maternal age, family living standards, maternal ethnicity), correlations between family life events and maternal reports of child-rearing problems were largely attributable to the mediating effects of maternal depression.

The authors stated that this finding could be the result of one of two different mechanisms. It is possible that children of depressed mothers react to the depression by developing an ever-increasing number of behavior problems. Thus, negative life events induce maternal depression, which in turn provokes child-rearing problems. Alternatively, it may be that rather than provoking objective changes in a child's behavior, depression changes the way the mother perceives her child's behavior. Thus, depressed women evaluate their children as being more troublesome than they would if they were not depressed.

Since this study relied on maternal reporting, it is impossible to say which mechanism is more likely. However, the results of studies such as that by Orvaschel, Weissmann, and Kidd (1980) strongly suggest that it is not merely maternal perception of the child's behavior that is changed by maternal depression. These researchers found that children with a depressive parent were significantly more likely to have some form of psychopathology than were children of normal parents.

The importance of the relationship between stress and/or maternal depression and children's behavior is further illustrated in a study by Huttunen and Niskanen (1978), who tabulated the frequency of psychiatric difficulties in children whose mothers had suffered the death of their husbands during pregnancy or during the first year of their children's lives. It was found that the children whose fathers died while they were still unborn had higher rates of psychiatric problems than those whose fathers died in the first year. Thus, it seems apparent that maternal stress plays a significant role in the development of the child, even before birth. Of course, this case was especially severe, since the stress of having to manage alone was combined with depression (grieving).

A great deal of work remains to be done in separating the effects of non-pathology-inducing stress from levels of stress that do generate maternal depression. More information about the various mediators of stress such as marital status, financial status, quality of the marriage, and availability of a confidante will help in this endeavor (Trad, 1988).

Parental Psychopathology. It is perhaps not surprising that overall childhood psychopathology increases in proportion to the number of family stressors to which the child is subjected. Rutter and Shaffer (1980) and Rutter (1981) have identified the following six significant family stressors:

1. The father's having an unskilled or semiskilled job.
2. Overcrowding in the home or a large family unit.
3. Maternal depression or neurosis.
4. The child's having at least one instance of being "in care."
5. Paternal conviction for a crime.
6. Marital discord.

Taken alone, none of these factors is significant. However, when two or more are present, the risk of emotional problems doubles or quadruples.

Shaw and Emery (1987) performed a study evaluating the impact on development of four of Rutter's factors—parental conflict, maternal depression, overcrowding, and family income—and obtained results similar to Rutter's. That is, grouping of stressors was associated with clinically elevated child behavior problems and below-average social competence and IQ.

In an attempt to isolate specific types of childhood pathology associated with specific parental behaviors, Lahey and colleagues (1988) conducted a study with 86 biological parents of outpatient children aged 6 to 13 years. They found that both mothers and fathers of children with conduct disorder (CD) were more likely to exhibit antisocial personality disorder. Fathers were more likely to abuse substances. Attention deficit disorder with hyperactivity (ADDH) was not associated with any parental disorder; however, the fathers of children with both CD and ADDH (a combination associated with greater aggression and persistent law breaking in children than in CD alone) were significantly more likely to have a history of aggression, arrest, and imprisonment. Thus, it seems evident that parental psychopathology, often involving drug abuse and chaotic family structure, increases the risk of childhood pathology.

Alcoholism and Substance Abuse. Another mediator of stress may be the use of psychoactive substances. For example, the association between depression and alcohol use has been known for many years. Data are just now beginning to emerge regarding the effects of parental drug use (especially alcohol) on childrearing. This is an important area of research because it is estimated that one of every eight children in the United States is being reared by an alcoholic parent, and only about 15% of these parents are under treatment for their addiction (McDonald & Blume, 1986).

Children raised in homes where one or both parents are chemically dependent are typically exposed to a very dysregulated family life, one that is lacking in consistency, stability, and emotional support. Perhaps the most problematic factor for the child, aside from lack of consistency, is the danger of being accidentally injured (either through a physical accident due to alcoholic negligence or through the disinhibiting effect of alcohol giving rise to violent actions that might otherwise be suppressed).

Cause for concern is further amplified by the fact that the number of women of childbearing age who are in need of treatment for drug abuse is increasing (Deren, 1986). This increase in maternal alcoholism and abuse of other substances may result in an increase in the number of addicted parents in the next generation since the potential for alcoholism, at least, is known to be genetically influenced (Schuckit, 1985). For instance, the frequency of alcoholism in adult offspring of alcoholics has been observed to increase with the number of affected parents (Earls, 1987).

Considering these epidemiological factors and the extra degree of chaos added to family interactions by alcohol or other drug use, the clinician should be sensitive to the possibility of substance abuse in any case, but especially in cases where maternal depression is evident. In cases where the origin of a child's problematic behavior is difficult to substantiate, it is advisable to consider maternal depression, with or without drug abuse, as a prime etiological factor.

Family History and Psychosis

The mediational role of parents in the development of their children is perhaps most powerful in the case of childhood psychoses. Not only may these children have a genetic deficit predisposing them to psycho-pathology, but they also may have little contact with persons who are more cognitively mature than they. In the absence of this contact, development is bound to be hindered (Trad, 1987).

Chandler (1978) has emphasized the role of parental egocentric thinking in the genesis of childhood psychopathy. Noting that egocentric thinking was prevalent in a population of mothers with histories of serious psychiatric disorders, Chandler administered a role- and perspective-taking test to their children. In this test a set of cartoon drawings is presented and children are asked to describe them from both their own perspective and that of other persons who are privy to less information than they. Intrusions of privileged information are marked as egocentric errors in distinguishing public from private information.

These children were slower to give up their own egocentric assumptions than were control children, and Chandler pointed out that these repeated egocentric errors were comparable to those observed in seriously emotionally disturbed children. Thus, there appears to be a pathological relationship between parental egocentric thinking and child development. Such parents are likely to have persistently egocentric children who are less alert to differences between themselves and their parents and so are less motivated to establish their separate existence. Therefore, in cases of suspected childhood psychosis, it may prove advisable to look first for signs of parental egocentrism.

However, there are many other elements of the environment that can enhance chances of pathological outcome. Environmental contributions to etiology have been receiving increased interest for some time in light of the moderate rates of concordance (40 to 60%) for schizophrenia in identical twins (Gottesman & Shields, 1982). The importance of environmental stressors in the etiology of schizophrenia is further emphasized by the fact that 88 to 90% of schizophrenics do not have a schizophrenic parent (Wynne, 1978).

With these considerations in mind, it seems clear that using parental schizophrenia alone as an indicator for future schizophrenia in offspring will prove woefully insufficient. Before discussing reports on the effects of other family-related risk factors on the development of schizophrenia, it is helpful to keep in mind possible contributions from the affected children themselves.

While data relating to high-risk infant temperamental factors independent of maternal behavior are extremely scarce, Walker and Emory (1983), in their extensive literature review, noted that many researchers have found a lower stimulus threshold in the children of schizophrenics when compared to children in control groups. Thus, as Walker and Emory have suggested, it is possible that regardless of whether a parent is schizophrenic, a child who is highly reactive when exposed to a stressful environment may develop a heightened central nervous system sensitivity to factors causing disequilibrium. The authors noted that this dynamic is in line with the postulation of Parmelee and Michaelis (1971), who conceptualized the infant vulnerable to schizophrenia as having a constitutionally based decreased threshold for central nervous system disequilibrium.

This hypothesis about the temperament of the vulnerable child can provide a heuristic framework in which to measure environmental contributions to the etiology of mental disorders. The results of an early study by Wolff (1961) are representative of the data being generated by many more recent studies. In this investigation, Wolff followed up 43 children under the age of 5 years who were seen in a child psychiatric clinic in 1952 and 1953. Those with diagnoses of organic brain disease, mental defect, epilepsy, or childhood psychosis were excluded from the study. At the times of admission, the children ranged in age from 2 years, 3 months to 4 years, 11 months.

In terms of the general social environment of the families, the children in the study group were no more disadvantaged than children in the general community who were born at a similar time and in similar parts of the country. Furthermore, neither the child's ordinal position in the family nor the age of the mother at the child's birth was discriminative in predicting the child's appearance at a child guidance clinic.

However, two factors were found to be significant in the background of the psychiatrically disturbed children, both of which pertained to their parents. These children had parents with a high incidence of psychiatric disturbance who had experienced deprivation in their own childhoods. While these figures have yet to be substantiated, Wolff has pointed out that, if accurate, the data would support Bowlby's (1951) contention that adults who are unable to make effective family relationships may themselves have been deprived of a normal home life during childhood.

The possibility that family interaction patterns have an etiologic importance comparable to that of genetic predisposition in the genesis of schizophrenia seems to be a strong one. In their comprehensive review, Walker and Emory (1983) found that pregnant women who have already experienced or will experience a schizophrenic breakdown are not at greater risk for prenatal medical complications than other pregnant women of comparable socioeconomic background. Therefore, schizophrenia in the mother apparently does not increase the likelihood of prenatal problems that could negatively affect the child's development.

Furthermore, Walker and Emory found no data to suggest that viable newborns who are at high risk due to having a schizophrenic parent show physical anomalies that set them apart from other children. Beyond the neonatal period, however, there does appear to be consistent reporting of retarded psychomotor development in high-risk infants.

Given these negative correlations and the positive correlations between schizophrenic development and depressed maternal mood, parental history of childhood impoverishment, and greater incidence of parental psychiatric disturbances, it seems that the greatest promise for developing predictive factors for development ramification of schizophrenia lies in studying pathological family interaction patterns.

One promising line of investigation in this regard was developed by Brown, Briley, and Wing (1972) and Vaughn and Leff (1976). Using the concept of expressed emotion (EE), these investigators found that measures of overinvolvement, hostility, and critical comments made by the patient's relatives (usually the parents) at the time the patient was admitted to the hospital carried strong prognostic information about the probability of relapse over a 9-month follow-up period. Pertinent to the comments about temperamental contributions of high-risk individuals, the findings of Vaughn and Leff suggest an exacerbated sensitivity of schizophrenic patients to certain discriminable attributes of family emotional environment (Goldstein & Doane, 1982). While these results apply to a much older age group, the strength of the findings gives hope that indexes of parental interaction patterns may one day be developed that will assist in detecting and intervening in an environment that may contribute to the later development of schizophrenia in particular and mental disturbance in general.

CONCLUSION

Psychiatric nosology in children is in a state of constant flux. Because young children move so quickly through time in terms of development and integration of the environment, the task of meticulously and globally assessing each child for possible etiologies is particularly crucial and at the same time very difficult.

Clinicians must guard against making the same associations between symptoms and disease states in children as they might in adults. Furthermore, it is vital to realize that in the 1,000 preschoolers psychiatrically hospitalized in 1975, and in all those treated since that time, the remission of psychiatric symptoms has depended on the establishment of a primary relationship with the therapist (Dalton, Pederson, & McEntyre, 1987).

While this often taxes clinicians and institutions to their limits and beyond, it is necessary to try to establish these primary relationships because lengthy hospitalizations have dire ramifications for young children in the absence of a bonding figure. For these and for children treated on an outpatient basis alike, the most important components of treatment are sufficient time, a global assessment of strengths and weaknesses within the social and developmental contexts, and the establishment of trust, both with the child and with the parent.

CHAPTER FOUR

Epidemiological Considerations for Assessment

Eden: Having Bad Feelings

Eden is a 4-year, 6-month-old Hispanic girl, who lives with her parents. She was born of an unplanned pregnancy, but her parents reported that they were happy about having a child. The pregnancy was interrupted 1 month early by cesarean section because her mother developed toxemia. She weighed 5 pounds 1 ounce and was kept in a hospital incubator for close to 3 weeks. All developmental milestones were reached within the expected age limits. Eden's parents reported longstanding marital problems. Her father, who works as a toll collector, is obese; he claims to have gained weight recently in response to increased marital distress. Her mother was diagnosed as having schizoaffective disorder. When Eden was 1 year old, her mother entered the hospital for a 2-month stay due to persistent feelings of hopelessness accompanied by auditory and visual hallucinations. During that time, Eden lived with her maternal grandparents and was visited frequently by her father.

Eden was referred for evaluation by the nursery psychologist, who noted that Eden had been having difficulties since she entered the nursery 16 months before. Her teachers reported that she had difficulty paying attention and she often daydreamed. In addition, Eden had shown signs of depression. According to her teachers, she always looked downcast and rarely smiled in class; moreover, she was reported to be an underachiever.

Assessment of Eden followed the standard procedure of a mental status examination. At the interview, she appeared well-groomed and looked her stated age. No abnormalities of physical features, posture, or psychomotor activity were noted. Eden's affective display was judged to be full range. Her mother was hospitalized when Eden was seen in the clinic, and, when discussing this, Eden began to cry and explained that she was "afraid" to tell people about her mother's hospitalization. At this time, Eden's underlying mood seemed to be depressed. She reported being "sad," and "having bad feelings." She denied auditory or visual hallucinations, although she did say that she sometimes heard her mother calling her, when in fact it was not her mother but someone else. Neither formal thought disorders nor unusual idiosyncratic speech patterns were noted, and Eden denied suicidal or homicidal ideation. Her insight and judgment were fair, and her adaptive functioning was assessed to be age-appropriate. Eden manifested a rich fantasy life and a vivid imagination. She reported daydreaming about being adopted by a "TV family" and then making up episodes with herself as a character. At no time during the interviews did she appear to lose reality testing. She gave the appearance of being suspicious, however, when she said she "needed" to see the evaluator's notes. Eden denied having any sleep, appetite, or somatic difficulties, and this was confirmed by her family and teachers. Eden's attention, concentration, and memory appeared intact; however, this one-to-one interview did not necessarily reflect her school performance in these areas.

Eden's symptoms, as well as the results of her assessment, pointed to a diagnosis of dysthymia. Her early separation from her mother (at age 12 months), her mother's psychiatric condition, and her parents' chronic marital discord were all contributing factors to this diagnosis. It was recommended that Eden be tested and be seen in individual exploratory psychotherapy twice a week in an attempt to rule out the possibility of other disorders.

INTRODUCTION

Problem behaviors in preschool children, as in the case of Eden, are far from infrequent, but differentiating between a problem that is likely to persist and cause increasing difficulties and one that merely represents a temporary surge of frustration or unhappiness in the course of normal development is one of the most difficult tasks facing parents, teachers, pediatricians, and psychiatrists alike. The difficulty derives from the lack of a coherent system that might be used to classify or at least describe behavioral and emotional problems in preschool children. Furthermore, there are few data pertaining to the prevalence of such problems and to the factors associated with their appearance and prognosis (Richman, Stevenson, & Graham, 1975).

The lack of reliable data regarding the relative pathogenicity that might be attached to any of the broad range of childhood behaviors is not difficult to understand. Richman and Graham (1971) have pointed out that the definition of any behavior depends on the particular social and cultural milieu as well as on individual cultural and familial expectations of what is appropriate or inappropriate for a given age.

In addition, there is tremendous variability among observer descriptions of so-called problem behaviors. In other words, the same behavior may be reported differently by different observers. In the preschool age group, the clinician almost always relies, at least in the beginning, on the description given by the mother, a person who has her own biases stemming from peer and cultural sources as well as from her own expectations of what her child should and should not be doing. In contrast to the mother's perceptions, a more objective clinical observer might well fail to see a problem in a child.

Discrepancies in assessment can occur even when a child is observed under controlled circumstances in the clinic. A consistent picture of behavior is difficult to formulate with a preschool child because normal development in this age group is accompanied by fairly extensive fluctuations in behavior from day to day. Thus, the reliability of diagnosis is negatively affected by variations in the child's response as well as by variations in the description given by the initial informant and the clinical observer over time. (Richman & Graham, 1971).

All these factors make it difficult to clearly define symptomatic behaviors in toddlers and preschoolers—to separate, for example, an attention deficit disorder from discipline problems and aggression, and to segregate from age-appropriate exploration and independence-seeking behaviors the many other symptoms that could prove problematic (Campbell, Ewing, Breaux, & Szumowski, 1986). Thus, a good deal of effort remains to be expended on investigating the differences between transient behavioral difficulties, those that persist, and those that recur for brief periods. In short, as Richman and Graham (1971) noted, "It would be most useful to know about the amount of variation which occurs in 'normal' children and the frequency of short-lived episodes of difficulty" (p. 21). Coleman, Wolkind, Pond, and Ashley (1977) addressed this problem, studying 100 3-year-old children in a London borough over a 2-year period. Their data (Table 4–1) give a broad but useful representation of the variations that may occur over time in the young child population.

Despite the lack of data regarding behavioral variation, the majority of investigators agree that the epidemiological pursuit of the distribution of maladaptive behaviors in children constitutes a potentially powerful tool in the attempt to diagnose and control psychiatric illness. This belief hinges on the following three assumptions:

1. Nonorganic types of psychopathology form during childhood in response to emotional conflicts and stress.
2. Without treatment these maladaptive defensive styles will persist into adulthood.
3. These psychopathologic systems will become more entrenched with time; thus they are more amenable to treatment at an early age than they are later on (Kohlberg, LaCrosse, & Ricks, 1972).

Before attempting to isolate the incidences of specific problems in the child population, it should be noted that most epidemiological data are derived from children between the ages of 6 and 18 years, probably due to the fact that data on preschoolers are difficult to obtain and interpret. In this age range, Garrison and Earls (1986) conservatively estimated that approximately 12% of children have a current diagnosable psychiatric disorder. In their review, the same investigators noted that more and more studies on preschool children are emerging and that, based on these studies, anywhere from 8 to 14% of preschool children in various samples across the Western Hemisphere have been reported to have psychiatric disorders.

Earls (1982) has noted that most definitions of psychiatric disorders in children so far have been based on symptoms and symptom clusters rather than on social and educational handicaps. He has also noted

Table 4-1.   Probability of Change, Over the 2-Year Period from Ages 3 to 5, of Nursery School Children Expressing Symptoms.

Symptom	3 yr	5 yr	Chi square	*p*
Taken into parents' bed	42	17	15.57	<0.01
Wet at night	35	17	13.13	<0.01
Nervous habits	65	45	11.03	<0.01
Wet in the day	17	3	9.39	<0.02
Fears	65	48	7.31	<0.02
Waking at night	45	29	5.61	*n.s.*
Temper tantrums	29	19	4.05	*n.s.*
Overactivity	35	25	3.37	*n.s.*
Difficulties with peers	53	39	2.03	*n.s.*
Management problem	41	33	1.75	*n.s.*
Difficulties over separation	16	12	1.60	*n.s.*
Unwilling to go to bed	36	33	0.59	*n.s.*
Worries	41	39	0.41	*n.s.*
Depressed mood	25	23	0.32	*n.s.*
Overdependence	28	26	0.28	*n.s.*

Note: Probabilities derived from one-tailed test.
Reprinted with permission from *Journal of Child Psychology and Psychiatry, 19,* J. Coleman, S. Wolkind, and L. Ashley, "Symptoms of Behavioral Disturbance and Adjustment to School," Copyright 1977 Pergamon Press plc.

that agreement across studies diminishes as soon as broad typologies of psychiatric disorders are abandoned and more specificity is sought. Nevertheless, at the present time, epidemiological studies on preschoolers, few as they may be, offer the most information about prevalence and variability of childhood problem behaviors. The ensuing discussion of epidemiological research on preschoolers will acquaint readers with the overall incidences, variabilities, and inherent predictability of potentially problematic behaviors among children of both sexes and in different cultures. Such information is necessary if a clinician is to arrive at an accurate assessment of the relative clinical importance of a given symptom in a given child.

EVALUATING THE PREVALENCE OF CHILDHOOD PSYCHIATRIC SYMPTOMS

Externalizing and Internalizing Symptoms

Before reviewing the relative frequencies of different symptoms, it will be helpful to discuss the general nature of preschool symptomatology. The lack of information regarding the etiologies of preschool disorders, combined with the previously stated problems of measurement, has led to a great deal of overlap between diagnostic groups. Even cluster analysis has provided heterogeneous diagnostic categories (Sherman, Shapiro, & Glassman, 1983).

Most recently, researchers in childhood psychopathology have attempted to describe aberrant conditions as being predominantly associated with one of two broad dimensions of behavior, the externalizing and internalizing dimensions. Internalizing behaviors exist along the continuum of being overcontrolled, withdrawn, and anxious, while externalizing symptoms are characterized by undercontrolled, aggressive behavior. This two-factor model of behavioral disorder forms the basis of DSM-III-R nosology.

The results of a study by Fischer, Rolf, Hasazi, and Cummings (1984) are representative of the findings to date from this factor-analytic approach. These investigators followed up 541 preschool children with second evaluations performed at ages 9 to 15 years. Their results supported those of other investigators such as Kellam, Branch, Agrawal, and Ensminger (1975) and Kohn (1977), who found continuity in either internalizing or externalizing behaviors across the period from preschool age to about 7 years later.

Angry-defiant behavior appeared to be more stable across time than apathetic-withdrawn behavior, suggesting that externalizing symptoms might be more indicative of later negative outcomes. These findings, however, are in opposition to those of Kellam and colleagues (1975), who found shy behaviors to be more stable than the externalizing-aggressive cluster. Furthermore, unlike the results of Fischer and colleagues, Kohn (1977) found that early shy behavior was the greater predictor of later social maladjustment than the angry-defiant behavior.

Rescorla (1986) ascribed this somewhat confused state of affairs to the fact that many disturbed preschool children exhibit both internalizing and externalizing symptoms. Therefore, in order to enhance observational perspective and provide additional information regarding the two-factor-analytic approach, Rescorla retrospectively studied the case records of 274 3- to 5-year-old children who had been evaluated prior to the publication of DSM-III.

The diagnostic categories used by the clinic to characterize these children were severe atypical development (21% of the sample; analogous to DSM-III pervasive developmental disorder-PDD); mild atypical development (13% of the sample; similar to DSM-III childhood-onset PDD); reactive disorder (44%; characterized by significant emotional or behavioral disturbance in the absence of signs of ego defect, psychosis, or any presumed constitutional vulnerability such as minimal brain dysfunction—these children had a wide range of behaviors from acting out to internalizing symptoms); and other (23%; including children with language delay, hyperkinetic syndrome, or minimal brain dysfunction in the absence of neurologic disorder).

Of the 274 children in the study, 34% were classified as atypical to some degree. However, contrary to the distinction in the DSM-III classification, the majority of children in both atypical groups clearly showed deviant development prior to 30 months of age. A large number of children from both of these groups were described by parents as exhibiting bizarre behaviors and autistic aloofness before age 30 months. Thus, the DSM-III method of distinguishing between different types of PDDs in terms of age of onset was not validated. Indeed, the revised version of DSM-III, DSM-III-R, drops this idea, recognizing autism as the only subcategory of PDDs and requiring only that childhood onset be noted if the condition existed prior to age 36 months.

Aside from illustrating the considerable heterogeneity of symptoms in children and the serviceability of more than one classification system, this study demonstrated a close interrelationship between aggressive-destructive behavior and feelings of anxiety, sadness, and emotional insecurity. This demonstrated that the DSM-III and DSM-III-R demarcation between acting-out problems such as conduct or oppositional disorder and internalizing syndromes such as anxiety disorders may not be accurate.

A further refinement in nosology is suggested by the fact that there was a very strong association between aggressive-destructive, acting-out behavior and problems of impulse control and attention: 40% of the girls and 45% of the boys scored high on both factors. Thus, contrary to DSM-III-R nosology, it seems plausible that impulsivity/hyperactivity is not distinct from conduct disorder. Rather, they may be two factors associated with the same disorder, as suggested by Quay (1979).

Individual Symptoms

Whether inside or outside the internalizing/externalizing dimension, it is advantageous to be acquainted with the general incidences of symptoms and disorders reported in young children for purposes of both clinical assessment and theoretical evaluation. Richman and colleagues (1975) studied the prevalence of different behavior problems in a random sample of 3-year-old children in London and found that the most frequent behaviors reported were bedwetting (44% of the boys; 30% of the girls) and daytime wetting (23% of the boys; 11% of the girls). Approximately 13 to 14% of the children had food fads, problems with settling at night, and night waking; 18% of the boys and 11% of the girls were reported with soiling; 3% of the overall sample were unhappy; and 5% demonstrated poor concentration and volatile tempers.

In another London survey by Richman and colleagues (1982), the most common clinical encounters were with children who were restless, sought attention, and proved difficult to manage. While there were more behavior problems among boys than girls, the difference was not significant.

Bentovim and Boston (1973), using a clinical population, studied 135 preschool children in a children's hospital day-care facility and found 30% to have severe management problems. Another 10% were highly anxious; 15% had primary retardation; 13% were autistic; and 11% had language and speech problems.

While these studies all pertain to Western culture and do little to assist in assessing the particular disorders and circumstances that may cause the most dire results, they do provide a general base for study, and they help acquaint clinicians with the broad pattern of psychiatric presentations in early childhood.

Screening for Symptoms with a Possible Organic Brain Etiology

There is still a good deal of debate about the psychological sequelae of brain damage in childhood. However, some progress is being made at the level of mild to severe brain injury. It is known that brain injury can result in mental retardation, but what is the extent of the connection between brain injury and the development of psychological disorder?

Rutter (1981), using comparison groups of children with physical as opposed to mental handicaps, established that psychiatric disorder is approximately twice as likely to occur in children with mental handicaps as in children with equally debilitating physical handicaps. However, this relationship only holds for children who have suffered a severe head injury (prolonged posttraumatic coma versus minimal or no coma). The effect of brain injury on the development of psychiatric illness appears to be indirect, since the relationship between brain injury and cognitive deficit was much stronger than that between injury and the development of psychopathology. Rutter pointed out that there have been other reports that duration of coma is associated with the severity of later educational difficulties. Among other things, these findings suggest that there is a difference between psychiatric disorder and intellectual impairment with respect to the etiological role of brain injury. Unfortunately, barring obvious gross intellectual impairment, neurologic etiologies are difficult to verify. For example, the cerebral damage or dysfunction underlying hyperactivity and learning disabilities is more inferred than demonstrated.

As Reed (1984a,b) has pointed out, the difficulty lies in the fact that changes in the performance on psychological tests of neurologically impaired children always reflect not only the effects of the brain damage but the effects of increasing mental capacity due to normal mental growth and development. The most effective way of circumventing this difficulty is to administer not one, but a comprehensive battery of psychological tests and to compare the performance of brain-lesioned children with standardized norms. In Reed's estimation, the most often used and validated scales and tests used in young children are the Bender Visual Motor Gestalt Test (1938) and the Weschler scales (1949).

A study by Hertzig (1982) investigated the occurrence and developmental course of nonfocal neurological signs in children in special education classes. The results revealed a decrease in some "soft signs" (impairments in motor coordination) over time, suggesting that they might be symptoms of developmental delays rather than evidence of central nervous system dysfunction. Another finding in this study was that children of lower-than-average IQ are more likely than children of average IQ to evidence different nonfocal neurological signs at different stages of development. This suggests that these signs might be reflective of central nervous system organization and development.

It is important to keep in mind that children with specific learning disabilities generally do poorly on group-administered tests of intelligence and that it is not accurate to reach a conclusion regarding the capacity of such a child using this technique. In terms of prevention, the importance of administering individual tests in order to clearly establish the presence or absence of minimal brain dysfunction in childhood is illustrated by the results of a study by Shaffer and colleagues (1985). They found that 17-year-old adolescents with early neurological soft signs exhibited lower IQ's and were more likely to have experienced a psychiatric disorder. In this investigation, 63 male and 27 female adolescents known to have had neurological soft signs at 7 years of age were compared with controls who had no soft signs at age 7.

All of the girls and 80% of the boys with early motor impairment exhibited psychiatric disturbances at age 17. In the boys, affective and anxiety disorders were prevalent, while the girls largely experienced anxiety disorders. While these results show a potentially useful sex differentiation and illustrate the high morbidity associated with early motor impairment, soft signs appear to be necessary but not sufficient for the manifestation of affective and anxiety disorders in adolescence, since a majority of children with early soft signs did not go on to develop affective or anxiety problems in late adolescence.

Cross-Cultural Data

In order to gain a better understanding of the behaviors that may actually prove problematic in preschoolers, it is useful to examine these behaviors in a way that is independent of cultural biases. When this is done, one of the first important discriminations to emerge is that of sex. However, while there are some categories of behavior that are more likely to be exhibited by males and others more likely to be associated with females, an excellent cross-cultural investigation by Whiting and Edwards (1973) has demonstrated that these sex-associated behaviors depend more on individual experience than might be generally assumed.

In their investigation, Whiting and Edwards studied the validity of the stereotypes of sex differences manifested in the behavior of children between the ages of 3 and 11 who were observed in six different parts of the world (Kenya, Okinawa, India, the Philippines, Mexico, and the United States). The children were studied individually for 5-minute periods in natural settings, usually their house or yard, an average of 17 different times over a period of 6 to 14 months.

The following twelve types of interactions that would indicate sex-stereotyped behaviors were selected for analysis:

1. Offering support.
2. Offering help.
3. Seeking help and comfort.
4. Seeking attention and approval.
5. Acting sociably.
6. Dominating.
7. Suggesting responsibility or prosocial dominance (suggesting that another change his or her behavior in such a way as to meet the rules of the family or group).
8. Reprimanding.
9. Seeking or offering physical contact.
10. Engaging in rough and tumble play.
11. Insulting.
12. Assaulting.

Whiting and Edwards used these summary categories to assess the validities of seven sex-associated stereotypic behaviors. The first, "girls are more dependent than boys," was measured according to scores on the categories of seeking help, seeking attention, and seeking physical contact. They found that the stereotype of female dependency holds across cultures for two types of behavior, seeking help and seeking or offering physical contact. However, this is particularly true of the younger age groups, since there was no significant difference in this behavior in the 7- to 11-year-old children. Furthermore, it was found that seeking attention was a male form of dependency in 7- to 11-year-olds.

The stereotypic assumption that girls are passive was assessed according to the measure of aggressive and dominant instigations. While boys were found to respond more aggressively than girls and showed a trend toward being less compliant than girls, these differences were not as great as many other authors have claimed.

In terms of the common assumption that girls are more sociable than boys, it was found that there was a slight tendency for this to be true, but it was not significant. In other words, behaviors of seeking or offering help were nearly equally distributed among the sexes.

In terms of the nurturance dimension, there were no significant differences found in the younger age group between the sexes in any of the six societies. However, by ages 7 to 11, girls were observed to offer help and support to a significantly greater degree than boys. Thus it appears that there may be no innate tendency in girls to be more supportive than boys, since there were no differences at early ages for this behavior.

In terms of whether or not girls are more responsible than boys, it was found that girls in the 3- to 6-year-old group offered responsible suggestions more often than boys in all samples. Again, however, there was a change in this behavior with age. By the ages of 7 to 11 years, boys increased markedly in making constructive suggestions, and the difference in this behavior between the sexes was eradicated.

Testing the stereotype that boys are more dominant than girls, Whiting and Edwards found that this appeared to hold true. Egoistic dominance was significantly greater in the boys than the girls in the early age group, but it was not greater in the 7- to 11-year-old sample.

Finally, the assumptions that boys are more physically aggressive than girls and girls are more verbally aggressive were tested. Boys were found to score higher than girls on all measures of aggression, but the differences were significant only for rough-and-tumble play and verbal aggression. Whiting and Edwards suggested that the sex differences that are greatest in the 3- to 6-year-old group may be the best candidates as innate sex-linked characteristics. If this is true, their results indicate that girls naturally tend to seek and offer physical contact while boys are less inclined to do so. Likewise, girls seem to be inherently more responsible (more socially aware) than boys. Nurturance, on the other hand, does not appear to be inborn, since this behavior increases greatly with age—especially in boys—probably in response to socialization pressure.

While it helps to be aware of the sex-specific trends in behavior, these trends are highly malleable and can be greatly influenced by environmental factors. For instance, Whiting and Edwards noted that the proportionate increase in self-instigated acts of boys may be the result of the fact that girls are generally assigned tasks that keep them closer to the house and to adults. Both of these factors are associated with more requests and demands from others.

Whiting and Edwards also pointed out that in societies where boys take care of infants, do the cooking, and perform other household chores, they tend to be less aggressive, seek attention less often, and are less egoistically dominant. Thus, children of both sexes are highly responsive to variations in social and environmental demands. For a summary of behavioral changes over time for the boys and girls in the Whiting and Edwards study, see Table 4–2.

To round out the picture, it may prove enlightening to review the results of a longitudinal study conducted by Wolff (1961) on a population of 43 clinic-referred British preschool children, since Britain was not included in the survey by Whiting and Edwards. In Wolff's study, the subjects consisted of 24 boys and 19 girls with a mean age of 3 years, 10 months. At follow-up, their mean age was 8 years, 10 months.

Wolff classified the presenting complaints according to five general categories: (1) complaints about the child's being bad or unmanageable; (2) complaints about the child's fearfulness; (3) complaints about habit disorders; (4) complaints about speech disorders; and (5) miscellaneous complaints about breathholding attacks, withdrawal, refusal to play with toys, nightly attacks of laughter, attacks of going stiff, and so forth.

These complaints were further broken down into three categories of general symptomatology: phobic symptoms (specific fears, night terrors, excessive timidity, excessive clinging to mother, severe food refusal); habit disorders (sleep disturbances other than night terrors; eating disturbances other than severe food refusal; enuresis—more than just "occasional"; encopresis; gratification habits—thumb-sucking, rocking, masturbation); and aggressive symptoms (disobedience or stubbornness, aggressivity recorded as such, cruelty, destructiveness, temper tantrums).

Results were similar to those reported by Whiting and Edwards. Aggressive symptoms were recorded more often in boys than in girls at

Table 4–2. Changes in the Behavior of Girls and Boys from Ages 3 years, 6 months to 7 years, 11 months.

Behavior	Girls	Boys
Offers help	+**	
Offers support	+*	
Responsibility		+***
Seeks or offers physical contact	−**	−***
Proportion of self-instigated acts		+*

Note: A (+) indicates an increase with age, a (−) indicates a decrease.
*$p < .05$. **$p < .01$. ***$p < .001$.
Source: Whiting, B., & Edwards, C. (1973). A cross-cultural analysis of sex differences in behavior of children aged 3–11. *The Journal of Social Psychology, 91,* 181. Reprinted with permission of the Helen Dwight Reid Educational Foundation. Copyright © 1973 by Heldref Publications.

the time of admission. Phobic symptoms, on the other hand, were more frequent in girls at the time of admission, but not significantly so. Habit disorders occurred with approximately equal frequency in both sexes. Interestingly, at follow-up, the incidence of aggressive symptoms was approximately the same for both sexes, as were symptoms of phobia and habit disorders.

Thus, in both the studies of Whiting and Edwards and of Wolff, there was a marked attrition in sex-specific symptoms over time, a dimension that will be discussed shortly in greater detail. On follow-up, it was found that boys were assessed as more disturbed than girls on all measures of outcome. Furthermore, outcome was impaired when the child came from a broken home, when there was open marital strife, and when the parents themselves had been treated for psychiatric disorders in the past.

The factors associated with poor outcome (i.e., risk factors) in Wolff's study have been noted frequently elsewhere as well. Sameroff, Seifer, Zax, and Barocas (1987) performed a 4-year longitudinal evaluation of pregnant women with varying degrees of mental illness beginning in the perinatal period. The effects of three sets of variables on their offspring were assessed after four years: (1) specific maternal psychiatric diagnosis, (2) severity and chronicity of the disturbance, and (3) general social status.

Interestingly, it was found that a specific maternal diagnosis of schizophrenia had the least impact on child development. Neurotic-depressive mothers, on the other hand, had the worst effect on the development of their children. Over all, children with high multiple environmental risk scores (maternal mental disorder, low socioeconomic status, family discord) displayed significantly worse outcomes than those with low scores. Thus, the relative risk that children of preschool age will develop behavior problems can be assessed at least partially in terms of parental mental health, degree of family discord, and socioeconomic status—findings that have been substantiated many times (e.g., Coleman et al., 1977; Richman, 1977).

STABILITY OF PRESCHOOL BEHAVIOR PROBLEMS

Studies Demonstrating Stability

The results just cited, which were obtained from cross-cultural analyses and those in Great Britain, are helpful in that they agree with one another to a great extent and therefore provide a background against which clinicians can view individual preschool patients. They are also encouraging in that they demonstrate the utility of epidemiological studies. There appears to be a good deal of stability across time from preschool to school age and beyond, in spite of the fact that the studies also agree that the number of problem symptoms tends to decrease with age (Wolff, 1961). A possible explanation for the observed stability of problematic symptoms in the face of an overall decline in the frequency of symptoms will be put forth shortly.

The stability of certain early childhood behaviors may be partially attributable to the stability of certain patterns of behavior. Waldrop and Halverson (1975) performed an intensive and extensive longitudinal analysis of peer behavior in 35 male and 27 female children from age 2 years, 6 months to 7 years, 6 months. Three indexes were used to measure peer behavior. The first, involvement with peers, was defined as "very aware of the other children; frequently intervening in their activities; seldom engaged in solitary play." The second dimension, friendliness, was described as "frequently took initiative in showing positive affect with peers, smiling, or attempting to be friendly in other ways, or showing awareness of the needs of peers by helping; in addition, responded positively to friendly overtures initiated by peers." The third measure, active coping when blocked by peers, was defined as "reacted to by immediate verbal and /or physical attack on the block, quickly resolving the conflict."

At the 5-year follow-up, when the children were 7 years, 6 months old, it was found that children of both sexes who were friendly, involved with peers, and able to cope with aggressive peers at age 2 years, 6 months tended to become socially at ease at 7 years, 6 months, spending a great deal of time with peers and deciding what and with whom to play. In short, sociability at 2 years, 6 months was predictive of sociability 5 years later. Furthermore, a child who was peer-oriented at 2 years, 6 months was likely to be energetic and relatively fearless at both ages. Thus, the relative sociability of a child may aid in assessing the potential severity of a given behavioral problem. That is, for example, a hyperactive child who is asocial may be at greater risk than one who demonstrates a high level of peer interaction.

Independent of the stability of peer interactions, Richman and colleagues (1975), in attempting to augment the literature on emotional disorders in preschool children, found a high degree of concordance between the rate of emotional and behavior disorders in preschoolers and in later childhood and adolescence. These investigators took a one-in-four random sample of children who were going to be 3 years old the following month in a single London borough ($n = 705$).

The children were assessed by survey and then by a trained interviewer visiting the home. The interviewer administered a semistructured screening interview assessing the child's health, development, and behavior and some social aspects of the family. Language was assessed as well. It was found, as in other studies, that boys were more often described as too active while girls, as is commonly the case, were described as being significantly more fearful. Over all, the rate of behavioral and emotional disorders in these preschoolers (7% moderate to severe; 15% mild) was found to be very similar to the rates reported in later childhood and adolescence (e.g., Rutter, 1979; Graham & Rutter, 1973).

This stability in behavioral traits from preschool to school age and beyond has also been demonstrated in a study by Coleman and colleagues (1977). These investigators studied 100 3-year-old children attending nursery schools in an inner-city London borough. The sample contained 51 girls and 49 boys who ranged in age from 3 years, 1 month, to 3 years, 11 months. Mothers were interviewed with a slightly modified version of the Richman and Graham questionnaire, and a short questionnaire on maternal health was also included—an abridged form of part of the Cornell Medical Index.

The results showed that overactivity at home among boys was linked to problems at school. Conversely, for girls, it was separation difficulties that were most closely associated with school problems. An added feature of this study was the calculation of the rate of change of symptom frequency with age for both sexes. It was found that not only did problem symptom frequency decrease with age for both sexes, but there were no significant differences between the sexes in terms of the rate of the decrease.

Again, there was a high level of stability from year to year for both girls and boys in terms of total symptom scores, but the stability was greater between ages 4 and 5 than between 3 and 4 years of age. This finding of a general decrease in symptoms over time brings up the question of what it is that might account for certain symptoms persisting over time while others simply dissipate and fail to cause lasting problems.

Stability of Hyperactivity (Attention Deficit Disorder)

A study by Campbell and colleagues (1986) may prove instructive in this regard. Noting that a number of recent studies had indicated that children with relatively high rates of externalizing symptoms at age 3 as reported by their parents, tend not to outgrow their problems (e.g., Bates, Camaioni, & Volterra, 1975; Richman, Stevenson, & Graham, 1982), Campbell and associates followed up 54 3-year-olds at age 6—21 problem boys, 12 problem girls, 10 control boys, and 11 control girls.

It was found that approximately half of these hard-to-manage toddlers and preschoolers continued to show clinically significant problems at age 6. The dominant symptomatology was inattentive and impulsive, aggressive, or both. One third of the children met DSM-III criteria for attention deficit disorder. These children were significantly more symptomatic at age 3 than problem toddlers who were later found to be improved. Thus, the authors concluded that stability of symptoms over time may be governed by the initial severity of the symptoms rather than the pattern of symptomatology.

CONCLUSION

The lability of behavior in the preschool period presents perhaps the major hindrance to early detection of significant problem behaviors. As Coleman and colleagues (1977) noted, "To believe in too much consistency or continuity, even of personality characteristics, leads to the danger of underestimating the importance of role-playing, as well as the critical significance of learning, in the determination of behavior" (p. 208).

Thus far the best rule of thumb emerging from the epidemiological literature is that of *additivity*. That is, the vulnerability to developing a psychiatric problem appears to be linearly related to the number of risk factors to which a child is exposed. The problem remains one of more clearly defining the risk factors and their potentials for inducing psychopathology.

Another area that needs increased attention is that of determining and measuring factors that protect the child from risk and mediate parental stress. Some of these include intelligence, financial and marital status, quality of the marriage, and protective relationships inside or outside the family.

Finally, epidemiological studies of behavioral symptoms would be of great use in helping to determine the boundary between what is normal and what is abnormal behavior—a boundary that is particularly hazy in reference to young children.

CHAPTER FIVE

The Mental Status Examination

Part 1: Structured Interview

Zachary: Bad or Ugly

Zachary is a 3-year-old male who lives with his older sister and their mother. Zachary's mother separated from his father while she was pregnant with Zachary. The full-term pregnancy and birth took place without incidence. Zachary's medical history is uneventful. All developmental milestones were reached within the appropriate age limits, with the exception of one. When he began to speak, Zachary's mother noted a pronounced lisp.

Zachary was referred by his teacher at the day-care center he attends. She reported that over the course of 1 year she had observed Zachary to be frequently abusive toward other children both physically and verbally. Zachary's mother reported that this problem behavior began when he was about 1 year old: "He hits me and curses at me and never does what I ask." Zachary's mother added that for the past year his sleep pattern had become erratic: "Sometimes, he'll stay up 'til real late; even if I lock him in his room he won't go to sleep. Other times, though, he just falls asleep right after dinner." Both Zachary's mother and his teacher claimed that Zachary did not respond well to limit setting and, when denied a request, tended to "throw a temper tantrum."

At the start of the interview, Zachary, a cute, neatly dressed boy, seemed eager to begin the play session. The mental status examination was employed during the psychiatric evaluation, and Zachary's appearance was noted to be within normal limits. He exhibited no abnormalities of either posture or psychomotor activity. It was noted that Zachary had difficulty articulating the letters *th* and *l*. His social relatedness was assessed to be normal. His affect, however, was constricted and mostly angry. Often during the interview he would hit the stuffed animals he was playing with. Zachary's mood was generally quite irritable and labile, with rapid changes between eagerness and irritability, depression and amusement. His thought content revealed a need for immediate gratification and wishes for affection and approval. No formal thought disorder was observed and Zachary denied having hallucinations or delusions. Zachary's responses to questions were quick and decisive and thus volition was noted to be within normal ranges. He exhibited no suicidal ideation or behavior. A low frustration tolerance was observed in that he would immediately become angry if his requests were not responded to. His judgment was limited by his deficient ability to endure tension; however, this in no way seemed to affect his adjustment to the interview.

Throughout the interview, it was observed that Zachary depended heavily on displacement as a defense mechanism, often channeling his anger through the play materials. Zachary displayed low to normal levels of self-esteem, at times referring to himself as "bad" or "ugly." There was no mention of abnormalities of either sphincter control or appetite. Zachary's mother did report, however, that in the past month, he had experienced difficulty falling asleep. Zachary did not manifest somatic complaints during the course of the interview, and reports from his pediatrician indicated no physical abnormalities. As determined by a standardized intelligence test, Zachary's intellectual capacity was in the normal to high range. He was alert and well-oriented, and his memory for immediate, recent, and remote past was intact. His attention and concentration spans were also within normal limits.

The results of the mental status examination, coupled with the reports from Zachary's mother and teacher, pointed to diagnoses of oppositional defiant disorder and developmental articulation disorder.

Although the features of conduct disorder are quite similar to those of oppositional defiant disorder, the former diagnosis includes violation of the basic rights of others and societal norms. Thus, it would be an inappropriate diagnosis in this case. The features of oppositional defiant disorder may also be seen in psychotic disorders such as schizophrenia; however, since Zachary displayed neither thought disorders nor transient psychotic symptoms, this diagnosis could be ruled out. Differential diagnosis could be made between Zachary's mood fluctuations and the chronic depression evident in dysthymia. Since intelligence testing revealed that Zachary did not fall into the category of mental retardation, this diagnosis could be ruled out as well. Furthermore, a diagnosis of pervasive developmental disorder could be ruled out because this would require certain behavioral abnormalities (e.g., severe difficulties in social functioning) not manifested by Zachary.

The Axis II diagnosis of developmental articulation disorder had to be made as well. It was discovered, through physical examinations and audiometric testing, that Zachary's articulation difficulties were not the result of structural abnormalities or hearing impairments.

Thus the diagnoses of oppositional defiant disorder and developmental articulation disorder were assigned. It was recommended that Zachary begin once-weekly sessions of individual psychotherapy immediately and attend speech therapy classes on a daily basis.

INTRODUCTION

The psychiatric examination, an example of which was given above, refers to a child's physical, behavioral, and psychological presentation. The mental status examination, in turn, is the tool used to elicit a child's emotional and cognitive states through behavioral manifestations. In other words, it is a method for detecting the signs and symptoms of a child's mental state. Signs, in the mental status examination, are those facets of the patient's presentation that are noted by the clinician during the examination. For example, the clinician may note that the child seems confused or is dressed in a certain way. Symptoms, on the other hand, are factors that are strictly limited to the patient's domain of existence—the complaints, explanations, and comments that patients make about themselves. The written summation of the mental status examination should note whether information was gathered from the patient history, clinical observation, or patient report. Speculations by the clinician about this information should not be included in the written report of the examination. The record should also reflect the patient's self-description.

The mental status examination serves as the baseline in the diagnosis and treatment of a child. Initial information from the examination is studied in terms of its diagnostic implications. The clinician is alert for disorders that have symptoms similar to those manifested by the patient. Historical, observational, and patient-reported information is then drawn on to aid in differential diagnosis. The use of all available information helps to reduce the possibility of an inaccurate description of a patient's possible disorder and proves invaluable in treatment. Thus, to ensure the varied utility of the mental status examination, the clinician must, without exception, administer it in its entirety. Knowledge of a patient's strengths and weaknesses is also of critical importance in the development of viable strategies.

In performing the mental status examination, it is important to follow certain rules. To avoid inadvertent failure to survey all relevant areas, symptoms and behaviors should be examined according to the order and guidelines addressed here. Shapiro (1979) cited four strategies, given in the following list, that can help clinicians reduce possible error in information collection and behavioral observation:

1. Strive to remain focused on the activity of the moment, rather than allowing concern about the development of a relationship with the patient to impinge on your alertness to present tasks.
2. If the child makes ambiguous or contradictory statements, do not merely record your inferences, instead ask questions that will lead to clarification.
3. Review information that was obtained while the interviewer was not clear or was stressed and therefore not able to interpret the child's intended meanings accurately.
4. The record should clearly differentiate between inferred and observed information. The psychiatric evaluation, then, includes every type of information in order to be an effective diagnostic tool and record of conditions, or predispositions to conditions, at a given point in time.

The following section on psychiatric evaluation can be used to ensure that all relevant information is elicited.

OUTLINE FOR THE PSYCHIATRIC
EXAMINATION

I. Identification of Patient.   Included is information on the patient's age, sex, date of birth, school, grade, and religious and ethnic background. The referral source is also included, and the reasons provided for the referral.

II. Presenting Problems.   The problems are listed and defined, and specific examples are given. Where possible, reports use a verbatim account of comments made by sources. Information is included on the date of onset, precipitating factors, course, severity, aggravating and reducing factors, associated problems, and previous treatment and its effect. The effect of the child's disorder on the family is also described. If necessary, a distinction should be made between the data provided by the referral source, the parents, or the child. The account also indicates why help is being sought now.

III. Family History.   A chronology of the family constellation, which includes a description of family members, is provided. The description of the parents includes their names, ages, marital status, occupation, and their relationship to the child. If the child is taken care of by a surrogate, then the surrogate's relationship to the child is specified. A description of the marital relationship is also included.

The cultural, psychological, social, occupational, and educational background of each parent should also be described. Information is included on their goals; their attitudes toward work, education, and family; their interests and activities; and their relationships with members of their original family. Any hereditary illness and constitutional factors should also be indicated.

The information on siblings includes their names, ages, dates of birth, sexes, marital status, and grade in school or occupation. The role of the patient in the family system should also be clearly defined. This may be determined by asking such questions as "Who does the child resemble physically and behaviorally?" and "How does the patient's ordinal position in the family relate to that of the parents in their original families?" It is especially important to compare the functioning and accomplishments of the siblings and to indicate parental differences in attitudes toward different children.

IV. Past History.   This section of the child's history includes an account of the different stages in the child's development including the prenatal, perinatal, infancy, early childhood, nursery school, school-age, puberty, and adolescent stages. It describes the course of physical, normative, and psychosexual developmental parameters and how these were influenced by family, illness, and traumatic events. The child's present functioning is analyzed in order to discern significant patterns of adaptive and maladaptive behavior. The origin and development of these patterns are also described.

The history begins with a note regarding the number of previous children or miscarriages, whether the pregnancy was planned, and the parents' expectations regarding the child. Information is included on any physical or mental problems of the mother during the pregnancy. Birthweight, complications during delivery, postnatal condition, and the length of the pregnancy are also indicated.

The evaluation provides a history of the child's feeding, sleep, activity level, and responsiveness. Developmental milestones are indicated, such as when the child first sat without support, walked without help, used meaningful words, began toilet training, and achieved consistent bowel and bladder control. Comparison with siblings, as well as any regressive trends and their causes, are also noted.

Early experiences such as whether a parent, close relative, or friend died or left for prolonged periods are indicated. The child's age at the time and his or her reaction to the event are noted. A history of the child's major behavioral, emotional, and cognitive characteristics is also provided, with particular attention given to changes in these characteristics, since the onset of the condition for which the child was referred. A medical history notes any pattern of illnesses, convulsions, injuries, and hospitalizations. Results of the most recent physical examination should also be included.

V. Current Level of Functioning.   The evaluation describes the child's habits and fears, personality characteristics, temperament, affective behavior, regularity of physical functions, sexual interest, sensitivity, adjustment and performance at school, aptitudes, skills, social relationships with peers, aggressiveness, interests, and sports activities.

The evaluation should also present an assessment to rule out neurological soft signs, and/or cognitive impairment. In particular, subcortical structures, cortical associational areas and their projections, and the possibility of lesions may be appraised.

VI. Additional Information.   Factual information on the child's school, physician, social worker, nurse, or hospital record should be provided. Sources of information and a statement regarding their reliability should also be noted.

VII. Mental Status Examination. The evaluation includes a detailed narrative account of all contacts between the evaluator and the child. It focuses on the child's ego functions, pertinent ideation content, and sensorium, and it should include verbatim accounts of conversations and responses to questions. A description of the child's physical appearance, movements, activity level, motor coordination, focus and span of attention, and language skills should be included. The child's way of interrelating, apparent affect and emotional reactions, way of thinking, intellectual functioning, external reality testing, manner of play, and self-concept should also be described. An account of the child's own report about himself or herself, and an interpretation of it should be provided. All observations and interpretations should be clearly attributed.

VIII. Psychometric Testing. Results of any previous psychological testing should be included.

IX. Diagnostic Impression and Differential Diagnosis. DSM-III-R (APA, 1987) diagnoses (including all five axes) and other possible diagnoses should be included.

X. Formulation. This section should give a brief identification of the patient, the nature and course of problem areas, areas of strength, constitutional factors, biological (physical/organic) factors, environmental factors, dynamic factors including level of psychosexual development, defenses, and prognosis.

An assessment is made of the child's activity level, motor skills, intellectual development, drive development, current level of ego functioning, superego development, character traits, and overall personality organization. The evaluation should comment on the influence of genetic and environmental factors.

XI. Indications for Further Diagnostic Procedures. Further diagnostic procedures (e.g., neurological evaluation) that might be useful in the case of this patient should be indicated.

XII. Recommendations for Treatment. The recommendation may suggest that immediate symptomatic relief is indicated, or it may propose certain environmental alterations. Whether the intervention should take the form of psychotherapy, medication, or education is specified, and alternatives are discussed with the child and the child's family. In addition, the treatment goals and a prognosis are included.

ELEMENTS OF THE MENTAL STATUS EXAMINATION

This section discusses the major symptoms and their associated disorders. It is limited to disorders that may be diagnosed by age 18. The suggestions regarding detection strategies merely provide a framework for investigation.

Physical Appearance.   In addition to taking note of a child's general physical characteristics, the clinician should note the presence of any physical abnormalities. The description should enable the reader to picture the child. The clinician should record, among other things, the patient's apparent age, the appropriateness of his or her dress, and his or her general demeanor during the interview. The description of physical appearance is based solely on observation during the interview.

Abnormalities of Posture.   Unlike a description of physical appearance, a description of abnormalities in the patient's posture refers only to the positioning of the child during the session. Abnormalities may include muscular rigidity or inflexibility, excitability, gesture repetition, or waxy flexibility. Detection is made on the basis of observation during the interview.

Psychomotor Activity.   The term *psychomotor activity* refers to the quality of the child's fine and gross movements during the interview. These may range from psychomotor agitation, as evidenced by overactivity, restlessness, repetitive movements, or inability to sit still, to psychomotor retardation, as evidenced by an overall slowness of movement. Psychomotor agitation and psychomotor retardation can occur simultaneously, and the existence of either can be determined using questioning, clinical observation, and reports from others. Appropriate questions include the following: "Do people often tell you to calm down?" "Do you feel that you must constantly do certain things?" "Is it hard for you to start talking?" "Do you get into many fights?" and "Do you feel like you don't have enough energy?" Observations of the following activities should also be included: fastening shirt buttons, tying shoelaces, putting puzzles together, copying figures and letters on paper, bouncing and catching a ball, and hopping on one foot.

Affect.   The term *affect* refers to a child's emotional state or mood during the interview. The affect may be apprehensive, joyous, aggressive, angry, sad, anxious, flat, or merely situationally inappropriate. It can be evaluated through observation of facial expression and through questions such as, "Is there anything that makes you scared?" "What makes you very happy?" or "Do you ever feel nervous or jumpy?"

Mood. Descriptions of mood, unlike affect, do not imply any external evidence of the emotion that is being experienced by a child. In fact, children's moods reflect their perceptions of their internal states. Abnormal moods include feelings of depression and hopelessness, feelings of elation, and labile feelings, which change rapidly, regardless of the situation. Although mood can be determined through observation, the child may display affects that do not accurately reflect his or her moods, and thus it is better for the therapist to supplement observation with reports from others and questions such as "Do you get the 'blues' often?" "Are there times when you feel almost too happy?" and "Do you feel that there is anything that can make you feel better? What?"

Speech and Language. Symptoms of deficiencies in the child's verbal communication skills include voluntary abstinence from speaking in certain situations, a continuous flow of sentences that are only tangentially related, abnormalities in articulation or rate of speech, or limitations in expressive language skills. Speech and language abnormalities can be detected by listening during the interview and by questioning the child and significant others. Appropriate questions include asking others "Are there some situations in which the child refuses to speak?" and asking the child "Are there some times (or people to whom) you do not talk? When?"

The interviewer may seek to determine whether or not the child

- Understands questions ("Where is the door?").
- Can follow directions ("Put the pen on the table").
- Can combine words (uses two- or three-word combinations).
- Can ask for what is needed (e.g., asks for water, or to use the bathroom).
- Can name objects (pointing to shoe, "What is that?").
- Can use pronouns (e.g., "my," "mine," "you").
- Can distinguish prepositions ("Put the pen under the table").
- Can recognize action (in a picture book, "Point out the people who are running").
- Can repeat a certain number of digits ("Repeat after me: four, seven, etc.").
- Can repeat sentences ("Repeat after me: I like to watch television").
- Can use plurals (passing two pens, "What are these?").

- Can converse in sentences (uses several sentences that are more than four words long).
- Can build sentences ("Make up a sentence about a doll, a child, and a bed").
- Can articulate sentences (i.e., correctly pronounce the consonants in the sentence).

Is the child able to write, and are attempts to read adequate? Can the child attempt to write his or her name? When given written material to be read, does the child hold the material at a normal distance?

Social Relatedness.   The term *social relatedness* refers to a child's level of adaptive functioning in social and occupational settings. It may involve a failure to develop friendships, a lack of sociability, an inability to sympathize or empathize with others, exhibitions of indiscriminate attachments, or abnormal responses to social stimuli. Such abnormalities may be discovered by observing the child's interactive skills during the interview, by reports of others, and by questions such as "Do you have any friends? How many?" "How do you feel about the other kids in your school?" and "What do you think they feel about you?"

Perception.   The term *perception* covers all functions related to the integration of external stimuli. Abnormalities of perception include misinterpretations or misrepresentations of environmental stimuli. Hallucinations are perceptions that occur in the absence of external stimuli; hallucinations in young children are not pathognomonic of psychosis, in fact more frequently than not they are associated with anxious states such as separation. They may be detected through reports from others who know the child, through evidence from the mental status examination, and through direct questioning of the child with such questions as "Have you ever seen a ghost?" "Have you ever heard voices that others don't hear?" and if the answer is yes, then "Do the voices tell you that you are not a nice _____?"

Content of Thought.   Abnormalities in thought content include delusions (judgments of reality that are at variance with social norms and are held despite evidence to the contrary) and obsessions (involuntary, intrusive ideas and thoughts or recurrent, inappropriate wishes, beliefs, or ideas, for example: excessive rumination, brooding, wishes of death, etc.). They can be detected through observation during the interview, through reports from others, or by asking the child such questions as "Do you ever think that you're being controlled by someone else?" "Do you often think the same thing over and over and feel like you can't stop?" "Do you have any secret thoughts, or some ideas that you don't tell anybody else because you think they won't understand?" and "Do you want to die soon?"

Comprehension. The term *comprehension* refers to a child's ability to correctly interpret unambiguous questions. Abnormalities in comprehension are detected from observation during the interview, reports of others, and by direct questioning of the child. Such questions might include "Who did you come with today?" "Working from left to right, describe the objects in the room." "What do we use our ears for?" "Put the pen on the table." and "Put your right hand on your left knee."

Word Finding. The term *word finding* refers to one aspect of the child's general language skills—the ability to find the correct word to describe something. Deficiencies in this skill can be detected from reports of others and by asking the child to name objects in the room or parts of his or her body.

Constructional Ability. Constructional ability is the ability to construct drawings of objects. Abnormalities are revealed through the reports of others and by either showing the child some drawings and asking him or her to reproduce them or by asking the child to draw an object such as a three-dimensional cube or a clock with its numbers.

Fund of Information. This term refers to the extent of the child's stock of knowledge. Abnormalities are detected from observation during the interview and reports of others. Questions may seek to determine whether the child

- Understands the concept of "one" ("Give me the pen").
- Understands notions about size (from a group of balls, "Show me the small, little ball").
- Understands use (from objects on a table, "Show me what we use to cut paper").
- Can distinguish body parts ("Show me the leg of the doll" and "Show me your own leg").
- Can name objects (pointing to table, "What is that?").
- Understands notions about length ("Show me the long pencil").
- Can recognize colors ("Which is the red ball?").
- Understands notions about weight differences ("Which is the heaviest ball?").
- Can distinguish and name coins ("Point to the quarter, the dime, etc.").

- Knows coin values ("How many pennies are there in a dime?").
- Can name animals (from a picture book, "Show me the horse," etc.).
- Can add and subtract numbers up to 10 ("How many pennies do you have left if you begin with six, and then take away three?").
- Knows his or her address and telephone number ("What is your address?").

Transient Psychotic Symptoms.   These are temporary manifestations of psychosis during which the child may experience delusions or hallucinations. Children with these symptoms typically feel that they are no longer in control of themselves. The presence of transient psychotic symptoms may be established from reports prepared by the patient and/ or from asking the patient such questions as "Do you ever feel from time to time like you are standing outside your body?" and "Do you ever feel as though you are a robot, or like one of your toys?"

Orientation.   *Orientation* refers to a child's ability to place himself or herself in time and place. Impairments in orientation may be detected through observation during the interview or by questioning the child about how much time has elapsed, or where the child is, where he or she came from, and where the child is going after the interview.

Volition.   Disturbances in volition, or will, include a child's inappropriate utilization of the power to decide and choose. The child may appear passive and avoid responsibility and confrontation or may consistently make choices that have negative outcomes. Disturbances in volition may be detected through observation during the interview, reports from the patient or others, or by asking the patient such questions as "What is the worst thing you've ever done?" "Did you think about the results before you did it?" and "If you think about it now, is there anything you did that you now think you shouldn't have done? What?"

Intentionality.   *Intentionality* refers to a child's awareness of people as agents who guide and control their own actions through intentional processes. This awareness is recursive when it is realized that knowledge of intention may be shared by others. Abnormalities of intentionality include an inability to regard intentions as causes of behavior and an inability to distinguish between intended actions and unintentional behavior such as mistakes, reflexes, and passive movements. These abnormalities may be detected through observation during the interview, reports by the child and others, and by asking the child such questions as "Why do you think your parents punished you?" and "Do you ever try to fool people about what you're up to?" To determine whether the child understands what the agents of action are, the interviewer can ask questions such as "Show me which one we cut with" (from a picture book).

Suicidal Ideation or Behavior. This term refers to persistent thoughts of or wishes for death or thoughts of killing oneself. It may also refer to a tendency to self-injurious behavior. The therapist should be aware of the difficulties in applying the concept to young children, many of whom are unable to grasp the meaning of death fully. The presence of suicidal ideation may be established through observation during the interview, from reports prepared by the patient or significant others, or from questioning the patient. Such questioning must first establish that the child understands the concept of death. Appropriate questions include "What happens when people die?" "Have you thought about dying?" "Have you ever tried to kill yourself?" and "What would happen if you died?"

Locus of Control. The term *locus of control* refers to the degree to which individuals perceive events to be contingent upon their own actions, rather than external forces. Children with an internal locus of control tend to be more goal- and task-oriented than those with an external locus of control. The locus of control may be determined from the reports of others and by asking the child such questions as "Tell me what makes you happy." "What makes your father happy?" "Do you find that no matter how hard you try, some people just don't like you?" and "Do you have a lot of bad luck?"

Impulse Control. Difficulty with impulse control usually manifests itself as a tendency to act quickly, without conscious thought. These actions are usually pleasurable and seemingly irresistible, but have harmful effects on the self. Impulsiveness may be evidenced through observation during the interview, reports by others, and asking the patient such questions as "Do you often do things without thinking about them first?" "Do you ever get into trouble for doing things that you don't think about ahead of time?" and "Do you ever have urges that you cannot control?"

Impulsivity. The term *impulsivity* is applied to people who make quick decisions in uncertain circumstances. The decisions are typically less appropriate to the circumstances than reflective decisions, which are made slowly. Fast, inaccurate decision makers are often anxious, very active, hypersensitive, and vulnerable. Impulsivity can be detected through observation during the interview, from reports by others, and by asking the patient such questions as "Do you need a lot of time be-fore making up your mind?" "What do you do if you're rushed to make a decision quickly?" and "Do you often find that your decisions are wrong?"

Judgment. The term *judgment* refers to the ability to select the best solution from among a number of options. Impaired judgment is re-flected in conflict between the choice and a given set of norms, values, and morals. It may be detected from reports from significant others and by asking the patient such questions as "What would you do if you found an addressed letter?" and "Have you ever hurt or killed an ani-mal? How often?"

Adaptive Functioning. A child's adaptive functioning refers to the ability to modify behavior to fit the environment. Deficits in adaptive functioning may be detected by observing how the child behaves during the interview, from reports by others such as teachers and parents, and by asking the child questions, that, for example, seek to determine whether the child can follow simple commands ("Put the pens in the box"); can comprehend physical needs ("What do you do when you are thirsty?"); is eager to try new activities; can tolerate frustration; can lis-ten before responding; is able to complete tasks; can play cooperatively; offers to help spontaneously; seeks help when appropriate; and re-sponds appropriately to the moods of other people.

Conception of Status and Role. Even young children have an aware-ness of their status and its implications, and they have some knowledge of role expectations and alignments. Confusion during role-play epi-sodes and poor socialization skills are signs of inadequate conceptual abilities in these areas. Such deficiencies are evidence of the child's in-ability to reflect on his or her actions from the viewpoint of others. The child's ability to correctly perceive status and role may be ascertained through observation, from the reports of the child and others, and by asking the child such questions as "When you're playing with other people, what role do you like to play?" "Do you like being a doctor, a teacher, a fireman, etc.?" "How do you feel when people tell you to do something?" and "What kinds of things do you do better than other friends?"

Repertoire of Activities and Interests. Abnormalities in a child's rep-ertoire of activities and interests typically manifest themselves in the form of resistance or exaggerated reactions to minor changes in usual activities or in exclusive interest in one kind of object or play. They may be detected using reports of others, observing during the interview, or by asking the child such questions as "When you are outside of school, what kinds of things do you like to do?" and "Are there things that you used to enjoy doing that you don't enjoy doing anymore?" "What?"

Defense Mechanisms. Defense mechanisms are unconscious processes that have the role of helping individuals deal with inner conflicts or anxiety. The defense mechanisms most often used by children are defined below.

Acting Out: The expression of unconscious feelings through behaviors and actions, rather than through words. These actions are generally impulsive and are carried out without regard for consequences.

Denial: The unconscious rejection of certain thoughts, beliefs, emotions, wishes, or obvious facts. This is indicated by omitting or forgetting information.

Devaluation: An overemphasis of the negative features of oneself and/or the surrounding environment.

Displacement: Feelings for some highly significant other are transferred onto someone or something that is less important or significant.

Dissociation: Separating one group of mental processes from the mainstream of consciousness. Behavior and thought may, consequently, lose their relationship to the rest of the personality.

Distortion: Misrepresenting or misinterpreting external stimuli in an attempt to meet internal concepts, needs, and beliefs. This is indicated by unusual or bizarre thought contents.

Idealization: Overemphasizing of the positive features of oneself, meaningful others, and/or the surrounding environment.

Intellectualization: Stripping ideas and thoughts of their emotionality.

Isolation: The separation of ideas from related thoughts and attitudes that may provoke anxiety or be considered unacceptable. This is indicated by a detached and literal attitude.

Passive Aggression: The manifestation of aggression through a lack of assertive behaviors.

Projection: The attribution to others of one's unacceptable feelings and ideas. This is indicated by a belief that others are to blame or that others have secrets.

Rationalization: Inventing a plausible reason for an action, thought, or emotion in an unconscious attempt to avoid confronting a real reason.

Reaction Formation: The manifestation of a behavior that is the direct opposite of unconscious feelings and wishes. This is indicated by exaggerated goodness, oppositional attitudes, and stubbornness.

Repression: Keeping thoughts, feelings, and ideas that may arouse anxiety from conscious awareness through control or restraint. This is indicated by overobedience, conformance, and statements such as "I didn't want it anyway."

Somatization: Excessive focusing on physical discomfort in the absence of any actual malady.

Splitting: The classifying of environmental and social stimuli as being either all good or all bad.

Undoing: Symbolically repeating a particular behavior in reverse in an attempt to relieve the anxiety brought about by the particular behavior. This is indicated by ambivalence or indecision and by statements such as "I would have done it, but. . . ."

The use of specific defense mechanisms may be detected from observation of the child, and from the reports of others.

Sense of Self.   This term refers to a child's perception of and feelings about himself or herself. Abnormalities in a child's sense of self may take the form of low self-esteem, oversensitivity to criticism, grandiosity, lack of self-confidence, or an inability to separate self from others. Disturbances in the child's sense of self may be detected from reports of others, observation during the interview, or by asking the child such questions as "How do you feel about yourself?" "Do you often worry about what others will think about you?" "Do you try to make everybody happy?" and "Do you think you are a better person than most people you know?" Whether or not the child refers to himself or herself by name should also be noted.

Body Image.   Body image refers to how a child perceives his or her body. A child may be overconcerned with physical appearance or may have a mistaken belief that he or she looks a certain way. Disturbances in body image are revealed through observation of the child's appearance during the interview and by asking the child such questions as "Could you describe to me what you look like?" "What do you think people notice about you when they meet first meet you?" and "Which do you think is more important, how a person looks or how he acts?"

Right-Left, Temporal, and Spatial Orientation.   These terms refer to the ability to correctly identify right from left, time sequences, and spatial dispositions. Abnormalities are revealed through reports of others, and by asking the child such questions as "Can you show me your left ear?" "Can you show me my right eye?" "Can you turn to the left?" "Can you tell me the days of the week?" "Can you tell me the seasons of the year?" and "Can you show me the right (or left) side of the room?"

Psychosexual Behavior. This term refers to sexual behavior that is guided by mental concepts, urges, and wishes. Abnormal psychosexual behavior may take the form of inhibition, discomfort with one's own gender, exposing one's genitals in public, or becoming sexually excited through inanimate objects, pain, or the induction of pain in others. Such disturbances may be detected through reports by the child or others and by asking such questions as "Are you a boy or a girl?" "Do you ever think that you should have been born a member of the opposite sex?" "How do you feel about being a _____?" and "Do you get excited when you put on (boys', girls') clothes?"

Sphincter Control. Sphincter control refers to control over elimination and excretion. Disturbances of sphincter control may be detected through observation during the interview, from reports by others, and by asking the child such questions as "Do you wet your bed often?" "Did you ever go to the doctor to find out about why you have those accidents? What did the doctor say?" and "Do you ever have bowel movements in places other than the toilet?"

Appetite and Eating Disturbances. Such disturbances may include severe changes in eating behaviors or some deviation from societal norms. Specific abnormalities include the consumption of massive quantities of food in a relatively short time span, repeated regurgitation without nausea or gastrointestinal disorders, ingesting nonnutrient substances, and refusal to eat. Eating disturbances may be detected from reports by the patient and others and by asking such questions as "Do you sometimes feel like you can't get full?" "Do you have to force yourself to eat at all?" and "How do you feel about your weight?"

Sleep/Awake Disturbances. The term *sleep disturbances* refers to a change in the child's normal sleep-wake patterns, persistent nightmares, inability to sleep, awakening in the middle of the night, and difficulty waking up. The presence of sleep disturbances may be detected from reports by the patient and others, or by asking the patient such questions as "Do you have difficulty falling asleep at bedtime? Waking up?" "After you fall asleep, do you sometimes wake up sooner than you want to?" and "Do you have a lot of nightmares?"

Somatic Complaints. Somatic complaints are complaints of physical pain and discomfort that are typically experienced in the presence of a specific environmental or social stimulus but have no explanatory physical cause. These may be reported by the child, or their presence may be detected through the reports of others. In addition, the child may be asked such questions as "Do you get many headaches? Stomach aches?" and "Do you feel sick like that on the weekend?"

Intellectual Functioning. Abnormal intellectual functioning refers to a level of intellectual performance that deviates from norms. It can be detected using standard intelligence tests, reports of parents and teachers, and clinical interviews.

Academic Performance. In contrast to the term *intellectual functioning, academic performance* refers solely to the child's accomplishments in school. Difficulties in academic performance are revealed in reports from teachers or other school officials and through a comparison of the child's results on skills and abilities tests with his or her general school performance.

Attention Span. This term refers to a child's ability to focus on a particular activity over a period of time. It can be judged from reports of others and through observations during the interview.

Concentration Span. In contrast to the term *attention span, concentration span* refers to the child's ability to make a conscious effort to engage in a particular activity for a period of time. This may be judged by reports from others and through observation during the interview.

Memory. Memory is a child's ability to correctly recall either new information or information learned in the past. The information may be either verbal or visual. In the case of patients with language difficulties, memory should be tested using visual memory tests. Memory skills can be measured through observation during the interview and by asking the patient questions regarding facts learned in the past or facts provided a few minutes earlier. Examples of such questions are "What is your mother's name?" "Can you tell me a rhyme or a song?" "How far back in time can you remember?" "What did I just say?" "Repeat the following sentence." "What were the numbers I just told you?" and "Tell me the names of some of your classmates." Visual memory can be tested by showing the child a group of objects and then 5 minutes later asking the child to name as many as possible. Is the child able to remember the properties?

Similarities. This term refers to the child's ability to recognize the essential similarity between objects, situations, or people that are overtly different. An inability to recognize similarities may be revealed by asking the patient questions such as "How are horses and dogs alike?" and "How are you and your parents alike?"

Opposites. The term *opposites* refers to the child's ability to recognize the essential likenesses or differences between objects, situations, or people. An inability to recognize these qualities may be revealed by asking the child a question such as "How are dolls and babies different?" and "How are boys and girls different?" The questions may also be framed as follows: "The elephant is big, the mouse is . . . ."

CONCLUSION

This chapter has provided a guide to the information that should be sought in order to evaluate a child's emotional and cognitive states. This information is the basis for diagnosis and subsequent treatment. Its breadth is indicative of the range of possibilities, and it is essential that the clinician touch on each area if an inaccurate description of the patient's possible disorder is to be avoided.

CHAPTER SIX

The Mental Status Examination

Part II: Play Interview

Brenda: Unusual Stereotypies

Brenda is a 3-year, 4-month-old girl who lives with her younger sister and their parents. Brenda was the product of a planned pregnancy; both pregnancy and birth had no complications. All developmental milestones were reached within the appropriate age limits. Brenda has a medical history of mild anemia, but she is otherwise healthy. There is no evidence of either neurological impairment or seizure disorder.

Brenda's mother brought her for treatment because of the presence of several unusual behaviors. Prior to falling asleep, Brenda sat on her bed and rocked from side to side. She then curled up in the fetal position, looked back and forth, pointed to the ceiling, made bubbles with her mouth, and emitted moaning or laughing noises. When someone entered her room, or called her name, Brenda immediately ceased this behavior pattern; however, when asked about it, she did not respond.

When called in from the waiting room to be administered the mental status examination, Brenda was observed to be playing energetically with her 20-month-old sister. Upon introduction to the therapist, however, Brenda became quiet and guarded. Throughout the interview, no abnormalities of posture were noted. Brenda's gross motor skills (e.g., running and walking up and down stairs) were performed without difficulty. Brenda's fine motor activity was tested and found to be well-coordinated. Furthermore, abnormal movements were not evidenced. Brenda frequently displayed anger throughout the session; however, this was only directed toward her mother.

Although fairly quiet during the interview, when Brenda did speak, it was in fluent, well-articulated Spanish. Her comprehension of English was exhibited by her nodding or shaking her head in response to questions posed in this language. With her mother translating, Brenda was able to name many animals and colors. When her mother left the room, Brenda became withdrawn and unresponsive; in later sessions, this behavior persisted.

No abnormalities in perception were noted; Brenda was aware of her surroundings and her thought processes were unremarkable. Brenda denied feeling sad or wanting to hurt herself or others. Her repertoire of activities and interests was restricted in that play appeared to be confined to a sensorimotor level (scribbling, piling up boxes). In addition, Brenda would not discuss her nighttime behavior and would turn away when questioned about it. Brenda displayed an intact sense of self, and her body image was not disturbed. Although Brenda's mother was concerned about Brenda's "sexual play and putting her hands in her pants," this behavior was not noted in any of the sessions. No disturbances of sphincter control or of eating patterns were reported, and sleep disturbances were limited to the behavior patterns mentioned previously. Brenda did not report somatic complaints throughout the interview.

Intellectual functioning was determined to be in the high range as determined by the use of standardized intelligence tests. No information was reported regarding Brenda's academic performance. Throughout the session Brenda displayed an adequate attention span and did not appear distracted or internally preoccupied. With the exception of Brenda's curling up in the fetal position on the couch next to her mother, none of the behaviors reported in the chief complaint were observed during the course of her interviews.

Although the pattern of behaviors or similar ones reportedly displayed by Brenda before she fell asleep were not observed during the interview, a tentative diagnosis of stereotypy/habit disorder was assigned. The consistent pattern of repetitive rocking and other behaviors displayed by Brenda at bedtime did not cause her injury; however, they did interfere with her ability to fall asleep and thus met the criteria for this disorder.

Self-stimulating behaviors (such as rocking before going to sleep) are common in normal infants and young children. However, the frequency with which Brenda manifested these behaviors and the fact that they were only a part of a pattern of behaviors (i.e., pointing, making bubbles, laughing or moaning) implied the presence of a disorder. Stereotyped behaviors such as these are also present in tic disorders; however, under such a diagnosis the behaviors would have to be intentional. Although patterns of nonfunctional behaviors are also a feature of pervasive developmental disorders, Brenda did not exhibit the qualitative impairment in the development of reciprocal social interaction that is an essential criterion for this diagnosis.

Thus, a diagnosis of stereotypy/habit disorder was assigned; however, both a diagnosis of tic disorder and one of pervasive developmental disorder would be considered during further assessment. For the time being, recommendation was made for Brenda to begin individual psychotherapy twice a week and for family counseling to take place on a monthly basis.

INTRODUCTION

Observations of play behavior, as in the case cited above, can be used to determine whether a child is meeting normal developmental-level expectations or is displaying a lack of developmental adaptation that may be indicative of psychopathology. The nature of the child's personal play styles and the choice of materials can also be examined. For example, Woltmann (1964) found that children suffering from psychosis seldom create patterns in their play, whereas obsessive-compulsive children may spend hours arranging and rearranging blocks or tiles in order to create geometric shapes and designs that are perfectly symmetrical. The therapist can observe whether the child's play schemes become alive in play situations that are either nonverbal and spontaneous or structured. When the child is provided with the structure of the play setting, spontaneous play can occur, which helps the child express himself or herself, thus enabling the therapist to better diagnose the child's mental status. Nonverbal play activities provide a means for diagnosing the young or impaired child who is unable to use verbal language for communicating thoughts and emotions.

The child's demeanor during play may aid the therapist in determining the child's attitude toward life in general. Moore (1964) stated that, in pretend situations, normal children are enthralled by their world, behaving like artists or scientists.

> *Regarding fantasy as a mere escape from boredom and frustration, is as one-sided as the opposite view that we are driven to face reality only as a refuge from an inner life which is primary but terrifying. The balanced individual should not only have come to terms with both worlds but should, at times in his life, have been an active explorer in the sheer joy of exploration.* (p. 35)

Pretending is not simply a means through which children express emotional conflicts or escape from boredom, it frees them to conjure up whatever images they are able to create.

Regarding the actual imaginative sequences, therapists must note the child's attitude toward his or her plans in order to determine the child's emotions as well as cognitive skills. A child may be playing skillfully at the appropriate developmental level, yet may not display joy or zest during this play activity.

The more unstructured the child's play situation becomes, the more likely the child is to release emotions and act out behaviors that may be beyond his or her control. Woltmann (1964) argued that the less structured the play materials, the greater the potential for projective communication and, therefore, the more definitive the diagnoses that can be derived from observations. Woltmann contended that nonverbal play activities are a language in themselves that replace verbal communications. The child's projections of self onto the materials provide a series of activities and creations available for interpretation.

Psychological disturbances place the child at risk for maladaptive and other damaging behaviors during pretend episodes. However, under specific therapeutic conditions, the play situation that may at one time represent a risk factor for the psychopathologically disordered child, may also provide the child with the means to alleviate distress (Barnett, 1984; Erikson, 1940; Freud, 1946, 1962; Waelder, 1933; Winnicott, 1971). The play environment should be safe and free from the immediate consequences of the real world, so that the child can concentrate more on play actions, and less on the outcomes of such actions (Bruner, 1972; Piaget, 1962; Vandenberg, 1968). In the case of aggressive/suicidal children, who lack the ability to regulate their behaviors, unstructured play situations carry the risk of self-damaging behavior.

Through play situations, the clinician can observe and consequently characterize the child's behavioral repertoire as it relates to a variety of diagnostic categories (Crowell, Feloman, & Ginsberg, 1988). Over time, qualitative and quantitative changes in play behaviors can be used to chart the child's mental status. This chapter outlines diagnostic corre-lates to play behavior that may become evident during unstructured play interviews and discusses their subsequent utility in identifying and/or validating diagnostic impressions.

DEFINITION OF PLAY BEHAVIORS

An all-encompassing definition of play does not exist. Piaget (1962) sug-gested that play activities are a means for children, from their own ego-centric perspective, to ascribe meanings and significance to people and objects. Vygotsky (1967), on the other hand, stated that play occurs wherever the child creates an imaginary situation. In this sense, play is an activity in which the child takes an experience from real life and transforms it into a symbolic, nonliteral representation. Vygotsky also argued that symbolic play catalyzes the transition from things as objects of action to things as objects of thought. Regardless of its definition, play provides developing children with the means by which they can rehearse the experiences that matter in real life.

SYMBOLIC MATURITY

Both language and symbolic play emerge during the child's 2nd year of life, a development that has been interpreted as the byproduct of com-mon representational processes (Casby & Della Corte, 1986; Lowe, 1975; Piaget, 1967). Pretend activities first appear during the 12th or 13th month of life (Fein & Apfel, 1979). They increase over the following 3 or 4 years and then begin to decline (Fein, 1981). Not surprisingly, a substantial difference exists between the frequency of pretend play in preschoolers and that in kindergarten groups; only 10 to 17% of pre-school children, as opposed to 33% of the older children engage in pretend play (Rubin, Maioni, & Hornung, 1976; Rubin, Watson, & Jambor, 1978; Singer, 1973). By the age of 4, however, 50% of the chil-dren's pretend activities are ideational in nature, and they do not de-pend on the presence of physical objects in their immediate environ-ment (Fein, 1981; McLoyd, 1980). Thus, if the action is directed toward the self, it is more likely for preschool children to gesturally represent an object (Overton & Jackson, 1973). Interactive pretend play increases between the ages of 3 and 6 years (Corsaro, 1979; Iwanaga, 1973). By 4 years of age, children can and are eager to describe their own pretend scenarios (Singer, 1973). This has great utility for exploring the child's mental status.

METACOMMUNICATION AND FANTASY

Metacommunication

During play the child must be able to discriminate the signifier from the object or its signified role, an ability that has been termed *metacommunication* (Bateson, 1955). The child who can recognize the symbol and/ or separate it from its referent is able to play adaptively, drawing upon a language of symbols to communicate thoughts and feelings. In sharp contrast, the child lacking metacommunicative skills may be at risk for acting-out, maladaptive behaviors. Failure to distinguish referents from symbols may lead the child to act out his or her immediate perceptions. Metacommunication, therefore, involves the child's ability to differentiate between play and nonplay states. Children develop the ability to frame their experience as well as its content, an activity that makes them adept at stepping in and out of the structural play frames (Bateson, 1955).

Fairy tales may be one means by which children recognize and master metacommunicative skills. Fairy tales are magical, timeless, and space-less stories that depict the growth of individuals through fascinating circumstances. Fairy tales may gratify children because they allow them to think that when they grow up they, too, will receive the fairy tales' promise of independence and a solid sense of self (Schwartz, 1964). Children are seeking solutions to their emotional conflicts; thus fairy tales aid their problem-solving efforts, giving them both magical and real answers that teach them how to master conflicts in the real world (Sullivan, 1953). They aim to enjoy the struggle of growing up and mastering conflicts.

Schwartz has stated that the heroes of fairy tales are like all people in the real world. However, these people live not in the real world, but rather in a supernatural world where anything can occur. Children who read fairy tales believe in this fantasy world. However, once the story concludes and the children are no longer caught up in its plot, they can recognize that although some elements of these stories do reflect real life, other elements are purely fantasy. Fairy tales have their origins in real life and reflect the culture from which they originate. However, although the morals in such tales may reflect those of real life, fairy tales are unrealistic in nature. The fairy tale world is governed by rules of magic in which anything can happen.

A very popular fairy tale is *Where the Wild Things Are*, by Maurice Sendak. In this tale, a young boy, Max, misbehaves, and as a result his mother sends him up to bed without his dinner. From his room, Max sets out on a journey to where the wild things are, where he cavorts and plays with the wild things, becoming their king. Max tires of this game and becomes hungry, so he returns home to find his dinner placed in his room by his mother. Metacommunicative skills are mastered through such stories. The child recognizes the reality of his self and recognizes the punishment inflicted upon him for misbehaving. The magic of the tale begins when Max sails away to the land of the wild things. At this point in the tale, the child must metacommunicate—the child believes that Max is able to make his fantastic journey because his anger, realistic in its force and recognizable to the child through his own experiences, finds resonant emotional expression through Max's trip. In it, Max can escape the object of his fury, wreak revenge, and assert control by conquering the monsters and making them his own. Having worked through these feelings, he can forgive, returning reconstituted and able, once again, to face the realities of his home situation. Through such a tale, the child learns that Max's journey is not realistic; however, Max's emotions can evoke an empathic response in the child, and thus appear to be more realistic.

Analysis of fairy tales can provide the therapist with clues to a culture, problems, solutions, and the elements of mental functioning. Schwartz has found that fairy tales can be analyzed much like dreams. He has defined seven characteristics inherent in the fairy tale situation. They (1) are symbolic; (2) contain hidden and obvious meanings; (3) are often structured around opposites (good versus evil; the giant versus the child); (4) distort and reinterpret reality; (5) contain elements of drama; (6) express wishes and desires; and (7) utilize the methods of condensation, substitution, displacement, devaluation, and overevaluation.

Since fairy tales, myths, and dreams employ elements the child encounters in reality, they may also serve to relieve the anxiety encountered during unsurmountable life episodes (Sullivan, 1953). However, whereas dreams meet the needs of one individual at one particular time, and this individual may retell the dream in order to confirm its validity, fairy tales serve a different purpose. Fairy tales are validated not by their culture but by the moral and problem-solving techniques given them by the culture. Sullivan contended that such tales encompass universal issues (love, war, etc.) that affect most people's lives. Therefore, these tales are embraced and passed down through generations, altered slightly to suit specific eras. Fairy tales serve as one means of metacommunication between a culture and its morals, both representing and rejecting the reality of the culture to which they refer. Children, whether they are conscious of such knowledge or not, are influenced by such fairy tales and learn to differentiate and assimilate their reality by rehearsing magical stories.

Scarlett and Wolf (1979) researched children's abilities to metacommunicate between fairy tales and real life, observing how children step within a fairy tale frame and yet hold onto the boundaries of real life and play situations. In play, children create imaginary situations in which they attribute meanings to objects and enact roles that suit their personal needs and desires. Play is an activity through which children can escape the confines of realistic thinking. The observation that children make what they know to be inanimate objects in reality into animate objects in play demonstrates their recognition that reality and play are separate, distinct worlds. Fairy tales, on the other hand, do not satisfy the same needs that play does. Scarlett and Wolf argued that fairy tales and real life overlap and intrude upon one another. They concurred with Sullivan (1953) and Schwartz (1964), who asserted that a culture and its fairy tales share many qualities—the culture rewriting the fairy tale over time, and the fairy tale influencing people's behavior patterns.

Scarlett and Wolf contended that the child has one foot in the storybook and the other firmly planted in reality. The child neither embraces nor rejects the story. The child must, therefore, be able to differentiate between the story and real life. Otherwise, the story itself, once heard, can become a reality. In addition, the researchers suggested that in order to solve any conflict within the story, the child must be able to refer back to real-life solutions. Thus, metacommunication involves the child's ability to relay information from within or outside the fairy tale back to reality. The child's learned ability to introduce reality-based knowledge into the fairy tale demonstrates the ability to comprehend the boundary existing between these two worlds.

Scarlett and Wolf argued that before the age of 3 years, children are incapable of making and comprehending reality-fantasy distinctions in stories because they have not yet acquired metacommunicative skills. They are only capable of making such distinctions in symbolic play activities. These researchers argued that the development of metacommunicative skills in play precedes that of stories, because pretend play is fluid in nature, whereas stories have a fixed, highly structured nature (see Table 6–1).

An awareness of play-reality distinctions develops between the ages of 3 and 5 years (Scarlett & Wolf, 1979), and children learn to organize and structure their play episodes and share them with others. This observation correlates with the recent research findings of Flavell, Green, and Flavell (1986), who found that by the ages of 4 to 5 years, children develop the ability to verbally announce object/role transformations

Table 6–1. *Distinctions Between Pretend Play and Story*

Pretend Play	Stories
Roles shift; the child may narrate as well as act the characters created.	Roles are fixed; the narrator is fixed, as are all the characters.
Events may occur in any sequence, however nonsensical it may be.	Events must realistically follow one another, and lead up to other events.
Problems may be resolved in any manner the child sees fit.	Problems must be solved from the narrative of the story alone.
The child may play with no regard as to how others construe his or her actions.	The narrator must always be aware of how listeners perceive the story.

Source: Scarlett and Wolf (1979)

prior to their occurrence. By 5 years of age, children have acquired the awareness that the objects they use in play are only symbolically transformed into other objects, and that these objects retain their reality-based characteristics. Children are now capable of framing their pretend episodes, and they subsequently develop the skill to step within the story frame and understand its literal and structured actions, just as they have already mastered pretend activities.

Children's ability to resolve story problems within their given boundaries depends on the extent to which they are capable of communicating the meanings of their own personal pretend episodes to others. Although action dominates the symbolic play activities of children from birth to age 4, 5-year-old children become increasingly more interested in using language to communicate the meanings of their play. As children grow adept at narrating the contents of their stories and metanarrating the stories in order for the audience to understand how they are to be interpreted, they learn to frame their play with story boundaries that contain all the elements necessary for resolving the problems in the stories. Once established, story boundaries provide a means through which children can organize, structure, and resolve conflicts within the story's autonomous world (Scarlett & Wolf, 1979).

Reading a story to a child may tap the child's ability to frame and resolve story/fantasy actions within their respective frames without bringing these unresolved problems back to the real environment. What the child is incapable of resolving in play, he or she may attempt to resolve in reality. Therefore, the ability to metacommunicate between the signifier and the signified object, as well as between the real world and the pretend world of a story, is intrinsic to healthy, adaptive play behavior. An inability to do so may place the child at risk for acting out potentially maladaptive and self-damaging behaviors either in play or in real-life situations.

Fantasy

One of the most important functions of play is to provide a means for the child to develop an ability to distinguish between fantasy and reality situations (Flavell, Green, & Flavell, 1986). Prior to the age of 2 years, during the vast majority of children's play, they use objects functionally. Field, DeStefano, and Koewler III (1982) studied children from three age groups (2–3 years, 3–4 years, and 4–5 years) and found that between the ages of 2 to 3 and 3 to 4, reality play activities decreased. In contrast, object-fantasy (the ability to transform an object into an absent object) increased with age. The 4- to 5-year-olds' object fantasy behaviors decreased and were replaced by person fantasy (role-playing) behaviors. Furthermore, these children were able to announce fantasy play (the child verbally announces the object/role transformation prior to its occurrence). Field and colleagues argued that the developmental change from reality-play to object-fantasy, and then onto announced and person-fantasy play is an age-related sequence. As children's cognitive abilities with regard to symbolic representations mature, they are able to create increasingly complex fantasies that can be predetermined and announced prior to their enactment. However, reality play, although decreasing between the age groups 2 to 3 and 3 to 4, remains a prominent behavioral feature in the 4- to 5-year-old child's overall play situations, comprising as much as 60% of the total play activity.

These findings are supported by Cole and La Voie (1985), who studied 2- to 6-year-old children in free-play episodes in classroom settings. The children were randomly assigned to play dyads and were observed three times a week for a period of 3 weeks in 15-minute free play sessions. The 2- to 3-year-old children played almost exclusively in either "attribution-of-function" use of objects (an attribution of function occurred when the child used the object for its functional purpose) or "other" play (other play being any play activity that did not include pretend behaviors). As well as playing in the attribution-of-function and other categories, the 4-year-old children manifested dimensions of imagery and role playing in their activities. The 5-year-old children demonstrated the widest array of play behaviors, engaging in all the play activities the researchers outlined except for the animation and attribution-of-function categories. The 6-year-olds decreased their play behaviors in all areas except the insubstantial situation and character-attribution play categories. Thus, fantasy play behavior becomes increasingly complex between the ages of 3 and 5, developing from a reality-based, functional use of objects into a fantasy play situation in

which objects can become other objects, people can become other beings, the supernatural can occur, and events are no longer bound by
the realities of time and space.

The ability to rehearse fantasy behaviors during play situations, as
distinct from real-life behaviors, is an activity that the child must master
in order to become aware of appearance-reality distinctions (Flavell,
Green, & Flavell, 1986). Flavell, Green, and Flavell (1986) found that
while 3-year-olds had almost no understanding of the appearance-reality
distinctions of dual-encoded objects (e.g., sponge painted to make it
look like a rock), 6- to 7-year-old children had acquired the appearance-
reality distinction, but found it difficult to verbalize such concepts. In
contrast, 11- to 12-year-old children had not only acquired the ability to
perform the specific tasks, but were also able to share such knowledge
with others. The researchers suggested that play may be the situation in
which the child acquires an ability to perceive the dual-encoding of objects and events.

Dual-encoding—the ability to perceive an object simultaneously as
being both what it appears and what it is in reality—is an inherent part
of the pretend situation. As children become more adept at distinguishing object/action, action/meaning, and role/person, the reality-pretend
distinction becomes clearer and better defined. As they gain knowledge
of this complex concept, they are able to decenter their play behaviors
and communicate with others in order to physically and mentally bring
them into their fantasy experience. Flavell, Green, and Flavell (1986)
suggested that once children have developed the ability to distinguish
dual-encoding of their play from real life, they may then be able to
apply this knowledge to the closely related appearance-reality and
perspective-taking concepts.

Once dual-encoding of appearance-reality has been acquired, a child
is able to process fundamental perceptual entities. The child should be
able to conceive the notion that the appearance of an object at the moment it is observed may not indicate the object's reality. The child realizes that things may not always be what they appear to be and that first
impressions may indeed be wrong. The researchers argued that "decentration largely means going beyond initial appearances" (Flavell, Green,
& Flavell, 1986, p. 64).

They contended that young children's difficulty with dual-encoding
tasks may have a great impact on their perceptions of self and others.
Young children who cannot conceive an object's being anything other
than what it presently appears to be, even though they have been shown
the object's reality status, may transfer this conceptualization into their
real lives. Although parents may always love their children, at the moment when children feel rejected they may have no conception that
their parents will continue to love them. Furthermore, common child-

hood fears may be more difficult to overcome. The child with a fear of the dark may overcome his or her anxiety one night, and then the following night, having no ability to conceive of both the appearance and the reality, may fear the dark as much as before (Flavell, Green, & Flavell, 1986).

> *Indeed, some of their "working through" of fears by acting out or otherwise cognitively reinstating something that frightens them may succeed because it helps them represent that thing's benign reality while experiencing its scary appearance.* (Flavell, Green, & Flavell, 1986, p. 64)

Morison and Gardner (1978) studied 20 children in kindergarten, second-, fourth- and sixth-grade levels in order to determine their ability to differentiate between fantasy and reality. Children were asked to perform two tasks. First, having been shown three picture items, the children were asked to create pairings and explain them. Second, the children were given 20 pictures and asked to separate the real from the pretend figures. The results indicated that the greatest increase in fantasy explanations occurred between the fourth- and sixth-grade groups. Fourth-graders gave only 17 fantasy explanations, in contrast to the 50 given by the sixth-graders. The researchers concluded that fantasy explanations and the ability to differentiate items based on reality-fantasy classification increase with age. However, they pointed out that this does not necessarily indicate that younger children, who spend a great deal of time in pretend play, cannot differentiate between reality and fantasy. Examining Morison and Gardner's findings in relation to Flavell, Green, and Flavell's (1986) study, it may be deduced that the younger children, although having an awareness of reality-fantasy differences, have not yet acquired the cognitive skills enabling them to conceptualize and transfer the play-reality behaviors they enact into other, non-play-oriented tasks. Perhaps the sixth-graders have acquired the ability not only to differentiate, but also to articulate the distinctions between fantasy and reality and can therefore perform such fantasy-reality tasks more adeptly.

Play may be the situation in which children, given the opportunity to divorce themselves from reality, can begin conceiving of the pretend-reality distinctions that act as the foundation for appearance-reality and perspective-taking dual-encoding concepts. Moore (1964) argued that fantasy play fluctuates from being realistic to nonrealistic in nature. He contended that as fantasy leaves real life behind and becomes freer, aggressive behaviors are also released. The resulting violent tendencies, in turn, arouse anxiety and fear within children and, as a result, their play turns back toward reality for the security and reassurance that fantasy play lacks. In order to alleviate the anxiety evoked by fantasy play, children may choose either one of two actions: they may reverse the fantasy back to concrete, real-life experience or referents, or they may halt play altogether, drawing conscious attention to the fact that they were only in a make-believe, fantasy situation (Moore, 1964).

Clinicians observing a child whose development of fantasy play deviates from the normal course may diagnose the potential for other consequent developmental deficits. For example, a child who fails to curb aggressive fantasy play activity may have trouble distinguishing fantasy play from real-life situations. The aggressive play the child enacts, if not eventually brought back to a realistic foundation, may place the child at risk for acting out self-destructive behavior. Clinicians must determine the cognitive developmental level of the child's fantasy play, plus the specific behavioral configuration within the fantasy situation that the child is representing. These may help define the child's full risk for potentially maladaptive behaviors.

MENTAL STATUS EXAMINATION

It is common to observe affective regulation that manifests itself by the predominance of positive affects and the ability to focus, concentrate, verbalize, and share with persistence during pretend/fantasy elaborations. Thus, the absence of any of these behavioral correlates, and/or the presence instead of dysregulated behaviors such as aggression is important for diagnosis. In addition, since the ability to engage in pretend play mirrors the degree of flexibility that a preschool child has in regard to cognitive, affective, and social regulation and in learning new information, the therapist should rule out such etiologies as disruptive home environment, anxiety, depression, or developmental lag that may hinder such activities. The therapist must be aware that during overt pretend activities, young children are likely to have imaginary companions, daydream, and/or withdraw from social exchanges (Moore, Evertson, & Brophy, 1974).

Behar and Rapoport (1983) reported that interviews should provide the child with the opportunity to demonstrate the following:

1. Nature of the interaction with the parent.
2. Separation reactions from the caregiver.
3. Nature of the interaction with the examiner.
4. Manipulation of toys during free play.
5. Spontaneous behavior during limit setting and without limit setting.
6. Play behaviors that are relevant and irrelevant to the working diagnosis.

The therapist should also take into account teacher and parent reports. These may disagree with what the therapist has observed. Behar and Rapoport contended that hypotheses concerning such matters are needed in order to prevent misdiagnosis. An incorrect diagnosis can also result from misinterpretation of the child's symbolic behaviors.

Symbolic play allows the therapist opportunities to observe the child's emotional life from the following four perspectives: (1) the child's self-representations, including the roles he or she assumes; (2) the child's representation of others; (3) the child's concerns, wishes, conflicts, and defense mechanisms; and (4) the child's perception of the world, habitual reasoning and thinking patterns (including intellectual capacities), and problem-solving skills (Irwin, 1983).

Review of Past History

During symbolic play, children reorganize and represent their past experiences via signifiers of the past events (Fein, 1979). The past experiences are divorced from their meanings, and the meanings are free to become attached to new, symbolic objects and actions that are representative of the past experiences. These actions, in turn, may depict present circumstances and predict future actions (Erikson, 1977).

Although many of these symbolic representations may be chosen arbitrarily by children, therapists should familiarize themselves with their patient's past histories, thus enabling them to observe how the children represent past experienced events in their symbolic play. This knowledge can also help a therapist understand what a particular child may be representing or avoiding during play. Careful observation of play may provide indicators of how the past experience has affected a child's current level of functioning.

Temperament

Lieberman (1965) and Singer and Rummo (1973) found that a playful temperament correlates with a child's play behaviors. The trait of playfulness is thought to be present when the child manifests a humorous attitude and is openly expressive, curious, imaginative, and interactive within the play situation. Singer, Singer, and Sherrod (1980) and Singer and Singer (1978) found that children who are like this display positive dispositions and are physically active. Singer (1973) found that playful children have greater imaginations and can use adaptive skills to cope better.

Earls and Cook (1983) examined the relationship between a 3-year-old child's play behavior and his behavior problems and temperamental characteristics. One month after the parents were interviewed, the child was observed in both a free play situation and a structured play situation. During these sessions, the child was asked to perform a number of developmental tasks based on the McCarthy Scales of Developmental Abilities (McCarthy, 1974). The researchers' data indicated that the temperamental dimension of approach/withdrawal showed the greatest correlation to play behaviors; high approach correlated with positive and imaginative play, whereas withdrawal correlated with the more negative and uninvolved pretend situations. Another interesting finding was that poor coping behaviors evidenced behavioral problems and were not positively correlated with temperamental traits. Earls and Cook stressed that one of the diagnostic potentials of play lies in its ability to reveal the child's coping and adaptive skills.

Observations of play may aid in defining a child's playfulness and, therefore, in defining the child's coping responses to stressful situations. It may also help in determining whether the child's temperamental characteristics are displayed positively or negatively during a free play situation. The ability to adapt and cope during play may have a direct bearing on the ways in which a child copes with developmental life stressors. For example, a child who cannot cope in a play situation may be at risk for acting out repressed conflicts and aggressive and/or suicidal behaviors. If unable to adapt and function in accordance with life's demands, the child may become isolated, withdrawn, and depressed, as opposed to being highly motivated to bring about changes and continue to learn from the environment.

Attachment and Prosocial Behavior

Play also provides the therapist with the opportunity to diagnose a child's attachment behaviors. As children's play behavior develops, so too does their desire to relate to their peers in a mutually agreed-upon play situation (Iwanaga, 1973; Parten, 1932; Piaget, 1965; Smilansky, 1968; Rubin, Maioni, & Hornung, 1976). Iwanaga (1973) studied the way in which 30 children ages 3, 4, and 5 structured their play interactions with peers during 1-hour spontaneous play periods over the course of 3 weeks. She noted the following stage-like progression in interpersonal play structures:

1. Independent structure: Play takes place without the involvement of others.
2. Parallel structure: Play takes place between two or more persons. The roles of the children are enacted independently of each other, and even though the children may remain in close, physical proximity, their roles are undifferentiated.

3. Complementary structure: Play takes place between two or more persons. Even though there is some degree of cooperation, the roles of such children are enacted independently of each other.

4. Interactive structure: Play takes place between two or more persons. Their roles, whether differentiated or undifferentiated, are enacted interactively upon each other during the course of their play together. Children focus on how their companions behave, becoming aware of the shifts in their peer's behaviors. Their respective roles take place interactively, and they continuously influence each other during the course of play.

In her study, Iwanaga noted that 3-year-olds can engage in independent and parallel interpersonal structures; 4-year-olds engage in independent, parallel, and complementary structures; and, in sharp contrast, 5-year-olds not only engage in the previous three types, but they also engage in the interpersonal interactive structure.

Cooperation, involving the child's ability to coordinate his or her behavior with others and to assess its degree of fitness to the goal, begins around the age of 4 years. Iwanaga's findings concur with those of Piaget (1951, 1965) that depict a transition from egocentrism to reciprocity, with the child's play developing from a state of social isolation to one in which the child seeks attachment through shared interactive play.

Play serves as a means through which the child can rehearse real-life schemata. For example, the 5-year-old, eager to play in isolation from his or her peers, may be lacking the social skills necessary for further development. The child's ability to manifest prosocial behavior in regard to others during a play situation may correlate directly with the ability to attach and relate to the environment.

Caregiving Environment

Singer (1973, 1979) has found that, among 3- to 6-year-olds, the degree to which the child displays pretend behavior relies heavily on the support and encouragement of caregivers. Caregivers provide children with the role models and themes of their pretend situations. The behaviors a child witnesses and is subjected to at home will invariably surface in social play behaviors (Rubin, Fein, & Vandenberg, 1983). A parent's ambivalence and/or outright disdain for the child's pretend behavior may have a direct bearing on both the child's fantasy behavior within the play situation and the child's ability and/or desire to initiate and act out imaginative representations. Rubin, Fein, and Vandenberg (1983) noted that the adult must give the child the freedom to play in any chosen manner. In order to play effectively, the child must have a play situation that is free of the stressors that may characterize his or her real life (Fein, 1981). Therefore, therapists should note the degree to which any event may override the child's ability to play freely. For example, the caregiver who impinges on the child's play situation may create a play situation that is more stress-provoking than stress-relieving.

Marshall (1961) and Rubin, Fein, and Vandenberg (1983) argued that the enactment of dramatic play in school relies heavily on the child's home environment. Marshall observed children from $2\frac{1}{2}$ to $6\frac{1}{2}$ years of age at home and at school.

Direct correlates were noted between children's use of language and hostility in play with peers. The more home experiences echoed the play topics in preschool, the more frequently children used dramatic play language and hostility with peers. Language and hostility were found to be directly related to a father's punitive and suppressive disciplinary actions. Marshall argues that these relationships suggest that play language and hostility with peers is necessary for peer interaction, is a desirable behavior for children, and relies heavily on the parents' beliefs concerning punishment, disciplinary behaviors, and possessiveness. The use of hostility with peers may be an indication of problems a child is experiencing with demanding, punitive, and suppressive parents.

Children who are subjected to suppression, deprivation, and over-possessiveness by their caregivers may need to establish dependent relationships with their teachers, thereby preventing themselves from engaging in peer interactions that would promote social skills. Thus, a healthy interaction between the child and his or her caregivers predicted the use of dramatic play, language, and hostility behaviors in a more adaptive fashion.

The home environment has a great impact on the child's play development. Hetherington, Cox, and Cox (1979) studied the developmental play levels of children from divorced homes in comparison with children from intact homes. The findings indicated that by 2 months after the divorce, the children displayed more functional and less dramatic play than their counterparts from intact homes. Two years after the divorce, the boys still displayed more solitary play than the boys from intact homes. Girls, however, were found to match developmentally after 2 years.

Since the child's play abilities rely so heavily on the home environment, the therapist must examine the caregiver's attitudes toward disciplinary actions and play behaviors and analyze the family's situation in order to better understand the child's role, or reality, use of language, and hostility. Without some knowledge of the home environment and the caregivers' thoughts, correlations cannot be made that associate the observed behaviors of the child in the playroom back to the home environment where they originated. Such correlations, once defined, can aid the therapist in understanding the complexity and scope of the child's developmental deficits in play.

Regulation of Aggression

A clinician who wishes to diagnose regulation of aggression in play must first be aware of the child's usual levels of aggression, since aggressive behaviors may be heightened during play situations. Although play may provide the observer with the opportunity to observe the child's aggressive behaviors, play itself does not alleviate the causes of aggressive outbursts.

Feshbach (1956) observed children ages 5 to 8 years who had been evaluated as either low-aggressive or high-aggressive by their teachers. The children were randomly divided into three groups: (1) an aggressive toy group (toys lending themselves to thematic aggressive play); (2) a neutral toy group (nonaggressive toys); and (3) a control group.

Permissive play failed to prevent the aggressive behaviors of the highly aggressive children. Furthermore, low-aggressive boys showed an increase in aggressive behaviors following the play sessions. Low-aggressive girls showed no increase in aggressive behaviors following permissive play. The results indicated that inappropriate aggressive behavior could be linked more closely to the use of aggressive toys than to the use of neutral toys. Feshbach concluded that play does not serve as a means for the catharsis of aggressive behaviors.

Self Versus Toy

Children move from a body-analogous interpretation of activities, evident at 16 months of age (Piaget & Inhelder, 1971), toward a decentered, object-related mode of interaction with the environment around the age of 2 years (Lowe, 1975). Watson and Fischer (1977) found that displays of body-analogous behavior decreased between the ages of 1 and $2\frac{1}{2}$ years while doll-referenced behaviors increased. At this stage, children are able to transfer the actions rehearsed on their body parts onto independent objects beyond themselves. A child who fails to do so may be suffering from a developmental deficit indicative of the inability to transfer inner thoughts and emotions onto external objects. The presence of a developmental lag is suspected if environmental circumstances exist in which the child feels threatened by the world outside of himself or herself. Children who (during play) fail to transfer feelings onto external objects may short-circuit these feelings by turning them onto themselves. Such a phenomenon suggests that these children may feel threatened by the toys themselves, or by feelings that they may want to express through the toys, or both. Children who display body-analogous play keep their feelings within themselves. This can result in directing harmful behaviors toward the self, instead of directing them toward the environment.

Superego

Moore (1964) argued that children do not always differentiate between their own superegos and authority figures. Children reared under strict disciplinary techniques often display the most hostility in play, and pent-up anger is often unleashed. Children who are angry with their parents may vent this hostility toward themselves in play. The existence of a developmental lag is suspected if a child feels threatened by the outside world. The therapist, observing aggressive behavior, may be able to discern regulating aspects of a child's superego from his or her behaviors. The child with aggressive outbursts may lack the ability to neutralize aggressive behaviors. This is evidence of the manner in which the child's superego restrains or allows the child's play behavior. Observations of how a child's superego regulates play may determine the child's risk for acting out aggressive behaviors.

Psychosexual Development

Peller (1954) correlated play stages with the child's psychosexual development. During the Oedipal stage (5 years), the child's play focuses on the anxiety-provoking conflict concerning fear of losing the love of the caregiver. The anxiety generated during the anal stage (2 years) is less than that produced by either the oral (1 year) or Oedipal periods. During the oral and Oedipal periods, the child is in a process of attachment and reattachment, respectively, to the caregiver. The anxiety felt is precipitated by processes of attachment that engender insecurity. Security is a fundamental element of the child's potential to engage in play behaviors (Fein, 1979), and, as a result, play may become disrupted at points during the pre-Oedipal and Oedipal periods when the child may no longer be able to represent attachment with the caregiver. Consequently, the child may feel insecure without the caregiver present and play activities may decrease. Erikson's (1951) examination of psychosexual development in play reveals that young boys create vertical structures that represent the penis, whereas young girls construct enclosures that represent their genitalia. This exemplifies children's use of play to express and work through current developmental issues.

Other behavioral differences by gender have been noted in the play activities themselves. A number of researchers have noted that sex differences in play may be evident at 2 years of age (Goldberg & Lewis, 1969). Boys have been shown to display roughhousing behaviors far more frequently than girls (Dipietro, 1981; Blurton-Jones, 1967; Smith & Connolly, 1972). However, accumulative research indicates that over the past 60 years girls have expressed more interest in and have participated in more boys' activities, while boys' activities on the whole have become less boisterous (Sutton-Smith, 1979).

The pattern of data shows that the attainment of gender constancy has special impact on sex-role development. According to Kohlberg (1966), when children develop the concept of a consistent, categorical gender identity, at about age 5, they become motivated to learn what behavior is "appropriate" for their gender and to act accordingly. Therefore, as cultural norms change, so do play behaviors considered appropriate for each sex.

State-Related Behavior

Peller (1952) contended that children's role-playing choices are founded upon their feelings toward people in real life. Children may take on the roles of people they love in order to achieve a feeling of security and goodness. On the other hand, they may imitate people they dislike in order to master their anxiety regarding such roles. When allowed to select what toys to play with, children tend to choose toys that are state-related (Gilmore, 1965, 1966). A child's anxiety can directly influence the child's choice of play materials. A child who is anxious about a visit to the doctor, for example, may prefer to play with toys reminiscent of medical instruments. Moreover, Gilmore posited that environmental influence can either increase or decrease the child's interest in toys relevant to the source of anxiety.

The child's selection of roles and toys can provide the therapist with a diagnostic tool for discovering the source of the child's feelings. Through observations, the therapist may be able to focus on the child's primary source of fears and concerns, in order to better understand and alleviate them.

Intentionality

Around the age of 3 to 5 years, children acquire the ability to differentiate between intended and unintended action (Shultz, Wells, & Sarda, 1980). Three-year-olds begin to view intention as a possible cause of actions. Furthermore, recursive awareness—the awareness that other people may be aware of one's own intended actions—develops around the 5th year of life (Shultz & Cloghesy, 1981). Recursiveness subsequently leads to the development of the child's ability to purposely hide and disguise his or her intentions from others (Schmidt, 1976; Shultz & Cloghesy, 1981). Children become aware not only of their similarity to other agents, but also that such social knowledge can be reciprocal.

Children who have developed recursive awareness have the ability to devise strategies by which they can consciously choose a specific behavior to achieve a specific end in any given situation. The ability to act upon intended goals represents a crucial aspect in children's play development. It marks the point at which a child no longer acts purely on unconscious emotions, but begins to play based on situations that he or she intends to communicate or hide from others. Five-year-olds, having developed recursive awareness, act with the knowledge that other people also know how they intend their actions and their resulting effects. Therapists should take note of their patients' intentions and attempts either to mask or reveal them as they develop play themes. For example, a child who intentionally acts self-destructively in a play situation may actually intend to hurt himself or herself either in life or within the play situation. Awareness of this intention should motivate the therapist to understand its origins. The clinician must differentiate between a child's intended and unintended acts in order to determine the true risk of such actions.

Unstable Representations

Play lends children opportunities to divorce the meaning of actions and objects from each other, thereby allowing the creation of an almanac of symbols that represent meanings. Furthermore, play acts as a vehicle through which children can use their symbols to organize higher levels of meaning (Fein, 1979). Developmentally, as Fein reported, only a few 7-month-olds can engage in two-object acts, but by 9 months of age almost all children can do so. By 13 months, children can perform simple object accommodative relations. By 20 months, children are able to manifest pretend behaviors. The 2-year-old child must have developed and coordinated adequate sensorimotor skills prior to acquiring the ability to symbolically represent objects and meanings, both of which are associated with the development of play behavior.

The child's ability to develop a stable representation of objects and meanings can be determined from the ability to adaptively fluctuate between real-life and pretend situations. The child must remain flexible in order to attribute an action to his or her signifiers—a milestone that has been termed by Golomb and Cornelius (1977) as *pseudoreversibility*. The child with a stable set of representations is able to attribute to the signifier his or her meaning, while the signifier's original state is simultaneously retained. On the other hand, unstable representations may prevent such flexibility. The child fails to acquire an ability to separate meaning from object, and such a deficit places the child in the sensorimotor level of play. Similarly, if the child is incapable of distinguishing play from nonplay, the child may have no sense of the object's potential for pseudoreversibility. Thus, such a child, whether interacting in play or in real life, is going to attribute meanings to the signifier as they are derived from the signified object.

Therapists, observing inadequate representational skills, may be able to determine why play does not give the child the opportunity to attain the higher levels of meaning necessary to facilitate further cognitive development. Even though play symbols can represent what is deeply felt by the child, in cases involving unstable representations children may not be able to express such powerful feelings. Finding no outlet in play, these emotions may surface in the child's real-life activities, possibly producing behaviors that may be damaging to others or to the child's own sense of self. The child's ability to develop stable object representations is one of play's most fundamental ingredients; thus, the prevalence of unstable representations may predispose the child to any number of cognitive, emotional, and interpersonal deficits.

Perspective Taking

Perspectivism is the ability to perceive an object or person as consisting of many separate, yet interrelated parts (Fein, 1979). The child must be able to take the perspective of an observer and regard objects and people as distinct from his or her perspective. Prior to the acquisition of perspectivism, the child's perceptions of the world are dominated by egocentric thought, which Sullivan (1953) characterized as both "unshared and unsocialized" in nature. Musatti (1986) concurred, defining egocentric thought in terms of an "unbalanced relationship between individual knowledge and socially shared knowledge" (p. 30).

Fenson and Ramsay (1980) studied infants ages 13, 19, and 24 months in order to determine the age at which children's self-centered acts become decentered. Self-centered acts usually appear at 12 months of age and refer to behaviors directed toward the self (e.g., eating, sleeping, drinking). Fenson and Ramsay defined the following three levels of decentration:

1. Passive decentered acts: acts during which an animate object or person receives an action from the child, with the animate object or person serving as the passive recipient of the action (e.g., a child swings a doll).
2. Active decentered acts: acts during which the child attributes "action potential" to a lifelike object (e.g., the child hands the doll a spoon, so that the doll can "feed" itself).
3. Object-directed acts: behaviors in which the child directs his or her actions at an inanimate object (e.g., stirring an imaginary pot of soup on a stove).

Fenson and Ramsay observed that around 13 months of age decentered acts are apparent. Multischemes (coordinations involving two or more actions instead of the repetition of one action) were not observed before the age of 24 months, indicating perhaps that other cognitive skills may need to be mastered prior to multischematic competency. Single-schema combinations also emerged concurrently with decentered acts at age 19 months.

Decentered children can separate themselves from actions and meanings (Fenson & Ramsay, 1980; McCune-Nicolich, 1981). Actions are no longer understood as being concretely bound to an individual, but become flexible and can be applied to other objects and people (McCune-Nicolich, 1981). Children who have the ability to transfer their emotions to other objects, whether they be animate or inanimate, are at a far lower risk for self-harmful behaviors than are children who remain self-centered and act out their emotions on themselves in a body-analogous manner. Indeed, Mead (1934) believed that play situations are essential for the development of a healthy sense of self-identity. Role playing and decentered acts provide a means through which children can view themselves as distinct from others. Failure to meet this developmental transition may indicate that a child fears external stimuli and prefers to remain withdrawn rather than interacting with the environment.

As children grow older and their cognitive thought processes develop, their egocentric thought recedes (Piaget, 1929, 1951). A reduction in egocentricity may be due in part to more frequent peer interactions, which have been found to increase a child's awareness of others' situations (Piaget, 1965). Vygotsky (1962) argued that egocentric thought does not really decline, but is metamorphosized into a form of private inner thought and language. On the other hand, Elkind (1976) contended that although egocentrism, as a whole structure of thought processes, may decline during the course of development, versions of egocentric thought exist in new forms. Such forms often pertain to the more specific and abstract elements of life (e.g., death).

Egocentrism is omnipresent in young children because they lack the ability to socially test the concepts and ideas they have been representing in their minds. The child's perspective of the world comes from creating an internal schema based on an external world. The internal schema is, in turn, used to further interpret the external world that generated the child's initial thoughts (Elkind, 1978). Thus, as Elkind contended, the development of concepts relies less on the process of assimilating new information than on the process of correcting past erroneous concepts. As the child becomes more adept at reorganizing past conceptions of the world, the egocentric thought processes have fewer opportunities to impose themselves on the child's perceptions.

Musatti (1983) found that 18-month-old children are able to share the meanings of their signified objects with others. From 18 months on, children are not only able to take others' perspectives in order to show them a picture, but they can also share their personal perspectives and meanings with others. Lempers, Flavell, and Flavell (1977) studied the perceptual awareness of children from 1 to 3 years of age. The researchers assessed the child's ability to take another person's perspective when given the task of showing another person an object. Results indicated that most 1-year-olds could point to another person when asked, but only 7 of the 12 could follow the pointing of the other. When given the task of showing the other an object, nearly half of the children did so by simply holding the object up.

The $1\frac{1}{2}$-year-olds were less egocentric in their behavior. When asked to show the other person a picture, most held the picture horizontally so that they and the other children could see the picture simultaneously. By 2 years of age, the children were able to show a picture to the other by turning it away from themselves, a movement that prevented them from continuing to see it. By the age of $2\frac{1}{2}$ years, children have begun to acquire the ability to both show and conceal an object from another's view. However, children at this age remain dependent on their ability to establish visual contact with the other. When asked to show an object to the other, when the other was behind a screen out of their visual field, half of the children could only do so by walking around the screen instead of holding the object up above the screen. The $2\frac{1}{2}$-year-olds' hiding ability appeared to have developed to the point where they could conceal objects from another by placing an obstacle between them. In addition, two thirds of the $2\frac{1}{2}$-year-olds could conceal themselves from another. In regard to the 3-year-old children, Lempers and colleagues noted that these children could easily perform all the tasks. They understood the function of their eyes, as well as the concept that just because the eyes are open does not indicate that total perception has been achieved. The 3-year-olds had arrived at the understanding that another person's visual perspective is independent of their own, and consequently they were able to perceive of, and take, another person's visual perspective.

In a later study concerning the perceptual abilities of children aged $4\frac{1}{2}$ to $5\frac{1}{2}$, Flavell, Flavell, Green, and Wilcox (1981) examined the development of the following three spatial perspective-taking rules:

1. An object will look the same if viewed from the same position by both oneself and another person.
2. A heterogenous-sided object (an object with an indistinct shape, in this case a clump of wire) will have different appearances when viewed by the self and another from two different positions.

3. A homogeneous-sided object such as a sphere will present the same appearance when viewed by the self and another from two different positions.

The researchers determined that rules 1 and 2 develop from $4\frac{1}{2}$ to $5\frac{1}{2}$ years of age and that $5\frac{1}{2}$-year-olds have acquired a good understanding of all three principles.

Therapists should examine both the child's ability to take another's perspective and the ability to communicate his or her own perspective. The child's ability or inability to do so may give the therapist the opportunity to understand the child's view of others as distinct from himself or herself, and allow the therapist to examine how the child attributes meanings to objects. The child begins accumulating knowledge of others and their individual situations, and thus develops the ability to anticipate specific outcomes from known actions and events as resulting from the nature of the objects and/or people themselves. Singer (1979) contended that both anticipation and expectation govern and direct much of a person's actions. Novel stimuli are matched toward past perceptions in order to guide further action. A child who lacks such anticipatory guidelines for novel stimuli may become frustrated or depressed. Play can act as the vehicle through which the child can transform overwhelming distressful stimuli into more manipulable forms (Singer, 1979). Children who are unable to relate past perceptions to novel stimuli may eventually give up, withdrawing from the novel stimuli or people and thus never achieving an ability to understand and share the perspective of another.

Speech and Language

Language represents one means through which children can communicate their thoughts and actions to themselves, caregivers, and peers. Piaget (1962) argued that language is one of a number of symbolic functions that emerge as a result of the child's maturation of his representational abilities. Having mastered and internalized his or her sensorimotor schemata, the young infant can and does commence symbolic play activities. Casby and Della Corte (1986) suggested that the language performance of young children is directly influenced by their nonlinguistic representational skills. Bates, Camaioni, and Volterra (1975) and Harding and Golinkoff (1979) found that a 10-month-old infant's prelinguistic language skills are directly related to stage V sensorimotor play development. One- to two-year-old children with advanced language development exhibit more symbolic play behaviors than children with a more standard language development (Rosenblatt,

1977). Thus, language development is considered to be a good indicator of the child's cognitive abilities. Some researchers argue that a child's language and symbolic play mirror the child's representational abilities (Bates, Camaioni, & Volterra, 1975; Brown, 1973; Casby & Della Corte, 1986; Harding & Golinkoff, 1979; McCune-Nicolich, 1981; Piaget, 1951; Singer, 1973; Werner & Kaplan, 1963; Zachry, 1978).

For example, children who can produce complex language combinations have been found to have greater representational abilities than those who cannot (Casby & Della Corte, 1986; Zachry, 1978). Research by Shore, O'Connell, and Bates (1984) has demonstrated that a child's mean length of language utterance correlates directly to the child's mean length of play episode. Correlations have been found to be stronger between language acquisition and level of play development than between language acquisition and the child's chronological age (Casby & Della Corte, 1986). Language acquisition may then be viewed as being inherently linked to other symbolic activities (e.g., play), each mutually facilitating and promoting the development of the other.

The child represents a meaningful action (eat, sleep) with the pretend action (pretending to eat or sleep). This correlates directly with language and thus with the child's awareness that words have specific meanings and can be used to represent and communicate thoughts and activities to others. McCune-Nicolich (1981) stated that "the evidence available suggests that symbolic play might provide a useful converging operation for identifying structural turning points in language" (p. 795).

Children who engage in fewer, less complex play sequences may be demonstrating their lack of representational and linguistic capacities. If language is linked to play development, a child's failure to engage in play episodes is indicative of his or her play age and may be evidence of the inability to communicate the representations formed within the child's mind. In addition, sociolinguists propose that through an analysis of the child's specific speech patterns during interactive play episodes an understanding of the child's mental representations of social roles can be achieved (Corsaro, 1979).

When defining contextualization cues, sociolinguists refer to the particular communicative aspects the child uses in role play by the paralinguistic features of intonation, gesture, and manipulation of objects, all of which function as a result of the child's view of social status and role. Corsaro (1979) typified linguistic contextualization cues into the following nine categories:

1. Imperatives: statements that control the actions of others (e.g., threats or commands).

2. Informative statements: statements that give knowledge to the other interactants concerning a shared activity.
3. Requests for permission: questions posed when the individual seeks permission for a specific activity.
4. Requests for joint action: questions posed when the individual seeks to join a group activity.
5. Answers: responses to the other interactant's queries or imperatives.
6. Direct questions: questions posed to direct another interactant to a specific activity.
7. Tag questions: questions indicative of a shared understanding of the situation (e.g., "We're eating now, right?").
8. Informative requests: questions posed to gain knowledge from other interactants about the group's ongoing activity.
9. Greetings: statements that serve to introduce another to the situation.

A child's actions and reactions to the statements of others reflect the child's awareness of the flexibility of social roles. Children who fail to mediate their behavior according to the responses they receive from others may be displaying signs of fixedness regarding the status of object relations. Children who are incapable of interacting except through imperatives, may become frustrated when confronted with situations that are beyond their control. This may indicate that they possess inadequate coping skills and therefore are at risk for acting-out, maladaptive behavior. On the other hand, children who only take orders from others, or constantly seek permission to participate in activities may be suffering from poor self-esteem—viewing themselves as of a lower status than their peers. Thus, the specific contextualization cues of language serve as a diagnostic tool through which clinicians can underscore how particular children relate to their peers and how they regard themselves.

Social Class

Rubin, Maioni, and Hornung (1976) examined social play behaviors in 3- to 4-year-old middle- and lower-class children. They found that lower-class children were more apt to display functional play behaviors than their middle-class counterparts, who displayed more constructive play behaviors. The researchers argued that middle-class children might have had more toys available to them at home and therefore were able to master the toys' functional aspects far sooner, thus expediting their development into constructive play structures. The lower-class children, on the other hand, most likely had no previous opportunities to use the toys, thus they had to begin fresh at mastering the toys' functional aspects.

Although social class alone may not correlate with a child's specific deficits, it may act as an indicator of access to toys and stimuli that can either enhance or hinder the child's developing cognitive and social abilities. Therapists should take note of their patients' social class, not only as an indicator of the children's access to the toys they need, but also in relation to their developmental level based on the toys that they do have at their disposal. Social class may have some degree of influence on a child's developmental play behavior, serving as an indicator of the environmental circumstances that may or may not place the child at risk for developmental deficits.

CLINICAL POPULATIONS

This section will focus on five groups known to suffer cognitive and emotional problems: children with separation anxiety, autism, suicidal play behaviors, conduct-disordered behaviors, and depressive behaviors. Although each of these populations at risk has distinct play behaviors that are indicative of their psychopathology, all of them are difficult to work with in the play therapy situation (Pfeffer, 1986b; Willock, 1983; Wulff, 1985), and their play behaviors must, therefore, be thoroughly understood prior to initiating therapeutic play treatment.

Separation Anxiety

Milos and Reiss (1982) studied the play behaviors of children aged 2 to 6 years whose teachers had noted them as suffering from separation anxiety. The children were placed in one of three thematic play groups: free play, directed play, or a modeling group. A nonthematic play condition was used as a control, so that pretreatment anxiety levels could be kept relatively equal. Lower levels of anxiety were reported in all three play groups on posttest anxiety speech disturbance scores, although this finding was not consistent with teacher ratings. The researchers found that opportunities to play with anxiety-relevant toys in permissive play, either directed or undirected by an adult, lowered the child's level of anxiety by enabling him or her to "work through" feelings of separation anxiety. Milos and Reiss suggested that separation anxiety feelings be explored in preschool and kindergarten classroom situations, particularly during the first week of school. Finally, children prefer to play with toys that are relevant to the origins of their anxiety (Gilmore, 1965,

1966). Therefore, teachers may introduce separation anxiety themes to the children through role-playing with dolls, thereby giving the children access to a method through which they can express and master their anxiety.

Autism

Autistic children have been shown to lag in their capacity to engage in symbolic play episodes (Kanner, 1943, 1973; Ungerer & Sigman, 1981; Wing, Gould, Yeates, & Brierley, 1977). Wing and colleagues found that none of the children with mental ages or language comprehension ages below 20 months could demonstrate any symbolic play behaviors. This concurred with Ungerer and Sigman's (1981) finding on autistic children with a mean chronological age of 4 years and a mean mental age of 2 years. Indeed, Kanner (1943, 1973) contends that the noted lack of pretend activities in early infancy may be indicative of autism. Ungerer and Sigman found that during spontaneous play sessions autistic children engaged in less symbolic play than when placed in highly structured play sessions with an adult. Wing and colleagues found that 67% of the autistic children exhibited no symbolic play and the remaining 33% engaged in stereotypical play involving simple sensorimotor manipulations of objects. However, among the mentally retarded children studied, 87% of the group demonstrated symbolic play behaviors, 2% engaged in stereotypical play behaviors, and only 11% displayed no symbolic play whatsoever.

Wulff (1985) stated that autistic children lack both symbolic play and verbal language systems. Wulff's contention may very likely be correct given the existing data correlating language acquisition to level of play achieved (Bates, Camaioni, & Volterra, 1975; Brown, 1973; Casby & Della Corte, 1986; Harding & Golinkoff, 1979; McCune-Nicolich, 1981; Piaget, 1951, 1962; Zachry, 1978). However, Sherman, Shapiro, and Glassman (1983) studied groups of mentally retarded, autistic, and developmentally atypical children and found that although play level and language development may be correlated to some degree in normal children, in these groups of children, adeptness at one did not necessarily correlate with competence in the other. Their findings indicate that peer play level among homogeneous groups of children serves as a better diagnostic indicator of development when coupled with measures indicating the child's linguistic competence.

Wulff argued that although play may be indicative of the child's level of cognitive development, for the autistic child, who lacks both verbal language and symbolic play capacities, play may not be an appropriate means through which to determine and alleviate the causes of distress. The autistic child's play can be regulated through interventions, and spontaneous play activities may increase, but without prolonged, re-peated therapy, developmental gains are quickly lost.

Neurologically Impaired/Learning Disabled

Increasingly, more children with learning disabilities are being identi-fied outside of the school environment. This benefits children by identi-fying at an early age those who have learning handicaps (Taylor & War-ren, 1984). Difficulties in assessment persist, however, particularly in differentiating between responses indicating emotional problems and problems resulting from neurologically based learning disabilities (Sil-ver, 1982). Because of this diagnostic confusion, Silver (1982) has cau-tioned that what is important is to make an adequate assessment of the child's behavioral, intellectual, and cognitive functioning as well as the child's family environment.

While multiple patterns of dysfunctional behavior exist for children with learning disabilities, all have similar groups of findings that can be assessed. All have one particular learning disability or more, but in addition about 40% show evidence of altered nervous system function-ing. This may be evidenced in play sessions by hyperactivity, distractibil-ity, or short attention spans that are not due to dynamically related anxiety.

In assessing learning disabled children, Silver (1982) has suggested that a four-step model should be observed. The first step is input: re-cording information in the brain. The second step is integration: orga-nizing and comprehending the received information. The third step is memory—the ability to store and then retrieve the integrated material—and the fourth step is output: the ability to communicate information from the brain to the environment (p. 715). Visual-perceptual and auditory-perceptual deficits are considered to be input disabilities. Chil-dren with visual-perceptual disabilities may confuse left with right, and top with bottom, may transpose letters when writing or drawing, or may read words incorrectly. Visual-motor tasks such as playing with puzzles, blocks, tinker toys, or other objects or catching a ball can be disrupted. Children with visual-perceptual disabilities become disoriented when confronted with problems of spatial relationships. They might confuse left with right or even appear dizzy or off-balance. Depth-perception problems may be evidenced by a child's tendency to misjudge distances, bump into things, or fall off chairs or hobbyhorses.

Auditory-perceptual disabilities may be inferred in different ways. A clinician should pay close attention to the child's ability to differentiate between subtle differences in sound. Does the child understand the therapist's verbalizations to him, or does he respond incorrectly? Does the therapist have to speak more slowly to be understood? Problems here may be indicative of an auditory lag.

Integration disabilities involve the sequencing and interpreting of information, and they can be visual, auditory, or intrasensory. Children with such problems may hear or see a story but confuse the beginning, middle, and end. In spelling, all letters might be there, but placed out of order. Another feature of integration involves the proclivity for abstract thought. This, however, is more difficult to assess through unstructured play, and it might better be assessed in the mental status examination.

Memory disabilities can be either short- or long-term. Short-term memory problems may be evident when a child fails to remember numbers needed for a game or has trouble learning a new song. A long-term memory problem, however, is a disability that so overwhelms learning processes that such children are more likely to be viewed as retarded than as learning disabled.

Output disabilities can be related to either language or motor activities. In the play situation, attention should be paid to both spontaneous language—when a child initiates a conversation, sings, or prattles to himself—and to demand language—how a child responds to situations when asked to respond verbally.

Motor output is quite obvious, and if the child has gross-motor disabilities he or she may stumble and seem clumsy. The child with fine-motor coordination disabilities might have trouble using drawing implements, doing puzzles, and playing with blocks.

In playroom diagnostic sessions, particulary unstructured ones, a clinician must be astutely observant—always keeping in mind the possibility of neurologically based learning problems. However, it is strongly recommended for this particular area of disability that any perceived problems be followed up by more finely tuned and specific neuropsychological testing.

Conduct Disordered Behaviors

Aggressive children, like suicidal children, often literally destroy their toys and environments. They consistently act so as to make themselves as difficult and unapproachable as possible. The therapeutic play of aggressive children, therefore, may be extremely difficult (Willock, 1983) and is usually doomed from the start (Berman, 1964). Yet, difficult as aggressive children may be in therapy, to ignore a population so bent on destroying the world is absurd. Aggressive children, like normal children, play, and play has been shown to alleviate distress. Through examination of the way the aggressive child plays, an understanding may be achieved of why this child's play does not alleviate his or her distress. Corrections can subsequently be made to make the play less stress-provoking and more distress-relieving.

Aggressive children's play behaviors typically include hitting, kicking, screaming obscenities, and throwing objects at the walls, floors, and therapist. They aim to create chaos. Play behaviors with such masked violent tendencies are indicative of a distorted awareness of object relations and interactive play development. Such play is not a situation from which the child derives pleasure, but it becomes a situation in which the child repeatedly encounters cognitive and/or emotional defeats.

Winnicott (1965) contended that traumatic life experiences occurring during the preverbal stage may only be expressed in action. Thus, aggressive children may be acting out in their play experiences that are haunting them from their past and present lives. In the therapy situation, aggressive children may become abusive in order to avoid talking about, and facing, their real-life problems. They act in order to gain control of the therapy situation, leaving the therapist with the problem of bringing structure back into the therapeutic environment (Willock, 1983). By creating an atmosphere in which there are no structures, aggressive children relieve themselves of the responsibility to answer the therapist. Whereas the play of normal children is governed by rules (Vygotsky, 1967), the play of aggressive children lacks any code of rules. Activities are carried out for the purpose of destroying order, thereby giving aggressive children a sense of control over their play world that they lack in the real world. Willock (1983) posited that aggressive children face problems and fear violent emotions and that the play situation may only act as a catalyst for their aggressive outbursts. Structured board games may be preferred by those children who fear their propensity to hurt the world.

Masked dependencies may be characteristic of aggressive children's play therapy sessions. *Masked dependencies* refer to the behaviors occurring during these children's outbursts. Such children behave as if their therapists are unwanted, yet they may be misbehaving so drastically because they either consciously or subconsciously want the therapists to intervene and save them from their behaviors. These children transfer so that their therapists are given the status of the parent figures who must be coerced into caring about their children. Thus, aggressive children in therapy may act as abusively as they can in order to win the attention and affection of their therapists. In addition, aggressive children in play may feel they have to perform in order to engage the interest and appreciation of their caregivers. The play experience, then, becomes less a situation in which these children can act for themselves, and more a situation in which they must compete with the rest of the world for the approval and love of their caregivers (Willock, 1983).

Suicidal Play Behaviors

The play behaviors of suicidal children are distinct from those of nonsuicidal children. If play is an activity in which the child acts unconsciously, solely for the purpose of the acts, and with no regard for the ends (Bruner, 1972; Dewey, 1938; Piaget, 1962; Vandenberg, 1978), then the suicidal child may be at risk for acting out potentially self-damaging behaviors with no knowledge of their acts' harmful ends. Pfeffer (1986b), after observing the play behaviors of suicidal children, grouped them into these four categories: responses to separation and autonomy, reckless and dangerous play, misuse of toys, and acting out of fantasies.

One behavior typical of the suicidal child's play is throwing objects out of windows. Pfeffer noted that throwing objects may be evident in nonsuicidal children's play; however, in suicidal children's play, the activity becomes repetitive and the emotional content of the act is significantly greater. These children also tend to have problems moving between play and real environments. Suicidal children may be incapable of playing in the play environment if they know that they may have to return to their stressful real life with its real-life consequences. Intervening in suicidal children's play is therefore more difficult. They may be unwilling to give up the play world where they believe they can act suicidally without having to accept the consequences of such behaviors. Pfeffer reported that jumping, throwing, and attempts at flying, as well as loss and retrieval themes, are the suicidal child's defenses against the realization that he or she is an autonomous, separate, and distinct person from all others—defenses against the fact that the child cannot control the world and his or her parents, and that the child has to rely on his or her self to succeed in this world.

Suicidal children's play has also been observed to contain reckless and harmful behaviors in which they use their bodies as the play objects. Such behaviors may be observed in their flying attempts, in which they leap off furniture, putting themselves in danger of being injured. These same children may take out their rage on their play objects, often throwing, breaking, and destroying the environment around them. Suicidal children transform the make-believe situation into an environment in which they blatantly act out what they feel. Pfeffer called this a form of ego-boundary diffusion. Such children may begin by throwing toys out of the window and then may transfer the action to themselves, throwing their own bodies out of the window, having lost the ability to differentiate between toys and body. Suicidal children do not have the power and control to destroy their real environment, but they can place them in the play situation, and given their inherent sense of being God, they will attempt to destroy the play environment as well as their "play" body.

The fourth play behavior Pfeffer observed is the acting out of powerful and threatening fantasies. She noted that suicidal children often play using superhero themes, yet heightening their behavior to such an extent that they become overly aggressive and sadistic. Violent emotions may be unleashed that these children cannot control and may not understand. Consequently, they may hurt themselves or other play partici-pants.

Just as with all emotionally disturbed children, the home life and stresses of suicidal children must be examined in order to gain a more thorough understanding of the origins and development of their sui-cidal behavior. Pfeffer (1986b) added that over the course of treatment the therapist should repeatedly ask such a child about his or her suicidal actions and fantasies. By giving the child an awareness of behaviors and intentions, the therapist may help the child begin to verbalize the emo-tions he or she acts out in pretend situations. Through an acquisition of awareness, the suicidal child may then use the play situation as just that—a play situation—rather than letting the play become the activity in which the child learns to cause his or her own destruction.

CONCLUSION

The therapist, making a diagnosis based on observation of play activi-ties, should always keep in mind the developmental context in which the child is imbedded. Changes in play behaviors over time can be used to chart the child's mental status. Sensorimotor play during the first year of life evolves from the purely manipulative use of objects and language—a transition that not only marks but also strengthens the ability to form internal symbols. Eventually, the child becomes more adept at differentiating, coordinating, and consolidating old and new information as it relates to the developmental nature of the child's role playing behavior. Therapists who factor such considerations into their diagnoses are less likely to make deficient diagnoses.

CHAPTER SEVEN

Psychological Assessment During the Preschool Years

Jimmy: Multiple Weaknesses

Jimmy is a 4-year, 3-month-old boy. He was born of a normal pregnancy and delivery. At age 3 days, Jimmy was adopted, and he now lives with his adoptive mother and her son, who is 2 years older than Jimmy. Jimmy has a history of ear infections. His developmental milestones were reportedly delayed—he walked independently at 16 months and his receptive and expressive speech were also significantly delayed.

His parents separated when Jimmy was 3, and his mother was concerned about the effects this would have on him. For this reason, she brought Jimmy in for a psychiatric evaluation. He had been having sleep difficulties and would wake up two or three times each night.

During the first evaluation, Jimmy, who was 3 years old at the time, interacted readily with the examiner and engaged in play activity. He displayed a healthy curiosity by examining the various toys and investigating the room. Although Jimmy's mother was present throughout the interview, she was unintrusive and the interaction between her and Jimmy was positive. Jimmy's mother was particularly concerned about his speech development.

Jimmy's results on the Stanford-Binet Intelligence Test yielded a mental age of 2.8 years. This placed him in the low-average range of intellectual functioning. His delayed language skills placed him at a distinct disadvantage. His receptive language, however, was less affected than his expressive language.

Jimmy's fine motor coordination appeared normal. He was able to identify objects by their use, and his short-term memory was adequately developed for a 3-year-old. Jimmy was able to relate appropriately to both adults and children. He was generally trusting of adults, and he accepted directions and limitations with little difficulty.

Jimmy's teacher reported that he helped with household tasks and was beginning to eat with a fork and care for himself when he used the bathroom. She also reported that Jimmy could put on and take off his coat but was unable to button it. Jimmy's score on the Vineland Social Maturity Scale placed him within the average range of functioning.

A recommendation was made for Jimmy to be enrolled in an early intervention program in his school and to begin speech and play therapy. The program was also to assess his developmental progress and growth. Jimmy's mother followed these suggestions. Jimmy participated in weekly play sessions and showed progress in his cooperative play ability. He also improved his ability to verbalize his needs, although he still had difficulty in this area.

At his second assessment (age 4 years, 3 months) Jimmy was again cooperative; he was friendly, outgoing, and eager to perform and succeed. He was not easily discouraged when encountering a difficult item. Jimmy's results on the Stanford-Binet Intelligence Test yielded a mental age of 4.0 (IQ of 94). His primary difficulty was in the area of language skills. Jimmy also displayed difficulty in motor planning, perceptual-motor organization, and visually discriminating between common items.

The results from the Vineland Social Maturity Scale supported the conclusion that weaknesses existed in the area of language development. For example, Jimmy's ability to label familiar objects at the 1 to 2 year level was still weak, and at the 2- to 3-year level he still had difficulty relating experiences verbally. Jimmy also had problems with perceptual-motor skills (such as cutting with scissors and buttoning.)

It was recommended that Jimmy be placed in a classroom setting in which his language difficulties could be addressed and remediated. He was also to undergo speech and language therapy five times a week and begin perceptual-motor training to develop his visual motor skills. Finally, a reevaluation in 1 year was recommended in order to assess Jimmy's level of progress and his remaining needs.

INTRODUCTION

A diagnostic formulation is achieved by combining information from a psychiatric history with the signs and symptoms garnered from observation and testing (Akiskal, 1986). Plenk and Hinchey (1985) have recommended that a complete evaluation should include standardized testing, behavior observation and rating, a developmental history, and a play interview. Once a firm understanding of the child's general character and functioning has been obtained, further evaluation is based on a clear knowledge of the developmental parameters involved. In many cases, a problem is perceived merely because a given behavior has persisted beyond an expected age (e.g., poor concentration, disobedience). In these cases the so-called problem may simply resolve itself with the passage of time. On the other hand, it may obstinately persist, and in the case of impaired or delayed development of attention, for example, there may be a resultant restlessness and frustration that interferes with both social and academic learning.

In addition to an awareness of delayed developmental sequences, it is useful to have a knowledge of the progressive stages of development and the psychopathologies possible at each. For example, Kashani and Carlson (1987) studied 1,000 preschoolers in a child development clinic. They discovered that the frequency of major depression increased with age and appeared to be uncommon in children of preschool age, even among those who were psychiatrically referred. Another finding that has proved useful for differential diagnosis in young children was that somatic complaints in association with depression occurred in all the depressed preschoolers studied and appeared to decrease with age.

The clinician who keeps abreast of the emerging trends in developmental dynamics will find it easier to keep in mind the overall developmental context in which a child is embedded. To further clarify the developmental perspective, the therapist should obtain a developmental history of the child, including information on the child's gestation and birth; physical and medical background; characteristics of infancy; attainment of motor milestones; self-help skills; nature of relationships with peers, siblings, and parents; and forms of discipline used by the parents. Such information helps the therapist perceive the developmental context of the child and is invaluable in weighing the probable causes of the symptoms.

This chapter outlines several features essential to an effective testing program and discusses the assessment of children's development, education, intelligence, personality, and neuropsychology. The more widely used tests in each area are also described.

TESTING

To maintain therapeutic neutrality, it is best that the therapist refer the child to an outside party for testing. Testing should be administered, scored, and interpreted by professionals who are specifically trained and skilled in each test. For proper diagnosis and use, it is especially important for the administrator to understand the theories and techniques of psychological functioning, adaptation, child psychopathology, and developmental psychology. To avoid misunderstanding and unnecessary exaggeration, results should never be discussed piecemeal. When results are discussed with a parent, teacher, or child, therapeutic issues must be considered. A feedback session can help prevent any harm to the child that might hinder further treatment. This fact should also be kept in mind when writing reports.

A test battery should be geared for the particular population it seeks to assess. Age, socioeconomic group, race, culture, primary language, and any known deficits or disabilities should be considered when choosing and interpreting a test battery. Only when such variables are considered is the adequacy and capacity of the tests' predictions clearly defined. Test batteries include an array of different tests. While specific tests are said to measure IQ, personality, organic damage, or deficits in language or perception, no one test should be used alone, because this can lead to partial, incomplete, and biased information. When a battery of tests is administered, however, a particular area of difficulty might be identified, indicating a need for further, more extensive, evaluation in this domain.

Good rapport is essential in testing a child because it ensures the child's best performance and, therefore, the most accurate assessment of his or her abilities. The examiner should exhibit a positive, playful attitude in order to elicit cooperation from the child. It is important to remain flexible throughout the testing procedures, as long as the quality of testing is not sacrificed. For example, difficult preschool children often have trouble sitting at a table for long periods. In such a case, the examiner can move to the floor to accommodate the child without losing test accuracy.

Tests that can be used in the psychological assessment of preschool children include the following:

Developmental Assessment:

- Gesell Development Schedules (4 weeks through 6 years)
- Bayley Scales of Infant Development (2 through 30 months)

Educational Assessment:

- Kaufman Assessment Battery for Children ($2\frac{1}{2}$ through $12\frac{1}{2}$ years)

Intelligence Assessment:

- Weschler Preschool Primary Scale of Intelligence (4 through 6 years)

Personality Assessment:

- Rorschach Test
- Child's Apperception Test (3 through 10 years)
- Vineland Adaptive Behavior Scales (birth to 18 years)
- Projective Drawings

Neuropsychological Assessment:

- Bender-Gestalt (4 through 12 years)

SPECIFIC ASSESSMENT PROCEDURES

Developmental Assessment

Methods for assessing a child's development usually assume that, while genetic endowment and environmental stimuli are definite influences, development is nonetheless a socially patterned process. It is this complex pattern that makes developmental assessment subject to differential diagnosis. This diagnosis generally focuses on adaptive behavior, gross motor behavior, fine motor behavior, language behavior, and personal-social behavior. The child's skills in these areas are measured against normal behavior patterns, which have been determined from systematic study of developmental patterns in healthy children. The child's measured performance is then converted into an age-equivalency level. Particular attention is placed on determining whether the developmental deficits are primarily caused by psychological impairment, brain dysfunction, or the child's environment. As the child becomes older, the predictive reliability of the assessment becomes greater, beginning by age 40 weeks, when the child has a large degree of control over his or her body.

The therapist should be wary of placing too much emphasis on particular items and should focus on patterns of performance, imbalances, and changes in the scores over time. The therapist should also take into consideration the influence of socioeconomic factors and recognize that many of the developmental norms were based on healthy, white, middle-class children. It is also important to use up-to-date normative data, because over time there has been an acceleration in the rate of maturation (Gesell & Amatruda, 1974).

Assessment requires detailed dated behavioral information for the child's entire history. This can be obtained from comprehensive interviews with parents, periodic screening examinations, or detailed formal examinations, which are essential when a differential diagnosis is required. According to Gesell and Amatruda (1974), the goal of the assessment is to

- Assess central nervous system function.
- Identify the presence of any neuromotor or sensory deficit.
- Discover the existence of treatable developmental disorders.
- Detect infants at risk of subsequent deterioration.
- Determine pathological conditions of the brain that preclude normal intellectual function, no matter how optimal the environmental circumstances.

Gesell and Amatruda (1974) also provided detailed tables specifying, in operational terms, skills a normal child should have mastered at key ages in the first 6 years of life. The skills are assessed using a variety of materials, each of which serves a specific purpose. These include catbells and tricolored rings, dangling rings, rattle, cup, cubes, pellet, pellet and bottle, formboard and blocks, small ball, picture book, paper and crayon, incomplete man, and colorforms.

As an illustration, a child who has just turned 3 would have normal visual-motor skills if the child could build a tower of 9 cubes, put 10 pellets into a bottle in 30 seconds, draw a copy of a circle, draw an imitation of a cross, be able to repeat 3 digits, and be able to adapt to the reversal of a formboard without error, or with immediate correction. Normal gross motor skills for this child include an ability to alternate feet while climbing stairs, ride a tricycle using pedals, and stand on one foot.

Moreover, this child has normal language skills if he or she uses plurals, can distinguish sex, is able to tell the action taking place in a picture book, can name 8 of 10 picture cards, understands prepositions such as "on" and "under" and can demonstrate them with a ball and a chair, and is able to give single-word answers using the appropriate nouns and verbs. Finally, normal personal-social skills exist if the child can feed himself or herself without spilling very much, pour well from a pitcher, put on shoes, undo accessible buttons, understand taking turns, and learn some rhymes.

To identify developmental deficits, the therapist needs a clear picture of the normal progression and timing of the development of a child's skills. Take, for example, the child's dressing skills, which are one element of personal-social skills. At 36 months, normal children can put on shoes and undo accessible buttons. By 42 months, they can wash and dry their hands and face. At 48 months, they can also brush their teeth and can dress and undress, provided they are supervised. By 60 months, no supervision or assistance is needed. Finally, at 72 months, they can tie their shoelaces.

Some of the more important developmental bridges normal children cross include the following:

- At age 30 months, they should be able to hold a crayon with their fingers, give their names in full, help put things away, and carry breakable objects.
- At age 36 months, they should be able to immediately adapt to reversals in a formboard without making mistakes, be able to ride a tricycle using pedals, use plurals in speech, and be able to feed themselves without spilling very much.
- At age 40 months, they should be able to name all picture cards, and associative play should have replaced parallel play.
- At age 48 months, they should be able to count three objects with correct pointing, be able to make running or standing jumps, cooperate in play with other children, and go on errands outside the home.
- At age 54 months, they should be able to make correct aesthetic comparisons, show off dramatically in play, tell fanciful tales, and be bossy and critical.
- At age 60 months, they should be able to draw the unmistakable

shape of a man, count up to 10 objects correctly, make descriptive comments about pictures, ask the meaning of words, and play by dressing up in adult clothes.

- At age 72 months, they should be able to stand on each foot with their eyes closed, and tie their shoelaces.

Two developmental tests, the Gesell Developmental Schedules and the Bayley Scales of Infant Development, are described briefly here.

Gesell Developmental Schedules.   Used on infants and young children from age 4 weeks through 6 years, these empirically derived, standardized measures reflect infant and early childhood development in motor, adaptive, language, and personal-social functioning. These schedules are observations of the child's activities compared to established norms, rather than purely objective tests. They also include the observations of the parent or caretaker. The Gesell is most useful as one measure in a battery of tests seeking to assess suspected neurological or organic disorders.

Bayley Scales of Infant Development.   Used for children between 2 and 30 months of age, the Bayley Scales assess mental, motor, and behavioral development. The Bayley is a standardized scale with well-established norms representative of the entire U.S. population. It is considered the most useful measure of infant development available, and it has satisfactory reliability and validity (Sattler, 1982). It should not be used with institutionalized children.

Educational Assessment

Achievement tests are used mainly to measure academic achievement, language skills, and cognitive abilities. The goal of academic achievement tests is to measure reading, mathematical, and spelling skills. They generally begin with a screening test, which is followed by a diagnostic test focusing on the possible deficiencies suggested in the earlier test. The results may be used in combination with intelligence tests to ascertain the extent to which the child is realizing his or her potential and to determine whether special training is required. Academic achievement tests suitable for use with preschoolers include the Woodcock-Johnson Psycho-Educational Battery (W-J) (Woodcock & Johnson, 1977), which is a screening test, and the Kraner Preschool Math Inventory (Kraner, 1976), which is a diagnostic test.

Tests of language skills focus on the child's ability to comprehend and use language. More specifically, they measure word knowledge, information acquired, ability to analyze and synthesize, and reasoning ability. Tests available for preschoolers include the Peabody Picture Vocabulary Test-Revised (Dunn & Dunn, 1981), which can be used as a receptive language test; the Slosson Intelligence Test-SIT (Slosson, 1963) and the McCarthy Scales (McCarthy, 1974), which can be used as expressive language tests; and the Detroit Test of Learning Aptitude (Baker & Leland, 1967), which can be used as a vocabulary and language association test.

Cognitive processing tests attempt to define the manner in which a child receives and remembers information. The efficiency of the child's auditory and visual processing and the extent of visual-motor integration are measured. Tests used on preschoolers include the Wechsler Preschool Primary Scale of Intelligence (WPPSI) (Wechsler, 1974) and the Detroit Test of Learning Aptitudes (Baker & Leland, 1967). One of the more commonly used tests, the Kaufman Assessment Battery for Children (K-ABC), is discussed below.

Kaufman Assessment Battery for Children (K-ABC). The Kaufman is used for children between the ages of $2\frac{1}{2}$ and $12\frac{1}{2}$ years. It was developed on a functional model of cognitive processes and pays particular attention to neuropsychological development. It is used for psychological and clinical assessment, psychoeducational assessment, and minority group assessment. It includes a nonverbal section for hearing- and language-impaired children, and for non-English-speaking children.

Its basic elements are the Mental Processing Scales and the Achievement Scale. The former assess the child's ability to solve problems, and the latter assesses the child's current level of academic knowledge. The subtests included in the Mental Processing Scales cover so-called *fluid* intelligence; that is, the type of mental functioning that relies on the nervous system and does not depend on formal training. The tests here relate to word order, number recall, spatial memory, and gestalt closure. The Achievement Scale is concerned with so-called *crystallized* intelligence, which is the product of the successful integration of fluid intelligence with environmentally acquired training and abilities. This group of tests relates to reading, arithmetic, riddles, and vocabulary.

Intelligence Assessment

Intelligence tests are used in making diagnoses, evaluating treatment progress, measuring developmental changes, and ascertaining the effects of psychopathology. They measure both verbal and nonverbal abilities. More specifically, intelligence tests have been used to assess children with learning disabilities, behavior disorders, mental retardation, brain damage, and psychosis.

While a score on an intelligence test is rarely a sufficient indication that a particular psychiatric disorder is present, there are important empirical regularities that can aid diagnosis and treatment. Learning disabilities may be indicated by, among other things, substantial differences between scores on intelligence tests and those on achievement tests. Children with behavior disorders do not have significantly different intelligence levels from those of normal children. However, delinquent children do tend to have better perceptual organization abilities than verbal comprehension abilities (Dehorn & Klinge, 1978; Sattler, 1982).

Other empirical regularities include the fact that brain-damaged children tend to have extremely high variability in their scores on different subtests (Rudel, Teuber, & Twitchell, 1974). In addition, psychotic children, on average, have lower IQ's than normal children, and in families with a predisposition toward schizophrenia, the child with the lowest intelligence is at greatest risk. Psychotic children with higher intelligence tend to have a better prognosis, as well as more complex symptoms. Finally, autistic children generally perform as poorly on intelligence tests as do mentally retarded children. They tend to have relatively good visual-spatial and memory abilities, but their language abilities are poor. It is also true that the lower the intelligence of the child, the more severe the symptoms tend to be.

In making inferences from test results, it is important to be aware of the impact of environmental and hereditary factors on intelligence. For example, heritability often accounts for between 40 and 80% of the variation in IQ levels, and perinatal factors, birth weight, malnutrition, cultural factors, and familial factors are also significant influences (Sattler, 1982). Scores may also be influenced by the degree of the child's willingness or motivation to participate and by temporary interferences with performance such as tiredness or stress.

Intelligence tests specifically designed for assessing preschool children include the Wechsler Preschool and Primary Scale of Intelligence (WPPSI) (Wechsler, 1967), the Merrill-Palmer Scale of Mental Tests (an extended version) (Stutsman, 1931; Ball, Merrifield, & Stott, 1978), the Bayley Scales of Infant Development (Bayley, 1969), and the Infant Psychological Developmental Scale (Uzgiris & Hunt, 1975). The WPPSI is discussed below.

Wechsler Preschool Primary Scale of Intelligence (WPPSI). The WPPSI assesses the intelligence of children ages 4 to 6. It should not be used as a simple IQ test, but rather as a descriptor of psychological functions whose impairment brings about lowered scores, which, in turn, affect recognition of the child's potential versus tested abilities. The WPPSI is a structured test consisting of numerous tasks divided into Verbal and Performance sections. Its structure is such that dynamic abnormalities that show up within the subtests, either in the answers themselves, the methods used to obtain answers, or comments the child makes while working, are viewed as being diagnostically significant. This contrasts with more unstructured tests such as the Rorschach, which attempts to reveal unconscious fantasies that may not evidence themselves in daily life and functioning.

Children who have been raised in a different culture, speak a different primary language, have grown up in poverty, or have been deprived of mainstream culture are at a decided disadvantage in this test. Such children might do poorly on the verbal subtests but achieve high scores on the performance section. In these cases, a combined IQ score is not properly representative, and it must be noted as such.

Freddy: Covered Up in Smoke

Freddy is a 5-year-old boy who was referred for evaluation in order to determine the basis of his emotional and interpersonal difficulties. He is prone to aggressive outbursts and is preoccupied with "rocketships and flying saucers."

Freddy, a handsome boy with blonde curly hair, was brought to the interviews by his mother. Although Freddy verbally expressed his discomfort with staying with the examiner, he neither clung to his mother, nor showed any tearfulness. Early on in the first session, Freddy announced that he did not want the examiner to tell him what to do and that he would choose the tasks to do. Freddy was unable to follow instructions for many of the tasks, and instead attempted to devise his own method of approaching each task. Efforts to set up materials for him were ignored or outwardly rejected. Freddy made little eye contact, spoke constantly about what he was doing or about fantasy material, and repeatedly used profane language. He attempted to rip the testing materials and, although informed that this was prohibited, continued his behavior. Several times throughout the session Freddy had to be physically restrained from ripping.

Results from the Rorschach test revealed Freddy's preoccupation with rocketships and monsters, as well as his limitations in reality testing. At times, Freddy did not even glance at the test cards, and thus his responses were more a reflection of his internal fantasies than of the task at hand. Freddy's use of profanity seemed to stem from the anxiety and anger aroused in him by the demands of the task and by the interpersonal nature of the situation. The examiner noted that Freddy was confused between what was within himself and what was external. For example, in his response to card seven, he explained that the examiner was unable to see the motorcycle because it was "covered up in smoke."

Personality Assessment

Objective tests, projective tests, and social adaptation tests are used to reveal personality characteristics of children. Such tests are used with children who are either unwilling or unable to reveal their thoughts or emotions in an assessment interview. They are rarely used in isolation, and they may not have diagnostic validity if this is done. Among the tests that may be used are the Rorschach test, the Child Appreciation Test (CAT), the Vineland Adaptive Behavior Scales, and Projective Drawings.

Rorschach. The Rorschach is an unstructured projective technique in which 10 ink blots are presented and the child states what he or she sees in each. The unstructured quality of the Rorschach is particularly helpful in elucidating a preschool child's inner world, because children's overt communications may not be developed enough to communicate the complexities of their inner psychological world, sense of relationships with others, and feelings about themselves. The Rorschach taps unconscious material that even the most willing and articulate subject could not possibly divulge. Making use of a gestalt imagery projection, the Rorschach can elucidate a child's characteristic perceptual processes and discover how these are shaped, distorted, and colored by the child's internal system of representations. The child's interpretations of the ink blots gives the clinician valuable information about the child's anticipatory and automatic interpretations of the world.

Diagnostically, the Rorschach can establish the existence of a current thought disorder and alert the therapist to the existence of fragile functioning or the danger of imminent episodes. Additionally, since the Rorschach gives information that is symbolic, deep-seated, and unconscious, it is particularly valuable in uncovering information indicating areas of emotional difficulty, as well as particular triggers. This information, which the child could not otherwise directly relate, might take years to obtain through therapeutic means. If a child is acting out, extremely depressed, in a borderline episode, experiencing school or separation anxiety, or the like, such information can rule out irrelevant hypotheses and help the clinician get to the heart of the matter.

The way in which the story is related, its internal consistency, the identification of protagonists and antagonists with whom the subject is identified, all give diagnostic information. Pathology can be seen in any disturbances in thinking processes that are evident, in preservation, or in losing the boundary of the cards. Affective tone is expressed through emotions described, distortions communicated, and which particular stimulus is being distorted. Defenses are revealed by how they are employed within the structures of the story. Finally, conflicts are evident from the content of the story and the level of defense employed in telling each story.

Child's Apperception Test (CAT). The CAT is a projective test used for young children. The test consists of a series of pictures that depict a story. Animals, rather than people, are portrayed, and the scenes are not complicated. The child is asked to tell a story of what is happening, what led up to it, and what will happen in the future. Each card is designed to elicit particular kinds of information; some simulate loneliness, some simulate aggressive fantasies, some the relationship between particular people such as father figure and son, mother figure and daughter, and so forth.

Vineland Adaptive Behavior Scales. This scale is used on children from birth to 18 years, 11 months. It assesses the child's personal and social sufficiency and capacity for self-care in an age-appropriate manner in terms of communication, daily living skills, socialization, and motor skills. It views the child's functioning as an important indicator of continued growth and development. It also indicates the child's ability to function adequately within the expectations and standards of societal norms.

Projective Drawings. In tests that use projective drawings, the child typically is asked to draw either a person, a house, or a tree, and deviations from a so-called normal drawing are noted. Of diagnostic importance are such graphomotor factors as erasing, placement, pressure, shading, and size, as well as factors such as detailing, distortions and omissions, symmetry, transparencies, and ground line treatment (Odgon, 1982). In drawings of people, the diagnostically important features are head characteristics, hair treatment, facial features, torso, anterior appendages, and so forth. In house drawings, they are usual modes of presentation, apparent distance, perspective, size and placement, and the like. Finally, in tree drawings, the characteristics to be noted are types of trees and their parts.

In each case, the drawing is viewed for the presence of abnormalities. Odgon (1982) listed drawing characteristics and noted studies that have offered possible interpretations of abnormalities in each. For example, a drawing of a person with an unusually small head suggests that the child has feelings of inadequacy or impotence. Odgon noted that it is reasonable to expect that the healthy child's drawing will contain some deviations from a normal drawing and, consequently, that individual signs are less reliable than the general configuration of signs.

Paul: Somehow Delayed

Paul is a 5-year-old boy who appears small for his age. He was referred for assessment by his pediatrician, who suspected the possibility of an emotional disorder. Paul's mother was concerned about possible learning disabilities since Paul "seems slow academically."

At the first two test sessions, Paul had difficulty separating from his mother; he claimed to be "scared that she won't be there when I get back." However, by the third session, Paul came to the testing room easily and was able to begin working without first playing with toys or refusing the task, as he had done previously. Once Paul became involved in a task, he was usually cooperative and was able to work for sustained periods of time. Although Paul was easily distracted and exhibited low frustration tolerance on some tasks, with encouragement and focused attention from the examiner he could be brought back to the task at hand.

Graphomotor tests indicated that Paul has some difficulty in this area. His drawings were executed in a fragmented fashion; he began with the feet, drew the head, and then drew connecting sections. On the Goodenough-Harris Draw-A-Man scoring system, Paul achieved a standard score of 70, which places him in the second percentile for his age.

Julie: Boo Boos and Wee Wees

Julie is a 4-year, 11-month-old girl who lives with her parents and her 2-year-old brother. Julie was the product of a full-term, uneventful pregnancy and was born with a faint heartbeat, jaundice, and cephalhematoma. Throughout her infancy, she frequently suffered croup and ear infections. The latter persisted into her childhood and resulted in a hearing loss, which was surgically corrected when Julie was 4 years old. Julie's speech and walking development were normal, although she currently withholds bowel movements. She also wanted to return to wearing a diaper when her brother was born. Julie does not have a history of separation anxiety. She enjoys being the center of attention and tries to take attention away from her brother. At age 2, Julie began a Montessori nursery program, and she reportedly did well until she was switched from her small class to a larger one. In the larger class, she began having trouble following directions and paying attention. Julie is generally more cooperative with her father than with her mother. She does best when those around her are calm, and she rebels against too much discipline. Julie is well liked, although she tends to play roughly with her peers.

Throughout the clinical interview, Julie was cooperative. She separated easily from her mother and was able to remain with the examiner without protest. Julie had slight articulation difficulties and sometimes exhibited a loosening of association. (When asked to define a "bicycle," she replied, "to pedal on, I know because my daddy told me . . . I have a sister.") Julie made continued references to an older sister, which she does not have, and throughout the interview reported herself to be a number of different ages (in high school, 6, 10). Julie exhibited a fascination with sexual topics. She made repeated references to "boo boos" and "wee wees," and expressed a desire to touch body parts. Her stories indicated some sadness over separation themes and concerns over being alone.

Julie's overall intellectual functioning was at the average level; however, her test scores ranged from low average to high average. This variability indicates her potential for higher functioning. When the Wechsler Preschool and Primary Scale of Intelligence was administered, Julie had notable difficulties on the subtests, which are designed to be sensitive to abstract reasoning. She had difficulty when asked to repeat, verbatim, sentences that were read to her. This is suggestive of problems with receptive language and processing. When asked, on the comprehension subtest, why sick children should stay home from school, Julie replied, "because they may be deaf ... and retarded." At other times, she spoke about an imagined sister or of going horseback riding with her father, both of which were irrelevant associations to the questions. This indicated that certain questions evoked personal concerns and made it seem as if she was not paying attention. Julie produced associations that resulted in poor concentration and interfered with information processing. Julie's full-scale IQ, on the Wechsler Preschool and Primary Scale of Intelligence was 97.

Julie's performance on the Peabody Picture Vocabulary Test was consistent. The Peabody requires that the child choose one out of four pictures to correctly identify a word or concept. It therefore minimizes demands on language and concentration. On this test, Julie obtained an IQ score of 114 (81st percentile).

Julie's developmental delays were evidenced by her difficulty in copying designs. She scored significantly below age level (3 years, 11 months) on the Beery-Buktenica. She could not draw a square, and her figure drawings were below age expectations. (They included facial features, but omitted arms and the lower body portions.)

Julie's performance on the Rorschach and the Children's Apperception Test was consistent with her results on the intellectual measures, insofar as her performance on the unstructured personality tests was marked by variability and a range of developmental levels. On all of the assessment measures, Julie showed a tendency to give the less common answer rather than the more typical and generally acceptable one. As situations became more personal and/or less structured, Julie became anxious and her reasoning seemed less organized. Although her anxiety was not overt, it was at these times that Julie turned to fantasy in order to feel safe and protected.

Based on Julie's results on the tests, it has been determined that she performs best in a structured, less stimulating environment. She should be spoken to in brief sentences and gently redirected when she seems to be off-topic or not paying attention. Julie should be guided gently toward performing appropriate behaviors, and frequent reinforcement for a range of behaviors (including merely staying on target, regardless of performance accuracy) is recommended. Exploratory psychotherapy was also recommended because of Julie's preoccupation with sexual themes, her tendency toward loose associations when upset, and her behavior problems (stool retention, stubbornness, etc.).

Neuropsychological Assessment

Neuropsychological assessment seeks to detect an underlying relationship between a child's behavior and brain damage or dysfunction. It is especially important when abnormal behavior could be due to either psychiatric or neurological causes. Boll (1983) suggested that there are several widely held misconceptions in this field. He argued that brain damage does not have a predictable effect on behavior characteristics. While there is an increase in behavioral variability, there is no clear pattern of behavioral deficits (Head, 1926). Similarly, while brain damage does typically result in a general reduction in cognitive functions, the extent of this reduction varies greatly, and there is no consistent pattern that can be said to be indicative of brain damage (Boll, 1983).

Brain damage frequently results in physical handicap, diminished intellectual skills, seizures, and abnormal brain electrical activity (Boll, 1983; Rutter, 1977). These factors, in turn, may contribute to emotional disorder, but they do not do so in a predictable manner. Boll (1983) also pointed to studies by Rutter, Graham, and Yule (1970), among others, and argued that, in contrast to common belief, hyperactivity is not commonly observed in brain-damaged patients.

Neurological functioning should be assessed in cases involving learning disabilities. Again, the therapist's aim is to weigh possible psychiatric causes against neurological causes. Children with brain lesions are also assessed using measures of language, perception, conceptualization ability, and motor skills.

Aside from diagnosis, neurological assessment is used to measure treatment progress with neurologically impaired children. This task is made particularly difficult by the need to disentangle the effects due to the treatment from those that are the natural function of normal growth and development.

The most widely used neuropsychological test for children is the Bender Visual Motor Gestalt Test (1938).

Bender-Gestalt. The Bender-Gestalt test consists of a series of nine geometric figures the person is asked to draw. In the first part of the test, the person is shown the cards and told to draw each geometrical figure as best he or she can. The second part of the test varies in its administration, but it most frequently is presented as a memory test, in which the subjects are asked to draw as many figures as they can remember.

The rationale behind the test derives from gestalt psychological theory. The perceptual-motor activities inherent in the test help delineate many important facets of individual neuromotor organization and functioning. How the child proceeds in organization and the manner and order in which the child draws help measure graphomotor control. Fragmentation of the gestalt figures, such as collisions, is significant and may be evidence of either visual-perceptual or psychodynamic disturbance. Further differential diagnosis using other tests is necessary. The size of the figures, and the quality of line—whether dark or heavy and boundary adding or edging—all impart information that can be useful in diagnosing depression, euphoria, expansiveness, grandiosity, or psychosis, among other things. Consistent difficulties usually signal visual-perceptual problems relating to convergence, left-right orientation, perpendicularity, and/or relationship. Variable functioning, which does not naturally coincide with the difficulty of the figures, usually indicates dynamic areas of difficulty. Perseveration, indicative of mechanical behavior, presupposes brain damage.

Interpretation of the figures is said to aid diagnostic confirmation of organic difficulties, mental deficiency, and sometimes schizophrenia or manic-depressive psychosis. Psychoneuroses are harder to discriminate using the Bender-Gestalt, but certain dynamic information and indication of emotional disturbance are thought to be interpreted through this measure.

The Bender-Gestalt test is most frequently used as an introductory test, and it can also provide an anxiety-reducing breather between the Rorschach and other tests, since children feel quickly reassured by their ability to copy simple figures. In addition, the test can help develop rapport between the child and the administrator.

CONCLUSION

Psychological testing should integrate psychological assessment into the more general goals of clinical treatment. Successful testing takes place within a contextual framework created to understand the whole child. This includes the child's present functioning; diagnoses of any disabilities or disorders; the child's potential abilities; his or her strengths, coping mechanisms, and defenses; and hypotheses seeking to explain unrealized potential. The results of clinical testing should significantly affect the course of clinical treatment by enhancing differential diagnosis and by aiding the monitoring and evaluation of interventions.

CHAPTER EIGHT

Pathological Correlates of Neuroendocrine Dysregulation

INTRODUCTION

Affective disorders in children have been under intense biological scrutiny for more than a quarter of a century. In addition to the mood disorders, the resultant body of literature has now begun to yield clues about the physiological relationships underlying the development of pervasive developmental disorders, schizophrenia, and anxiety disorders.

The shift toward attempting to identify the biological bases underlying the causes and risk factors for affective and other disorders is largely attributable to two factors: the development of highly sophisticated biophysical techniques for studying psychopathology and the emergence of the notion of neuroendocrine dysregulation as a correlate of studying psychopathology.

While disorders of schizophrenia, autism, and anxiety are possibly the result of disturbances in neuroendocrine regulation, they do not often result in the kinds and/or severity of dysregulation that are seen in the most extreme cases of depression—cases in which the primary complication is suicide. The taking of one's own life very likely represents dysregulation at its peak. Therefore, this chapter discusses the neuroendocrine correlates of suicide since this phenomenon provides a "worst case" scenario, or endpoint of dysregulation, against which the lesser or different dysregulation underlying other forms of psychopathology can be compared.

Conditions such as high cortisol levels, low levels of 5-hydroxyindoleacetic acid (the principal metabolite of serotonin) in cerebrospinal fluid (CSF), low monoamine oxidase platelet activity, and a blunted response of thyroid-stimulating hormone (TSH) to thyrotropin-releasing hormone (TRH) have been found to correlate with suicidal dysregulation. However, it can only be said that these may be state (i.e., current) markers—not necessarily trait (i.e., enduring) markers—indicating hormonal dysregulation. Abnormalities in cortisol levels and a blunted TSH response are regarded as indicating dysregulation within the hypothalamic-pituitary-adrenal (HPA) axis, the site of emotional mediation. If there is a single major neurophysiological mechanism behind suicide (and, by inference, extreme neuroendocrine dysregulation), the most likely candidate at present appears to be hypoactivity of central serotonergic function (Banki, 1985; Banki & Arato, 1983).

Asberg and Traskman (1981) have proposed that it might be possible to further refine the understanding of serotonergic influence on suicidal behavior. In their view, it might be more accurate to say that, while hyperserotonergic function and suicide do appear to be linked in many cases, the actual relationship may be between serotonin turnover and some personality trait that, under adverse conditions, renders the individual more vulnerable to suicidal impulses. Aside from having the potential to reveal the intermediary mechanisms between serotonergic function and suicide/dysregulation (if it exists), this latter interpretation also allows researchers to bring to bear the construct of temperament.

By defining temperament as a constitutional difference in self-regulation and reactivity to stress, Derryberry and Rothbart (1984) have provided a potentially powerful tool for investigating suicidal behavior. The concept of temperament provides a valuable means of studying the development of normal and abnormal affective states (Chess & Thomas, 1984; Chess, Thomas, & Hassibi, 1983). Self-regulation and reactivity to stress reflect multiple neuroendocrine functions that can be observed behaviorally from infancy through adulthood. If trait markers for suicidal behavior are to be found, they will most likely be identified as a result of early longitudinal investigation into the interactions of early neuroendocrine functions with the environment, as manifested by the dimensions of temperament.

This approach appears to be feasible because many researchers on temperament agree that the inborn reactive and regulatory capabilities of an infant continue to change and develop after birth (Rothbart & Derryberry, 1982; Thomas & Chess, 1984).

As higher-level neuroendocrine control mechanisms develop, the more primitive reflexes are neutralized. This process has become known as *inhibitory maturation*, and study of the monoamine systems (principally serotonin, dopamine, and norepinephrine) in the early developmental period has documented the fact that the maturation of these systems gradually inhibits the newborn's excitatory tendencies (Pradhan & Pradhan, 1980). Serotonin again comes to the fore because it has been implicated as a primary inhibitor or modulator of behavior, exerting its effect as early as the 15th day of life in rats, for example (Lidov & Molliver, 1982; Mabry & Campbell, 1974; Pradhan & Pradhan, 1980).

To reiterate, the child who is unable to regulate affective changes is at a higher risk for developing depression/suicidal ideation/suicidal behavior in response to repeated blows to his or her sense of self. At present, research attention is largely focused on serotonin because it is known to be a major regulator of neuroendocrine rhythms—especially cortisol secretion—beginning very early in life (Heninger, Charney, & Sternberg, 1984). In addition, the general effect of serotonin from birth onward is to inhibit nearly every type of motivated and emotional behavior, including negative emotions such as fear and anxiety (Lidov & Molliver, 1982; Panksepp, 1986). Thus, from the viewpoint of temperament as well as from the empirical standpoint, serotonin appears to be the link between childhood and adulthood in terms of HPA regulation.

Panksepp (1986) has stated that as yet there is no taxonomy sufficient for describing the basic behavioral control processes of the brain, but that this can be remedied if psychobiology becomes a more theoretical science. In examining serotonergic influence on the development of temperament, this chapter will attempt to provide fresh insight regarding the origins of pathological behaviors.

NEUROENDOCRINE DETERMINANTS OF AFFECTIVE STATE

Fundamental Relationships

Physiologically, the primary areas involved in mediating the individual's interaction with the environment are the limbic system and the adrenal glands. Collectively, this interconnected network is referred to as the *hypothalmo-pituitary-adrenal (HPA) axis.* While no unitary concept of limbic function has yet emerged, it can be said that the internal and external states of the organism become superimposed within the limbic circuitry (Carroll, 1972; Iverson, 1982). In terms of the internal state, the hypothalamus, along with the brain-stem extensions, regulates homeostatic and autonomic functioning and interacts with the pituitary to modify endocrine activity. Incoming sensations from the environment are processed primarily in the amygdala and hippocampus (Guillemin & Borgus, 1972; Schally, Arimura, & Kastin, 1973).

Within the HPA axis, it appears that the brain monoamines, especially serotonin, norepinephrine, and dopamine, are major determinants of mood and behavior (Davis, 1970, in Janowsky, El-Yousef, & Davis, 1974). However, the cholinergic transmitter acetylcholine and the endorphins, as well as a growing number of amino acids and nonopioid peptides, have been implicated in the mediation of affective state (Janowsky et al., 1972, 1973; Panksepp, 1986).

If one or more of these neurochemical systems is deranged at birth or becomes unsynchronized in response to environmental stress, the individual may react inappropriately to incoming stimuli. Decreased or exaggerated responses to stimuli result in an inability to cope properly, which leads to dysphoric feelings that can culminate in a depressive or even suicidal state.

The involvement of the biogenic amines in the depressive disorder was accidentally discovered prior to 1950 when several investigators noticed that a significant number of hypertensive patients receiving reserpine developed severe depressive reactions (Freis, 1954; Jenson, 1959). The relationship between reserpine and depression proved to be a strong one. The severity of induced depression was found to depend on the dose of reserpine administered. Furthermore, the incidence of depression among hypertensive patients receiving reserpine was significantly greater than among those receiving other antihypertensive medications. Finally, the depressive state cleared when reserpine was discontinued and resumed upon reinstatement of the drug (Bunney & Davis, 1965).

Subsequent investigations revealed that reserpine and related compounds caused a definite reduction in serotonin, norepinephrine, and dopamine in the brain and peripheral tissues (Bunney & Davis, 1965; Carlson, Lindvist, & Magnusson, 1957; Jenson, 1959; Pare & Sandler, 1959). Thus, the effect of reserpine not only served to suggest that depression can have a chemical basis but helped to reveal the involvement of the biogenic amines in affective states.

The Biogenic Amines and Depression

Schildkraut (1965) was the first to postulate an association between depression and low levels of catecholamine, particularly norepinephrine. In his catecholamine hypothesis of affective disorders, Schildkraut also suggested an association between manias and abnormally high levels of norepinephrine. However, he was the first to point out that the catecholamine theory did not account for all the endocrine activity relating to depression.

Subsequent to the catecholamine hypothesis, the indoleamine hypothesis was presented, which postulated that a shortage of serotonin results in a depressed state. The exact role of serotonergic hyper- or hypoactivity in depressive and manic states remains somewhat ambiguous (Meltzer, Peline, Tricou, Lowry, & Robertson, 1984a,b). However there is a great deal of biochemical and pharmacological evidence showing a relationship between depression and hyposerotonergic function (Asberg & Traskman, 1981; Braverman & Pfeiffer, 1985; Lopez-Ibor, Saiz-Ruiz, & de los Cobos, 1985).

In addition to involvement of the catecholamines and indoleamines in affective state, acetylcholine and the endorphins should also be mentioned. Evidence of cholinergic involvement in depression was reported by Gershen & Shaw (1961), who observed the development of depression in individuals poisoned with cholinesterase-inhibitor insecticides. A later study reported the induction of anergy and depressed mood in patients who received a cholinesterase inhibitor. Presumably, an increase in acetylcholine results in a depressed affect (Bowers, Goodman, & Sim, 1964; Janowski et al., 1974).

The discovery of three separate families of endorphin-like compounds in the mammalian brain has generated many—and as yet mostly unanswered—questions regarding their possible neuropsychiatric functions (Berger & Barchas, 1983). The most obvious hypothesis would be that mania is associated with the hyperactivity of endorphinergic systems, while depression results from hypofunction of these systems.

However, studies with naloxone, an endorphin antagonist, do not reliably demonstrate induction of depression in normal individuals, nor does naloxone reproducibly alleviate mania (Emrich, 1982). Nevertheless, the overall effect of morphine on mood and behavior strongly indicates a possible involvement of the endorphins in psychiatric disturbances. This is especially true in light of the fact that the endorphins are known to play a role in neuroendocrine regulation, stimulating the secretion of hypothalamic-releasing hormones (Agren, Terenius, & Wahlstrom, 1982).

Specifically, the endorphinergic pathways are known to play a part in the regulation of adrenocorticotropic hormone (ACTH). Morphine administered acutely triggers the release of ACTH, while chronic administration blocks the release of ACTH that would normally occur in response to a broad range of stressors. However, since opiate antagonists such as naloxone do not block stress-induced release of ACTH, the endorphin system is unlikely to be the essential mediator of ACTH regulation (Reichlin, 1985).

Regardless of the specifics, the interaction between the biogenic amines and affective state is a crucial one, not only because of impairment of function due to depressed state but also because of a probable additional interaction either between depressed state and immune function or directly between the biogenic amines and immune function. Many studies have documented an association between bereavement—generally regarded to be the most severe of affective disturbances—and morbidity and mortality. For example, Young and colleagues (1963, in Irwin, Daniels, & Weiner, 1987) studying mortality among widowers, found that of 4,486 widowers aged 55 and older, 213 died within the first 6 months following loss of a spouse. This represented an increase of about 40% over the expected mortality rate for married men of the same age.

While the relationship has not been studied in any great detail, it seems reasonable to postulate that neuroendocrine changes might play a role in mediating changes in immune function subsequent to bereavement. In attempting to further define these relationships, Irwin and colleagues (1987) reviewed and integrated the existing literature and concluded that

> women who experience the death of spouses show increased plasma cortisol levels and reduced immune function. In distressed women anticipating the death of their spouses, NK (natural killer cells) activity is similarly reduced even though plasma cortisol levels remain unchanged. The reduction of NK activity during anticipatory and actual bereavement cannot be explained solely on the basis of increased cortisol secretion. (p. 462).

The Dysregulation Hypothesis of Affective Disorders

The complexity of neuroendocrine response to environmental stress has given rise to a more integrated model of the neurochemical correlates of affective states. Siever and Davis (1985) have pointed to the fact that the catecholamine and indoleamine theories, as well as the poorly understood endorphinergic influences, are far from adequate in describing affective disorders. The bioamine theories are based on the assumption that these neurochemical systems are either overactive or underactive in affective disorders. Rather than limit observation to this simple perspective, Siever and Davis have devised a formulation based on the operational dynamics of neurotransmitter systems.

These dynamics center around time- and stimulus-dependent regulation of neuroendocrine systems, which in turn are mediated by multiple, hierarchically arranged control systems. In contrast to simply observing the level of a given system's activity, irregularities in bioamine or endorphinergic neurotransmitter systems can be regarded within the broader context of malfunctioning in the regulation or buffering of these systems. Dysregulated neurotransmitter systems do not respond appropriately to external stimulation and may be highly unsynchronized from normal periodicities.

Siever and Davis (1985) have provided six criteria for use in testing for pathophysiology of affective disorders based on time- and stimulus-dependent regulation of neurotransmitter systems. Dysregulation of affect may be present if any of the following are found:

1. Impairment of one or more regulatory or homeostatic mechanisms.
2. Erratic pattern of basal output in the neurotransmitter system.
3. Disruption in the normal periodicities of the system, including circadian rhythmicities.
4. Diminished selective responsiveness of the system to external stimuli.
5. Sluggish return of the system to basal activity following a perturbation.
6. Restoration of efficient regulation by pharmacologic agents demonstrating clinical effectiveness.

The dysregulation model of affective disorders agrees with what is known about the relationship of neural systems to animal models of depression induced by learned helplessness and with the clinical signs, symptoms, and courses of the affective disorders in humans (Seligman, 1975; Siever & Davis, 1985; Weiss, Glazer, Pohorecky, Bailey, & Schneider, 1979). In addition, because behavioral regulation is a central premise of temperament theory, this model promises to be most useful in achieving a developmental understanding of depression if it is used in conjunction with measures of temperament.

The Dopamine Hypothesis of Schizophrenia

Consonant with the neuroendocrine dysregulation hypothesis of affective disorders is the mounting evidence implicating dopamine in the etiology of the schizophrenic disorders. While the affective disorders seem most influenced by norepinephrine and serotonin, the principal sources of evidence to indicate dysregulation of dopamine in schizophrenics derives from the fact that neuroleptics almost universally act to inhibit the action of dopamine in the CNS (Freedman, Adler, Waldo, Pachtman, & Franks, 1983). Furthermore, the induction of paranoid psychotic symptoms by amphetamines has also long been known to be alleviated by neuroleptics acting to reduce dopamine in the brain (Hughes, Preskorn, Adams, & Kent, 1986). However, data are not limited to these findings.

The neurosciences have so greatly advanced in recent years that attention has been expanded beyond neurotransmission at the synapse to include the extra cellular fluid in the brain in its entirety, including all the known neurotransmitters, peptides, and ions involved in neuronal communications. Evidence from these studies suggests the following three possible alternatives regarding the nature of dopamine dysregulation in schizophrenia:

1. Elevated levels of dopamine may be available to dopaminergic synapses.
2. There may be an increased sensitivity of these synapses.
3. Re-uptake at nerve endings may be impaired (Barnes, 1987).

Weiner (1985) has further noted that an increase in dopamine could be the result of a decrease in the conversion of dopamine to norepinephrine by dopamine-beta-hydroxylase (DBH). While there has been some postmortem evidence in schizophrenics supporting this hypothesis, it has yet to be confirmed by further research. In any event, Weiner has pointed out that, regardless of the strong evidence in favor of the role of dopamine in the pathophysiology of schizophrenia, the dopamine hypothesis has not yet been proved.

It may be more accurate to say that, while dopamine plays a role in schizophrenia, it may not be a causal one. One argument supporting this contention is that the brain may react to neuroleptics that block dopamine receptors by generating more receptors to override the block. Weiner has also pointed out that there may be a reduction in the number of receptor sites in the brains of untreated schizophrenics since the Parkinson-like symptoms seen in schizophrenics are likely the product of neuroleptic drugs. Noting that autism has been considered to be the earliest expression of a schizophrenic process, Goldberg, Maltz, Bow, Karson, and Leleszi (1987) studied dopamine activity as manifested in blink rate in 15 autistic children with a mean age of 9 years. These investigators found elevated blink rates among the autistic children and concluded that "the data suggest that catecholamine abnormalities may be associated with autism and that there may be points of commonality between child and adult psychosis" (p. 337).

Involvement of Endogenous Opioid Peptides in Schizophrenic Disorders

A further example of the complexity involved in tracing the etiology of mental pathology stems from the possible involvement of the endorphins and enkephalins in the origins of both schizophrenia and affective disorders (see the discussion of anxiety disorders in this chapter). As Brambilla, Genazzani, and Facchinetti (1984) pointed out in their extensive review, both of these substances can act as neurotransmitters whose functions could alter the actions of certain neuronal enzymes.

As examples, changes in the levels of beta-endorphin could play a causal role in the development of mental diseases by interfering with the activity of classical neurotransmitters such as serotonin, dopamine, or acetylcholine. As a further example, enkephalins have been observed to inhibit the release of acetylcholine in the hippocampus and noradrenaline, dopamine, and adenylate cyclase in the entire brain (Kosterlitz & Hughes, 1975, in Brambilla et al., 1984).

In terms of the affective disorders, it has been hypothesized that beta-endorphin is elevated in mania, leading to the suggestion that naloxone therapy might be beneficial in these cases. As noted previously, this conclusion resulted from findings that beta-endorphins in some cases induce a euphoria similar to that seen in mania (Byck, 1976; Kline et al., 1977; both in Brambilla et al., 1984). Manic patients also have been reported to feel less pain than normal subjects (Davis et al., 1978, in Brambilla et al., 1984). However, despite these indications, treatment with endorphin antagonists has met with mixed results.

Progress has also been limited in building treatment schemes for schizophrenia based on evidence about the action of the endorphins and enkephalins, despite strong evidence for their involvement in the pathophysiology of the disorder. For example, results with naloxone and naltrexone have failed to show consistency in alleviating auditory hallucinations (Gitlan & Rosenblatt, 1978; Kurland et al., 1977; Volavka et al., 1977; all in Brambilla et al., 1984).

Brambilla and colleagues concluded that alterations in blood levels of opioids are insufficient to wholly explain the etiologies of schizophrenia and affective disorders. At this juncture, it seems that the most accurate statement that can be made is that changes in opioid levels are among the many causative biochemical factors that occur and interact to produce affective and schizophrenic disorders as a result of neuroendocrine dysregulation.

Serotonin in Obsessive Compulsive Disorders

Several lines of investigation have implicated serotonergic hyperfunction in the etiology of obsessive-compulsive disorder (OCD). The so-called serotonin hypothesis of OCD has been generated from studies showing an improvement in symptoms on treatment with clomipramine, a serotonin reuptake inhibitor (e.g., Thoren et al., 1980, in Zohar, Mueller, Insel, Zohar-Kadouch, & Murphy, 1987).

A recent study by Zohar and colleagues (1987) has added further credence to the role of serotonin in OCD. Metachlorophenylpiperazine (mCPP), a serotonergic agonist, was administered to 12 patients and 20 controls in a single dose of 0.5 mg/kg. Following administration of the mCPP, but not following placebo, patients experienced a marked exacerbation of OCD symptomatology. While this result agrees with the serotonin hypothesis of OCD, it is not conclusive because the drug was not given to patients with other psychiatric conditions. Therefore, it is not clear whether mCPP induces specific exacerbation of OCD symptoms or general aggravation of symptoms associated with other psychopathologic disorders.

Despite the difficulties inherent in proving that serotonin plays a role in the genesis and/or maintenance of OCD, the preponderance of research seems to favor such a conclusion as time goes on. For example, essentially the same mechanism of serotonergic hyperfunction was found in children with OCD in a recent study. Flament, Rapoport, Murphy, Berg, and Lake (1987) administered clomipramine hydrochloride, a potent inhibitor of serotonin reuptake, to 29 adolescent patients with OCD in a double-blind, placebo-controlled trial over a course of 5 weeks.

Compared with the placebo groups, patients receiving clomipramine experienced the expected decrease in platelet serotonin concentration and also showed significant improvement in their OCD symptoms. The authors noted that their biochemical findings in adolescents agreed with the findings of others in adults along the following three parameters:

1. There was an overall lack of biochemical differences between untreated OCD patients and normal controls.

2. Clomipramine treatment significantly affected serotonergic function and the change in serotonin was closely related to the therapeutic response.

3. Clomipramine, in addition to influencing serotonergic function, also had an impact on peripheral measures of the noradrenergic system, an effect consonant with its known neuropharmacologic properties.

Thus, there seems to be some continuity between adult and adolescent biochemical underpinnings of OCD. Whether or not this extends to younger children awaits confirmation.

Pervasive Developmental Disorders

PDD and Autism. Thus far the discussion has centered around the etiology and treatment of affective disorders and schizophrenia in adults. However, when the focus is shifted to the early onset of these disorders in children, the picture becomes even further obscured. As Weiner (1985) has noted, aberrations in brain chemistry and/or structure do not necessarily occur solely as a result of genetically controlled defects in neuroenzymes or anatomy. These alterations can just as plausibly result from early experience.

In fact, much of the problem in identifying these disorders stems from the fact that the DSM-III-R predominantly assumes mental conditions in adults to exist in a relatively stable social, cognitive, and biological environment. While this frequently may not be the case in reality, it almost certainly is never the case for the relatively few children afflicted with these disorders, who inevitably experience rapid and powerful developmental influences (Prior & Werry, 1986).

Despite the confusion of labeling such as *psychotic-retarded-autistic* that is found throughout the literature because of problems of diagnosis and detection, the study of pervasive developmental disorders has progressed a great deal from the time when autism was regarded as signifying the infant's rage reaction against the mother, who unconsciously wished that her child did not exist (Ciaranello, 1982; Mikkelsen, 1982). There are now some indications that autism responds to neuroleptic therapy. Anderson and colleagues (1984) performed a double-blind, placebo-controlled study involving 40 autistic children using haloperidol. No adverse effects were found, while notable gains were made in facilitation and retention of discriminative learning.

While there have been no neuropathologic findings to date that are strongly associated with autism, a limited number of studies with fenfluramine have suggested that there might be a hyperserotonergic mechanism underlying this disorder. Fenfluramine acts to reduce brain serotonin and its major metabolite, 5-hydroxyindoleactic acids while it increases levels of homovanilic acid, the major metabolite of dopamine.

In a trial by August and colleagues (1984), 10 autistic patients, 5 to 13 years of age, were treated with fenfluramine. After 4 months, blood concentrations of serotonin decreased an average of 60%. The reduction was accompanied by decreases in motor activity, distractibility, and mood disturbances. Since the clinical reaction to fenfluramine was not related to initial serotonin blood levels, the investigators speculated that the effect of fenfluramine might be one of symptom relief, rather than proving serotonin as a causative factor in autism.

Interestingly, in a later study with 10 autistic outpatients who were 4 to 14 years of age, August, Raz, and Baird (1987) achieved results with fenfluramine similar to those of previous studies in autistic children. However, a subgroup of high-functioning autistic children were included in the later study. In these children, fenfluramine was observed to significantly improve social awareness as measured by parent ratings on the Social Awareness Rating Scale. Since there was no indication that short-term fenfluramine administration enhanced intellectual functioning, the authors concluded that fenfluramine might exhibit a more specific clinical effect in higher-functioning autistic subjects whose better functioning may be attributable to lack of complication by mental retardation.

Ciaranello (1982) has suggested two possible mechanisms by which serotonin might influence autism. First, elevations in serotonin might interfere with the function of other neuronal systems; alternatively, it might regulate neuronal morphogenesis. Both hypotheses await further testing.

As with the adult forms of affective and schizophrenic disorders, the endogenous opiates have also been implicated in childhood disorders. Gillberg, Terenius, and Lonnerholm (1985) measured the cerebrospinal fluid concentrations of endorphin fractions I and II in 20 autistic children ages 2 to 13 years, comparing these levels with those of matched normal controls. Significantly higher levels of fraction I and II endorphins were found in the autistic children. While these results are preliminary, the endorphins do appear to play a role in the early development of psychosis, as do the biogenic amines.

Attention Deficit Disorders

The biological understanding of attention deficit disorders is in its early stages. However, the fact that aberrant behaviors such as hyperactivity are observed across situations argues in favor of a neuroendocrine mechanism, since this demonstrates that ADD symptoms are not solely an artifact of situational demands (Raskin, Shaywitz, Shaywitz, Anderson, & Cohen, 1984).

There is good evidence that catecholamines, specifically dopamine, are involved in attention deficit disorders just as they appear to be involved in many other psychiatric manifestations of dysregulation. The principal evidence regarding hypoactivity of dopamine function lies in the fact that children with ADD are frequently treated beneficially with either dextroamphetamine or methylphenidate, both of which act to block the reuptake of dopamine and increase presynaptic release of catecholamines.

Further recent evidence supporting the hypoactivity of dopamine has come from Sokol, Campbell, Goldstein, and Kreichman (1987), who reported four cases in which hyperactive children taking high-side doses of methylphenidate began exhibiting sterotypic behaviors typical of those seen in laboratory animals with increased levels of dopamine. Furthermore, when Pliszka (1986) compared the efficacy of tricyclics against stimulants in the treatment of children with ADD, the stimulants were found to be generally more effective except in cases where underlying mood disorder might have existed.

Interestingly, the findings regarding the relationship of dopamine to attentional parameters might also have some application to the etiology of schizophrenia. Asarnow, Sherman, and Strandburg (1986), in reviewing the literature on the psychobiological substrate of childhood-onset schizophrenia, found that schizophrenic children suffered from impaired controlled attentional processes, while their more automatic modes of attending were essentially intact.

Anxiety Disorders

The somewhat hazy definitions of childhood psychopathy allow a plausible connection to be made between the childhood phenomenon of anxiety (e.g., separation) and the childhood schizophrenic diagnostic category of schizoid disorder. This disorder is characterized by vestigial interest in social contacts "without any schizophrenic type symptoms and without any necessary ultimate connection with schizophrenia" (Prior & Werry, 1986, p. 184). Rather than being viewed as schizophrenic, children displaying these symptoms may more accurately be viewed as exhibiting extreme withdrawal that is possibly prompted by loss or elevated levels of expectations regarding performance (DSM-III-R).

The preponderance of data implicates elevated levels of epinephrine in anxiety states in adults. As an example, Charney and Heninger (1986) decreased noradrenergic function in 21 healthy subjects and 26 drug-free patients with agoraphobia and panic attacks by administering clonidine hydrochloride. It was found that the primary metabolite of epinephrine, MHPG, was more significantly reduced in the anxious patients compared to the controls.

Nevertheless, results such as these fail to answer the question of whether internally dysregulated noradrenergic function predisposes the individual to anxiety or whether external events promote increases in norepinephrine. In light of the powerful developmental forces— both environmental and biological—experienced by young children as compared to adults, children may conceivably be vulnerable to both processes. Thus, children may be highly prone to developing anxiety— anxiety that could produce deficits in coping ability sufficient to induce depression in some cases.

The foregoing discussions of childhood schizophrenia and affective and anxious disorders have illustrated not only the associations between certain neuroendocrine substances and the pathologies subsequent to their dysregulation but also the high degree of children's vulnerability to these HPA axis dysregulations. Attention will now be focused primarily on the affective disorders, since these seem to have the potential to disrupt neuroendocrine regulation most seriously—a disruption so severe that its endpoint could be manifested in the death of the individual at his or her own hands.

Norepinephrine as a Possible "Umbrella" Neuromodulator in Psychopathologic Conditions

Recently, Potter (1986) has attempted to explain the efficacy of antidepressant drugs in the treatment of conditions such as panic attack, attention deficit disorder, and others. He has postulated an underlying mechanism based on the fact that the tricyclics are especially potent in terms of inhibiting either norepinephrine or serotonin uptake, whereas MAO inhibitors are less specific in their effect, acting on all three major neurotransmitters (norepinephrine, serotonin, and dopamine). Thus, efforts to understand antidepressant effects focus on the serotonin and norepinephrine systems.

Of these two, the norepinephrine system plays a major role as a modulator of incoming signals, increasing the signal-to-noise ratio of incoming messages. Norepinephrine apparently has a focusing function for other neurotransmitter systems, suppressing spontaneous neuronal firing and causing the response of a neuron to incoming signals to have greater specificity. Thus, any drugs affecting the noradrenergic system will have numerous effects on several other systems as well. This might provide, to some degree, a rationale explaining the usefulness of antidepressants in a variety of syndromes in addition to depression.

Kagan, Resnick, and Snidman (1987) have posited noradrenergic function to be instrumental in explaining individual temperamental differences in the threshold of responsivity in limbic and hypothalamic structures to unfamiliar (i.e., stressful) stimuli. They have postulated that individual differences in response to unfamiliarity, threat, or challenge are due, at least partially, to tonic differences in the threshold of reactivity of parts of the limbic lobe—in particular, the amygdala and hypothalamus.

One possible explanation of these differences might lie in the relative levels of central norepinephrine, since this bioamine amplifies the brain's reaction to novelty by suppressing background neural activity, thereby enhancing the psychological importance of, and reaction to, an incentive stimulus. While this remains highly speculative, it does demonstrate the type of interactions and effects that will have to be unraveled before a clear picture of neuroendocrine relation to psychological state can be obtained.

MANIFESTATIONS OF DYSREGULATION IN DEPRESSION

Hierarchical Nature of Limbic Function

The various chemical and psychological effects of neuroendocrine dysregulation independent of the issue of suicide will be discussed first, since suicide in many cases represents the endpoint or extreme limit of the depressive condition. The chemical state or trait markers present in suicidal individuals with or without depression will be presented in the next section. Before either topic is discussed the underlying order of limbic function should be emphasized. As is true for the developmental measures of temperament, limbic function is ordered hierarchically. Although the functional specifics are still incompletely understood, environmental stimuli trigger a series of endocrine reactions in stepwise fashion; that is higher control mechanisms modulate the reactive state of subordinate neuroendocrine systems (Akiskal & McKinney, 1975).

As a broad example, the hypothalamus reacts to external stimuli by secreting corticotropin-releasing factor (CRF), which in turn causes the pituitary to release adrenocorticotropic hormone (ACTH). The ACTH in turn stimulates the adrenal cortex to release cortisol, the level of which is thought to be closely related to the degree of stress or a strong sign of dysregulation (Anders, Sacher, Kream, Roffwarg, & Hellman, 1970; Goodman & Gilman, 1970; Pfohl, Sherman, Schlechte, & Stone, 1985; Tennes & Carter, 1973). Under normal conditions the level of cortisol is controlled by means of a negative feedback loop in which an elevated level of cortisol inhibits the release of CRF (Yates & Maran,

1974). It is also important to realize that the endorphins are involved in the secretion of ACTH and that serotonin is a major determinant of cortisol release (Heninger et al., 1984; Puig-Antich, 1986).

Cortisol

One of the strongest indicators of depression produced by dysregulation is the occurrence of abnormally high serum cortisol levels in patients with major depression. Such elevations are found in approximately 40% of these patients as measured by the dexamethasone suppression test (DST) (Halbreich, Asnis, Schindledecker, Zumoff, & Nathan, 1985; Pfohl et al., 1985).

The overnight dexamethasone suppression test was originally devised to screen for Cushing's disease, but it was adopted for psychiatric use when hypersecretion of cortisol was detected in severely depressed patients. The usual procedure for administering the DST involves oral administration of 1 mg dexamethasone at 11:00 P.M. Blood samples for plasma control are then taken at 4:00 and 11:00 P.M. the following day. A plasma cortisol concentration of 5 ug/dl in either sample is taken as an abnormal, or positive, result (Carroll, 1984).

An abnormal DST result indicates disinhibited function of the HPA axis, because under normal conditions dexamethasone suppresses the production of cortisol for at least 24 hours. As this test continues to be used, its diagnostic value is regarded as useful but somewhat limited, having an average sensitivity of approximately 50% (Asnis et al., 1981; Fang, Tricou, Robertson, & Meltzer, 1981; Poznanski, Carroll, Banegas, Cook, & Grossman, 1982). *Sensitivity* is a measure of the number of positive tests among patients with clinical signs of depression. Specificity of the test, defined as the rate of negative tests in a control population, typically ranges from 85% to 100% (Baldessarini, 1983). Carroll, Greden, and Feinberg (1981) have claimed an overall specificity of 96% and a sensitivity of 43% for the DST. Generally, it is felt that the DST is not suitable for screening unselected patients, but it can be of use when the clinician is attempting to answer a specific diagnostic question (Carroll, 1984).

The biological markers of depression in children have not been studied as intensively as those in adults (Geller, Rogol, & Knitter, 1983). Kashani and Cantwell (1983) found that when adults with major depressive disorder of the melancholic subtype are compared with similarly diagnosed children only about half as many children as adults can be shown to hypersecrete cortisol. This might be a reflection of the presence of an age effect. However, Klee and Garfinkel (1984) made the observation that the specificity of the DST might actually be somewhat better in children than adults due to the fact that, aside from the depressive condition, cortisol nonsuppression has been associated with a number of conditions that are usually absent in early childhood—for example, anorexia nervosa, bulimia, and opiate addiction.

In one study, the DST was administered to 30 children, of whom 7 were diagnosed with major depression, 6 with dysthymia, and 17 with nonaffective disorders (Petty, Asarnow, Carlson, & Lesser, 1985). The children were hospitalized for psychiatric reasons and ranged in age from 5 to 12 years. Each child either met the DSM-III criteria for major depressive disorder or dysthymic disorder or clearly did not meet the criteria for either of these disorders.

Similar rates of nonsuppression were found in the major depressive group (6 of 7, or 86%), in the dysthymic group (5 of 6, or 83%), and in a subgroup of the controls diagnosed as "definitely not depressed" (5 of 6, or 83%). In this study the DST had a good sensitivity for major depression (87%), but its specificity was low (53%).

As a rule, the limited but significant number of trials to date have demonstrated that the DST can be useful in the detection of depression in children (Branyon, 1983; Geller et al., 1983; Klee & Garfinkel, 1984; Weller, Weller, Fristad, & Preskorn, 1984). In another study, Poznanski and colleagues (1982) used the test in 18 dysphoric children aged 6 to 12 years and concluded that endogenous depression is not rare and is neurophysiologically similar to the adult disorder. This study and the others discussed support the validity of DSM-III-R nosology, which applies essentially the same symptomatology to adults and children alike for detecting affective disorders.

Cortisol-Serotonin Interaction

In terms of hierarchical control mechanisms, cortisol release is largely dependent on serotonergic function in the HPA (Heninger et al., 1984). The strong relationship between serotonin and cortisol release is illustrated by a study performed by Meltzer and colleagues (1984a) in which a 200-mg dose of 5-hydroxytryptophan, the metabolic precursor of serotonin, was administered orally to 25 patients with major depression, 6 schizoaffective depressed patients, and 16 bipolar manic patients. Subsequent to the administration of the precursor, serum cortisol levels were significantly higher in depressed patients than in the controls.

The increase in cortisol levels was also positively correlated with Hamilton ratings of depressed mood, worthlessness, and helplessness (Hamilton, 1960). Interestingly, a positive correlation was discovered between suicidal behavior and the 5-hydroxytryptophan-induced increase in cortisol. Furthermore, the highest cortisol response was observed in the one patient who later succeeded in committing suicide.

In a second study, Meltzer and colleagues (1984b) measured the efficacy of antidepressant drugs in the eight unipolar and seven bipolar depressed patients and the seven manic patients who were involved in their first study. After 3 to 5 weeks of treatment with lithium carbonate or a monoamine oxidase (MAO) inhibitor, the mean cortisol increase induced by the 200-mg dose of 5-hydroxytryptophan was increased. When patients were treated with tricyclics and second-generation antidepressants, there was a reaction in mean cortisol response in those with major depression.

Thus, the tricyclics and second-generation antidepressants appeared to normalize the cortisol response to serotonin. This is an indication that these treatments facilitate serotonergic action, which produces a down regulation of serotonin receptors.

The data produced by Meltzer and colleagues (1984a,b) point to a permissive role of serotonin in which abnormally low levels of serotonin may make an individual more vulnerable to depression.

The hierarchically controlled distribution of cortisol by serotonin appears to be in evidence at a very early neonatal stage. Gunnar, Fisch, and Malone (1984) performed a study with 18 healthy newborn boys age 2 to 5 days who were about to undergo circumcision. Half were assigned in random fashion to a group that was given pacifiers during the procedure. The other half, who served as controls, were given no pacifiers. Blood samples for cortisol were taken just before circumcision and 30 minutes after. Pretrial cortisol levels did not differ between groups. The investigators made behavioral observations 30 minutes before, during, and after the procedure. While the experimental group experienced a reduction in crying of about 40% induced by the pacifier, serum levels of cortisol after circumcision did not differ between groups. However, there were marked elevations of cortisol in both groups 30 minutes after the procedure.

These data lend further support to the plausibility of using measures of adrenocortical activity to detect variations in response to stressful events in neonates. Observation of both adrenocortical and behavioral responses to stress seems to be a useful way of examining stress and coping mechanisms in the newborns (Gunnar et al., 1984).

In an effort to extend knowledge about the secretion and circulation of cortisol, Gunnar and colleagues (1984) performed another experiment using circumcision performed without anesthesia as an aversive experience to newborns. Baseline cortisol concentrations were taken after 30 minutes of observation in 80 healthy newborns age 2 to 3 days. After circumcision without anesthesia, the newborns were assigned to one of four treatment groups in which blood sampling was performed 30, 90, 120, and 240 minutes after the start of the procedure. The behavior of the infants was monitored during the procedure and for 30 minutes after.

The newborns reacted to the combined blood sampling and circumcision with transient but intense distress. Cortisol production increased markedly in response to the stress, but normalized by 150 to 250 minutes following circumcision.

Cortisol response to stress in children was studied by Knight and colleagues (1979), who examined the anticipatory impact of elective surgery in 19 boys and 6 girls between the ages of 7 and 11. While they were in the pediatric ward prior to elective surgery, their cortisol response to stress was measured at three different times.

The first measurement (Time I) occurred when the children had just been told to return for surgery in 2 weeks. In an effort to assess coping ability and to determine the types of defense used (using the defense effectiveness scale), an extensive interview was conducted with each child. In addition, the children were instructed to collect urine samples during two 24-hour periods over the following weekend.

Time II occurred on the day following admission to the hospital. The hospital and the prospect of surgery became very real at this time, and urine samples were collected over a 24-hour period. During this time, the children were again interviewed by a clinician who was blind to the outcomes of the previous interview.

Time III was the day following surgery, during which the child remained in the hospital. No urine samples for cortisol assay were taken.

At Time I there was no correlation between cortisol production and scores for defense effectiveness. However, cortisol production rates and defense effectiveness scores changed significantly between Time I and Time II. Knight and co-workers found that increased cortisol levels were negatively correlated with efficacy of defense. Children had higher cortisol levels when they used denial and displacement to defend against the stress of hospitalization than when they used intellectualization or a mixed pattern of response.

In a different study on catecholamines and cortisol in 30 second-grade children, Tennes, Kreye, Auitable, and Wells (1986) obtained results suggesting that these neuroendocrine substances might be related more strongly to certain personality traits than to specific defense mechanisms. Baseline catecholamines and cortisol levels were taken on 3 regular school days at intervals of 1 or 2 months and on 2 days during which achievement tests (the stress inducer) were given at the end of the school year.

While the mean cortisol value was higher on test days, Tennes and colleagues found that the variance in cortisol was more closely related to personality and behavioral variables than to the academic stressor. The same appeared to be true of variance in epinephrine levels. That is, 41% of the epinephrine variance was related to two behaviors, the frequency of social approach by peers and the frequency of small extraneous movements. (For example, children who engaged in tapping a pencil or swinging their legs rather than concentrating on school work had lower overall epinephrine levels.)

Over all, children with higher levels of excreted cortisol and epinephrine were more socially engaged and less aggressive than those with cortisol and epinephrine levels in the lower ratings. Noting that levels of cortisol excretion are very stable from infancy onward, Tennes and colleagues pointed out that this might be one measure of temperament, since stress induces fluctuations from a basic level of physiologic functioning (manifested in the inherent cortisol level) typical for each individual.

Regardless of individual differences, studies such as those performed by Gunnar and colleagues (1984) and Knight and colleagues (1979) have demonstrated a remarkable capacity for coping in children, and especially in newborns. Healthy newborns are not only capable of enduring the strain of minor surgery, but are able to eat and interact normally with their mothers within minutes after cessation of the procedure.

The early sophistication of the HPA axis is also revealed by in-vitro studies. Yanaihara and Arai (1981) found that even in the fetal stage the HPA axis can respond to ACTH release induced by stress and is able to secrete steroid precursors of sex hormones. Furthermore, during delivery, the anterior pituitary of the fetus releases increasing amounts of ACTH as delivery progresses. Thus, it appears that the fetal adrenal axis is active during the delivery process and during the switch from intra- to extra-uterine life (Arai, Yanaihara, & Okinga, 1976).

Other studies have pointed to the fact that the chromaffin tissue of the adrenal glands is capable of responding to the stress of hypoxia by releasing catecholamines into fetal circulation. This results in stimulation of alpha receptors and peripheral vasoconstriction producing an increase in perfusion of the fetal heart and brain (Behrman, 1970; Goodwin, 1976; Meschia, 1978; Sheldon, Peeters, Jones, Makowski, & Meschia, 1979).

Serotonin/Cortisol and Temperament

The hierarchically controlled distribution of cortisol in response to stress interfaces with the study of temperament (reactivity and self-regulation), which is also a hierarchically interlocked system (higher-level processes of self-regulation modulate the reactive state of the somatic, endocrine, automatic, and central nervous systems) (Derryberry & Rothbart, 1984). The correlation of neuroendocrinological differences with observed differences in temperament at an early age would be a valuable tool for studying the development of depression and suicide.

A major step in this direction was taken by Tennes, Downey, and Vernadkis (1977). Urinary cortisol secretion rates were determined during 8 hours for 3 days in 20 infants age 11 to 13 months. Baseline cortisol levels were obtained on the first day. Stress was induced on the second day by separating the infants from their mothers for 1 hour. Responses of the infants were then monitored.

Those who reacted with fear or anxiety when their mothers left were found to have higher levels of cortisol than those who did not react fearfully. It is important to note that members of the fearful/anxious group had chronically higher levels of cortisol than members of the other group.

Among members of the fear/anxiety group, there were two distinct subgroups. Response to separation by one group was marked by easily quantifiable affective reactions (crying or making movements directed toward retaining the mother). However, members of the other group became immobilized and exhibited a passive withdrawal that might have been a physiological regression to a drowsy state allowing them to withdraw from interaction with the environment. Psychological regression to an earlier state of helplessness may have been involved as well.

Members of the latter group had lower levels of cortisol both chronically and in association with the stress event than did those who exhibited more overt reactions. It thus appears that hyperactivity and hypoactivity, as well as normal functioning of the neuroendocrine system as measured by urinary cortisol excretion rate, may be used to predict two different types of behavioral reactivity to stress.

Another dimension of temperament as revealed by differences in neuroendocrine function also emerged from this study. The infants were categorized according to their response to toys during a play session: happy, indifferent, or fearful. It was found that the infants categorized as happy or indifferent had cortisol levels similar to control levels. On the other hand, infants who reacted to the toys with fear exhibited cortisol levels on a par with those seen in infants who experienced anxiety on being separated from their mothers.

The reactions of infants described in this study are essentially analogous to those observed to occur in similar stress situations in the Ainsworth Strange Situation Procedure (Ainsworth & Wittig, 1969). In this paradigm, infants whose attachment behavior to their caregivers is seen to be resistant or ambivalent typically display a reluctance to engage in exploratory behavior or play with toys and show active or passive distress at being separated from their mothers. These widely observed correlations between types of reactivity to stress and specific affective state are compelling. Both the fact that Ainsworth's behavioral findings corroborate those of Tennes and co-workers and the strength of the latter researchers' physiological data indicate that certain affective states are positively correlated with relative levels of serum cortisol.

Tennes and colleagues (1977) reached the conclusion that cortisol levels are associated with psychological variables by 1 year of age. Certainly this result raises curiosity regarding the extent to which interaction with caretakers affects the hormonal response pattern of infants. It is also interesting to know the degree to which infants' temperaments (the constitutionally determined capacity to regulate their own neuroendocrine systems) affect their relationships with caregivers.

Serotonin/Cortisol and Separation

In the study by Tennes and co-workers (1977), it is possible that the infants with low cortisol levels who displayed little or no emotion were relatively serotonin-deprived and thereby made more vulnerable to stress. This hypothesis is supported by the finding that the antidepressant imipramine, whose action is to selectively block serotonin reuptake, appears to reduce the intensity of despair responses in infant rhesus monkeys (Suomi, Collins, & Harlow, 1976).

The fact that psychoendocrine correlates in 1-year-old infants who were separated from their mothers for 1 hour are similar to findings in highly emotional versus more reserved adults is another indication of the rapidity with which neuroendocrine systems mature and points to the potential value of studying the attachment bond in infancy. Severance of this bond might well provide a useful paradigm of depression in infancy, especially in light of the intensity of the despair response and the physiological changes known to occur upon traumatic separation, for example, negative changes in sleep patterns, monoamine systems, immune function, body temperature, and endocrine function (Kalin & Carnes, 1984).

Endorphins and Separation

To emphasize the probable active role of endogenous opiates, Herman and Panksepp (1978) arrived at an interesting postulation about the association of endorphins with separation distress. These investigators studied the effects of morphine and naloxone on attachment behavior—specifically separation distress and approach—finding that distress on separation was alleviated by morphine and potentiated by naloxone. This result led them to hypothesize that an endorphin-based process analogous to addiction may provide the neurochemical basis for social attachments. Thus, separation distress may be a reflection of endogenous opiate withdrawal.

OTHER PHYSIOLOGICAL MARKERS FOR DEPRESSION

TRH-TSH Test

The response to stress of increased amounts of cortisol by newborns and children is parallel to that seen in adults. Other physiological indicators also point to the continuity of affective disorders from childhood to adulthood (Puig-Antich, 1986). In addition to the dexamethasone test, which tests for dysregulation of the serotonin-cortisol dynamic, the TRH-TSH test also provides a measure of HPA dysfunction, in particular the pituitary-thyroid axis (Lingjaerde, 1983).

This procedure measures serum thyrotropin response following a dose of thyrotropin-releasing hormone (TRH). Measures at baseline of serum thyroid-stimulating hormone (TSH) are taken prior to intravenous administration of TRH, and more samples are taken during the next 2 hours (Loosen & Prange, 1982). Under normal circumstances there is a dramatic increase in TSH, which peaks 30 minutes after injection.

A decreased, or blunted, TSH response has been observed in approximately 25% of adult patients with primary endogenous depression. But as is true for the DST, decreased responses have also been noted in patients with alcoholism and anorexia nervosa (Loosen & Prange, 1982).

Neither the DST nor the TRH-TSH test is capable of differentiating between unipolar and bipolar endogenous depression, but unlike nonsuppression in the DST, a blunted TSH response sometimes continues after remission. Thus, the TSH response may be more trait dependent, while the DST is largely state dependent.

Growth Hormone

One of the most dramatic relationships between endocrine function and affective disorder is reflected in the distribution of growth hormone (GH). Neglected children frequently experience a decrease in GH secretion that leads to a significant stunting of growth. There is strong evidence that a direct cause-and-effect relationship exists between emotional abuse and deficiency of growth (Powell, Brasel, & Blizzard, 1967). This disorder is frequently referred to as *psychosocial dwarfism* or *nonorganic failure to thrive* and typically begins before 8 months of age. Its etiology is probably associated with lack of one or more positive elements between caregiver and child. In short, this disorder is caused by a disturbance in the attachment bond.

It is significant that this cause-and-effect relationship appears to be reversible in some cases. Powell and colleagues (1967) noted an absence of growth hormone release in a cohort of emotionally deprived or abused children and then observed a rapid recovery of the GH deficiency when the children's environment was changed. Thus, it appears that reduction in GH output, like the increase in cortisol production, is more a state marker than a trait marker of depression.

Sleep EEG

While much of the physiological evidence supports the continuity of depression in childhood and adulthood, which provides the basis for the use of adult criteria for childhood depression in DSM-III-R, there are age-related differences in physiological manifestations of depression. These probably are reflected most clearly in polysomnographic markers from childhood to adulthood.

Several investigators have found adult major depressive patients to exhibit a decreased latency to the first rapid eye movement period (REMp) as well as decreases in time spent in low-wave sleep and overall sleep efficiency. Increased REMp density and an irregular temporal distribution of REMp have also been reported (Kerkhofs, Hoffman, De-Martelaere, Linkowski, & Mendlewica, 1985). However, none of these indicators has been seen to be consistently associated with depressive episodes in prepubertal children (Puig-Antich, 1986). However, Puig-Antich, Goetz, Hanlon, Tabrizi, Davies, and Weitzman (1983) reported a highly significant shortening of the first REMp latencies and an increase in the number of REMp's in 28 fully recovered prepubertal patients who had been diagnosed previously as having major depressive disorders. It is possible that these characteristics are markers of a past depressive episode or are actual trait markers in prepubertal children who are likely to develop depressive disorder.

IDENTIFYING BIOLOGICAL MARKERS OF SUICIDE

Metabolite Studies: A Methodological Problem

While aberrations in cortisol, thyroid-stimulating hormone, growth hormone, and other brain substances do appear to be strongly related to HPA dysregulation and hence depression and suicide, there is a methodological problem relating to these findings. Aside from the dexamethasone suppression test, all these correlations are the product of metabolite studies. Such urine or cerebrospinal fluid (CSF) metabolites may not be accurate representations of the actual metabolism that occurs in the brain (Blomberg, Koplin, Gordon, Markey, & Ebert, 1980).

It is difficult to accurately assess the relation of the rate of metabolic turnover to the functional state of the neuroendocrine system (Kelly & Stinus, 1984; Wilk & Watson, 1973). As an example, the blood brain barrier inhibits the escape of serotonin. Additionally, serotonin metabolism is very sensitive to tryptophan in the diet (Van Praag & de Haan, 1980). Similar difficulties exist with regard to norepinephrine metabolism. Thus, the excretion rates of the amines, endorphins, and other neuroendocrine hormones may be a loose reflection of the central and peripheral metabolism.

The area of urinary metabolites is particularly problematic in this regard. For instance, MHPG is the primary metabolite of brain norepinephrine, but the exact fraction of urinary MHPG directly derived from brain norepinephrine is still unknown (Deleon-Jones, Maas, Dekirmanjian, & Sanchez, 1975; Maas, DeKirmanjian, & Fawcett, 1971; Schatzberg et al., 1981).

TEMPERAMENT AS AN INVESTIGATIVE TOOL

As Linnoila and colleagues (1983) have pointed out, prospective studies are needed to definitively isolate biological markers of depression and/ or suicidal behavior. The use of temperament measures may be helpful in this regard. Close examination of the literature reveals that the longitudinal stability of temperament characteristics makes it possible to use temperament data in the attempt to identify infants and children who are at risk for developing behavioral disorders (Carey & McDevitt, 1978; Chess & Thomas, 1984).

The study of temperament is of course closely allied to the nature-nurture controversy. The role of heredity versus that of experience in determining behavior has long been debated. However, only two methodologically sound techniques have emerged that might help resolve this issue: cross-fostering studies and studies of monozygotic and dizygotic twins (Lester, 1986).

Cross-fostering studies focus on cases in which the offspring of mothers with the condition to be studied (e.g., schizophrenia) are removed and raised by other mothers. If the condition arises in the offspring, the role of genetic influence can be assumed to be real. To date no such studies have been performed for the condition of suicidal ideation/ behavior. However, some studies of twins have been done.

Evidence in monozygous versus dizygous twins indicates a strong genetic coherency of temperamental variables over time (Plomin, 1982).

Torgeson and Kringlen (1978) studied the genetic aspects of temperamental differences in 53 same-sex infant twin pairs using a parent-interview protocol and item-scoring method for the period of infancy. Nine dimensions of temperament were evaluated from maternal interviews when the infants were 2 months and 9 months old.

The monozygous twins were more alike than the dizygous same-sex twins for all nine dimensions. At 2 months the greater similarity in the monozygous as compared to the dizygous twins was statistically significant for rhythmicity, threshold, and intensity. At 9 months the greater similarity in monozygous twins was significant for all nine categories.

When data were obtained on these same twin pairs 6 years later, the effect of inherent constitutional differences was present but dissipated compared to that at the 9-month testing (Torgensen, 1981). At 6 years of age, genetic influence was highly significant for the categories of activity, approach–withdrawal, intensity, and attention span/persistence. Thus, while environmental factors did have some impact on these qualities of temperament, genetic factors appeared to be stronger.

The three traits that displayed the least evidence of genetic influence at age 6 years, and hence might have been most susceptible to the vicissitudes of the environment, were regularity, adaptability, and mood. Torgensen pointed out that these were the traits that have been identified as risk factors for the development of behavior disorders. Irregularity, low adaptability, and negative mood along with withdrawal and high intensity are thought to constitute the characteristics of the difficult child at high risk for behavioral disturbance (Chess & Thomas, 1984; Thomas et al., 1968). These findings suggest that the environment is a strong, but not the only, influence in the development of behavior disorders in infancy and early childhood—an influence that, in some cases, may be strong enough to cause dysregulation of the HPA axis.

The New York Longitudinal Study, in which the behavioral development of 133 subjects was followed from infancy to early adulthood, also monitored variables of temperament (Chess & Thomas, 1985). Six of these subjects developed depression subsequent to infancy. While temperamental characteristics per se did not appear to be a pathogenic factor in the patients with major depression, the four cases of depressive neurosis or adjustment disorder with depressed mood were highly associated with a particular temperamental trait or constellation of traits. In one case the trait was extreme persistence, in another it was marked distractibility and short attention span. Two of the subjects exhibited the difficult temperament pattern.

For purposes of isolating early biological markers for depression/suicide, the prospective nature of the study of temperament is of major importance. A study by Carey and McDevitt (1978) illustrates the value of this approach. They compared the individual temperament profiles of 187 children in infancy with similar ratings in early childhood (3 to 7 years).

They found a strong environmental influence on the development of temperament in that the majority of difficult infants became less difficult over time. These investigators have pointed out that the infant temperament characteristics associated with the few subjects who remained difficult are of greatest clinical interest. The difficult infant with either high activity or extremely negative mood is apparently more likely to remain difficult in early childhood than is a difficult infant with moderate ratings in these categories. Behavioral disorder is not guaranteed in such cases, but follow-up might be advisable in cases in which intra-family difficulties exist.

Temperament and Serotonin

Prospective follow-up of infants with very difficult temperaments is also advisable for purposes of potentially identifying biological trait markers for depression/suicide. Serial serum assays in these individuals might yield a wealth of information about the onset of depression.

One specific area of study that might prove useful in this regard emerges from the consistent reporting of the association of extreme negative mood with difficult temperament. The strong relationship between hyposerotonergic function and depression has already been discussed. Intensified investigation of serotonergic function in infants and children with difficult temperament has the potential to yield valuable developmental data regarding depression. The value of this approach was highlighted by Asberg, Bertilsson, and Martensson (1984) who pointed out that the association between low levels of serotonin and suicidal behavior has also been seen in patients who did not fulfill DSM-III-R criteria for major depressive disorder. Therefore, the link between serotonin and suicide might better be sought within the context of personality or temperament variables.

ISSUES MEDIATING THE IDENTIFICATION OF MARKERS FOR SUICIDE

State and Trait Markers

Puig-Antich (1986) has provided some useful definitions of state and trait markers. Their necessary rigor illustrates the difficulty of finding either kind of marker. Identifying a state marker not only requires finding an abnormality closely associated in time with the onset of the depressive episode, but also requires that the abnormality normalize in step with affective recovery.

A marker that is still abnormal after full recovery is not necessarily a trait marker. A true trait marker is an abnormality that may have been present for a long time prior to the onset of the first depressive episode and may have remained unaltered during the entire lifetime of the patient. This may not always be true of abnormalities that remain after recovery, since the patient may be still too close in time to the clinical endpoint of the prior episode. It may also be that the abnormality thought to be a trait marker actually first occurred during the first depressive episode and never normalized following recovery.

Behavioral Components of Suicide

The situation is further complicated by the existence of a number of dimensions to suicidal behavior. There are violent and nonviolent categories of attempted and completed suicide, and these are linked to such temperamental characteristics as impulsive versus nonimpulsive and aggressive versus nonaggressive tendencies. Despite these variables, there is a general consensus that suicidal behavior is related to a disturbance in central serotonergic function (Asberg et al., 1984; Banki, 1985; Linkowski et al., 1984). The results obtained by Banki and Arato (1983) are typical, and they support the general concept that suicide is an extreme case of depression.

Banki and Arato (1983) measured levels of serotonin metabolite (5-hydroxyindoleacetic acid, 5-HIAA) in the cerebrospinal fluid (CSF) of 62 female inpatients. Of these studied 19 were diagnosed with major depression; 18 with schizophrenic disorder; 13 with alcohol dependence; and 12 with other disorders. Nineteen of these patients had attempted suicide just before admission, and 6 of the attempts had been violent.

Levels of CSF 5-HIAA were significantly lower in the patients who had made violent suicide attempts but did not differ between those who had attempted suicide by taking drugs and those who had not attempted suicide.

The Marke-Nyman Scale was used to measure personality dimensions, and findings showed that validity was lower and stability higher in suicidal patients and that both these dimensions were more pronounced in the violent attempter group, thus illustrating a further possible relationship between serotonin and difficult temperament (Sjobring, 1973).

Another important finding of this study was that those who attempted suicide by violent means formed a separate subgroup because of their simultaneously low CSF 5-HIAA values and Marke-Nyman validity scores. This evidence of a bimodal distribution of CSF 5-HIAA in depression has been demonstrated in other studies that showed suicide attempters had 5-HIAA values in the lower mode and that violent attempters and those who made repeated attempts had the lowest 5-HIAA concentrations of all (Asberg et al., 1976; Traskman et al., 1981; both in Banki & Arato, 1983).

SUICIDE AND THE DST

While the results summarized here appear to reflect the general relationship between serotonin and suicidal behavior, there are a number of factors preventing the rapid identification of specific trait markers. A number of psychiatric conditions carry an increased risk for suicide relative to the nonpathologic population. Schizophrenia (narrowly defined) and unipolar and bipolar affective illness all carry the same risk of death from suicide in spite of the fact that these illnesses are clearly distinct from each other (Coryell & Schlesser, 1981).

Furthermore, the concatenation of psychological and physiological occurrences that culminate in suicide is likely to vary across diagnoses. For this reason, predictors of suicide would also be expected to vary according to diagnosis. Unfortunately, little is known as yet about what the specifics of these variations might be.

Banki and Arato (1983) measured CSF 5-HIAA in 57 drug-free female patients, of whom 14 had DSM-III-R diagnoses of major unipolar or bipolar depression, 18 had schizophrenic disorder, 13 had alcohol dependence, and 12 had other disorders. Of these patients 14 had attempted suicide immediately before admission—4 of them by violent methods. The DST was administered to all patients immediately after lumbar punctures. The severity of the depression regardless of diagnosis was assessed for all patients on the 24-item Hamilton scale.

While no significant differences in amine metabolite or postdexamethasone plasma cortisol concentrations emerged in this study, partial correlations revealed that suicide attempts, but not depression, were significantly correlated with CSF 5-HIAA.

Coryell and Schlesser (1981) studied 243 inpatients with unipolar depression who had received DST's. Among those with primary depression (205), the 4 who later committed suicide were among 96 who had registered abnormal DST results. This result led Coryell and Schlesser to conclude that there may be a subtype of primary depressive illness that is more likely to involve suicide than other types.

Aggressiveness and Impulsivity

Not all patients with suicidal thoughts are at equal risk for future attempts (Robbins & Alessi, 1985). Given the likelihood of the existence of subtypes of depression that are more apt to result in suicidal acts, criteria are needed that can be used to define these subtypes. The fact that serotonin has been linked to both impulsivity and aggressiveness makes these traits logical candidates for study.

Banki, Arato, Papp, and Kurcz (1984) studied 141 female psychiatric inpatients with major depression, schizophrenia, alcohol dependence, or adjustment disorder, of whom 52 had been hospitalized following suicide attempts, 18 of them employing violent means. Levels of CSF 5-HIAA were tested in all patients.

In the violent attempters, CSF 5-HIAA was significantly lower in all four diagnostic categories. The authors pointed out that since these biochemical observations were essentially independent of the clinical diagnoses, further exploration into the nature of human aggression and suicide is a viable research direction.

Linnoila and colleagues (1983) studied the relationships of impulsive and nonimpulsive violent behavior to CSF 5-HIAA in 36 violent criminal offenders. Their study revealed a difference between those who had premeditated their acts and those who had not. The premeditating offenders had relatively normal levels of 5-HIAA in contrast to the impulsive offenders, who had relatively low levels. The specific involvement of serotonin was evidenced by the fact that other CSF monoamine or metabolite concentrations were not significantly different between the two groups.

Another interesting finding of this study was that the lowest levels of 5-HIAA were recorded in impulsive violent offenders who had attempted suicide. Thus, Linnoila and co-workers concluded that very low levels of CSF 5-HIAA concentration may be a marker for impulsivity rather than violence.

A later study by Linnoila and colleagues (1984, in Lopez-Ibor et al., 1985) corroborated these results, demonstrating that violent, impulsive offenders have lower CSF 5-HIAA concentrations compared to offenders who have planned their violent criminal action. These studies illustrate the fact that serotonic transmission is integral to behaviors that may be related but are nevertheless very different, such as suicide, aggressivity, and lack of control of impulses. These results also make clear the kind of issues that must be resolved before a clear state marker of suicide, if such exists, can be identified.

The Episodic Dyscontrol Syndrome

One promising area that might be studied in order to further understand the contribution of the aggressiveness component to suicide-like behavior is the episodic dyscontrol syndrome. While this syndrome is relatively rare in children, it is characterized by episodic bursts of extreme aggressive behavior with minimal provocation. Onset is often marked by anticipatory fear, and extreme remorse is experienced following an episode. As Nunn (1986) pointed out, the fact that the individual is not susceptible to influence during an attack and the episodic nature, anticipatory fear, and later remorse strongly indicate HPA dysregulation manifested in an inability to control aggressive urges.

Patients who have experienced these episodes from childhood generally amass a backlog of arrests, divorces, and lost jobs. The severity of aggressive behavior associated with this condition, along with the fact that medical and surgical treatment in adults has met with some success, give promise that this syndrome may provide relatively unconfounded cases of aggressive behavior that are more clearly associated with biological concomitants. Nevertheless, as Maletzky (1973) has noted, the episodic dyscontrol syndrome has been used to describe extreme aggressive behavior resulting from not one but many different sources.

Hellman and Blackman (1966) described a relationship between extreme aggressiveness/criminality in adulthood and the childhood triad of enuresis, fire starting, and cruelty to animals. These investigators attributed the evolution of this behavioral triad to loss of or rejection by a parent, which produces aggressive behavior as a means of achieving reunion. However, this interpretation does not preclude possible contributions from HPA dysregulation.

In their assessment of 130 patients whose chief complaint was explosive violent behavior, Bach-Y-Rita, Lion, Climent and Ervin (1971) found a high incidence of histories including birth injuries, mental retardation, coma-producing diseases, head injury with prolonged unconsciousness, and febrile convulsions in infancy. However, these were not the sole contributing factors in most cases. The psychosocial histories of most patients showed childhood deprivation and social maladjustment reflected in work and family instability. The majority of patients had lower-middle-class jobs with home situations that were tenuous and emotionally impoverished.

Bach-Y-Rita and co-workers noted that their patients could be viewed as having inadequate ego defenses. The resulting poor ability to cope with stress leads to loss of control and disorganized thinking and behavior. What distinguished these patients from others with poor ego defenses was that they reacted to stress with violence rather than withdrawal.

While the extremely violent behavior displayed by these patients qualified them as being susceptible to episodic dyscontrol of aggression, the many related causes of this behavior led Maletzky (1973) to attempt to better differentiate individuals with poor ego control who react violently from those who do not. Maletzky studied 22 subjects over a 2-year period, all of whom fit the general description of episodic dyscontrol.

Since not everyone who displays extreme aggressive behavior suffers from episodic dyscontrol, patients were excluded if their aggressive behavior occurred under conditions of schizophrenia, temporal lobe epilepsy, acute drug reactions (excluding alcohol), and pathological intoxication. A control group was not employed due to the ethical restrictions on withholding therapy from someone who might hurt others.

Of the 22 patients studied, 14 had seriously injured someone and 5 had committed homicide; 14 had engaged in acts of violence that appeared totally unprovoked. In all instances, victims had difficulty defending themselves due to the swiftness and unpredictability of the attack. The duration of the violent outburst varied from 10 minutes to several hours.

The attacks appeared to be related to convulsions in a number of ways, including accompaniment by aurae of hyperacusis, visual illusions, numbness of the extremities, and nausea. Headaches and drowsiness were reported to follow the attacks in 50% of the cases. Seventeen of the patients also reported severe headaches at times other than those corresponding to the episode.

All patients included for study were males in the lower socioeconomic groups. Most appeared for treatment in their 20's and early 30's and were rarely educated beyond grade school levels. In keeping with the results of Bach-Y-Rita and co-workers (1971), childhood psychopathology frequently appeared in the histories of these patients, of whom 16 were hyperactive as children, 12 reported febrile convulsions, 5 had histories of enuresis, and 4 had engaged in cruelty to animals.

It is important to note that the etiology of this syndrome is not unaffected by family characteristics. Of the patients studied, 19 had fathers prone to acts of aggression, 9 of whom had left home before the child was 2 years old. While no consistent pattern of psychopathology was detectable in female relatives, they were frequently described as anxious, depressed, and passive. Ten patients had male relatives with epilepsy, three had female epileptic relatives, and two had both male and female relatives with this condition.

Thus, the origin of the episodic dyscontrol syndrome appears to have a strong basis in neurochemical or neurostructural pathology with contributions from physical, genetic, and environmental sources, all of which may interact to one degree or another. The multifactorial nature of the etiology may not seem surprising in light of the severity of the aggressive behavior under discussion. An individual may have to receive contributions from many sources before such severe dyscontrol results.

Ounsted (1969) has pointed out that rage is a natural part of an infant's behavior. This behavior is a powerful signal that results through the bestowal of simplified social signals of reassurance by parents. It is when this behavior continues past the point of inability to do harm that pathology can result.

Delgado (1969, in Nunn, 1986) showed that radio stimulation of the amygdala, hypothalamus, septum, and reticular formation led to aggressive behavior in monkeys and chimpanzees, but this behavior did not exceed the bounds of the group's dominant-submissive hierarchy. Whether this is, as Nunn (1986) has suggested, the result of insufficient gross pathology or it demonstrates an insufficient accumulation of genetic, environmental, and physical factors, the continued behavior of uncontrollable aggression toward loved ones and others in the environment can lead to suicidal ideation and acts in childhood or adulthood. It is perhaps significant that 8 of the 22 carefully screened patients in the study by Maletzky (1973) had made at least one suicide gesture prior to the study.

While the multiple etiology of the episodic dyscontrol syndrome complicates the task of identifying a specific cause or causes, there is some evidence linking low levels of CSF 5-HIAA with dyscontrolled acts of aggression directed outward (van Praag, 1986). Thus, a key area in which to continue investigation would be to test the effects of serotonin precursor therapy in cases of childhood episodic dyscontrol.

Aggression/Impulsivity and Serotonin

Lopez-Ibor, Jr. and co-workers (1985) have pointed out that suicide can be viewed as a form of self-aggressivity, which can include a heteroaggressive component such as committing suicide for the purpose of revenge. Brown and Goodwin (1986) attempted to further refine the relationship between aggression and suicide by pointing out that researchers linked serotonin with aggressive behavior in animals prior to the hypothesis of its relationship to suicidal behavior in humans. These investigators suggested that a portion of suicidal behavior may comprise a specific kind of aggressive behavior in humans.

Van Praag (1986) acknowledged the strong role of serotonin in aggressive/impulsive behavior and suicide by citing the work of Asberg and colleagues (1981) in which CSF 5-HIAA was found to be prognostically valuable. That is, low levels of 5-HIAA augured an increased risk of subsequent suicidal behavior. Van Praag (1986) also acknowledged the dilemma posed by the fact that lowered CSF 5-HIAA has been reliably reported in both depression and aggression disorders without concomitant depression. Van Praag suggested that the serotonin-depression hypothesis should not be discarded in order to establish a serotonin-aggression hypothesis. Instead, it might be more reasonable to hypothesize that disturbances in serotonergic regulation can bring about both mood and aggressive disorders. Such a hypothesis provides a biological explanation for the clinically observed fact that these disorders often occur together.

Evidence for the validity of van Praag's hypothesis can be found in a study by Pfeffer, Zuckerman, Plutchnik, and Mizruchi (1984) with 101 randomly selected preadolescent school children in which aggressivity/impulse control was not significantly different between suicidal and nonsuicidal subjects. However, the suicidal children were significantly more depressed than the nonsuicidal students.

This study was unique in two respects. A number of studies have succeeded in relating certain factors to suicide in child psychiatric inpatients, but the study by Pfeffer and co-workers (1984) observed suicidal factors in nonpsychiatric patients. Furthermore, this sample was systematically compared to a group of child psychiatric inpatients from a previous study (Pfeffer, Solomon, Plutchnik, Mizruchi, & Weiner, 1982).

The 101 randomly selected school children were between 6 and 12 years of age. The students were segregated according to age, sex, and racial/ethnic background and compared to 65 children in a voluntary child psychiatric hospital. Each child and a parent (usually the mother) were interviewed at the school the child attended by either an experienced child psychologist or a child psychiatrist. Measurement instruments included a Spectrum of Suicidal Behavior Scale, a Spectrum of Assaultive Behavior Scale, a Precipitating Events Scale, Affects and Behavior Scales (recent and past), Child Concept of Death Questionnaire and Scale, Family Background Scale and Questionnaire, Ego Mechanisms Scale, Ego Defense Scale, and Medical-Neurological History Questionnaire. Each child was also given the Bender-Gestalt test to measure perceptual-motor functioning.

Of the 101 school children, 11.9% were found to have suicidal ideas, threats, or attempts. This contrasted greatly to the inpatient population, in which 78.5% were found to have these factors. The majority of suicidal tendencies among the school children were suicidal ideas, whereas among the inpatients there was an equal distribution of suicidal ideas, threats and attempts. Behavior spectrum scores between boys and girls were not significantly different.

Of the 12 school children who had suicidal tendencies, 5 had no concrete ideas about a plan or method for suicidal action. The mothers of suicidal children had suicidal behavior scores that were significantly higher than those of mothers with nonsuicidal children. The suicidal behavior scores of fathers of suicidal versus nonsuicidal children did not differ significantly.

Overall, 11 differences emerged between the suicidal and nonsuicidal children in this study. The suicidal children were higher on nine variables, in particular preoccupation with death, recent depression, Bender-Gestalt score, tendency to use introjection as a defense, depression in the child's past history, tendency for the mother to have suicidal thoughts, and recent and past signs of general psychopathology. As mentioned previously, measures of impulse control/aggressivity were not significantly different between the suicidal and nonsuicidal students.

The randomly selected group of school children showed lower mean scores than inpatients on variables such as recent and past aggression, recent and past antisocial behavior, recent depression, total ego defenses, and parental separation. Factors of childhood depression, preoccupation with death, introjection, and parental suicidal tendencies were higher for suicidal than for nonsuicidal children in both the school population and the inpatient group.

In terms of the hypothesis of van Pragg (1986) it is significant that when hospitalization status was held constant, children with suicidal ideas had significantly higher scores on both recent aggression and recent depression. It appears that any consideration of the behavioral dynamics of suicide will have to include the possibility of either depression, aggression, or both. Thus, it seems prudent to incorporate a theory such as that of van Pragg (1986) in which serotonin is regarded as mediating both mood and aggression, either of which alone or in combination could give rise to suicidal behavior.

CONCLUSION

At the present time the most conservative interpretation seems to be that dysregulation of the HPA axis increases the risk of psychopathology along a number of dimensions, the most serious of which may result in suicide. A central neurotransmitter dysfunction, primarily associated with serotonin, may reduce the capacity of these patients to resist acting on suicidal impulses. Neuroendocrine disturbances in dopamine have been noted to have schizophrenic and learning disorder consequences, while norepinephrine dysregulation has been implicated in anxiety disorders. While the consequences of these perturbations can be severe, they apparently are less life-threatening than are cases of depression associated with serotonergic dysregulation.

Disturbances in serotonin regulation may give rise to the dysregulation of impulse control or aggression as well as affect, since low CSF 5-HIAA has been found in depressed patients without a suicidal history and has been seen to be lowest in depressed patients who have made violent suicide attempts.

Prospective studies in larger groups might confirm the high incidence of HPA disturbances in depressed patients with a past history of violent suicidal behavior. If such confirmation occurs, gradations in the indoleamine (serotonin) and catecholamine dysfunctions involved may serve as true biological trait markers for suicide—the most advanced manifestation of depression.

Another necessary step toward identifying trait markers for suicide will be a further refinement in the definition of affective disorders. The continued study of temperament and attachment behavior will contribute to this effort by prospectively identifying the developmental antecedents of disordered personality.

One development that might come to pass is the use of two or more biological tests as a definitive marker of depression. Preliminary results of studies in the adult psychiatric population indicate that the combined use of the DST and TRH tests may identify major depressive disorder with a sensitivity of 67 to 84% and a specificity of 92 to 98% (Chabrol, Claverie, & Moron, 1983).

Perhaps the most promising investigative direction that could be taken at present would be to integrate prospective temperament and attachment measures into studies of the behavior of depressed patients with suicidal tendencies and low CSF 5-HIAA after treatment to improve or enhance the metabolism of serotonin.

Part III

Clinical Syndromes

CHAPTER NINE

Pervasive Developmental Disorders and Their Differential Diagnosis

Nicholas: An Inexplicable Child

Nicholas is a 4-year-old boy who lives in a house with his mother, his maternal aunt and her husband, and his maternal grandparents. His mother and father were never married, although they did live together for a year before Nicholas's birth and for 7 months after, before Nicholas's mother returned to her parents' home with Nicholas. The grandmother and grandfather are first cousins, and Nicholas's mother's brother—after whom he is named—is mentally retarded and institutionalized. Nicholas's mother stated that she believed that Nicholas's father had a mentally retarded brother who died of pneumonia. Nicholas's confusion of his aunt, his mother, and his grandmother may be attributable to their constant interchange in and out of the role of his mother. Family members' reports were confusing and indicated limited intellectual capabilities.

Nicholas's caretakers reported that his developmental milestones were delayed, although the ages his mother provided for his initiation of different activities were judged as normal by developmental standards. He was bottle-fed until age 2. As a toddler, he spit out his food, and he has remained a very picky eater who restricts his diet to a few select foods. All of his caretakers reported that Nicholas had no favorite toy as a baby and that he did not use a pacifier. Nicholas is afraid of the dark, but sleeps well with the light on. Urinary continence was achieved by age $2\frac{1}{2}$, but encopresis persists. Nicholas was medically evaluated for physical problems that might be causing his severe stomach pains while defecating and his resistance to toilet-training. Nicholas's mother stated that the doctor thought Nicholas had "acquired constipation" and placed him on a mineral-oil regimen that was not adhered to. Nicholas's bowel incontinence is a family focal issue; his mother, aunt, and grandmother cooperatively administer enemas according to a system they have adopted, but his constipation and encopresis have not improved as a result of their treatments. Nicholas's first words were at 14 months, and his speech patterns never progressed beyond one- or two-word combinations.

Nicholas's mother first noticed that Nicholas was perhaps "not normal" when she took him on vacation and they were surrounded by other 3- and 4-year-olds. She heard the other children using more complex speech patterns and not merely mimicking or delivering one- or two-word commands, as did Nicholas. Nicholas also failed to initiate or participate in play with other children. His nursery school teacher commented that he plays best when alone and can play in groups only when he uses the other children as agents within his solitary play themes. His teacher added that he does not try to make friends and that his activities involving the few children he does interact with reveal his ignorance of how to interact with his peers. For example, he sometimes uses his classmates as inanimate objects in play. At school, Nicholas's use of speech is severely limited, and his activity often is focused on one thing for extended time periods. Often, this activity entails repetitive movements of a single part of his body. At home and at school, Nicholas shows no interest in symbolic play or in role-playing activity. His behavior is described as disorganized, impulsive, and abusive.

Nicholas was referred for evaluation upon the nursery school's recommendation. Although Nicholas initially displayed interest in the meeting, this was rapidly lost. His response to the therapist's questions were delivered in one to three poorly articulated words, and only after prompting. His motor coordination appeared to be impaired, and he held his hands at an odd angle throughout most of the interview. Other elements of the mental status examination were within normal ranges. He repeatedly referred to a wish to be "adopted"—a concept that he failed to truly comprehend. Intelligence testing yielded a determination of a full-scale IQ of 80. Nicholas's symptoms, as derived from histories from several family members and from the assessment interview and observation, indicated that he has autistic disorder.

His inability to interact appropriately with other children, his grossly impaired communication skills, restricted range of interests, lack of imaginative activity, stereotyped movements, odd posture, and unusual eating habits are all symptoms commonly found in autistic disorder. The chaotic home environment likely plays a role in the precipitation and/or continuation of Nicholas's symptoms. To verify the diagnosis of autistic disorder, a differential diagnosis was performed. Nicholas's IQ score indicated that he is not mentally retarded, and the absence of any apparent delusions or hallucinations ruled out the diagnosis of schizophrenia. Physical examination revealed no hearing acuity deficit, and Nicholas did not display a desire for normal social interaction that would be evident if his difficulties were due only to specific developmental disorders. Similarly, if Nicholas had a tic disorder or stereotypy/habit disorder, he would not have such grossly impaired reciprocal social interactions.

Thus, a diagnosis of autistic disorder was made with recommendation for therapeutic nursery placement. Weekly therapy for household family members was also part of the treatment plan.

INTRODUCTION

Classically, preschool children like Nicholas who have severe speech impediments, disturbed social relations, and behavioral and emotional abnormalities have been regarded as having pervasive developmental disorder (PDD) or being schizophrenic or brain damaged (Sanua, 1983). The confusion resulting from the interchangeability of these terms has led to a new nosological system, put forth in DSM-III-R, in which autism is a recognized subcategory of PDD and schizophrenia is held clearly separate. In differentiating between autism and other PDD conditions, DSM-III-R proposes the use of pervasive developmental disorder not otherwise specified (PDDNOS).

In DSM-III-R, both autism and PDDNOS, with their qualitative distortions of normal development, are distinct from the other developmental disorders, mental retardation and specific developmental disorders (academic skills disorders, language and speech disorders, etc.).

Autism and PDDNOS must also be differentiated from possible organic brain syndromes. Therefore, the diagnostic task is one of differentiating between autism and PDDNOS, between autism/PDDNOS and schizophrenia, and between autism/PDDNOS and mental retardation and organic brain syndromes.

It is not difficult to see from this decision tree that much of differential diagnosis of childhood disorders relies on a clear understanding of pervasive developmental disorder apart from the relatively easily recognized autistic disorder. Unfortunately, definition of this pathology has consistently resisted investigative efforts. However, since autism is widely viewed as the prototypic PDD, predictive diagnostic efforts can begin with a search for autistic symptomatology. If insufficient symptomatology is present to warrant a diagnosis of autism, the PDDNOS diagnosis can be made only after the other conditions previously listed have been eliminated. Because of the many conditions that have symptom complexes similar to those seen in autism—and because of the lability that is currently associated with nosology in the area of PDDS—the characteristics and possible etiologies of autism will be presented prior to the discussion of differential diagnosis.

INFANTILE AUTISM: CHARACTERISTICS AND CONCEPTS

Because autism is likely the most severe form of PDD (DSM-III-R) and comprises the nosological keystone for differentiating between the various childhood onset disorders, a clear understanding of this condition is essential. Autism, also known as infantile autism, is estimated to occur in four to five children in every 10,000, whereas the prevalence of PDD (autism and PDDNOS) is estimated to occur in 10 to 15 children in every 10,000 (American Psychiatric Association [DSM-III-R], 1987). Furthermore, autism is between three and four times more frequent in males than in females (DSM-III-R).

Studies of mono- and dizygotic twins have suggested that there may be a genetic basis for the inheritance of infantile autism (Ritvo, Ritvo, & Brothers, 1982; Ritvo et al., 1985). There is also some evidence indicating that autistic children tend to be first-borns and have a lower incidence of parents with psychopathology than do child schizophrenics (Despert, 1961; Kanner & Eisenberg, 1956; Sanua, 1983).

Despite these indications, disagreement about the nature of the pathology underlying autism continues to be widespread, although a primary psychogenic etiology has generally been rejected along with the idea that deviant childrearing patterns are causative (Christian, 1982; Volkmar & Cohen, 1986). While genetic research is moving toward identification of a genetic marker for autism—perhaps the fragile X syndrome—and there has been evidence for autosomal recessive inheritance (Ritvo et al., 1985), there is still no definitive marker or proven mode of genetic transmission.

Definition of Autism

The DSM-III-R classification for autistic disorder requires onset during infancy or childhood and the presence of 8 of 16 criteria listed under three different categories. Two of the following five criteria must be present from Category A—Qualitative Impairment in Reciprocal Social Interaction:

1. Marked lack of awareness of the existence or feelings of others (e.g., remains unaware of another person's distress; treats another person like a piece of furniture).
2. No or abnormal seeking of comfort at times of distress (e.g., fails to come for comfort when sick or hurt; seeks comfort in a stereotyped way such as repeating the same word over and over when hurt).
3. Lack of or impaired imitation (e.g., does not wave bye-bye; mechanically imitates the actions of others out of context).
4. No or abnormal social play (e.g., does not actively participate in simple games; involves other children only as "mechanical aids").
5. Gross impairment in the ability to make peer friendships (e.g., exhibits no interest in making peer friends; despite interest in making peer friends, demonstrates lack of understanding of conventions of social interaction, for example by reading a phone book to a disinterested peer).

One item must also be present from Category B—Qualitative Impairment in Verbal and Nonverbal Communication, and in Imaginative Activity:

1. No mode of communication such as communicative babbling, facial expression, gesture, mime, or spoken language.
2. Markedly abnormal nonverbal communication, as in the use of eye-to-eye gaze, facial expression, body posture, or gestures to initiate or modulate social interaction (e.g., does not anticipate being held; stiffens when held; does not look at the person or smile when making a social approach; does not greet parents or visitors; has a fixed stare in social situations).

3. Absence of imaginative activity such as playacting or adult roles, fantasy characters, or animals; lack of interest in stories about imaginary events.

4. Marked abnormalities in the form or content of speech, including stereotyped and repetitive use of speech (e.g., immediate echolalia or mechanical repetition of a television commercial); use of "you" when "I" is meant; idiosyncratic use of words or phrases (e.g., "Go on green riding" to mean "I want to go on the swing"); or frequent irrelevant remarks (e.g., starts talking about train schedules during a conversation about sports).

5. Marked impairment in the ability to initiate or sustain a conversation with others despite adequate speech (e.g., indulges in lengthy monologs on one subject regardless of interjections from others).

Finally, one item must be present from Category C—Markedly Restricted Repertoire of Activities and Interests:

1. Stereotypic body movements (e.g., hand-flicking or -twisting, spinning, head-banging, complex whole-body movements).

2. Persistent preoccupation with parts of objects (e.g., sniffs or smells objects, repetitively feels texture of materials, spins wheels of toy cars) or attachment to unusual objects (e.g., insists on carrying around a piece of string).

3. Marked distress over changes in trivial aspects of environment (e.g., when a vase is moved from usual position).

4. Unreasonable insistence on following routines in precise detail (e.g., insists that exactly the same route always be followed when shopping).

5. Markedly restricted range of interests and a preoccupation with one narrow interest (e.g., is interested only in lining up objects, in amassing facts about meteorology, or in pretending to be a fantasy character).

Social Abnormalities in Autism

The single most important component in diagnosing autism and differentiating it from other childhood psychopathologies is that of *social behavioral deficit*. In his original work, Kanner (1943) suggested that the primary defect of autism was the loss of affective contact, or social withdrawal. He felt that this primary abnormality was what produced the concomitant language and cognitive impairments. Rutter (1982) has summarized the evidence to the contrary, pointing to studies that separate cognitive dysfunctions from social withdrawal and to the existence of biological impairments that cannot be explained by social withdrawal. Nevertheless, the social deficits in autism are so specific that any theory of underlying pathology must account for them as primary effects if not causes.

The distinctive social abnormalities are beginning to be studied systematically. A foremost feature, evident in the preschool years, is the inability to develop specific attachment relationships (Sorosky, Ornitz, Brown, & Ritvo, 1968). Autistic children show no real preference for mother over other adults. They do not commonly follow their parents around the house as normal children do, and they do not seek comfort or cuddling as readily. While they may not physically withdraw, they do not seek contact; this may be evident in the first year, when anticipatory gestures of reaching to be picked up or held do not develop. Mothers report that their infants feel "stiff" in their arms and often are not comforted by being held (Lee-Dukes, 1986). There is a lack of eye-to-eye gaze that is distinguishable from the gaze avoidance of anxious children. In autistic children, eye contact occurs but is not harmonious with social intentions—the gaze is not used to gain attention or communicate as with normal children, nor is it simply avoided in intense social situations, as with shy children.

In later development, earlier patterns of social withdrawal surface in the form of a clear lack of empathy: Autistic children have difficulty conceptualizing or perceiving others' feelings. The result is a lack of reciprocity in social interactions with other children, preventing the development of cooperative play and the growth of personal friendships. The social interaction of autistic adolescents does sometimes improve, but affectional bonds are more likely to develop with parents or other family members than with peers (Rumsey & Rapoport, 1983). Wing and Gould (1979), in their study of children with social impairments and associated abnormalities, developed a structured schedule, the MRC Children's Handicaps, Behavior, and Skills (HBS). This schedule was used to structure interviews in order to obtain the relevant clinical information in critical areas of functioning: quality of social interaction; abnormalities of symbolic, imaginative activities; stereotypes; and overall pattern of interests. Their breakdown of social impairments may be widely applicable to determine the presence of the full syndrome of autism or other pervasive developmental disorders.

Wing and Gould rated social behavior under the following four headings:

1. *Social aloofness*—the most severe impairment, including children who evidenced aloofness or indifference in all circumstances.

    Some physical contact may be sought, but without interest in the social aspects of interaction.

2. *Passive interaction*—including children who did not seek social contact, but did not necessarily resist the approaches of others.

3. *Active but odd interaction*—including children who made spontaneous approaches, but whose needs were characterized by some repetitive, idiosyncratic preoccupation. They lacked empathy and identification in their approaches and were therefore less socially accepted than the passive group.

4. *Appropriate interaction*—covering those children whose social intercourse was deemed appropriate for their mental age. As mentioned, this category resulted in the classification "sociable, severely mentally retarded."

Wing and Gould concluded that such a system, based on severity of social impairment, yields the most statistically significant associations with behavioral, psychological, and medical variables—more than just presence or absence of a history of autism. The autistic children in their study had better nonverbal skills than the other socially impaired children, yet were generally differentiated from the others by the idiosyncratic speech patterns (pronominal confusion, repetitive routines, etc.) and by categorization in the "social aloofness" category (32 of 37 with a history of autism were so classified).

Surprisingly, the various subgroups of "socially impaired" did not differ significantly on the speech patterns and behaviors typically associated with autism, but they did differ with regard to many other cognitive and behavioral variables measured. On this basis, the authors called for descriptions of socially impaired children based on severity and quality of the social abnormalities, intelligence, language comprehension age, and development of symbolic activity, along with the standard clinical history and demographics. They went further in calling for a lexicon no longer reliant on the restrictive terms *autism* and *psychosis*. Suffice it to say that the more recent classifications of PDD have begun to rectify the limitations of the older nosology, but Wing and Gould's HBS schedule, particularly their rating system of quality of social interaction, can be useful in diagnosis and treatment strategy for a range of disorders, including PDD's, autism, and retardation. Rapoport and Ismond (1984) have provided a list of observations demonstrating the *lack of social responsiveness* characteristic of infantile autism:

- Failure to cuddle.
- Lack of eye contact.
- Lack of facial expression.

- Indifference or aversion to affection.
- Indifference or aversion to physical contact.
- Treating adults as interchangeable.
- Mechanical clinging to specific adult.
- Failure to develop cooperative play.
- Failure to develop friendships.

Older children may attain a level of *superficial sociability*, such as:

- Awareness of parents or familiar adults.
- Attachment to parents or familiar adults only, but failure to relate to others.
- Passive involvement in games or physical play.

The attempt to comprehend the social disabilities of autism continues unabated. Theories of cognitive deficiency and its putative neuropathological underpinnings must be broad enough to include an explication of the specific disorders of social interaction and communication. Hobson (1984) conducted an innovative study of autistic children's responses in a picture-matching paradigm. Using videotapes portraying people, emotions, and objects in terms of visual and aural stimuli, he found that autistic children evidenced an abnormality in the comprehension of objects and were unable to differentiate varying emotions or distinguish between people (for example, in terms of gender). His findings and those of others (e.g., Langdell, 1978; Rutter, 1983) suggest a lapse in the capacity to process affective information and social stimuli.

Cohen, Paul, and Volkmar (1986) have proposed a scheme for assessing a child suspected of being autistic based on this primary feature of impaired social functioning. In their scheme, assessment takes place along three parameters: (1) sociability and social communication; (2) comprehension and expression of emotions; and (3) attachment behavior. The first category, sociability and social communication, is concerned with measuring the degree to which the potentially autistic child might prefer objects over people. This feature could be measured in terms of consistency of response and attention to people, time spent looking at people rather than objects, and interest in peers as opposed to adults.

The second dimension, comprehension and expression of emotions, could be assessed in terms of the relative ability to express normal emotions in their appropriate context. There may be difficulty in making the transition from a state of calm to activation and arousal, and empathy may be lacking, showing failure to recognize that other people have feelings. Finally, attachment can be assessed for autistic traits by looking at such factors as whether or not the child prefers parents to strangers, shows indifference at the parents' absence, or becomes more distressed when separated from a favorite object than when separated from parents or familiar others.

Amin: Silent by Choice

Amin, age 5, recently moved from a suburban community to an urban area with his mother, his older sister, and his younger brother. His father has not lived with the family since Amin was 2 years old, and he is now in prison. Not long ago, however, Amin's father contacted his wife and children through a letter in which he apologized for deserting his family and attributed his past transgressions to "spiritual illness" (Amin's family members are black Muslims). In their new environment, Amin attends a public school and was placed in a gifted program after tests revealed that he is cognitively advanced for his age. Before the move, Amin attended three different schools. The first was a private school, where teachers described Amin as shy, but without developmental or academic problems. Amin was moved to a public school the next year, when his mother encountered financial difficulties. Teachers there described Amin as bored. They also noted that Amin spent 15 to 20 minutes deciding what to do and usually chose from a limited few activities such as painting, blocks, and puzzles. Since it was surmised that Amin's play was constricted, he was placed in his third school, a Montessori school. At the Montessori school, Amin excelled at structured tasks, and he showed significant improvement in his social skills as well. Amin left this school when his family moved away.

Since his move to the urban area, Amin's behavior includes combativeness and jealousy toward his younger brother, who is physically handicapped. At school, Amin is stubborn, he refuses to talk to teachers, he opposes rules, and he assumes an appearance of inattention. At home, Amin sometimes is nonresponsive to his mother and unwilling to speak to her; he also wastes time and lingers in the morning when he should be preparing for school. Lately, he has been refusing to go to school. Amin was referred for evaluation when his mother expressed worry that these difficulties might interfere with his academic growth.

During the initial assessment, Amin remained close to his mother, was electively mute, and showed little emotion. He smiled only once during the assessment, when his father was being discussed. After the interview, Amin was placed in a diagnostic play group, during which his behavior was more revealing. At first, while the interviewers were present, Amin remained electively mute, but he did engage in a game with a boy 2 years his senior. As soon as the interviewers left the play area to observe behind a two-way mirror, Amin's entire demeanor and affect changed remarkably. Suddenly, he spoke noisily and without hesitation, and he trotted about the room and played freely with the other child. Nothing in Amin's speech, content of thought, or behavior indicated psychosis. His fine and gross motor skills were judged age-appropriate, and he appeared to be cognitively advanced for his age. Other elements of the mental status examination were assessed to be within normal ranges. When the interviewers returned to the room where Amin was playing, Amin suddenly calmed down and resumed his initial demeanor.

No doubt, the stressors experienced by Amin—repeated moves between schools, a regional move, the departure of his father, the birth of a physically handicapped brother (which was preceded by his mother's temporary incapacitation), and the recent communication from his father—contributed to his aggressive and oppositional tendencies. Interestingly, reports from his mother and teacher and the diagnostic assessment revealed a restriction of oppositional behaviors to situations involving interaction with adults, and virtually no abnormality was observed when Amin was playing with an unknown child in the absence of adults. Amin's behavior toward his teacher and his mother indicate a desire to annoy and defy them. Manifestations of anger, resentment, and spitefulness are all evident in Amin's provocation of conflict with his brother. It is common in elective mutism—and is apparent in Amin's case—for the child to limit characteristic disordered activities to school or to other specific situations such as interactions with adults.

Before assigning an elective mutism disorder diagnosis, the patient's assessment was viewed within the contexts of mental retardation, autism, and developmental expressive language disorder. Mental retardation was ruled out because Amin's demonstrated academic accomplishments eliminated the possibility that his intellectual functioning was significantly impaired. Although Amin did exhibit characteristic aggressive activity that is also sometimes found in autism, this diagnosis was ruled out because Amin's language comprehension was normal, his play patterns were adaptive and sociable, and his use of language, though restricted by choice, was of normal character and appropriate for his developmental stage. Characteristic symptoms of developmental expressive language disorder—constricted vocabulary, difficulty learning new words, and general delays in speech development and progress—were not present in Amin's receptive, expressive, and written language, and thus a diagnosis of developmental expressive language disorder was ruled out.

Therapists concluded that Amin was suffering from elective mutism, with several stressors contributing to the accompanying manifestations of aggressive and oppositional behaviors. Weekly play therapy for Amin with parent counseling every other week was recommended.

Language Deficits

While deficits in social functioning may provide the best comprehensive means of diagnosing autism, assessment of language impairment can be helpful in substantiating—or in Amin's case, nullifying—the diagnosis. The language impairments characteristic of autism have been viewed variously as central to the full syndrome (Churchill, 1972), as secondary to cognitive defects, or as secondary to social impairments. This kind of paradigm appears now to be reductionist. Language deficits may be a central feature of autism, but they are not the core pathology and are not inextricably related to the full range of cognitive and social abnormalities, both in terms of neurophysiological and psychological causes and effects. The fact that dysphoric and autistic children share a number of the same defects in language acquisition, but that dysphoric children evidence few of the social and behavioral characteristics of autism, supports this view (Rutter, 1982).

It is probable, however, that cognitive deficits underlie the language disorders of autism, and that language disorders contribute to impoverished social interaction. If any realm can be seen as representing the core pathology, it is the cognitive realm, although a functional relationship exists among all three realms.

The statement "language is the common denominator for the early detection of developmental disabilities" (Capute, Palmer, Shapiro, Wachtel, & Accardo, 1981) sums up the significance of language impairments. The first and foremost sign of a problem is the delay in speech acquisition, although a small percentage of autistic children have a normal sequence of language development until sudden regression occurs between 18 and 30 months of age. When language does develop, it is abnormal in a number of striking ways (DeMyer, Hingtgen, & Jackson, 1981). These abnormalities are more specifically characteristic of autism than the delay in acquisition per se.

Pronominal confusion is a very common language abnormality, usually in the form of confusing "I" and "you." Early psychogenic theories of autism posited distorted self-conceptualization as the cause, although more recent studies demonstrated that the absent or insufficient use of "I" can be reversed when statements are systematically made to the child with the "I" used at the end of the sentence. This clearly indicated the essentially echolalic property of pronominal reversal (Bartak, 1978; Christian, 1982).

Of course, imitation is a proper function of normal acquisition. The key here is inappropriate, delayed, or peculiar echolalia. In a sense, the echolalia of autism is distinctive by virtue of its developmental deviance; rather than advancing communication or the acquisition of normal speech patterns, it specifically frustrates them. Immediate echolalia is the instant repetition of all or part of a speaker's statement; delayed echolalia involves complete imitation of the statement(s) verbatim, including content, tone, and rhythm.

Other typical language disorders of autism include disorders of receptive language, abnormalities of speech rhythm and melody, the use of stereotypes and neologisms, and improper or disordered syntax and semantics (Cantwell, Baker, & Rutter, 1985; Cantwell, Rutter, & Baker, 1978; Simmons & Baltaxe, 1975). Langdell (1980) and Rutter (1985) have argued that the language deficits of autism should be viewed not as syntactical or semantic, but rather as pragmatic, and that the underlying incapacity is contextual and conceptual. Again, this implies the relative primacy of cognitive dysfunction.

Autistic children have as much difficulty understanding spoken language as they have in acquiring it. Nonverbal gestures and cues are often required to elicit a response. Just as they lack reciprocity in social relations, they lack reciprocity in the language exchange occurring in normal conversation; indeed, these two lacks are analogous and interrelated. These developmental disorders with regard to language have been distinguished through comparison with the language disorders of aphasic children. Autistic children's symbols of speech tend to be invested with idiosyncratic meanings; words are no longer used as referrants and, over all, there is a total or near-total absence of communicative intentions—features that are seldom shared by aphasic children. The characteristic oddities of inflection and tone are far less common among aphasic children. In terms of language comprehension, autistic and aphasic children are both limited in their capacities. However, a study by Freidlander, Wetstone, and McPeek (1974) found that selective listening performance was more disturbed in the developmentally disordered children. They responded similarly to intelligible and unintelligible sounds, whereas aphasic children would often reject nonsense syllables.

Regardless of the degree to which language disorder is considered the core pathology of autism, it is still a critical measure of initial severity and prognosis—perhaps *the* critical measure. To that end Fish, Shapiro, and Campbell (1968), Shapiro and Fish (1969), Shapiro (1979), and Shapiro, Chiarandini, and Fish (1974) have focused on language development as the criterion for classification and prognosis. They developed new rating scales for language skills including measures of speech morphology (intelligibility) and speech function, the latter emphasizing degrees of communicativeness. Their scales were based on detailed classification of speech events on a molecular level. For example, a child's utterances would be tape recorded while activities and behavioral context would be recorded in notes by a second observer in the room (Shapiro & Fish, 1969). Careful criteria were set for intelligibility and communicativeness; the latter would be rated by observers after matching taped utterances to context notes.

Shapiro and colleagues (1974) applied their method to a group of 30 severely disturbed children, enabling them to classify according to three groups: (1) children who are severely retarded (based primarily on the intelligibility rating); (2) children who are comparatively more verbal than group 1, but whose communicative speech is markedly deviant (including speech patterns such as echolalia and inappropriate context); and (3) retarded children who evidence the beginnings of largely communicative speech. The latter group could be predicted to have the best outcome. The researchers stressed that the type of molecular analysis of language they employed can be used to make accurate prognoses of eventual outcomes at 3 years, 6 months old rather than at 5, as had been previously presented.

Play and Other Behaviors

The play of autistic children is fraught with expressions and signs of developmental disability. It is also, however, an arena within which they can be better understood and approached by others (parents, other children, therapists), despite the myriad obstacles resulting from social deficiencies. It therefore offers the psychiatrist, therapist, or counselor a naturalistic setting for diagnostic investigation and therapy.

Ritualistic phenomena are characteristic of the play of autistic children. Repetitive movements or actions, unusual hand or finger mannerisms, and whole-body movements such as spinning are common (Bartak & Rutter, 1976). Patterns of play are rigid and sometimes compulsive; autistic children rarely engage in symbolic activities with others involving a play of the imagination. In general, creativity is superseded by an almost mechanistic repetition. Preoccupations with memorizing numbers, patterns, and colors are common, for example, the information of bus routes. Intense attachments to peculiar objects may occur, and these children will often protest vehemently if such objects are taken away. A typical example of how autistic children relate to toys is the child who is fascinated with one wheel of a toy truck, spinning it endlessly, but who never plays with the toy as a truck (Lee-Dukes, 1986).

Other unusual behaviors sometimes associated with autism include the following:

- Extreme negative reactions to changes in the environment.
- Making bizarre sounds or noises.
- Facial grimaces.
- Marked overactivity.
- Self-injuring actions (head banging, biting of arms, wrists).
- Extreme food fads.
- Short attention span.
- Pronounced fears, extreme aggression, or tantrums.

The deficits in play are not just a result of language abnormality, even though they are most evident among children with the most retarded language skills (Sigman & Ungerer, 1984). They are certainly also a direct expression of social deficiencies. The strange physical behaviors, which are regressive in nature, must be viewed as resulting from disturbances in neuromuscular functioning and central nervous system (CNS) development.

DIFFERENTIAL DIAGNOSIS OF AUTISM, SCHIZOPHRENIA, AND OTHER CHILDHOOD DISORDERS

Sally: Progressive Dissolution

Sally is a 6-year, 3-month-old girl who lives with her younger brother and her parents. Her father has changed jobs four times in the past 4 years, and her parents are currently in the process of divorcing. Sally was born of a normal pregnancy, but her heartbeat at birth was weak. She also had jaundice. Her past medical history indicates that she had frequent ear infections that resulted in some hearing loss. An operation to restore her hearing was performed when Sally was $4\frac{1}{2}$ years of age. Sally reached developmental milestones at normal ages. She was toilet trained at age 2 years, 4 months, but she expressed a desire to return to wearing diapers. In addition, Sally has recently begun withholding bowel movements.

Sally began a Montessori nursery school 3 half-days each week, reportedly because her mother was too tired by her pregnancy to take care of her. Sally's school performance was satisfactory until the following year, when she was promoted to a larger class. At this point she regressed and exhibited loss of bladder control. It was also at this time that Sally had her ear operations. When she entered kindergarten, it was reported that she acted up in school, frequently interrupting the class and fighting with other children. To discipline her, Sally's teacher taped her mouth shut and supposedly threatened to put her in a dark closet. Over the course of that year, Sally's parents began divorce proceedings.

Sally was referred for evaluation by her teacher, who noted that she had marked academic difficulties and a short attention span. In addition to this, for several weeks Sally maintained that Sally had died and that now she was "Jenny." Sally also frequently complained of headaches, stomachaches, and "things crawling on me." Sally's parents reported that she had frequent angry outbursts and temper tantrums and was overtly jealous of the attention given to her younger brother. Sally has tried to harm her brother. She is afraid of "monsters" and of being alone at any time. She is also terrified (almost phobically afraid) of closed doors.

During assessment, Sally appeared well-groomed and alert. She exhibited no separation anxiety and was both cooperative with and responsive to the evaluator. Although her vocabulary was good, she had slight verbal articulation difficulties and her expressive language seemed somewhat disjointed. Loosening of associations were evident in Sally's stream of thought. Her mood throughout the assessment was cheerful. This affect, at times, was inappropriate because of its lack of adaptive range; she specifically stated that she did experience feelings of hurt or sadness. Intelligence testing revealed average intellectual functioning with greater potential than was being exhibited. Sally appeared to be fully aware of her environment, and reality testing proved normal.

Sally's symptoms are indicative of schizophrenia, disorganized type. Although there is no evidence of hallucinations, Sally did, for more than 2 weeks, insist that she had died and currently asserts that she has an older sister. These episodes are indicative of delusions. Sally has exhibited a marked loosening of associations as well as inappropriate affect. Her behavior does not meet the criteria for schizophrenia, catatonic type, because she is not preoccupied with systemized delusions or with frequent auditory hallucinations related to a single theme. The fact that Sally's symptoms have been present for more than 6 months and that she has shown impairments in academic achievement further support a diagnosis of schizophrenia, disorganized type.

Medical examination of Sally's sensorium ruled out the possibility of an organic mental disorder. A differential diagnosis of mood disorder can be made on the basis that although Sally was inappropriately cheerful at times during the evaluation, a diagnosis of a manic episode cannot be superimposed on a diagnosis of schizophrenia. Sally cannot be considered as having a psychotic disorder not otherwise specified because she, in fact, exhibited a clear decline in functioning from her previous level. Although in autistic disorder there often are disturbances in communication and in affect that suggest schizophrenia, the additional diagnosis of schizophrenia made on the basis of prominent delusions preempts both a diagnosis of autistic disorder and a residual diagnosis of pervasive developmental disorder not otherwise specified (PDDNOS).

Children in chaotic environments may appear to have difficulty in sustaining attention and in goal-directed behavior. In such cases, as in the case of Sally, it is difficult to determine whether the disorganized behavior is primarily a function of the chaotic environment or whether it is due largely to psychopathology.

Sally's behavior does, however, meet the criteria for a diagnosis of attention deficit disorder with hyperactivity. Her symptoms have been present for more than 6 months, she is younger than age 7, and her maladaptive activities are similar to those specified as necessary for a diagnosis of attention deficit disorder (difficulty sustaining attention, easily distractable, interrupts or intrudes on others, etc.).

A diagnosis of schizophrenia, disorganized type (and attention deficit disorder with hyperactivity) was therefore assigned, and it was recommended that Sally be placed in a small, highly structured class. Sally was referred to individual psychotherapy twice a week, along with family counseling once weekly.

Autism Versus Schizophrenia

The differential diagnosis of autism/PDDNOS should proceed stepwise, starting with application of the criteria for autism, followed by a ruling out of psychotic disorders, primary (but not secondary) mental retardation, organic brain syndromes, and a host of other psychiatric conditions such as reactive attachment disorder and the specific developmental disorders listed in DSM-III-R.

With regard to schizophrenia, there are differing opinions about whether or not this condition can arise at all before 30 months of age, and this issue has yet to be resolved (Cantor, Evans, Pearce, & Pezzet-Pearce, 1982). In the interim, childhood schizophrenia arising after 30 months, and more commonly after the age of 5, does have an established clinical picture, despite early confusion. Sally clearly demonstrates this fact.

The main problem originated 2 decades ago when the term *childhood schizophrenia* was used to denote almost all childhood psychoses. A reaction against this tendency began with the findings of Kolvin and colleagues (1971), who uncovered and described critical differences between early-onset and late-onset childhood psychoses. This research was later widely supported by other investigators (Eisenberg, 1971; Makita, 1966; Rutter, 1982). Characterization of early-onset and late-onset psychoses, the differentiation of infantile autism from other psychiatric conditions, and later, the development of the diagnostic category of pervasive developmental disorders, were all major advances in the classification, diagnosis, and understanding of childhood psychopathology. On the other hand, the understanding of what childhood schizophrenia is and the clarification of its utility as a diagnostic category became obfuscated. However, despite the confusion, there is still active speculation about the relationship between the PDD phenomenological spectrum and the development of schizophrenia. Results of investigations into the characteristics of atypical children and prospective studies of schizophrenic patients from childhood suggest the possibility that levels of developmental impairment short of full-blown autism may be etiologically related to schizophrenia.

For example, both Rescorla (1986) and Sparrow and colleagues (1986) have studied atypical children in comparison with normal and autistic children. They found that in comparison with controls, children with nonautistic PDD show deficits in cognitive achievement areas as well as poorer motor development and relatively impaired social functioning. However, even in the severe atypical categories, not every child was mentally retarded.

Results such as these naturally stimulate curiosity about the long-term effects of nonautistic types of PDD. Certainly it seems likely that these children will suffer pervasive decrements in coping and learning abilities, but in what way? One prospective study, at least, reports a case in which a child with atypical developmental characteristics experienced an acute schizophrenic break at age 19. Fish (1986) studied 12 offspring of schizophrenic mothers from birth. Only one child, a boy, subsequently developed schizophrenia, but this child demonstrated an early onset of social-affective and cognitive dysfunction.

Affect in this boy was noted to be odd from the earliest examination, even though parenting was judged to be warm and demonstrative. His expression was habitually solemn, and the angles of his mouth were turned down from the first day following birth. Subsequent analyses revealed a continuous path toward depersonalization and derealization culminating in a psychotic breakdown at 19.

While all children with early atypical developmental characteristics certainly do not become schizophrenic in later life, it is perhaps not surprising that some do, since their rarified sense of connectedness to others and the environment could easily lead to isolation and obsession with internal phenomena. It may be that children with atypical development may be at risk of later schizophrenic decompensation, especially in the presence of a family history of the disorder.

Returning to the issue of diagnosis at the present time, DSM-III-R not only rules out the possibility of childhood schizophrenia arising before 30 months, it also recommends that schizophrenia occurring in childhood be diagnosed by the same criteria as schizophrenia in adulthood (Beitchman, 1985); meaning that delusions, hallucinations, incoherence, or marked loosening of associations must be present. Hence, autism or PDDNOS may resemble childhood schizophrenia without hallucinations, delusions, and so forth. This is still a sticking point for many clinicians who believe that these symptoms may be present but not in the form that is readily detectable or verifiable. The following are the DSM-III-R criteria for schizophrenic disorder:

Diagnostic Criteria for Schizophrenia

A. *Presence of characteristic psychotic symptoms in the active phase: either (1), (2), or (3) for at least one week (unless the symptoms are successfully treated):*
   (1) two of the following:
      (a) delusions;
      (b) prominent hallucinations (throughout the day for several days or several times a week for several weeks, each hallucinatory experience not being limited to a few brief moments);
      (c) incoherence or marked loosening of associations;

(d) *catatonic behavior;*

(e) *flat or grossly inappropriate affect.*

(2) *bizarre delusions (i.e., involving a phenomenon that the person's culture would regard as totally implausible, e.g., thought broadcasting, being controlled by a dead person);*

(3) *prominent hallucinations of a voice [as defined in (1)(b) above] with content having no apparent relation to depression or elation, or a voice keeping up a running commentary on the person's behavior or thoughts, or two or more voices conversing with each other.*

B. *During the course of the disturbance, functioning in such areas as work, social relations, and self-care is markedly below the highest level achieved before onset of the disturbance (or, when the onset is in childhood or adolescence, failure to achieve expected level of social development).*

C. *Schizoaffective Disorder and Mood Disorder with Psychotic Features have been ruled out, i.e., if a Major Depressive or Manic Syndrome has ever been present during an active phase of the disturbance, the total duration of all episodes of a mood syndrome has been brief relative to the total duration of the active and residual phases of the disturbance.*

D. *Continuous signs of the disturbance for at least six months. The six-month period must include an active phase (of at least one week, or less if symptoms have been successfully treated) during which there were psychotic symptoms characteristic of Schizophrenia (symptoms in A), with or without a prodromal or residual phase, as defined below.*

   Prodromal phase: A clear deterioration in functioning before the active phase of the disturbance that is not due to a disturbance in mood or to a Psychoactive Substance Use Disorder and that involves at least two of the symptoms listed below.

   Residual phase: Following the active phase of the disturbance, persistence of at least two of the symptoms noted below, these not being due to a disturbance in mood or to a Psychactive Substance Use Disorder.

   Prodromal or residual symptoms:

(1) *marked social isolation or withdrawal;*

(2) *marked impairment in role functioning as wage-earner, student, or homemaker;*

(3) *markedly peculiar behavior (e.g., collecting garbage, talking to self in public, hoarding food);*

(4) *marked impairment in personal hygiene and grooming;*

(5) *blunted or inappropriate affect;*

(6) *digressive, vague, overelaborate, or circumstantial speech, or poverty of speech, or poverty of content of speech;*

(7) *odd beliefs or magical thinking, influencing behavior and inconsistent with cultural norms, e.g., superstitiousness, belief in clairvoyance, telepathy, "sixth sense," "others can feel my feelings," overvalued ideas, ideas of reference;*

(8) *unusual perceptual experiences, e.g., recurrent illusions, sensing the presence of a force or person not actually present;*

(9) *marked lack of initiative, interests, or energy.*

   Examples: Six months of prodromal symptoms with one week of symptoms from A; no prodromal symptoms with six months of symptoms from A; no prodromal symptoms with one week of symptoms from A and six months of residual symptoms.

E. *It cannot be established that an organic factor initiated and maintained the distur-*
   bance.

F. *If there is a history of Autistic Disorder, the additional diagnosis of Schizophrenia is*
   made only if prominent delusions or hallucinations are also present. (DSM-III-R, pp.
   194–195)

It seems clear that the differential diagnosis of autism and PDDNOS
from schizophrenia hinges on the determination of presence or absence of delusions, hallucinations, or marked loosening of associations.
Symptoms of thought disorder apparent in organic mental disorders
are extremely random and haphazard, without evidence of systematization—the point of departure from schizophrenia.

There has been criticism from several quarters that standard diagnostic practices have ignored childhood schizophrenia, not only in terms
of its existence but in terms of a fine delineation of its differences from
and similarities to adult schizophrenia. Only in the last few years has
there been some investigation of these issues.

There is no doubt that schizophrenia in childhood, to the extent that
it is recognized as such, arises most often after 5 years of age. Beyond
the question of whether schizophrenia can ever arise in infancy, there
is still the unresolved question of whether or not conditions originating
before the age of 3 that are classified as autism or psychosis are simply
the early manifestations of childhood schizophrenia, which becomes
full blown later when characteristic symptoms such as thought disorder,
loosening of associations, hallucinations, and so forth develop and are
detectable. (Clearly, few reliable clinical measures exist for thought disorders at the preverbal level.) While the evidence has been mixed, a
handful of prospective studies have shown that a small subset of children designated autistic in early childhood does go on to develop
schizophrenia in later childhood, adolescence, or adulthood (Bender &
Faetra, 1972; Brown, 1963, 1969; Dahl, 1976; Reiser & Brown, 1964).

On the other hand, in her longitudinal study of the development of
schizophrenia, Fish (1987) found no cases of autism in any of the children considered at risk due to having severely schizophrenic mothers.
However, schizotypal symptoms did appear in a number of the at-risk
children. While this study only encompassed 12 experimental and 12
control individuals, its longitudinal span (35 years) was extensive and
the trends revealed are instructive. In five of the risk subjects, a drop in
the Weschler Comprehension Subtest score of 2 to 7 points was noticed
between 10 and 15 years of age, and this was correlated with the author's
nonblind evaluation of an increase in schizotypal behavior. Of these
five children, two were hallucinating at 14 to 15 years. Two others began
to show withdrawal and acting-out behavior at 13 years, and one, at age

15, blocked so completely that the TAT (Thematic Apperception Test) had to be terminated.

Fish found that three of the infants who were later to develop psychiatric disorders exhibited an abnormally quiet state in the first month of life. This included a distinctive depression of arousal limited to gross motor, proprioceptive, and vestibular responses. This condition appeared to be related to their later affective blunting. Fish noted that this general dysfunction may not prove to be specific for schizotypal infants. However, she speculated that intervention to reduce early impairments should improve the quality of subsequent premorbid adaptation. In terms of development, Fish's experience with the six children who were most affected by schizotypal symptoms convinced her that once a child is 3 to 6 years of age, the chances of preventing cognitive and social-affective impairment are nearly nonexistent, at least in the case of some genetically vulnerable children.

This issue of familial contributions to schizophrenia is important, not only in terms of etiology but for purposes of diagnosis and nosology as well. In a recent and comprehensive review of the literature that was integrated with the results of two new family studies and one twin study, Kendler, Tsuang, and Hays (1987) found there was no strong or consistent relationship between age at onset of schizophrenia and the risk of recurrence for schizophrenia in relatives. The age at onset of schizophrenia was modestly correlated between pairs of affected siblings and highly correlated between concordant, monozygotic twin pairs.

These results led Kendler and colleagues to conclude that early- and late-onset adult schizophrenia appear to be the same disorder when viewed from a family perspective. Furthermore, in cases where the individual does develop schizophrenia, familial predisposing factors do appear to influence the age of onset of the condition. Thus, it appears that, while family history of schizophrenia is an important piece of diagnostic information, it can hardly be taken as predictive—especially in light of reports such as the one by Ritvo and colleagues (1987) in which one family with four autistic siblings and four families with three autistic siblings are described. It would be valuable indeed to discover the differences between these genetically vulnerable autistic children and those who are vulnerable to schizophrenia due to familial predisposition.

Part of the difficulty in interpreting familial vulnerability to schizophrenia has its roots in nosological confusion, as suggested by the results of a study by Burd and Kerbeshian (1987). In attempting to establish prevalence rates for various DSM-III diagnoses throughout North Dakota, they found that among 47 children between the ages of 2 and 12 years with an early history of DSM-III ODD, none met DSM-III criteria for schizophrenia. The authors concluded that either the diagnostic criteria applied to this age group had little validity or schizophrenia in childhood is far rarer than autism or PDD. In the face of the foregoing discussion, it seems that, while the DSM-III-R technique of segregating autism and PDDNOS from each other is a step in the right direction, much nosological clarification remains to be done.

In an attempt at such clarification, specifically the delineation of the difference between autism and PDDNOS (or DSM-III childhood-onset PDD and atypical PDD), Burd, Fisher, and Kerbeshian (1987) once again turned to the childhood population of North Dakota. At the time of the study, there were 180,986 children in the state between the ages of 2 and 18. More than 200 of these children and adolescents were evaluated subsequent to reports by relevant health personnel that they had autistic symptoms.

After evaluation, 21 cases of autism were diagnosed, along with 36 cases of atypical PDD and 2 of childhood-onset PDD. The preponderance of atypical PDD cases was dictated by the DSM-III requirement of onset after 30 months. The prevalence for infantile autism was 1.16 per 10,000, and for both PDDs (presumably the DSM-III-R PDDNOS) it was 1.99. Thus, the DSM-III-R separation of autism and PDDNOS, subsequent to the elimination of the age-at-onset requirement, seems appropriate, both in light of the genetic evidence regarding the variability of the age-at-onset criterion and because two discrete populations do seem to exist without this requirement. Volkmar, Stier, and Cohen (1985) suggested that it may be more appropriate and diagnostically useful to use the term *age of recognition* rather than *age at onset*, since symptoms almost invariably exist some time prior to psychiatric evaluation.

Debby: Willing But Unable

Debby is a 3-year-old girl who lives with her mother, her father, and her two older sisters. Debby's father is an attorney, and her mother is an architect who returned to work when Debby began nursery school a few months ago, after an 8-year break during which she stayed home to rear her daughters. Debby's parents and her sisters describe her as a very happy, good-natured child. Debby feeds and dresses herself, but she is not toilet-trained. Debby began talking at around 14 months of age; however, her vocabulary has not developed significantly, and her speech is limited to one- or two-word phrases. Debby's parents were concerned about this failure of language to increase, and they sought assessment when her nursery school teacher expressed similar concerns.

In addition to concerns about Debby's limited speech, her teacher noted that Debby's attention span is extremely short. During school activities, Debby sometimes hits other students for no apparent reason, with no evidence of anger or other precipitating cause for her aggression. She also latches on to other students or to the teacher during games and seems unable to function alone. Debby has trouble understanding instructions and learning new concepts. The teacher recommended assessment when Debby recently spent much of a school day biting her own arm.

During the assessment interview, Debby separated from her parents easily. She was found to be an unusually attractive girl, dressed in age- and gender-appropriate clothing. Speech articulation was slightly slurred, and expressive language consisted of infrequent one- and two-word phrases. Debby's motor coordination was limited, assessed to be of a developmental level of 22 months. Cognitive ability was judged to be at about the 21-month level. Debby's attention span was extremely short, and she was highly distractible during the entire evaluation process. She indicated interest in other people and communicated with other children in a play group. Overall, Debby was assessed to be operating at a developmental level of about 20 to 22 months. A physical examination yielded that she was in good general health, and no organic factors that could be causing her symptoms were found.

The pervasive delays in Debby's development, as opposed to specific difficulties with speech or motor coordination, indicate that she suffers either from mental retardation or from a pervasive developmental disorder such as autistic disorder. Debby's interest in others and her impatient attempts to communicate, however, suggest that she is not harboring the deficits in reciprocal social interaction that would support a diagnosis of autistic disorder. Reports of other characteristic symptoms of autism such as abnormalities in sleeping and eating and so forth are also absent. Tests indicate that, cognitively, Debby is functioning at a developmental level appropriate to someone 14 months younger than she. The nature of her clinical presentation is that she is at an earlier developmental stage than would be expected for her age. This is characteristic of individuals with mental retardation. Individuals with pervasive developmental disorders, on the other hand, do not behave as though they were passing through any normal or average developmental stage; their symptoms indicate departures from normal—or even merely slowed—socioemotional development.

Thus, a diagnosis of mental retardation was tentatively made pending further testing to rule out borderline intellectual functioning. Tests to determine whether Debby has borderline intellectual functioning, (IQ 71–84), or mental retardation, (IQ below 70) will be done when Debby reaches a developmental stage at which IQ testing is possible. Recommendation was made for periodic assessment and for placement in an early intervention preschool program.

Autism Versus Mental Retardation

According to DSM-III-R, the essential features of mental retardation are (1) significantly subaverage general intellectual functioning, accompanied by (2) deficits or impairments in adaptive functioning, with (3) onset before age 18. The diagnosis is made regardless of whether or not there is a coexisting physical or other mental disorder. The DSM-III-R codes for mental retardation are as follows: (1) mild (IQ 50–55 to approximately 70); (2) moderate (IQ 35–40 to 50–55); (3) severe (IQ 20–25 to 35–40); and (4) profound (IQ below 20–25).

Autism/PDDNOS often coexists with mental retardation, but, as can be seen with Debby, those who are mentally retarded clearly differ from those with autism due to their sociability and ability to communicate (even if nonverbally). Differential diagnosis is most difficult in cases of profound mental retardation. In general, a singular diagnosis of mental retardation is appropriate either when there are no other behavioral symptoms or when the behavioral symptoms present do not match the essentials of the clinical picture of infantile autism or PDDNOS.

It is often justified to diagnose autistic children as also mentally retarded when they have an IQ below 70. It is reported that 40% of all autistic children have IQ scores lower than 50 (Rapoport & Ismond, 1984), whereas approximately 25% of autistic children have IQ's in the normal range. The basic features of mental retardation, in addition to having an IQ below 70, include impaired adaptive behavior and onset before age 18 (later onset is considered justification for a diagnosis of dementia). In distinguishing mentally retarded individuals from those with PDD or PDD/mental retardation, it is important to determine whether development, while lagging far behind age expectations, nevertheless proceeds in stages despite its slower than normal rate. For children with PDD's—with or without mental retardation—there is little regularity to the staging of intellectual and social development.

The IQ scores of autistic children should have the same implications as for other children. One special consideration is that very low IQ scores are associated with increased risk of epileptic seizures during adolescence (Rutter, 1982). A number of investigators have theorized that among autistic children who are also mentally retarded a form of organic brain damage is responsible for both the social impairments and the arrestment of intelligence and that region(s) of the brain responsible for social interaction, symbolic imagination, and certain cognitive skills are affected (Wing & Gould, 1979). This is supported by the belief that in children with multiple diagnoses the autism and mental retardation form part of the same disorder (Rutter, 1982).

Wing and Gould (1979) developed a rating system of behavioral variables designed to determine degree and quality of social impairments among children with social, emotional, and intellectual abnormalities. They applied their criteria to a group of 132 selected children under age 15 from a working-class section of southeast London. Rigorous application of structured interviews with the disturbed children resulted in a determination that 58 of them displayed social interaction that was appropriate for their mental age. They used the term *sociable, severely retarded* to classify this group—a useful way to denote mental retardation without autism or PDDNOS, and a means of indicating the social potential of mentally retarded individuals.

Autism Versus Specific Developmental Disorders

DSM-III-R discusses difficulties in academic performance, language and speech problems, and impairment or deficit in motor skills under the category of specific developmental disorders. The inadequate development of specific academic, language, speech, and motor skills under this heading must not be due to demonstrable physical or neurologic disorders, a PDD, mental retardation, or deficient educational opportunities. All of the specific developmental disorders are associated with impairment in academic functioning in children who are in school. The impairment is most pronounced when language is affected. If the child is not in school, there is impairment in daily living activities.

Fundamentally, the pervasive developmental disorders can be differentiated from the specific developmental disorders by means of the sociability factor. Disorders involving only sensory and perceptual impairment can be differentiated from PDD's not only by the presence of social interaction but also by the desire for communication appropriate to the child's mental age.

Autism Versus Reactive Attachment Disorder of Infancy and Childhood

The symptoms of reactive attachment disorder can easily be mistaken for autism unless the etiology of the symptoms is closely scrutinized. As in the case of autism, children with this disorder exhibit a markedly disturbed social relatedness in most contexts beginning before age 5.

The symptoms of reactive attachment disorder can either take the form of autistic-like characteristics such as a persistent failure to initiate or respond in an age-expected manner to most social interactions or (in an older child) there may be indiscriminate sociability such as excessive familiarity with relative strangers.

The DSM-III-R criteria for reactive attachment disorder of infant or early childhood are as follows:

A. *Markedly disturbed social relatedness in most contexts, beginning before the age of five, as evidenced by either (1) or (2):*
   (1) persistent failure to initiate or respond to most social interactions (e.g., in infants, absence of visual tracking and reciprocal play, lack of vocal

> *imitation or playfulness, apathy, little or no spontaneity; at later ages, lack of or little curiosity and social interest)*
>
> (2) *indiscriminate sociability, e.g., excessive familiarity with relative strangers by making requests and displaying affection*
>
> B. *The disturbance in A is not a symptom of either Mental Retardation or a Pervasive Developmental Disorder, such as Autistic Disorder.*
>
> C. *Grossly pathogenic care, as evidenced by at least one of the following:*
>
> (1) *persistent disregard of the child's basic emotional needs for comfort, stimulation, and affection.* Examples: *overly harsh punishment by caregiver; consistent neglect by caregiver*
>
> (2) *persistent disregard of the child's basic physical needs, including nutrition, adequate housing, and protection from physical danger and assault (including sexual abuse)*
>
> (3) *repeated change of primary caregiver so that stable attachments are not possible, e.g., frequent changes in foster parents*
>
> D. *There is a presumption that the care described in C is responsible for the disturbed behavior in A; this presumption is warranted if the disturbance in A began following the pathogenic care in C.* (DSM-III-R, p. 93)

As stated previously, a critical difference beteen reactive attachment disorder and PDD is its direct attributability to inadequate caretaking (Rapoport & Ismond, 1984). The condition can be improved by enhancing caretaking by such means as providing a proper and nurturing environment. Following this measure, affectionate bonding will usually develop and the symptoms partially or totally remit.

A favorable response to treatment is considered by some to confirm the diagnosis of reactive attachment disorder, but others claim that this is an improper retrospective form of differential diagnosis (Rapoport & Ismond, 1984; Rutter & Shaffer, 1980). Regardless of this issue, the early onset of symptoms and social withdrawal exhibited by those with reactive attachment disorder, while they do resemble the characteristics of autism, are only some of the specifics of reactive attachment. The others, as listed, can be used to achieve differential diagnosis.

CONCLUSION

Much of the future understanding of childhood psychoses will depend on a clearer understanding of infantile autism. Is autism caused by genetic make-up? Is it the result of a traumatizing environment? Or, as seems most likely, is it the result of a combination of both temperament and environment to one degree or another (Trad, 1986)? Another question that must be definitively answered is whether or not autism should be classified under childhood schizophrenia.

With regard to the first issue, Tinbergen and Tinbergen (1972; Tinbergen, 1974) posited a scheme in which nature and nurture interact to produce autistic behavior. As the Tinbergens viewed it, autism is predominantly an emotional disorder—an anxiety neurosis—that is produced when children with an inherently timid temperament are exposed to an increasingly crowded and stressful world (and are being raised by parents who must also contend with that world). The anxiety, which could start well before verbal communication develops, prevents or slows the formation of bonds between infant and parent and child and peers. Socialization is thus impaired, and this impedes the development of speech and other learning processes.

If this explanation of autism is accepted for the sake of argument, the children for whom the DSM-III-R diagnosis of PDDNOS is applicable might be those for whom the anxiety is not quite so profound as in the case of full-blown autism. If the attendant anxietal state is not completely paralyzing, the signal function of anxiety may eventually develop, at least to some degree, allowing these children to learn, grow, and change. Alternatively, a child with this lesser, but still severe, degree of inherent anxiety or fearfulness might exhibit the full autistic symptomatology if reared in an abusive or emotionally impoverished environment.

Another interesting notion of how autism might develop has been reported by Bemporad, Ratey, and O'Driscoll (1987). Drawing on the work by Buck (1984) regarding the communicative function of emotion, Bemporad and co-workers proposed that autism develops as a result of an inability to perceive the emotional state of others through facial expressions and body language. The lack of ability to perceive the caretaker's nonverbal signals could easily produce the eventual lack of eye contact noted in autistic children. Since there is no information in the caretaker's facial expression, there is little motivation to watch the face.

The innate inability to understand facial expressions and gestures could putatively result in arousal and frustration in a way analogous to that which occurs in aphasic children in response to language. Thus, Bemporad's construct provides an etiological framework in which symptoms of autism may be seen to arise as the result of the innate deficit, defenses that develop in response to the negative effects of the deficit, and impoverished social experiences arising from the deficit and defenses alike.

Regardless of etiology, research directed at answering the question of whether or not autism is a form of schizophrenia seems to be accumulating evidence in favor of separating the two—this in spite of the fact that overt signs of psychosis such as hallucinations are not always specific to schizophrenia (Asaad & Shapiro, 1986). However, in order to further define the autistic condition, more study is needed of the nature of the social deficits accompanying this disorder.

Sigman, Mundy, Sherman, and Ungerer (1986) have taken a step in this direction by demonstrating that the most salient feature of the social behavior of autistic children appears to be their infrequent sharing of attention with their caregivers. While this is of great value in differentiating autism from mental retardation, its applicability to differentiating schizophrenia from autism is less clear. Therefore, it might be beneficial to study the specifics of social interaction in children diagnosed as schizophrenic more closely, since comparisons of these behaviors might provide further grounds for differentiating this condition from autism.

CHAPTER TEN

Developmental Learning Disorders and Their Differential Diagnosis

Steve: The Pain of Learning to Learn

Steve is a 5-year-old boy who lives with his mother, his older brother, and his younger sister. Although his parents are separated, his father lives in the same apartment building. The father frequently visits the mother in their apartment at night. Steve's mother describes him as a happy child, and has no memory of developmental abnormalities. She reports no temper tantrums, and she has remarked that Steve can spend very long periods of time at solitary play or singing and dancing. In nursery school, Steve is described as having both a hard time focusing on specific tasks and a short attention span. When faced with frustration or denial, he becomes angry and violent toward others. Steve was referred for assessment because of these difficulties and because of speech deficits.

During assessment, Steve was well-behaved and, at first, rather shy. His speech was difficult to understand because of poor articulation and because it was delivered in almost a whisper at times. Speech evaluation indicated expressive language difficulties, including a problem with the concepts of *between, after,* and *before* and pronominal reversal. His play was normal, and no indication of psychoses was encountered. He seemed intelligent, and his cognitive capabilities appeared intact. Steve could copy shapes and follow directions in an age-appropriate manner without difficulty. Intelligence testing revealed normal intelligence, and the elements of the mental status examination were developmentally appropriate.

Steve's difficulty with language construction and speech articulation indicated two possible diagnoses, developmental expressive language disorder and developmental articulation disorder. Further testing was done to assess these diagnostic categories. Hearing tests revealed auditory discrimination difficulties, which might be judged the cause of his articulation and language difficulties. No other physical abnormalities were found, and Steve's IQ score disqualified a possible diagnosis of mental retardation. Symptoms of pervasive developmental disorder, such as pervasive behavioral abnormalities (Steve's are limited to situations in which he is frustrated or angry) and a restricted repertoire of interests and activities, were not documented. No injury has been recalled that coincided with the onset of problems, and Steve does not have episodes of elective mutism.

Thus, Steve's clinical picture is indicative of speech delays and learning disabilities that may be caused by his auditory discrimination deficits. Behavioral problems such as his angry outbursts when he must repeat himself to be understood are not unusual within the context of specific developmental disorders. A comprehensive speech, hearing, and language evaluation was recommended before a treatment would be formulated.

INTRODUCTION

The diagnosis and treatment of learning disorders is widely recognized as one of the most important goals of pediatric medicine. However, as in all areas of mental dysfunction, definitional issues complicate both diagnosis and treatment. This is acknowledged in DSM-III-R, which admits that the inclusion of categories of learning impairment in a classification of mental disorders is somewhat questionable since some learning impaired individuals experience no other signs of psychopathology. This is suggested by the slowly emerging results of prospective studies such as that by Spreen (1981), who found that the presence of learning disability did not produce an increased likelihood of encounters with police or a greater-than-average number of antisocial incidences. Steve seems to be a good candidate for a positive outcome in this regard if he is given early assistance in his learning attempts.

By definition, half the students in any school system perform at below-average levels. Helveston (1986) has estimated that 20% of these students (10% of the general school population) operate well below the expectations of their families and that an unspecified fraction of these conceivably fit into the category of learning disabled. In providing some idea of the size of the problem, Gearhart and Weishahn (1976) have estimated that 3.5 to 5% of the school population have speech or language disorders, 2.5 to 3% are mentally retarded, and 2.4% have other learning disabilities.

Thus, excluding the mentally retarded, 6 to 10% of school children may be learning disabled. This relatively high prevalence of learning difficulties in the general population has prompted many independent and government-sponsored investigations that have given rise to numerous measurement scales attempting to detect the deficits present in learning ability. However, as the categories chosen by Gearhart and Weishahn illustrate, it is difficult to isolate specific etiologies for areas of dysfunction in learning ability, and, as Lotstein (1984) has pointed out, a given individual may well have more than one problem area. Furthermore, learning problems can appear without significant behavioral, social, or motor problems, or one or more of these can accompany the impairment (Culbertson & Ferry, 1982).

Given these many possibilities, diagnosis must first be guided by the realization that there is no single standard classification fitting every child. The heterogeneity of learning disorders dictates that a given child be recognized as having a wide range of learning skills, more than one of which can be impaired at some point in time. Learning problems can occur in a single area, such as dyscalculia, or several functions can be affected, such as language, spelling, and reading.

Since the possible areas and combinations of areas in which learning problems can occur are so numerous, it is appropriate to attempt to detect a learning deficit before postulating a psychosocial cause for poor performance. Children who have difficulty learning are prone to feelings of shame and inadequacy and are likely to experience an increasing sense of frustration and humiliation as failure continues from year to year. If the learning disability is not detected early enough, these feelings may erupt into intractable adjustment problems and mood disturbances—an outcome clearly demonstrated in a study by Berman and Siegal (1976).

These researchers studied 45 boys from 15 to 18 years of age, who resided in a correctional facility for delinquents. While a matched control group demonstrated few if any learning deficits, 70% of the delinquents were found to have measurable learning disorders. Even though it is not possible to determine the degree to which the learning deficit factor resulted in incarceration, there is little doubt that it had a significant contributory role.

Compounding the importance of early intervention is the fact that treatment for these disorders in adulthood usually meets with poor outcome, due in part to the effects of repeated academic failure. Futhermore, because human and animal studies suggest that the nervous system is more malleable and open to change during the period of maturation when behavior is less differentiated (Caldwell, 1968), early recognition and treatment appear to be crucial.

Once it is determined that learning impairment is not secondary to emotional disturbance, the clinician must look for other possible primary causes such as neurological or physical disorders, mental retardation, pervasive developmental disorders, or inadequate schooling. This topic will be explored more fully in the remainder of this chapter. For the moment, it is sufficient to say that batteries of tests exist that are directed at detecting the presence of mental retardation and that attempt to screen for the specific area or areas of disturbance (e.g., language disorder of an expressive or receptive nature). Unfortunately, the validity of some of these tests remains questionable (Lawson & Inglis, 1985; Lindquist, 1982).

The third, and very difficult, diagnostic step is to determine whether the primary learning deficit exists in isolation or is accompanied by one or more disorders of learning, development, behavior, or mood. The DSM-III-R correctly points out that a learning disorder does not, a priori, preclude the existence of other conditions such as mental retardation, inadequate schooling, pervasive developmental disorder, and so forth.

In order to fulfill this requirement of the diagnostician's task, it is useful to refer to the theoretical analysis of Lotstein (1984) regarding the hypothetical models of Satz and Fletcher (1981). Both Lotstein and Satz and Fletcher recognized the importance of the developmental context in assessing learning disabilities. "Because interpretations of performance differences between disabled and nondisabled learners form the inferential basis for these theories (of the cognitive and cerebral organization of disabled learners), the developmental context becomes crucial" (Lotstein, 1984, p. 64).

Beyond the importance of the developmental context, these investigators recognized the confusion regarding the operational definition of the constructs commonly used to describe the performance patterns of children with learning impairment. Such terms as *deficit, lag, delay,* and *rate* are used throughout the literature on learning disorders with little attention being paid to standardization or consistency.

This situation prompted Satz and Fletcher (1981) to attempt to better define these crucially important terms within a developmental context. Specifically, they undertook to standardize the use of *lag, deficit, delay,* and *rate* by first postulating that for any behavior there is an initial level—the zero level—where all groups are equal and the behavior is not measurable. Second, they hypothesized that there is a maximum level, or ceiling, where the individual's performance will no longer increase (the 100% level). (It may be useful here to note that the concept of a ceiling to intellectual functioning may prove valuable in conceptualizing and diagnosing mental retardation.)

With these logical postulations in place, Satz and Fletcher proceeded to define *lag* as a difference between two individuals or groups in performance level on a particular behavior at one time in development that diminishes later when the lower-performing individual catches up and attains the 100% level of the higher group.

Accordingly, *deficit* describes the situation in which there is a difference in performance level on a given behavior between two individuals or groups that continues to exist when they are both at their respective 100% levels. In this case, the lower group never catches up and the degree of development is different. This term is meant to be used primarily as a descriptor and thus does not include any of the connotations of abnormal processes with which it has previously been associated.

Delay is present when the point of departure from the zero level of performance occurs later in one group than in the other. In other words, the age of onset is not simultaneous for both groups.

Finally Satz and Fletcher defined *rate* as the case in which, after initial onset, the change in level of performance over time is different for the individuals being compared. Since the differences between the individuals are changing over time, comparisons at the same age will reveal variations in performance-level differences.

Once these terms have been given a consistent interpretation, it is possible to construct five models of primary types of learning dysfunction. In the first, the *lag-rate model*, both individuals achieve the same level of 100% performance, and the onset of the behavior is the same for both as well. However, the learning disabled person or group acquires the behavior at a slower rate. Thus, the person with learning disability catches up with the so-called normal individual, and same-age comparisons during development will show variations in performance-level differences.

The second, or *Type 2 model*, describes the situation in which the onset of the given behavior occurs later in the learning impaired group. However, once the behavior occurs, learning proceeds to the same 100% level at the same rate. Thus, disabled learners would catch up with the controls, and same-age comparisons of performance level differences between the two would not be different over time. In this instance, the impaired learners would acquire the same degree of mastery as the controls, but at a later age.

Type 3 is described as a *deficit-rate model* in which the two individuals or groups experience the same onset of the behavior, but the rate of learning in the disabled group is slower and its final maximum performance is less than the 100% level of the control group. Thus, the disabled learners would not catch up, but same-age comparisons between the two groups would reveal variations in performance-level differences.

The Type 4 model, or *deficit-delay*, describes the situation in which behavioral onset begins later for the learning disabled group. Subsequently, the performance of the behavior proceeds at a rate similar to that of the control group but reaches a lower final maximum level. In this case, the lower group would never catch up and the same-age comparisons would show no variations in performance-level differences.

The fifth model of primary deficit, Type 5, is termed *deficit-unexpected*. In this case, the two groups experience the same onset of the behavior and also share the same rate of acquisition until, at some point in development, the behavior is suddenly arrested in one group. This may be caused by a random event such as brain damage.

While the foregoing five types of learning disorders describe a system whereby learning impairment might be categorized, Satz and Fletcher pointed out that many other combinations might occur. These "hybrids" can be generated by combining additional delay or rate factors with the five primary types. As an example, there might be another lag model in which the manifest onset occurs later in the learning impaired group but, once it appears, proceeds to the same 100% level as the control group at a faster rate. In this case, the model would be classified as a *lag* (main type), *delay* (main mechanism), and *faster rate* (method used to catch up) type. However, both learning disabled and normal children learn in manifold ways, and they might not fit into any of these categories in clinical assessment.

Faced with numerous possibilities, it may be difficult for the clinician not to despair. However, a systematic approach should yield enough information at least to allow initiation of therapy in most cases. The first step should be to check for etiologies of an emotional nature or of inadequate schooling, followed by the elimination of organic causes, mental retardation, or other developmental disorders such as autism.

Next, the primary learning deficit should be identified through interviews with teachers and parents and diagnostic testing of the child. Once therapy is initiated based on the primary learning disorder, it is possible to monitor progress and test for possible secondary or concomitant learning deficits.

Toward an Integrated View of Learning Disorders

The work of Satz and Fletcher is helpful in that it helps the clinician keep in mind the heterogeneity of learning disorders and the many possible combinations of deficits that can exist in a given case. However, their scheme does little to explain the underlying etiologies of learning impairment. When the question of etiology is raised, answers invariably are couched within the particular research approach of the investigator. There are, for example, brain process models, neurological models, and genetic schemata, as well as etiologic paradigms based on developmental trends, test classifications, and co-morbidity profiles.

Johnson and Myklebust (1967) have proposed a process model of learning disorders in which children are viewed as having a psychoneurological learning disability. Thus, learning problems result not from a generalized incapacity to learn but from disturbances in behavior resulting from brain dysfunction. This fits well with the neurological model proposed by Shapiro, Palmer, Watchel, and Caputo (1983) in which it is hypothesized that early maturational delays in neural development might be the underpinnings of specific learning disorders. If this is the case, the mechanisms underlying these delays could be predictors of learning problems.

However, results of research into the feasibility of identifying predictors have not been promising. Prospective studies have largely failed in their attempts to isolate predictors. For example, Spreen (1981) followed up 203 adolescents and young adults who had been referred to a neuropsychiatric clinic between the ages of 8 and 12 due to learning difficulties. These individuals and 52 matched control subjects were evaluated in terms of offenses, encounters with police, and penalties received from social enforcing agencies. It was found that the presence of a learning disorder failed to indicate an increased likelihood of police encounters or a greater number of offenses.

The inability to find predictors with regard to learning disorders extends even to adult populations who had learning problems as children. Watson, Watson, and Fredd (1982) reviewed follow-up studies of children and adolescents with specific reading disabilities and found that test results of these children failed to predict reading outcome 4 to 5 years later. These investigators concluded that current research is inadequate to the task of predicting the reading skills of adults who were identified as reading disabled during their school years.

Much the same conclusion was reached by Horn, O'Donnell, & Vitulano (1983) in their extensive review of the prospective literature on learning disabilities. Reviewing literature published after 1960 that dealt with long-term outcomes of learning disabled persons, these investigators found a variety of conflicting results, many of which were attributable to the variety of variables used to assess outcome. If test functioning was used as the most important indicator of outcome, learning impaired people appeared to experience lasting deficits. However, if measures of educational and vocational attainment levels were taken as a powerful indicator of progress, people with learning problems did not appear to have an especially poor prognosis. In this review, as in those by Spreen and Watson and co-workers, no reliable predictors of learning problems emerged.

Given the lack of success in finding behavior and/or test predictors of learning disabilities (LD), the goal of finding and defining underlying neural mechanisms seems distant indeed. It is hardly feasible to isolate an underlying mechanism for LD in the absence of predictors.

While attempts at explaining the etiologies of LD by neurological means have been largely unsuccessful, attempts to arrive at etiological explanations via other routes have not been especially helpful either. Hartzell and Compton (1984) and others (e.g., Baker & Cantwell, 1987a,b; Beitchman, Nair, Clegg, Ferguson, & Patel, 1986; Cantwell & Baker, 1980; Munir, Biederman, & Knee, 1987) have performed assessments of co-morbidity variables in an attempt to discover patterns of association between LD and other psychological and physiological conditions that might provide some clues about the genesis of learning problems.

Grounds for this approach come from the widely reported association between learning difficulties and other debilitating conditions including psychiatric disorders. The extent of this association is indicated by studies performed by Baker and Cantwell, who demonstrated that approximately one-half of children presenting for first evaluations to a community speech clinic had at least one psychiatric disorder (e.g., Baker & Cantwell, 1987a).

As examples of some of the associations between LD and other conditions, Munir and colleagues (1987) studied 22 children with attention deficit disorder and compared them to 20 normal control subjects. ADD patients were found to have significantly increased rates of learning disorders as well as higher incidences of conduct disorder, oppositional disorder, major affective disorder, non-Tourette tics, and encopresis.

In terms of psychiatric co-morbidity, Beitchman and colleagues (1986) studied a representative sample of 5-year-old kindergarten children who were assessed for speech and language disorders and found three significant differences between controls and children diagnosed as having a learning problem. The children with speech/language impairment (1) showed behavioral disturbances according to teachers and a parent; (2) were diagnosed as having some DSM-III Axis I disorder, especially attention deficit disorder; and (3) suffered from psychosocial stressors.

The importance of the association between LD and psychiatric disorder is demonstrated in a study by Baker and Cantwell (1987a), who followed up 300 communication impaired children who had been evaluated 5 years before. These investigators found that, while there were improvements in some areas, there was a significant increase not only in psychiatric disorders but also in developmental disorders and disorders of language usage and processing. Superficially, at least, these data lend further support to the importance of early intervention and treatment of learning disabilities. However, it is still not known conclusively that learning problems lead to psychiatric difficulty. The reverse may be true; psychiatric disorder may produce learning deficits.

Baker and Cantwell sought to solve at least this small part of the puzzle in another study (1987b). The backgrounds and developmental and psychosocial aspects of children with different types of psychiatric disorders and associated speech or language disorders were examined. Four groups were isolated for study: (1) psychiatrically well children ($n = 298$); (2) a behaviorally disordered group ($n = 142$); (3) an emotionally disordered group ($n = 92$); and (4) a mixed group having both an emotional and a behavioral disorder ($n = 11$).

After comparison of these groups for a number of variables, Baker and Cantwell concluded that the most likely sequence of events is the one in which psychiatric disorder is indirectly produced by the communication disorder. In nearly every case the communication problem set in before the psychiatric disorder. Also, there was a very low prevalence of psychiatric conditions having a communication problem as a core part of the symptomatology (e.g., elective mutism or pervasive developmental disorder). While these findings regarding the direction of the interaction between learning problems and psychiatric conditions are certainly helpful, they represent only the beginning of the search for an etiological explanation of learning disorders by assessment of co-morbidity patterns.

The co-morbidity model, along with schemes based on brain processes, neurological events, developmental trends, and genetic and test score assessment, provides only an incomplete picture of possible etiologies for learning disorders. The disagreement about how to understand the origins of LD clearly stems from the particular approaches of the researchers involved. Unfortunately, it is not yet possible to construct a unitary model at this point.

George: Multiple Problems

George was a muscular, 4-year, 10-month-old black boy who appeared older than his age. At the time of referral, his general behavior seemed to be governed by hyperactivity, poor impulse control, aggressiveness, and lability of mood. George attained a verbal IQ of 90 (average), a prorated performance IQ of 104 (average), and a full-scale IQ of 96 (average). Eye-hand coordination and color matching were average (animal house), while perceptual and visual-motor organization (geometric design), visual planning ability and problem solving (mazes), and visual acuity (picture arrangement) fell within the bright normal range.

George was referred by the therapeutic nursery he had been attending because of aggressive, overtly assaultive behavior. He would attack, unpredictably and without provocation, by kicking, punching, scratching, and spitting at children who even got near him. The incident precipitating referral was an attack in which George attempted to blind another child with a pair of scissors.

At the time of referral, George was living in a run-down apartment house, eating and sleeping in the same room with his mother, two siblings, and a father who had been unemployed for the past year and a half. The father, a heavy drinker and suspected IV drug user, would often come home late at night, wake up the mother to demand sex, and beat her in front of the children when she refused.

When George was able to persist in working at a task, he took great pleasure in his accomplishment. However, he was easily frustrated and quickly became oppositional. He frequently became angry and explosive when requested to comply with rules. The frequency of incidences of frustration was increased by the fact that he often had to repeat himself to be understood. He had mild auditory discrimination difficulties and a speech articulation disorder in which he exhibited pronominal reversal, reversing the usage of "me" and "I." He also showed difficulty in discriminating between the concepts of *between, after,* and *before.*

While his fantasies during play situations did not contain any bizarre or psychotic content, his behavior appeared to be governed by the fact that he perceived aggression as the only mode of expressing his feelings—probably due in large part to having seen his father behave in this way.

Accordingly, George was diagnosed (with DSM-III criteria then in use) as having conduct disorder, undersocialized, aggressive. On Axis II, he was classified as mixed specific developmental disorder. Attention deficit disorder with hyperactivity was ruled out, as was dysthymic disorder.

George illustrates the heterogeneity encountered in children with learning disabilities. Clearly, all facets of the situation must be taken into account—social and environmental, as well as developmental and specific functional deficits. In this case, the prognosis was relatively poor, less because of any learning disability than because of protracted exposure to violence and lack of structure in his life.

DIFFERENTIAL DIAGNOSIS OF LEARNING DISORDERS

Broad Classification of Learning Dysfunctions

While Satz and Fletcher (1981) have presented five theoretical schemes to conceptualize levels of learning sequences, Culbertson and Ferry (1982) have adopted a somewhat broader approach in their descriptions. However, it is interesting that both systems are comprised of five categories of impairment that may encompass inhibited information processing.

The five categories adopted by Culbertson and Ferry are (1) disorders of verbal and nonverbal learning; (2) disorders of input and output; (3) disorders of perception and perceptual-motor learning; (4) disorders of memory; and (5) disorders of thinking. It seems likely that verbal disorders have the highest potential for limiting learning ability. Inability to read and speak language undercuts the potential for learning across the spectrum. However, nonverbal impairments such as an inability to maintain time or spatial orientation, or confusion between left and right, will also significantly hinder learning.

The inability to receive input from the environment or express information is also damaging. Input disorders can negatively affect such things as vocabulary recognition, discrimination between similar characters or phonemes, and the ability to discriminate one voice (the teacher's) from among many. Difficulties with output generate problems with speaking, writing, and the performance of coordinated motor activities.

The detection of disorders of perception and perceptual-motor learning are especially crucial for proper treatment. Perception is the manner in which a child understands information received through the senses. Perceptual and perceptual-motor deficits must be distinguished from deficits in visual and auditory acuity, and the perceptual modalities, or combination of modalities, that are strongest or weakest for a given child should be determined through testing.

Memory disorders are a fourth way in which learning can be hindered. Deficits in memory ability frequently emerge in tasks requiring short- or long-term storage, retrieval of previously learned information, or attempts to recall a series of facts in proper order.

Finally, disordered thinking, as illustrated by failure to understand the relationships among objects or concepts or an inability to perceive associations among facts, will also impede learning. These disorders, like verbal disorders, tend to be global in their effects, manifesting themselves in more than one academic area.

The systems of Satz and Fletcher and Culbertson and Ferry may not be parallel or even related. However, it will prove interesting to see whether any of the lag-delay-rate-deficit models of Satz and Fletcher apply specifically to one or more of the learning dysfunction classifications put forth by Culbertson and Ferry.

DSM-III-R Classifications: Specific Developmental Disorders

Perhaps reflecting an effort to increase diagnostic specificity, the DSM-III-R system has opted for an approach to learning disabilities that is more segmented than that of Culbertson and Ferry. The DSM-III-R category of developmental language disorder has been divided into developmental expressive language disorder and developmental receptive language disorder in the model of the aphasias. A new category, developmental expressive writing disorder, has been added. In general, however, all of the specific developmental disorders have the concomitant of impairment in academic functioning in school children. Furthermore, in these classifications, impairment is most marked when language is affected.

Developmental Reading Disorder

Commonly referred to as *dyslexia*, marked impairment in the development of word recognition skills and reading comprehension is the hallmark of this academic skills disorder. With an onset usually from birth but most evident by age 7, it is estimated that 2 to 8% or more of school-age children are afflicted with this condition. Reading comprehension is subnormal and oral reading frequently reveals omissions, distortions, and substitutions of words, as well as slow, halting reading.

Because verbal ability is so central to the acquisition and use of information, children with developmental reading disorder commonly have deficits in expressive language and speech discrimination. If these are severe enough, concomitant diagnoses of developmental expressive or receptive language disorder, and even developmental expressive writing disorder, may be warranted.

The DSM-III-R diagnostic criteria for developmental reading disorder are as follows:

A. *Reading achievement, as measured by a standardized, individually administered test, is markedly below the expected level, given the person's schooling and intellectual capacity (as determined by an individually administered IQ test).*

B. *The disturbance in A significantly interferes with academic achievement or activities of daily living requiring reading skills.*

C. Not due to a defect in visual or hearing acuity or a neurologic disorder.
(p. 44)

Learning to read entails the acquisition of strategies that allow for integrating ever larger patterns of invariance. However, as Satz and Fletcher (1981) pointed out, developmental changes can be observed in the type and size of the attributes being processed. In the beginning, readers pay attention mostly to graphological and phonological attributes of single words. As the process of comprehension evolves, these features recede into the background and irregularities in syntax and vocabulary become the focus of attention. This progression marks the emerging use of different systems for efficiently processing informational units that are larger than a single word. In effect, aberrations or delay in this larger system comprise a clear indication of developmental problems or stagnation.

In making a differential diagnosis based solely on the presenting reading and/or writing impairments, the clinician may find it difficult to determine whether a child has an organic brain problem, is emotionally disturbed, or is suffering from inadequate schooling. However, an intelligence test is central to discovering whether or not the poor performance is directly related to overall reduced ability. In the case of an individual with mild mental retardation who is reading well below the expected level, a concomitant diagnosis of developmental reading disorder should be made, because treatment of the reading disability will greatly improve the child's chances for employment in adulthood.

In addition to mental retardation, it is also vital to test the efficiency of hearing and vision, which, if flawed, could be responsible for the reading deficit. Finally, if inadequate schooling is at the root of subnormal reading levels, the child's history will frequently reveal a number of school changes or absenteeism. If the school itself is at fault, the majority of children in the school are likely to exhibit similar problems.

Developmental Expressive Writing Disorder

This comprises the second of the academic skills disorders subcategory of specific developmental disorders given in DSM-III-R. This is a new entry, not included in DSM-III, which is meant to identify a developmental disturbance in which writing skills are significantly below normal given the child's schooling and intellectual capacity.

Thought to be as prevalent as developmental reading disorder, this condition tends to be associated with a greater number of other disorders, namely, developmental reading disorder, developmental expressive and receptive language disorder, developmental arithmetic disorder, developmental coordination disorder, and disruptive behavior disorders. The disorder is apparent in severe cases by age 7. However, if less severe, the disorder may not be noticed until age 10 or later.

The diagnostic criteria for developmental expressive writing disorder as given in DSM-III-R are as follows:

A. *Writing skills, as measured by a standardized, individually administered test, are markedly below the expected level, given the person's schooling and intellectual capacity (as determined by an individually administered IQ test).*

B. *The disturbance in A significantly interferes with academic achievement or activities of daily living requiring the composition of written texts (spelling words and expressing thoughts in grammatically correct sentences and organized paragraphs).*

C. *Not due to a defect in visual or hearing acuity or a neurologic disorder.* (p. 43)

Differential diagnosis requires screening for a possible primary contribution from mental retardation. In cases where mental retardation is the cause, the difficulty in composing written text is commensurate with the overall performance deficiency.

However, as in the case of developmental reading disorder, when the level of writing is below expectation for a mildly retarded child, the additional diagnosis of developmental writing disorder is made in order to institute correction of the writing disabilities. In addition to tests for mental retardation, audiometric or visual screening tests can be given to rule out sensory impairment, and a history of many school changes will likely accompany the child whose inadequate schooling is primary to the disability.

Developmental Arithmetic Disorder

The third, and final, academic skills disorder in DSM-III-R is developmental arithmetic disorder. This condition, believed to be somewhat less prevalent than developmental reading disorder, is intended to describe a significant impairment in the evolution of arithmetic skills which, like the other academic skills disorders, cannot be attributed to mental retardation, sensory defects, or inadequate schooling.

With an age of onset as early as 6 years, there are a number of functions that, when impaired, contribute to the failure to attain age-appropriate levels of arithmetic skill. Among these are (1) linguistic skills in which the individual may not be able to comprehend the naming of mathematical operations or terms; (2) perceptual skills in which the ability to recognize numerical symbols or to cluster objects sharing a common trait into groups is impaired; (3) attention skills in which the individual may fail to copy figures correctly or observe operational signs or add in carried numbers; and (4) mathematical skills in which there is a deficit in the ability to count objects, follow the sequences of mathematical steps, or learn the multiplication tables.

Not surprisingly, there are a large number of conditions that are potentially related to this disorder, all of which can contribute to the severity and type of mathematical impairment. The associated features listed by DSM-III-R are developmental receptive language disorder, developmental reading disorder, developmental expressive writing disorder, developmental coordination disorder, and memory or attention deficits.

Specifically, the DSM-III-R diagnostic criteria for developmental arithmetic disorder are as follows:

A. *Arithmetic skills, as measured by a standardized, individually administered test, are markedly below the expected level, given the person's schooling and intellectual capacity (as determined by an individually administered IQ test).*

B. *The disturbance in A significantly interferes with academic achievement or activities of daily living requiring arithmetic skills.*

C. *Not due to a defect in visual or hearing acuity or to a neurologic disorder.* (p. 42)

As with the other academic skills disorders, the elimination of mental retardation is crucial to differential diagnosis. In cases of mental retardation, the deficit in mathematical ability is on a par with the overall impairment in functioning. If arithmetic ability is significantly lower than the levels of other skills in a mentally retarded individual, it may be helpful to bestow on the individual the additional diagnosis of developmental arithmetic disorder and to offer remedial mathematics training.

Audiometric and visual tests can be given to eliminate possible deficits in sensory function that might be causing below-normal levels of learning. Finally, if inadequate schooling is the root cause, a history will usually reveal many changes in schools, or, if this is not the case, other students in the school will show similar deficits in learning.

Developmental Expressive Language Disorder

Like the academic skills disorders listed in DSM-III-R, the language and speech disorders are separated into three categories: developmental expressive language disorder, developmental receptive language disorder, and developmental articulation disorder. All three of these disorders require the same exclusion criteria (mental retardation, sensory/neurologic impairment, inadequate schooling) as the academic skills disorders. However, when dealing with language and speech disorders, there is an additional potential cause that must be ruled out, pervasive developmental disorder (autism).

In developmental expressive language disorder, there is a significant deficit in the development of expressive language that is not attributable to any of the exclusion criteria given above. The extent of the linguistic abnormalities depends on the severity of the disorder and the age of the child. There may be difficulty in acquiring new words, a limited vocabulary, errors of vocabulary involving substitutions or overgeneralizations, simplified grammatical structures, omissions of critical parts of sentences, and so forth.

The specific diagnostic criteria for developmental expressive language disorder are as follows:

A. *The score obtained from a standardized measure of expressive language is substantially below that obtained from a standardized measure of nonverbal intellectual capacity (as determined by an individually administered IQ test).*

B. *The disturbance in A significantly interferes with academic achievement or activities of daily living requiring the expression of verbal (or sign) language. This may be evidenced in severe cases by use of a markedly limited vocabulary, by speaking only in simple sentences, or by speaking only in the present tense. In less severe cases, there may be hesitations or errors in recalling certain words, or errors in the production of long or complex sentences.*

C. *Not due to a Pervasive Developmental Disorder, defect in hearing acuity, or a neurologic disorder (aphasia).* (p. 47)

In making the differential diagnosis in terms of mental retardation or auditory acuity, tests can be administered and results interpreted in much the same way as for the academic skills disorders. In the case of pervasive developmental disorders, there is usually a noticeable lack of effort directed at communication of any kind, verbal or nonverbal. Elective mutism is manifested in reduced expressive output, but it can be distinguished from developmental expressive language disorder by tests showing age-appropriate levels of comprehension.

Developmental Receptive Language Disorder

This condition is defined as a marked impairment in the development of language comprehension that cannot be attributed to the same exclusion criteria as given for developmental expressive language disorder. As with the latter condition, the degree of deficit depends on the severity of the disorder and the age of the child. In severe cases, there may be multiple problems, including an inability to understand basic vocabulary or simple sentences and deficits in various areas of auditory processing such as the association of sounds and symbols, storage, recall, and sequencing.

The disorder often appears before the age of 4 years. In severe cases it is noticeable by age 2, while milder cases may not manifest until age 7 or older. This condition can be accompanied by developmental articulation disorder and/or developmental expressive language disorder, as well as the academic skills disorders.

The diagnostic criteria for developmental receptive language disorder are as follows:

A. *The score obtained from a standardized measure of receptive language is substantially below that obtained from a standardized measure of nonverbal intellectual capacity (as determined by an individually administered IQ test).*

B. *The disturbance in A significantly interferes with academic achievement or activities of daily living requiring the comprehension of verbal (or sign) language. This may be manifested in more severe cases by an inability to understand simple words or sentences. In less severe cases, there may be difficulty in understanding only certain types of words, such as spatial terms, or an inability to comprehend longer or more complex statements.*

C. *Not due to a Pervasive Developmental Disorder, defect in hearing acuity, or a neurologic disorder (aphasia).* (p. 48)

In making the differential diagnosis, the considerations are much the same as for developmental expressive language disorder. If mental retardation is present, the reduced degree of language comprehension is on a par with the overall intelligence deficit. Hearing can be tested to detect possible contributions from this source. In pervasive developmental disorders, there is typically little or no effort to communicate through nonverbal means when there is impairment in language comprehension. If elective mutism is the source of an apparent language comprehension deficit, formal testing will reveal comprehension to be within normal limits.

Daniel: Nothing Good to Say

Daniel is a 4-year, 2-month-old boy who has been living with his 10-year-old sister and their paternal grandparents for the past 4 months. Daniel's mother, a chronic substance abuser, moved in with Daniel's father 11 years ago, when she was 16. She died after overdosing with sleeping pills 8 months ago. Daniel's father was adopted when he was 7 months old. He rocked repetitively as a child and had severe learning disabilities. He is now on welfare. He is a heroin addict who is currently on methadone maintenance and was declared negligent by social services when neighbors reported finding the apartment "a mess and without food." Daniel's sister seems to have been his primary caretaker. According to Daniel's paternal grandfather, Daniel's mother was using Valium and cocaine throughout her pregnancy. Daniel was born "sleepy and unresponsive, with an immature cry." He was also "not reactive to sounds." Other than this, Daniel's medical history has been unremarkable. Daniel's developmental milestones are unknown.

Daniel was referred for evaluation by his day-care teacher and by his grandfather. Both sources noted that Daniel's expressive language skills are poor. In addition, he is preoccupied with death and abandonment. He also has a very short attention span. Daniel has exhibited tendencies to be explosive (on two occasions, when frustrated, he attacked his companions). Daniel's grandfather noted that he refuses food when he is upset and that he is extremely dependent on his sister (Daniel can only sleep when she is near).

During assessment, Daniel's gross motor movements appeared clumsy (e.g., he could not zip his pants easily). His speech was significantly slurred and his sentences were both abbreviated and awkward. Daniel's receptive language, however, was normal. His affect was labile: he seemed frightened initially, but later he was quick to attach himself and cling to the evaluator. Daniel lacked reciprocity in play, and his moods fluctuated rapidly. He had no delusions or hallucinations and denied the presence of suicidal or homicidal thoughts. Daniel exhibited impulsivity throughout the session.

Daniel's symptoms led to a diagnosis of developmental articulation disorder: a consistent failure to use developmentally expected speech sounds that is not due to a pervasive developmental disorder, mental retardation, a deficit in hearing acuity, disorders of oral speech mechanisms, or a neurological disorder.

A diagnosis of a pervasive developmental disorder could be ruled out on the basis that Daniel does not exhibit "qualitative impairment in the development of social skills and imaginative activity." Furthermore, it was clear to the evaluator that Daniel, in spite of his difficulties, had both the desire and intention of communicating with the evaluator. He did not engage in the stereotyped and repetitive actions that are common to children with a pervasive developmental disorder. Neither auditory nor oral abnormalities were noted in a physical examination: thus a diagnosis of disorders of oral speech mechanisms was not applicable. The fact that Daniel's receptive language skills are normal indicates that he has no defect in hearing acuity.

Thus the diagnosis of developmental articulation disorder was given. Individual psychotherapy and parental counseling were recommended, as was further neurological examination. Daniel's father was referred for individual psychotherapy.

Developmental Articulation Disorder

This condition represents a state in which there is consistent failure to make correct, age-appropriate, articulations of speech sounds. In Daniel's case it is easy to see how difficulty in communicating can lead to further isolation, frustration, and rage. Individuals with this disorder are frequently described as using "baby talk," since misarticulations, substitutions, or omissions of speech sounds occur. The most frequently misarticulated sounds are *r, sh, th, f, z, l,* and *ch*—all of which are acquired later in the developmental sequence of language acquisition.

Not surprisingly, there are a number of specific developmental disorders that may coexist with developmental articulation disorder. Among these are developmental expressive language disorder, developmental receptive language disorder, developmental reading disorder, and developmental coordination disorder. Some children may also have functional enuresis and others may experience a delay in reaching speech milestones such as "first word" or "first sentence." Onset is usually evident by age 3 in severe cases and by age 6 in milder cases.

The specific diagnostic criteria for developmental articulation disorder as given in DSM-III-R are as follows:

A. *Consistent failure to use developmentally expected speech sounds. For example, in a three-year-old, failure to articulate p, b, and t, and in a six-year-old, failure to articulate r, sh, th, f, z, and l.*

B. *Not due to a Pervasive Developmental Disorder, Mental Retardation, defect in hearing acuity, disorders of the oral speech mechanism, or a neurologic disorder. (p. 45)*

The differential diagnosis with regard to mental retardation is identical to that for the other disorders discussed. In pervasive developmental disorders there will be behavioral abnormalities that are not present in children with developmental articulation disorder.

Speech impediments caused by physical abnormalities or hearing impairment are usually easily ruled out by physical examination and testing. In cases of dysarthria or apraxia, there are muscular weaknesses, oral mechanism defects, or there may be a neurological disorder accompanied by drooling, chewing, or sucking and problems with rate of speech.

Motor Skills Disorder (Developmental Coordination Disorder)

Deficits in motor function can readily impede the learning process. In developmental coordination disorder there is a significant impairment in the development of graphomotor coordination. The condition typically is recognized when the child first attempts such tasks as running or holding a fork or knife. These difficulties may be accompanied by clumsiness and delays in tying shoelaces, buttoning shirts, assembling puzzles, building models, and printing or writing. Developmental articulation disorder and developmental receptive and expressive language disorders may accompany the condition.

The specific diagnostic criteria for developmental coordination disorder that are given in DSM-III-R are as follows:

A. *The person's performance in daily activities requiring motor coordination is markedly below the expected level, given the person's chronological age and intellectual capacity. This may be manifested by marked delays in achieving motor milestones (walking, crawling, sitting), dropping things, "clumsiness," poor performance in sports, or poor handwriting.*

B. *The disturbance in A significantly interferes with academic achievement or activities of daily living.*

C. *Not due to a known physical disorder, such as cerebral palsy, hemiplegia, or muscular dystrophy.* (p. 49)

In reaching a differential diagnosis, there is definite neural damage and abnormal neurological findings if the clumsiness is attributable to specific neurological disorders such as cerebral palsy. Distractibility and impulsiveness can be looked for in children who bump into things or fall down as a result of attention deficit hyperactivity disorder. In mental retardation, the impairment is in line with the overall deficit in functioning, and in pervasive developmental disorders an abnormal gait and/or delays in motor functioning are congruent with a pervasive history of abnormal development.

Philip: Blocked at Every Turn

Philip is a 6-year-old boy who lives with his mother and his maternal grandparents, all of whom work. He has never met his father, for the parents divorced while Philip's mother was pregnant. Philip entered a mainstream kindergarten class 2 months ago after attending an early-intervention nursery school program for developmentally delayed children. He had been placed in that nursery school program when, in a regular nursery school, it was noted that he was behind in average skills and progress. Philip's developmental milestones were all slightly delayed, as assessed prior to placement in the early-intervention program. Testing was done when Philip was 28 months old, and a tentative diagnosis of borderline intellectual functioning (IQ between 71 and 85) was assigned based on Philip's assessed developmental level of 20 months.

Philip is able to dress and feed himself, and toilet-training was completed at age 4 years. Philip is a highly social child who enjoys playing with other children. Although he is sometimes aggressive toward other children and has a low frustration tolerance, he was placed in a regular kindergarten because it was determined that the environment would provide the greatest stimulus for his further development. Upon school entry, Philip was placed in speech therapy for articulation difficulties (he had speech therapy in nursery school as well). His kindergarten teacher noticed that he seems to understand what others say most of the time, but that he is very restricted in his own use of expressive language. She felt that the disparity between apparent language comprehension and language expression was great enough to warrant assessment.

During assessment, Philip, an attractive little boy, separated without incident from his mother. His motor coordination appeared to be developmentally average. He displayed a full range of affect and immediately attached himself to the clinician in a dependent manner. He was friendly toward the clinician, although his attention span was very short and he was highly distractible. It was also noted during assessment that Philip's self-esteem was deficient; when asked to draw a picture, he insisted that he could not draw well and that he could not do it even though he wanted to. The clinician found that he attempts to communicate with others even though his speech is limited.

Testing was done to determine the cause of his difficulties in articulation and expression. Results revealed that his IQ is approximately 60 to 65. At his age and measured IQ, Philip's speech delays are not unusual and would not be diagnosed as speech articulation or developmental expressive language disorder. The IQ assessment points to mental retardation as an appropriate diagnosis because Philip's IQ is below the established maximum (70) for individuals with mental retardation.

More specifically, his impairment would be labeled mild mental retardation (IQ between 50–55 and 70). Further testing of speech and expressive language should be performed to rule out diagnoses of developmental speech articulation disorder and developmental expressive language disorder, in addition to the diagnosis of mild mental retardation. The previous tentative diagnosis of borderline intellectual functioning was ruled out, based on IQ test results. A diagnosis of pervasive developmental disorder was considered and subsequently dismissed as a possibility because Philip's reciprocal social interaction and verbal communication skills are appropriate for the delayed developmental stage he is passing through. In pervasive developmental disorder, the absence of reciprocal interaction and the restricted range of imaginative and social activity would not be considered normal within any developmental stage.

Thus, a diagnosis of mild mental retardation was assigned. Recommendation was made for further evaluation of speech difficulties, in order to assure proper attention to these deficits. It was also recommended that Philip remain in a mainstream kindergarten class, as opposed to a class for children with mental retardation, because his impairment is mild and interaction with children of normal IQ is likely to best stimulate his learning. It was suggested that Philip be placed in a class with fewer students, however, so that he will receive more personal attention.

Differentiating Learning Disorders from Mental Retardation

In thinking about Daniel's case, it is important to note that the language and speech disorders, as well as developmental coordination disorder, appear to bear out the definitions of delay, lag, rate, and deficit put forth by Satz and Fletcher (1981). The course of these disorders, if treatment is rendered, is more positive than negative. Therefore, it appears that there may be at least some basis for the rationale that although learning impaired children lag behind the normal group in acquiring language and speech, they may proceed to catch up at either a faster or slower rate.

If this is the case, it is little wonder that mental retardation poses the most difficult barrier to differential diagnosis, since even with severe degrees of mental handicap the same order of phases of development may occur. However, it appears that the rate at which these phases progress is much slowed (Woodward & Stern, 1963). Thus, learning disorders may easily appear to be mental retardation because both involve deviant levels and rates of learning. Therefore, Daniel's diagnosis could be made only after extensive testing and examination.

In attempting to construct a developmental neuropsychological model of central processing deficiencies in children, Rourke (1982) noted that three principal neurological axes must be examined: the progression from lower to higher centers, the progression from the posterior regions of the cerebrum to the anterior regions, and the right hemisphere-left hemisphere interaction.

Focusing initially on the right-left hemisphere dimension, Rourke posited the existence of the following five neurological phenomena that may well have importance in relation to children with processing deficiencies, regardless of whether they are mentally retarded or have a learning disability:

1. The ontology of brain development causes a progression from the salience of right-hemisphere functioning to that of the left hemisphere.
2. Children's conceptualizations range from global to specific, which reflects the right-to-left hemispherical development.
3. The development of right hemisphere systems is required before there can be adequate development of left hemisphere systems.
4. In the normal course of developing constructs and concepts, the right hemisphere organization provides the content for concepts,

while the left is more geared to their articulation, elaboration, and application.

5. With respect to the development of maladaptive or insufficient abilities, reduced access to or disordered functioning of right hemisphere systems is especially debilitating.

In this scheme, the left cerebral hemisphere is more oriented toward performing unimodal processing, motor processing, and storing codes, whereas the right hemisphere is more oriented toward intermodal integration, processing novel stimuli, and handling complex information. Thus, the left hemisphere would be superior in tasks requiring fixation on a single mode of representation or execution, while the right hemisphere would be better at processing many modes of representation within a single cognitive task such as, initially, reading.

More recent brain research has uncovered a number of interesting findings regarding the development and use of language. It has been long known that speech is primarily under control of the left hemisphere, a fact associated with anatomical, chemical, and electrical asymmetries in the brain. In some individuals, however, the right side gains partial dominance, and these individuals are at higher risk of having language-related learning disorders. Also, there are sex-related differences in brain structure pertaining to language development. Males are generally more likely to have anomalous dominance for speech, to be left-handed, and to have speech-related learning disorders. There has been speculation that the factor that might be most significantly involved in these sex differences is testosterone (Marx, 1983).

These findings illustrate the great number of areas in which the neurological system can be altered detrimentally. Pennington and Smith (1983) elaborated on the consequences of this fact by noting that the absence of a clear etiology for learning disorders or mental retardation greatly complicates early detection, intervention, and prognosis. In looking at possible genetic contributions to learning disabilities, they first cited a number of environmental factors that could have etiological importance: prenatal exposure to alcohol, postnatal exposure to lead, and reduced parental and environmental stimulation.

Pennington and Smith attempted to unravel some of the causes and relationships of learning disorders by applying the approach taken to resolve some of the genetically homogenous subtypes of mental retardation. They postulated that some learning disabilities and speech and language disorders represent the tail of the normal distribution of a specific cognitive or linguistic trait, such as verbal processing ability, which is essential for academic skills and normal development of speech and language.

These investigators concluded that since the cognitive systems involved in speech and learning are so numerous and interrelated and since these systems can be interrupted at any number of levels, either singularly or plurally, a much better nosology of developmental language and speech disorders is needed. Such an improved nosology, based on a clearer understanding of the cognitive processes involved, would allow the identification of clear subtypes of disorder, isolated to a specific area or areas of functioning.

However, such an accurate nosology does not yet exist, either for mental retardation or for learning disorders. Therefore, the first steps to take in focusing on the possibility of mental retardation are to obtain a history of the child's pre-, peri-, and postnatal life, investigate the family background, and clinically assess the child. When evaluating this information, especially if a learning disorder is suspected, it is essential to realize that for differential purposes there are two basic populations of mentally retarded individuals, the mildly retarded in one group and the moderately, severely, and profoundly retarded in the other (Clarke & Clarke, 1978; Kirman, 1985). Another way to conceptualize the situation is that anyone with an IQ under 50 has a definite handicap. Clearly, then, it is those children who are only mildly retarded who pose the greatest difficulty in terms of diagnosing a learning disorder.

Taking a history and being aware of the existence of mildly retarded children is especially important in light of the fact that relatively few cases of mental retardation can be categorized to form a recognizable syndrome. Despite the difficulties, however, an exhaustive determination including, if necessary, laboratory tests such as the Guthrie or amino acid chromatography is more than worthwhile. Perhaps the question most frequently asked by a new mother pertains to the so-called normality of her child. Certainly this question requires an informed answer.

CONCLUSION

The fact that children with learning disabilities are at risk not only of failing to achieve competitive levels of learning, but of developing emotional problems as well, emphasizes the importance of early detection and treatment. Unfortunately, attempts at isolating predictors of learning dysfunction, while they have not been wholly unsuccessful, are in need of further attention.

One hindrance to obtaining early predictors is the relatively long period of time required for differentiating between lags (normative maturational changes) and deficits. For example, in relating the classic work of Morley (1965) to the operational definitions of Satz and

Fletcher (1981), Orsini, Fletcher, and Satz (1984) found that there was a significant difference in the rate of onset of intelligible speech between boys and girls. In normal children at age 2 years, 55% of boys possess intelligible speech compared to 82% of girls. If assessment had not continued for a sufficient period of time, an erroneous conclusion might have been reached in which the later-learning boys would have been judged to have a deficit.

The picture is further obscured by the fact that, as Orsini and colleagues (1984) observed, "performance differences between disabled and nondisabled learners have many interpretations" (p. 83). In order to reach a consistent body of knowledge it will first be necessary to answer the question of whether performance differences represent variations on normal development or are in fact distinctly divergent from the course of normal development.

In order to answer this question, a developmental approach will be essential, a fact acknowledged by Shapiro and co-workers (1983), who suggested that motor development may be a good place to begin the search for early predictors. Observing that motor attainment is the major focus of development during the first 18 months of life, "disordered motor development may be a presenting sign for children who have other developmental disabilities without major motor handicaps" (p. 18). Thus, Shapiro and co-workers suggested that it might be possible to detect specific learning disabilities before school age by focusing on deviant neurodevelopment rather than waiting for academic underachievement to emerge.

This strategy, while it is not new, represents a refreshing alternative to the techniques used previously. The majority of investigations into the problem of learning disability have relied on comparisons in levels of performance on one or a number of variables between normal and learning disabled subjects. As Fisk and Rourke (1979) pointed out, this strategy implicitly assumes that children who are learning disabled are members of a homogenous population in terms of their adaptive structures. Given the vast arenas of brain functioning and the richness of environmental possibilities, this hardly seems a viable assumption.

While the process of treatment and diagnosis of learning disorders continues to evolve, Hartzell and Compton (1984) have provided an example of the variables that influence outcome at the present time. In their prospective 10-year follow-up study of 114 children treated for learning disabilities, they found that while there was no difference between the test group and controls in terms of job satisfaction, the learning disabled group achieved significantly lower levels of academic and professional achievement.

The factors found to be most beneficial to outcome of the learning disabled individuals were high IQ, less severe learning disability, effective family function and support, high occupational level of the family wage earner, and high level of education of the mother. Also, the availability of early remediation was crucial for positive outcome. Negative factors included a more severe degree of learning disability, the presence of hyperactivity, and a concomitant disability in mathematics.

While these results are hardly cause for jubilation, one can be grateful that these individuals received early evaluation and treatment. It is almost certain that their histories would have been far worse in the absence of intervention.

CHAPTER ELEVEN

Personality Traits and Disorders and Their Differential Diagnosis

Sam: Aggressively Lost

Sam was a 4-year-old black boy, who lived with his mother, his older brother, his younger sister, and his father, who was only occasionally present. His father was violent, drank heavily, and was an intravenous drug user. Sam witnessed the abuse of his mother by his father and saw his parents engage in sexual relations. The family moved back and forth between Chicago and New York several times. Sam's mother reported no abnormalities or difficulties in Sam's development and asserted that Sam had never been the victim of physical abuse, although Child Protective Services had been involved in the past in order to investigate the possibility of abuse. His mother described Sam as a "happy child" who enjoyed playing with other children. Sam was referred for assessment by the nursery school he attended, after his repeated, escalating manifestations of aggression. Examples of Sam's aggressive behavior included pushing and spitting at children who came near him, in the absence of provocation. In one incident, Sam tried to blind another child with a pair of scissors.

During assessment, it was noted that Sam appeared to be older than his stated age, with increased physical activity but no abnormal mannerisms. When initially approaching others Sam acted shy but he soon warmed up and engaged in parallel play, with which he was able to occupy himself for extended periods of time. If Sam was confronted with rules or was denied something, he became angry and attempted physical assault. When asked to do something, he usually said, "no," but he would later comply. Examination yielded some difficulties with speech intonation and articulation, mild auditory discrimination difficulties, and some expressive language impairment to a moderate degree. Indications of attentional deficits and hyperactivity were also noted. Other elements of the mental status examination were within normal range. Sam was preoccupied with aggressive, violent ideas, and he was at risk for both aggressive and suicidal behavior. While Sam exhibited symptoms of several disorders, it was judged that the symptoms of borderline personality disorder were most pervasive and that this was the most appropriate diagnosis.

Sam's aggressive behaviors were exhibited during group therapy, at which time he was confronted about such activities. After that, he began adjusting, finding more acceptable ways to make requests of others, other than through physical assaults. Because he often had to repeat himself to be understood by others, Sam became frustrated and his attention deficits and hyperactivity surfaced. His frustration tolerance was very low, and he lacked the ability to control his resulting behavior. The apparent behavior problems, the intensity and fluctuation of Sam's moods, and the contribution of these factors to the impairment of Sam's social relationships pointed to a diagnosis of borderline personality traits. A look at his family situation confirmed the likelihood of borderline personality disorder. Sam's father was often absent and was ineffective when present; he, too, exhibited some characteristic borderline traits, including abuse of alcohol and drugs and episodic aggressive behavior. Sam's mother was inconsistent in her interactions with her children, and she had difficulty setting limits on Sam's behavior. Such a constellation of family elements is commonly associated with a diagnosis of borderline personality disorder.

A diagnosis of identity disorder was ruled out because Sam's symptoms indicated that the disorder was not likely to be limited to a single developmental stage, and also because the disturbance was pervasive and persistent. A diagnosis of cyclothymia was also considered but rejected upon revelation that Sam's mood shifts were not associated with characteristics of the hypomanic episodes found in cyclothymia such as racing thoughts and less need for sleep.

Thus, a diagnosis of borderline personality traits was assigned, and Sam was referred for residential therapeutic placement so that he would be in an environment where external structure and limit setting would help him to develop internal controls. His treatment recommendations included individual psychotherapy and involvement of his mother in a parent-child group and a parent's group.

INTRODUCTION

The diagnostic constructs of *neurotic* and *psychotic* suggest the existence of an intermediary construct, one that delineates a personality structure associated with a degree of dysfunctionality more severe than that seen in the upper range of neurosis but less severe than seen in psychosis. It seems evident that Sam's behavior reflects a personality existing in this range. However, all analyses and discussions of this area must allow for the fact that the term *borderline* does not impart any more meaning, in and of itself, than do the terms *neurotic* or *psychotic*. As Pine (1986) has noted, the "borderline" individual is not a phenomenon that already exists in nature. If this were the case, it would be detectable through the isolation of an independent variable, like the micro-organism responsible for pneumonia.

The fact that the borderline construct is a kind of nosological "child" to the diagnostic categories of neurosis and psychosis is evidenced by the relatively late date at which the borderline diagnosis began to be used clinically. The concept of borderline was posited at least as early as the late 19th century (Grinker, Werble, & Drye, 1968), but it was not until the 1950's that "borderline" came to be used as a diagnosis (Knight, 1953). From that time to the present, attempts to define this syndrome have been an imprecise mix of developmental psychology, nosological systems of psychopathology, and psychoanalytic theory (Greenman, Gunderson, Cane, & Saltzman, 1986).

Nonetheless, the existence of clinical personalities characterized by dysfunctionality that is profound but not immediately apparent is now well documented (Barasch, Frances, Hurt, Clarkin, & Cohen, 1985; Pine,

1982 a,b; Verhulst, 1984). This is true for adults, and there are indications that it may be true as well for children and adolescents (Aarkrog,
1981; Kernberg, 1975). However, applying the borderline diagnosis to
children is complicated by the fact that this condition is usually more
difficult to identify in younger individuals. Since discontinuity of cognition and emotion and lack of personality integration are normal developmental hallmarks of childhood, detecting a truly borderline level of
personality development can be a difficult task (Trad, 1988).

Regardless of the difficulty inherent in applying adult criteria to
childhood borderline states, one thing seems clear: The borderline condition in adulthood represents—perhaps to an even greater degree
than that seen for neuroses and psychoses—the endpoint of pathological childhood development (Holman, 1985). Thus, the task is to isolate
characteristics that are universal to both adults and children who have
been diagnosed as borderline. Attempts to discover the etiology of these
debilitating characteristics are also useful, but in the absence of longitudinal data, these attempts must rely on retrospective analyses—a serious
limitation.

It should be made clear that this discussion will largely focus on borderline characteristics with a predominantly developmental etiology.
Recent work by Andrulonis, Gluek, Stroebel, and Vogel (1982) and
Andrulonis and Vogel (1984) has persuasively argued in favor of the
contention that, rather than being descriptive of only one type of
personality disorder, the term *borderline* can be broken into several subcategories, depending on etiology.

In the first, or so-called developmental borderline category, the individual has failed to successfully resolve the separation-individuation
stage of development. In the minimal brain dysfunction subcategory,
the individual has evolved a borderline structure as a result of the onset
of earlier emotional and functional difficulties that may be based, at
least in part, on a constitutional deficit. The last subcategory of patients
are those with more severe and definite organic brain trauma—patients
who may respond to lithium carbonate and/or anticonvulsant medications.

The developmental borderline individual is one who fails in the task
of self-expansion as a result of missing the early foundations of self-
experience, depriving him or her of positive self-esteem. Pine (1982b)
suggested that the early foundations of experience which, if lacking in
the individual's history, may lead to pathology are (a) ease/continuity, the
continuity of being when the mother's ministrations protect the infant
from excessive intrusions; (b) activity/effectiveness, the bodily and rela-
tionally derived gratifications that provide the infant with a range of
affects; and (c) self-esteem, the sense of being an operative agent in the
world upon the establishment of quiet exploratory play.

The developmental borderline person, lacking in one or more of these essential components of early childhood (and therefore lacking in feelings of worthwhileness), has difficulty incorporating elements charged with conflict. Rather than recognizing a conflictual feeling and allowing it to co-exist in the psyche until a resolution can be worked out, the borderline individual will attempt to deny its existence through such defenses as repression or splitting. This difference between the borderline and the nonborderline state illustrates the crux of the issue. The integrated personality is able to exist within broad boundaries. The borders of the self contain an area that is large enough to hold many different feelings and conflicts within the self-experience. In the borderline individual, the boundaries of the self are much more constricted.

Even when the discussion is limited to the borderline disorder resulting from unresolved separation-individuation (developmental borderline), it is not an easy task to find phenomena that link all the manifestations of borderline personality organization (Pine, 1974, 1982, 1986). However, as Schmideberg (1959) has stated, the paramount reason for viewing the borderline personality as a clinical entity is that these individuals remain "stable in their instability" because they are largely unable to learn from experience. Thus, the question becomes one of when and why these persons lost their capacity to grow and mature, to establish adequate ego stability and object relations. If the hallmark of the adult borderline individual is an inability to integrate the self with the environment, the implication is that, at least for the developmental subgroup, the primitive coping strategies in childhood were somehow "frozen" in place, preempting further development of mastery. This, indeed, is the consensus of most researchers; i.e., that there is inadequate resolution of the normal developmental conflicts in separation-individuation during the toddler phase (Mahler, 1975). In short, the fundamental childhood dynamic underlying the development of a nonorganic borderline personality appears to occur as follows: Trauma upon separation gives rise to anxiety, which quickly escalates to panic or triggers massive regression (Ekstein, 1980).

The remainder of this discussion focuses on the differences and similarities between adult and childhood borderline conditions and on the seminal experiences in childhood that give rise to the development of nonorganic borderline pathology. The excellent work of Pine (1974, 1986) is of particular value, positing as it does three discrete elements integral to the development of borderline personality structure: early trauma, deficits in development, and primitive coping strategies.

However, Pine was the first to point out that, beyond these elements, it is still necessary to employ descriptions that are highly individualized to each patient. Furthermore, as Aarkrog (1981) noted, borderline types are probably as well understood in terms of ego-psychology as they are within the framework of object relationships. Ekstein (1980) has posited that borderline states can be conceived as members of a continuum of borderline conditions from one extreme to the other. The nature of the continuum can then be related to a given developmental scheme. The continuum might represent the area between primary or secondary process; between autism, symbiosis, and object-self differentiation; or between a chaotic ego and an organized, mature ego. While all of these approaches are useful, the following discussion of nonorganic borderline conditions will center on the readily identifiable criteria posited by Pine (1986) as seminal in the development of a borderline personality state: *early trauma, deficits in development,* and *primitive coping strategies.* These criteria not only provide a testable base, but also supply a flexible but durable system capable of incorporating analyses from both the developmental and psychodynamic perspectives.

DIFFERENTIAL DIAGNOSIS OF BORDERLINE PERSONALITY ORGANIZATIONS

DSM-III-R Criteria

DSM-III-R depicts the borderline personality as a pervasive pattern of instability of self-image, mood, and interpersonal relationships. Common to borderline structures are persistent identity disturbances manifested in such areas as confusion as to which values to adopt as part of the self, sexual image, and long-term goals. Affective instability is also prevalent, appearing as marked shifts in mood from baseline to depression, irritability, or anxiety. These mood shifts last anywhere from a few hours to a few days. Overidealization and devaluation are common, as is an inability to control anger.

Specifically, according to DSM-III-R, a diagnosis of borderline personality disorder can be made if at least five of the following eight characteristics are present:

(1) *a pattern of unstable and intense interpersonal relationships characterized by alternating between extremes of overidealization and devaluation*

(2) *impulsiveness in at least two areas that are potentially self-damaging, e.g., spending, sex, substance use, shoplifting, reckless driving, binge eating (Do not include suicidal or self-mutilating behavior covered in [5].)*

(3) *affective instability: marked shifts from baseline mood to depression, irritability, or anxiety, usually lasting a few hours and only rarely more than a few days*

(4) *inappropriate, intense anger or lack of control of anger, e.g., frequent displays of temper, constant anger, recurrent physical fights*

(5) *recurrent suicidal threats, gestures, or behavior, or self-mutilating behavior*

(6) *marked and persistent identity disturbance manifested by uncertainty about at least two of the following: self-image, sexual orientation, long-term goals or career choice, type of friends desired, preferred values*

(7) *chronic feelings of emptiness and boredom*

(8) *frantic efforts to avoid real or imagined abandonment (Do not include suicidal or self-mutilating behavior covered in [5].)* (p. 347)

Differential diagnosis requires the exclusion of other psychiatric conditions that carry some of the same symptomatology. Identity disorder presents perhaps the most extensive symptom overlap. This condition is characterized by severe subjective distress regarding uncertainty about a variety of issues relating to identity, including three or more of the following: (a) long-term goals; (b) career choice; (c) friendship patterns; (d) sexual orientation and behavior; (e) religious identification; (f) moral value systems; and (g) group loyalties.

Also present in identity disorder is an impairment in social or occupational (including academic) functioning stemming from the symptoms just mentioned. It is not difficult to see the similarity in presentations between this condition and the borderline disorder. However, a diagnosis of borderline preempts the diagnosis of identity disorder if the borderline disturbance is pervasive and persistent and is not limited to a developmental stage.

Aside from the obvious similarity of the identity disorder to borderline conditions, features of many other disorders can accompany the borderline state. For example, affective instability is also present in cyclothymia, but (in the absence of a coexisting mood disorder) there are no hypomanic episodes in borderline personality disorder. The DSM-III-R points out, however, that in some cases both cyclothymia and borderline personality may be present.

Another condition that can accompany borderline states is depression, or major depressive episode, which is characterized by dysphoric mood or loss of interest or pleasure in nearly all usual activities and pastimes. Persistent sadness, hopelessness, and irritability are the hallmarks of this condition, and it is not difficult to understand why they may accompany a disorder such as the borderline condition in which coping ability is severely and chronically impaired.

Akin to major depressive episode and cyclothymia is dysthymic disorder, in which, for the past 2 years, the person has been bothered most or all of the time by symptoms characteristic of the depressive syndrome but not quite as severe. The DSM-III-R lists other possible disorders whose features can be similar to those of the borderline state such as schizotypal, histrionic, narcissistic, and antisocial personality disorders. While these features may be subsumed under the borderline condition, it is often the case that more than one diagnosis is warranted.

Shared Characteristics of Adulthood and Childhood Borderline States

There does appear to be some value in applying adult criteria to the borderline conditions of childhood. In their study of 86 children, Greenman and colleagues (1986) cited the work of Petti and Law (1982), who found that DSM-III adult criteria for borderline and schizotypal personality disorders could distinguish the two disorders in 10 latency-aged children with borderline psychotic psychopathology. Also, Pfeffer, Plutchnik, and Mizruchi (1983), in studying 102 children, found that 54% of those who showed suicidal and assaultive behavior fulfilled the DSM-III criteria for borderline personality.

Greenman and co-workers expanded this work by retrospectively examining the charts of 86 children aged 6 to 12 years. These investigators engaged in an exhaustive analysis using the Diagnostic Interview for Borderlines (DIB) adapted for retrospective use (DIB-R) developed by Armelius, Kullgren, and Renberg (1985). Making the group particularly likely to possess borderline characteristics, 57 of the 86 children selected for study had either threatened or attempted suicide. The remaining 29 were nonsuicidal children who had been admitted to the same facility over the same period of time (7 years). There were no significant differences between the two groups in mean age, male-to-female ratio, or socioeconomic status. The sample was largely white, middle-class, and male (72%), with a mean age of 9.9 years. Greenman and co-workers assessed 30 other variables in addition to those specified in the DIB-R, some of which were presumed related to the borderline condition in adults and some in children. The diagnosis and degree of improvement on discharge also were recorded.

In this comprehensive study, 27 subjects (31%) were found to be borderline according to criteria of the DIB-R. The most frequent DSM-III diagnoses given to those classified as borderline included conduct disorder (37%) and other personality disorder (15%). The percentage of borderline patients in the suicidal group (33%) was in fact not significantly higher than the percentage in the nonsuicidal group (28%).

In summary, this study revealed that a sizeable proportion of a selected nonpsychotic child inpatient sample met adult criteria for borderline personality disorder. However, as Greenman and co-workers pointed out, the evidence was not overly strong in support of the contention that adult borderline personality criteria define a clear and meaningful syndrome in children. They concluded that still more effort is needed to build a discriminative method for identifying shared characteristics of borderline children. In addition, they stressed the need for studying the predictive validity of these diagnostic criteria for children, that is, whether patterns of behavior seen in these children will predict future behavior.

ELEMENTS CONTRIBUTING TO THE DEVELOPMENT OF THE BORDERLINE DISORDER

Dynamics

The characteristics of the borderline state in childhood are more difficult to define because childhood is the period of both genesis and gestation for the events and reactions to these events that come to shape the borderline personality. Therefore, the results of Greenman and co-workers are to be expected, at least with respect to the relatively greater difficulty in identifying the features of childhood borderline states when compared to those of adulthood. In order to answer the question posed by Greenman and co-workers as to whether or not patterns of behavior seen in borderline children are predictive of adult patterns, it is first necessary to discern what recognizable patterns there may be in childhood borderline states. The search for patterns begins with an understanding of the etiology of the condition.

The single factor that seems most prominent in linking childhood and adulthood borderline conditions is a pervading sense of *desperation*. Desperate (i.e., primitive) measures are taken to forestall desperate feelings. Two defensive dynamics in particular—panic and splitting—are associated with the alleviation of these intensely threatening feelings.

Panic.   As early as 1933, Freud noticed a failure to achieve the function of anxiety as a signal in borderline children. Normally, relatively early in development, the child will begin to anticipate the occurrence of an anxiety-inducing situation on the basis of memory. The mild anxiety accompanying the anticipation causes mobilization of defenses such as flight, seeking the caregiver, or intrapsychic defenses if these exist. The ability to activate these defenses requires significant developmental achievement. The infant or the grossly underdeveloped child feels helpless in the face of anxiety—a feeling that can quickly escalate the anxiety to panic proportions. In order to reduce the panic, the underdeveloped or aberrantly developed child resorts to primitive mechanisms such as regression to a less integrated state—one that may resemble psychosis in certain aspects.

The inability to use anxiety as a signal to mobilize effective defense strategies indicates more than just a failure in development. It is also a major roadblock to the further development of mastery. Thus, it appears that the failure to achieve the signal function of anxiety is a prime contributor to the adult borderline state in which these individuals are seen to be unable to learn from experience.

Splitting.   Another defense mechanism that appears to be continuous from childhood to adulthood is splitting. Splitting marks a failure to integrate the "good" and "bad" elements of the self and others into a workable, functional image. As Pine (1974) pointed out, splitting may have dire consequences when it occurs in the borderline adult. The child who appears "sweet" or good in the classroom may well be harboring violent and destructive fantasies—fantasies which, as adults, these individuals may act out.

Etiology

Organic Borderline.   As Andrulonis and colleagues (1982) have observed, there has been much attention paid to developing a multidimensional model of the borderline personality disorder. The assumption is that there may be limbic dysregulation such as episodic dyscontrol or minimal or mild brain dysfunction that contributes to the evolution of borderline personality.

In attempting to discover the feasibility of this hypothesis, Andrulonis and Vogel (1984) compared 106 patients fulfilling the DSM-III classification of unstable borderline personality disorder with 55 schizophrenics and 55 patients with affective disorders. Data taken included sex, age on current admission, age of problem onset, admission weight, IQ, EEG, past medications, current medications, history of psychiatric difficulties, family psychiatric history, organicity, minipsychotic episodes, eating disturbances, and previous psychiatric hospitalizations.

Depending on the analysis from a previous study (Andrulonis et al., 1982), the 106 borderline patients were divided into one of three categories: (1) developmental or nonorganic borderline patients with no past or current history or major or minimal brain dysfunction; (2) those with a past history of significant head trauma, encephalitis, or epilepsy; and (3) those with attention deficit disorder/learning disabilities (ADD/LD).

Data from this study and from the previous investigation confirmed the existence of four primary borderline subgroups. The first subgroup, nonorganic or developmental borderline patients, were observed to have a typical history of acting-out behavior, depression, alcohol/drug abuse, and a family history of depression. These individuals, predominantly females, were on a continuum with affective disorders, schizoaffective psychoses, cycloid psychoses, or atypical psychoses.

The second group was an affective disorder subcategory that overlapped with constitutional/genetic depressive illness. The third group, those with minimal brain dysfunction (ADD/LD), showed primarily constitutional etiologic components, a finding that was also true of the fourth group, who had suffered trauma, encephalitis, or epilepsy. Interestingly, those with organic brain involvement tended to be males, while members of the first two categories tended to be females. In these two studies and in other studies (e.g., Baron, Gruen, Asnis, & Lord, 1985) it was found that while there was some overlapping between borderline personality disorder and affective states, there was little if any confounding between borderline personality disorder and schizophrenia.

Developmental (Nonorganic) Borderline.   There are several points from which the borderline personality can originate, not the least of which pertain to the child's temperament. For example, a child who is temperamentally more reactive to stress may be more prone to elevated levels of anxiety that give rise to desperate adherence to primitive coping mechanisms. In addition, there is a general consensus that the dynamics of borderline constructs can be traced to developmental arrest or aberrant development in various aspects of object relationship or ego functioning, which are largely secondary to inadequate resolution of the normal developmental conflicts of separation-individuation (Aarkrog, 1981; Holman, 1985; Mahler, Pine, & Bergman, 1975 in Holman, 1985; Pine, 1974). However, as Pine (1974) noted, it is not always easy to differentiate between what is normal development and what is only a semblance of normal development.

Pine (1986) cautioned further that the term *borderline* is analogous to concepts such as transference or regression, which are merely "terms that serve communication through consensus" (p. 450). With this caveat in mind, Pine (1974, 1982, 1986) erected a developmental model depicting the genesis of borderline personality constructs. This model posits the existence of three elements in borderline etiology: early trauma (experiences of being overwhelmed), evolution of developmental deficits, and desperate reliance on such ultimately maladaptive coping mechanisms as splitting and panic.

For his first tenet, early trauma, Pine drew on work by Chethik (1986), who found that early trauma (physical illness and pain) experienced as an aggressive attack from the external world was common in the infancy and childhood of his sample of borderline children. It was Pine's contention that these early negative experiences "create too much noise in the psychic system." They interfere with the creation and maintenance of certain elements of early development. This "noise" is experienced by the young infant in an undifferentiated way that prevents mastery through repetition.

Here again there is potential for input into the system from the child's temperament. An active and stimulating mother, if her infant is also active and fast-paced, may overstimulate and push the child into too tense a state (Trad, 1986, 1987). Alternatively, what is experienced as too much aloneness or neglect can have the effect of overwhelming the child with isolation and need. It is always the child's *experience* of the stimulus, and not the external perception of it, that must be considered.

Developmental Deficits. The most fundamental deficit in development resulting from overwhelming negative experiences is the failure of development of trust in the caregiver and thus in the world at large. Pine suggested that this failure to develop trust may underlie every other failure in development. This is due to the fact that lack of trust prevents the formation of the expectation that gratification will eventually occur. It is this expectation that allows for delay in the face of distress, a period in which much learning normally takes place. Thus, lack of trust formation may contribute to the absence of the signal function of anxiety. The fear that gratification will not be forthcoming can rapidly escalate from a state of anxiety to panic, eclipsing the possibility of self-control.

A second type of developmental failure resulting from early negative experiences is the inability to move from indiscriminate, need-fulfilling relationships to the association of need satisfaction with specific desirable others. In the perceived absence of reliable others, the need remains paramount and the specific object (need satisfier) is less important than the negative, internal need state. It is perhaps this failure in development that is primarily responsible for the manipulative behavior seen in many adult borderline personalities.

A third deficit in development stemming from early trauma is lack of integration and control of aggression. The loving and angry images of the self fail to become integrated. This sometimes occurs when reactive rage in the unsatisfied infant overwhelms the infant's more positive feelings. As a result, defensive splitting occurs, which further prevents integration of loving and hate-filled images.

Pine also pointed out that flexibility in the development of defenses can be impaired by early trauma. When the child feels flooded, the first reaction is to cling to early-developed defenses, regardless of the fact that these are frequently unsuccessful and almost certainly maladaptive.

Finally, as a result of these deficits, positive self-esteem fails to develop fully. Positive self-esteem is inconsistent with the level of subjectively perceived negativity and failure. There is little inward experience of the "good" self.

Desperate Reliance on Primitive, Maladaptive Coping Mechanisms. The many developmental failures listed here result in the child's having little chance of being able to handle stress effectively. Nevertheless, the child must employ some survival technique if he or she is to survive. As a result, early primitive defense mechanisms such as splitting and regression are mobilized at the first sign of anxiety. Pine contended that these unstable and maladaptive coping mechanisms, in addition to the developmental failures secondary to trauma, comprise the category of borderline personality.

Patterns of Borderline Personality Organization

Pine (1986) concluded that the term *borderline* is best viewed as a "loose supraclassification under the rubric of a broad overall definition (early trauma, developmental deficit, survival technique) with highly individualized description beyond that" (p. 456). However, he did identify personality patterns of development stemming from this broad definition.

Chronic Ego Deviance.   In terms of diagnosis, this is the parent to all the other permutations or patterns of borderline pathology that develop. Children with chronic ego deviance are deficient in the development of object relationship, reality testing, synthetic function, and proper use of age-adequate defenses. Since there is failure to establish the reality principle, inability to perceive the signal function of anxiety, and fluidity in object attachments, these children lack the fundamental stabilizers of functioning necessary to normal development. They have no reliable anchor in external reality. Thus, these children may grow up to be odd adults—borderline schizoid or worse.

Shifting Levels of Ego Organization.   One of the most dramatic aspects of borderline conditions is the ego's shifting levels of organization. This type of pattern causes fluctuation back and forth from orientation toward reality to idiosyncratic fantasy. These children go from near-autistic unrelatedness on the one hand to true object relationship on the other. Thus, ego organization is achieved, but on two levels—a mixture of partial organization along with what appears to be attentional interruptions and occasionally panic.

Internal Disorganization in Response to External Disorganization. Schmideberg (1959) referred to internally disorganized children as being "stable in their instability." These children frequently come from extremely destabilizing environments containing such elements as prostitution, drug use and dealing, and child abuse. The traumatizing environment produces reactive disorganization, leading to behavioral pathology. These children, in the clinical setting away from the destabilizing home environment, usually integrate quite well. However, their recovery is greatly hampered by their return home after hospitalization.

Incomplete Internalization of Psychosis.   Children with this pattern of development are reactive to a disorganized environment in which the love object is also disorganized (i.e., psychotic). Thus, problems of separation-individuation are particularly salient.

Ego Limitation.   Very early restriction of ego development marks these children. One cause may be deprivation. Further growth is stunted, as are later elaborations of thought, modulation of affect, and enrichment of object relationships.

Schizoid Personality.   These children have isolated personalities with aberrations of thought and fantasy life. Affective range and expression are blocked, so they tend to remain emotionally distant from others. Their character structure is stabilized at the cost of isolation and strangeness.

Mistrustful Personality (Paranoid Character).   Here, patterns of suspiciousness and rigidity of thinking are the hallmarks. There is failure in the development of object relations and in the attainment of a clear boundary between self and others. This category is rarely observed in a stable state prior to preadolescence. In childhood, according to Pine, these children manifest tendencies toward intellectualization, omnipotence, projection, and splitting. Therefore, as adults, these children may tend toward paranoid character.

From the foregoing discussion it is evident that the etiology and dynamics inherent in the development of a borderline personality are extremely diverse, leaving much room for individual adaptation dependent on temperament and many other factors. As Pine (1982) noted, "Our diagnostic terms are discontinuous, whereas human phenomena are continuous" (p. 865). Nevertheless, as Pine and others have demonstrated, it is possible to perceive broad patterns within borderline organization.

Carryover of Borderline Development into Adolescence

What is the consequence in adolescence of the various childhood patterns of borderline personality organization? As Kernberg (1975) has pointed out, the borderline states in childhood and adolescence can be defined more in terms of developmental level than in terms of an intrinsic type of psychopathology. Theoretically, the characteristics of borderline states—lack of internal integration of aspects of the self and confusion about object relations—should tend toward stability, since early defense mechanisms are seized upon and retained at all costs, including the cost of further development. In support of this contention, the same brittle defenses used by borderline children have been noted in borderline adolescents, but with a somewhat more refined ability to mobilize them into action (Rosenfeld & Sprince, 1963).

These considerations notwithstanding, the question of the stability of borderline states is an important one. The following discussion centers on the stability of the borderline condition in adolescence and on the validity of diagnosing children as borderline as opposed to some other psychiatric condition.

VALIDITY AND STABILITY OF BORDERLINE STATES IN CHILDREN AND ADOLESCENTS

Greg: Very Troubled But Not Borderline

Greg is a 4-year, 2-month-old boy who lives with both of his parents. His father works full time as a businessman, and his mother works part time selling real estate. Greg attends nursery school and is going into a class for 4-year-olds. He was held back for a year when he was 3. Greg's parents adopted him when he was 5 days old; they could not have children due to a combined subfertility of both parents. Greg lives with no brothers or sisters, and he has stated a desire for siblings.

Greg's parents have noted no abnormalities in his speech or motor development. Greg was bottle-fed, and he took the bottle to bed until age 4. His parents have commented that Greg is not especially curious; they feel that they often tell him more than he is interested in learning. His parents, teachers, and camp counselors all have noted an absence of attention at times; Greg will stare into space and detach himself from environmental happenings. When Greg is angry, he leaves the situation instead of confronting issues or initiating conflict. If he becomes frustrated in play, he may speak to his toys or smash them together. Greg has only one friend, a girl who is a year younger than he; Greg idolizes her and believes everything she tells him. In school, Greg has difficulty paying attention to assignments or class activities. In groups, with other children, he tends to be disruptive and silly. He tries to avoid new situations and becomes very quiet when confronted with new people, especially adults.

Greg's teacher noted that Greg has begun to have trouble pulling his pants up after using the bathroom. His parents added that he avoids getting dressed in the morning and has an especially difficult time putting on his pants (to the extent that his parents must help him). Greg runs awkwardly, holding his hands flush to his sides. If he is being particularly slow or recalcitrant, Greg's mother will tell him that she is leaving. When used by his mother or by his teachers at school, this technique invariably serves to motivate Greg to do whatever task is demanded. Greg responds to others' demands by pouting and staring at the floor, which his teacher has described as "putting up a wall." Although Greg does function better in small groups than in large groups, he has never avoided school, and he seems to want to be with other children.

Greg was referred for evaluation because his parents and teacher thought it would be important to assess the possible future implications of this combination of characteristic behaviors. During the interview, Greg demonstrated clear thought processes and the ability to differentiate between right and wrong. His speech and range of affect were assessed as normal. While his mood was generally good, it was variable, with downturns when he was asked to do something he did not want to do. Greg responded negatively to requests by assuming a demeanor that almost suggested he was in another world. Greg did respond positively to a request to draw, after much coaxing and after checking with his mother. However, he displayed extreme concern that he could not draw well and was unable to even draw an "X." Greg would not talk about his worries that he was unable to draw; instead, he became silent and refused to acknowledge his concerns. Greg has no known physical problems, but does complain of frequent stomachaches for which a doctor could identify no explanatory physical cause. Other elements of the mental status examination were judged to be developmentally appropriate.

A first consideration in Greg's case is the apparent lag in development of motor coordination. His awkward stance while running, his inability to dress himself, and his inability to draw even a simple letter indicate impairment in the development of fine motor skills. These symptoms indicate a diagnosis of developmental coordination disorder because Greg has no explanatory physical problem and because the motoric skills deficiency interferes with his participation in group and individual activities. Greg's expression of fear with regard to his inability to draw was followed by avoidance of admission of a problem. Greg's usual pattern of response to fear (e.g., of meeting new people), coupled with his wishes to have social relationships (as expressed by his desire to attend school), implies an additional diagnosis—avoidant disorder of childhood. In the assessment interview with a clinician who was a stranger, Greg was embarrassed and, at points, withdrawn.

In differentiating Greg's symptoms, it was determined that his avoidance is not due to social reticence, since he does not seem to be able to warm up to new people even after some time passes. Separation anxiety disorder was also ruled out because Greg displays only slight difficulties in departing from his major attachment figures and because he displays no other associated symptoms. The social isolation and withdrawal he occasionally effects are specific to situations in which there are new people, and they are not generalized as they would be if Greg were suffering from depression or dysthymia. Adjustment disorder with withdrawal was also ruled out as an associated diagnosis because there was no identifiable stressor within 6 months prior to the manifestation of the abnormal behaviors.

Examination of criteria indicating a diagnosis of overanxious disorder did not rule out this disorder as an associated diagnosis. Greg does seem to have excessive anxiety regarding fears of abandonment, as indicated both by the nature of his responses to the threat of someone leaving and by his need to check with his mother before agreeing to draw during the interview. Greg's stomachaches that arise when he is faced with the challenge of meeting new people might also be explained as a response to his anxiety about social competence. Greg's worries about being unable to draw convey self-consciousness, and his response to a request to draw that came only after receiving his mother's approval and repeated assurances from the therapist that he could not do it wrong indicate an excessive need for assurance and approval of others.

A differential diagnosis of overanxious disorder in addition to that of avoidant disorder included an examination for symptomatology of attention deficit hyperactive disorder. This was ruled out based on the absence of indicators of hyperactivity in Greg's behavior. Greg's anxiety was not related to an identifiable stressor, nor to a psychotic or mood disorder, so adjustment, psychotic, and mood disorders were all ruled out.

The assessment, then, points to a three-part diagnosis: developmental coordination disorder, avoidant disorder of childhood, and overanxious disorder. It was recommended that more neurological and cognitive testing be done to ascertain whether the abnormalities might be genetically related (e.g., fragile-X chromosome syndrome). Future interactions with Greg must include attempts to clarify whether Greg's difficulties are centered around specific fears such as fear of growing up and being independent or fear of being unable to complete a task successfully.

Validity of the Borderline Diagnosis in Children

The complexities in arriving at an accurate diagnosis in Greg's case demonstrate that the scheme presented by Pine (1986) and the schemes of many others (e.g., Ekstein & Wallerstein, 1954; Greenman et al., 1986; Weil, 1956), while logical and elegant, require a final test of validity for the diagnosis of borderline disorder in children through empirical research. Verhulst (1984), noting the lack of controlled studies in which borderline children are compared to children with other diagnoses, undertook to make this comparison.

Verhulst evaluated many diverse studies and selected a set of 28 items that was used to differentiate borderline children from neurotic and overtly psychotic children. Child psychiatrists in Holland were sent questionnaires, and information was received on 57 borderline children, 69 neurotic children, and 47 children who were diagnosed as psychotic. In keeping with the noted failure to develop the signal function of anxiety, anxiety was the main affect reported for borderline children that distinguished them from neurotic children. The best criteria for overall detection of borderline children were demanding, clinging, and unpredictable relationships; primitive defense mechanisms; shifting levels of ego functioning; micropsychotic states; suspicious or paranoid behavior; and marked fantasy activity.

An interesting outcome of this study was that the difference between neurotic and borderline children was much more definite than that between the borderline and psychotic children. Compared to the psychotic children, the borderline children were more unpredictable in their private day-to-day functioning and their interpersonal relationships. Also, the borderline children did not insist as stridently on sameness and withdrawal from contact as did the psychotic children.

It is interesting to note that, in support of his analysis, Pine (1974, 1982) previously made the observation that the distinction between borderline disorder and psychosis is less clear than the one between borderline and neurosis. Thus, while there is good evidence from this study supporting the autonomous existence of the borderline syndrome, it appears that the diagnosis of chronic psychosis versus borderline disorder is a more difficult differential diagnosis.

Stability of Borderline States from Adolescence to Adulthood

Given the results of Verhulst and the consistency of systems worked out after exhaustive observation by Pine and others, it appears that the borderline state describes a true clinical category in much the same way as do the terms neurosis and psychosis. However, to date there has been little or no definitive research delineating subclassification of the borderline state, nor has the stability of this condition been adequately tested.

An excellent start in describing the stability of the borderline diagnosis has been made by Aarkrog (1981), who evaluated 50 borderline adolescents at the time of hospitalization and 5 following discharge from an adolescent ward. Of these patients, 29 had been psychiatrically examined during childhood as well, while the remainder had not. Of 11 children diagnosed as having infantile borderline psychoses, 9 (82%) retained this diagnosis in adolescence. One was diagnosed in adolescence as having a pseudoneurotic borderline state and the other was diagnosed with pseudopsychopathic borderline state. In terms of the predicted diagnoses at discharge, of 43 adolescents who were admitted with borderline conditions, 30 (70%) were assessed as being borderline 5 years later. Given the very high stability of borderline personality organization observed in this study (82% from childhood to adolescence and 70% from adolescence to early adulthood), this diagnostic category clearly warrants the considerable attention it is now receiving.

CONCLUSION

In terms of diagnosing and treating children with borderline personality organizations, it is best to keep in mind that the characteristic feature of a borderline individual is comprised not of his or her symptoms, but of the severe disturbance of the personality structure. Rather than arrested development, there is skewed development. This perturbation in the natural evolution of personality is evident during the school-age period because the expected degree of character stability and socialization is absent.

Most critical is the necessity of recognizing the interference of primitive defense mechanisms in developing the signal function of anxiety. In order to reinstitute growth in borderline individuals, reactive panic must be eliminated or at least greatly reduced. Thus, it is necessary not merely to educate but to undo and resolve character pathology and conflict configurations. This undeniably takes time, as was evidenced in the study by Verhulst (1984) in which prolonged contact with borderline cases was necessary just to arrive at the diagnosis.

There are few data on how best to treat certain types of borderline patients because these types are still in the process of being described. Nevertheless, Pine (1974) observed that for children evidencing internal disorganization in response to external disorganizers, rescue is the first line of treatment. That is, these children must be removed from their disorganizing environment. Beyond this step, therapy remains difficult.

Perhaps the most promising therapeutic technique was illustrated by Holman (1985). Holman set up a time-limited treatment program with mothers diagnosed as borderline who had toddlers. Because of the strong contribution to borderline states from early difficulties in separation-individuation, the focus of the work with the toddlers was on expanding their efforts to master tasks and relationships outside the mother-child dyad. Therapy for the mothers was centered on their difficulties with emotional separation-individuation and on strengthening ego function. For example, the mothers were encouraged to recognize that their own feelings of rage on termination of therapy mirrored the current attitudes of their children.

Certainly, such intervention programs promise to lessen the likelihood or severity of borderline development. Considering the stubbornness of this condition to diagnosis and treatment, prevention seems a much easier and more promising route than does prolonged therapy.

CHAPTER TWELVE

Affective Disorders and Their Differential Diagnosis

Mary: Pervasive Sadness

Mary is a 5-year-old who lives with her grandmother because her mother feels that she already has enough children to care for. Mary's father is a substance abuser who sees his daughter sporadically. During the past 5 years, Mary has been in and out of foster homes and has lived with friends of her mother and with her father for a very brief period. Mary's grandmother was in the process of gaining legal custody when Mary called her to say that her father had left her alone for a day. It was then that Mary's grandmother removed Mary from her father's care.

Mary's grandmother did not have information about Mary's developmental milestones, but Mary is in kindergarten and is currently doing satisfactorily. Mary's grandmother brought Mary for assessment because she noticed a change from her granddaughter's previously predominantly "happy, carefree mood" and because she felt that Mary has experienced much emotional upset as a result of her unpredictable environment. Her grandmother described Mary's behavior during the past month as changed from before, with recent whining and crying, a decreased appetite, trouble falling asleep, and frequent vomiting after meals. Her teacher reported that Mary cries at school and is unable to share. Mary has trouble responding when the teacher or her grandmother set limits, and lately she has begun pulling her hair out.

During assessment, Mary appeared neat and clean and was dressed in appropriate clothing. Her speech was very quiet and somewhat childish. Mary displayed a full range of affect, with immediate attachment to the therapist and sadness and crying at the session's close. No suicidal tendencies were elicited, and attention and memory were assessed as normal, as were other elements of the mental status examination.

Mary's dramatic change in mood and the concomitant emergence of problems at school point toward the characteristics of a major depressive episode. Her irritability, quiet speech, decreased appetite, and recurrent insomnia are all symptoms commonly found in major depression. The evidence of somatic difficulties (her vomiting after meals) and the psychomotor abnormalities evidenced (pulling out her hair) are particularly characteristic of depression in prepubertal children. To confirm the diagnosis of a major depressive episode, other differential diagnoses were ruled out. The stresses of repeated moves and of separation from both of her parents, which could cause Mary to feel rejected or unwanted, are likely risk factors for the development of her depression.

The absence of an organic factor that could have initiated and maintained Mary's depressed mood rules out the diagnosis of organic mood syndrome with depression. Schizophrenia and schizoaffective disorder were both ruled out because Mary revealed no psychotic symptoms. Uncomplicated bereavement was also ruled out as a part of Mary's depressed mood because there was no actual or perceived death to which she was reacting. A diagnosis of a major depressive episode was thus assigned, and further history taking with Mary's biological parents was recommended as well as subsequent individual twice-weekly therapy for Mary.

INTRODUCTION

Classically, the dysphoria noted in depressed individuals has been ascribed either to endogenous or to exogenous (including neurotic) sources. In Mary's case, the latter seems to apply. Prior to effective drug therapies, individuals with endogenous, or psychotic, depression were hospitalized, while those with nonendogenous depression were treated with psychotherapy. Following the advent of chemical treatments for depression, many of those who were previously hospitalized were effectively treated on an outpatient basis, while exogenous depression, viewed as being caused by psychosocial stressors, continued to be treated with psychotherapy—sometimes in conjunction with antidepressant medication. Regardless of this trend in treatment, diagnosis remains somewhat confounded by the fact that judgments regarding situational depression and those pertaining to endogenous states are still held to be independent. Therefore, criteria for both diagnoses may easily be met simultaneously (Hirschfeld, Klerman, Andreasen, Clayton, & Keller, 1985).

Subsequent to the radical improvements in antidepressant treatment in the 1960's, theorists have been caught up in the process of deciding whether the discontinuous endogenous–exogenous formulation is in fact correct or whether the various depressive states might be placed on a continuum from endogenous to nonendogenous. For purposes of detecting and treating depressive mood in children, it may be that neither case applies. During childhood, it is possible that depression, in its general form, is associated with a series of symptom complexes whose manner of expression is tied to the level of the child's development.

In adults, as described in DSM-III-R, there is an implicit assumption of continuity among depressive states, since dysthymic disorder (nonendogenous depression) is defined essentially as a less severe form of major, or endogenous, depression. However, due to the intensity and rapidity of physiological and psychological developmental events, it is much more difficult to make the supposition of continuity of mood disorders in children.

Recent studies do suggest, however, that developmental changes over time may only have mild to moderate effects on the expression of affective symptoms. For example, Ryan, Ledger, and Weed (1987) compared symptom frequencies in two clinically referred samples of 95 children and 92 adolescents. The age range of the patients was from 6 to 18 years.

For the majority of depressive symptoms there were no significant differences between the two groups. However, prepubertal children were observed to have greater depressed appearance and more somatic complaints, psychomotor agitation, separation anxiety, phobias, and hallucinations. Adolescents, on the other hand, showed greater anhedonia, hopelessness, hypersomnia, weight change, and lethality of suicide attempt.

Results such as these do not support the assumptions of most of the preceding 20th century, when the mere idea that children could experience debilitating depression was unacceptable to psychologists and laymen alike. The understanding that children do suffer from mood disorders comparable to those of adults has only gradually come to be accepted over the past 20 years. Since this recognition is relatively new, the diagnostic criteria for adult depression as outlined in DSM-III-R are still the primary means used to diagnose depression in children.

The standardization achieved by the application of DSM-III-R criteria to all depressive states is beneficial; however, the specific criteria fail to adjust sufficiently for the differences between the adult and childhood states. These differences may arise from the interaction of a consistent dysphoric syndrome with developmental changes in physiology, biochemistry, and psychology, or the nature of depressive disorders themselves may undergo developmental age and stage changes (Trad, 1986, 1987).

Thus, it may actually prove counterproductive to make any assumption regarding the continuity or duality of affective disorders in children. In the absence of supporting evidence for either case, the most productive approach appears to be the one in which particular developmental milestones are measured and taken into account when analyzing a given set of symptoms that are suspected as being indicative of depression. This is the approach attempted by most of those who have studied the nature of depression in childhood.

While use of the full DSM-III and DSM-III-R criteria for adult depression can prove useful in diagnosing depression in children, Kashani, Ray, and Carlson (1984); Kashani, Carlson, Horwitz, and Reid (1985); Kashani, Holcomb, and Orvaschel (1986); Kashani, Horwitz, Ray, and Reid (1986); Kashani and Ray (1987); and Kashani and Carlson (1985) have concentrated on symptoms that are clearly measurable in childhood. Symptoms such as simple sadness are indicative of depression in children, even though they would be insufficient to diagnose major depression according to DSM-III-R criteria in adults. This approach seems to be particularly justified in the case of preschool-age children. Not only are children in this age group difficult to assess in terms of mood, they are highly energetic and have a limited ability to conceptualize and express their feelings.

Clearly the task of finding certain clusters of symptoms that describe a depressive syndrome is more feasible, or at least simpler, when applied to mature (i.e., developed) individuals than when applied to children. Therefore, when diagnosing and treating children at this point in nosological development, it seems wiser to follow the course of Kashani and others, concentrating on symptomatology alone and attempting to isolate depressive symptoms that may be intrinsic to the developmental stage of the child. Not only is there insufficient information to define discrete depressive syndromes in this age group, but the superimposition of adult criteria would very likely result in failure to diagnose children who are depressed but do not exhibit traditional (i.e., adult-like) symptom complexes (Kashani et al., 1984).

As an example, severe dysphoria in adults may be accompanied by anhedonia, sleep and appetite disturbances, loss of energy, psychomotor retardation or agitation, feelings of self-reproach or guilt, and inability to concentrate. While these symptoms describe major depression in adults, there is some evidence suggesting that it is not sadness alone but anger that is the predominant feeling of a depressed preschooler (Kashani & Carlson, 1985, 1987; Kashani et al., 1986).

Obviously, the features associated with sadness are different from those that accompany anger, yet both, depending on the developmental stage of the individual, may be indicative of depression. Therefore, it is important to remain free of adult biases regarding the nature of depression in children. While the ensuing discussion will begin with DSM-III-R criteria for adult depression, some of which may in fact generalize to at least certain age categories of children, epidemiological and longitudinal studies will be examined in an effort to define differences in the depressed state between adults and children and between age groups of children.

DIFFERENTIAL DIAGNOSIS OF DEPRESSION

Definitions: DSM-III-R Criteria

Major Depressive Episode. The chief feature of an episode of major depression is dysphoric mood or loss of pleasure in all usual activities and pastimes (for children and adolescents depressed mood may be signified by irritability, and in children under 6 dysphoric mood may be expressed by persistently sad facial expression). The dysphoric mood may thus be characterized by such symptoms as being "down in the dumps" or irritable.

The mood disturbance must be prominent and relatively persistent, but it need not be the most dominant symptom. The diagnosis of a major depression does not include momentary shifts from one dysphoric mood to another affective state (e.g., anxiety to depression to anger, such as seen in states of acute psychotic turmoil).

At least five of the following nine symptoms must have been present concurrently, nearly every day, for a period of at least 2 weeks. Also, at least one of the symptoms must be either depressed mood or loss of interest or pleasure.

(1) *depressed mood (or can be irritable mood in children and adolescents) most of the day, nearly every day, as indicated either by subjective accounts or observation by others*

(2) *markedly diminished interest or pleasure in all, or almost all, activities most of the day, nearly every day (as indicated either by subjective account or observation by others of apathy most of the time)*

(3) *significant weight loss or weight gain when not dieting (e.g., more than 5% of body weight in a month), or decrease or increase in appetite nearly every day (in children, consider failure to make expected weight gains)*

(4) *insomnia or hypersomnia nearly every day*

(5) *psychomotor agitation or retardation nearly every day (observable by others, not merely subjective feelings of restlessness or being slowed down)*

(6) *fatigue or loss of energy nearly every day*

(7) *feelings of worthlessness or excessive or inappropriate guilt (which may be delusional) nearly every day (not merely self-reproach or guilt about being sick)*

(8) *diminished ability to think or concentrate, or indecisiveness, nearly every day (either by subjective account or as observed by others)*

(9) *recurrent thoughts of death (not just fear of dying), recurrent suicidal ideation without a specific plan, or a suicide attempt or a specific plan for committing suicide* (DSM-III-R, pp. 222–223)

People experiencing a major depressive episode commonly describe their mood as depressed, sad, down, or hopeless, but some do not consciously recognize their sadness and instead describe their mood as "not caring anymore." Appetite disturbances usually take the form of loss of appetite, but overeating may occur in some cases. Similarly, sleep disturbance is usually in the form of insomnia or early waking, but may on occasion manifest as hypersomnia.

Psychomotor agitation involves restlessness; pacing; hand-wringing; rubbing of hair, skin, or clothing; or vocal outbursts. Conversely, psychomotor retardation may be evidenced in slowed or blurred speech, excessive pauses in conversation, or slowed body movements.

A diagnosis of major depression precludes bizarre behavior or preoccupation with a mood-incongruent delusion in the absence of the affective syndrome. Also, the depression cannot be due to any organic mental disorder or uncomplicated bereavement, nor can it be superimposed on either schizophrenia, schizophreniform disorder, delusional disorder, or psychotic disorder.

Major depression may also occur with psychotic features and/or melancholia. Psychotic features, indicative of gross impairment of reality testing, include delusions or hallucinations or depressive stupor. The psychotic features may be either mood congruent or incongruent. Mood congruent delusions or hallucinations are those whose content is entirely consistent with the themes of either personal guilt, inadequacy, disease, death, nihilism, or deserved punishment. Mood incongruent features, on the other hand, are signified by delusions or hallucinations not involving these themes but instead including such symptoms as persecutory delusions, thought insertion, thought broadcasting, and delusions of control.

Exclusion Criteria for Major Depression. In DSM-III-R, major depression is defined as much by what it is not as by what it is. A diagnosis of major depressive episode requires that the possibilities of an organic factor or uncomplicated bereavement be eliminated. Organic mental syndromes may be confused with depression principally in the area of delusional content. Organic mental syndromes are marked by hallucinations, delusions, and disordered thinking and speech. In delirium, for example, these symptoms are random and haphazard, without evidence of systematization. The course fluctuates, and there is evidence of a clouded state of consciousness with global cognitive impairment. Finally, in delirium there is often a generalized slowing in EEG background, indicating an organic etiology.

More generally, in the organic mental syndromes as a whole, there are disorientation or impairment of memory and clinical features that develop over a short period of time (hours or days) and tend to fluctuate over the course of a day. Finally, there must be evidence from the history, physical examination, or laboratory tests of a specific organic factor judged to be etiologically related to the disturbance.

Thus, it is apparent that the delusions or hallucinations that may accompany some cases of major depression are, as a rule, accompanied by less overall impairment of function than is seen in cases of organic mental syndromes. Futhermore, if organic mental syndromes are suspected, laboratory tests and EEG measurements will likely prove more definitive than these tests for major depression.

Differentiating major depression from uncomplicated bereavement is simpler than differentiating it from organic mental disorders, since there is a clear loss preceding the bereaved state. This loss is commonly associated with guilt about things that were done or not done prior to the time of death of the loved one. Reaction to the loss may not be immediate, but it rarely occurs later than 2 or 3 months following the loss. The duration of normal bereavement varies considerably among different subcultural groups, but usually does not extend beyond 6 months to a year. However, morbid preoccupation with worthlessness, suicidal ideation, marked functional impairment, or psychomotor retardation may indicate bereavement complicated by major depression.

In addition to eliminating the presence of bereavement and organic brain syndromes, DSM-III-R requires that the possible presence of a less severe form of unipolar depression—dysthymic disorder—also be ruled out when making a diagnosis of major depression. Furthermore, there can be no delusional episodes.

The essential features of dysthymic depression or depressive neurosis are a chronically depressed mood and anhedonia that are not sufficiently intense to qualify as a major depressive episode. This mood may be continuous or intermittent with periods of normal mood and functioning. If the periods of normal functioning with absence of depression last more than 2 months, dysthymia cannot be diagnosed.

During the depressive periods, at least two of the following six symptoms must be present: (1) insomnia or hypersomnia; (2) low energy level or chronic tiredness; (3) low self-esteem; (4) poor appetite or overeating; (5) decreased attention, concentration, or ability to think clearly; and (6) feelings of hopelessness.

While dysthymic disorder is a unipolar condition and must be differentiated from major depression (which is also unipolar), it is further necessary to establish that the major depressed state is not in actuality one phase of a bipolar disorder. Information regarding the nature of childhood depressive disorders is scarce, and information regarding bipolar mood disorders in children is even more sparse. The DSM-III-R classifies bipolar disorder into three categories—mixed, manic, and depressed—and there is mounting evidence showing that bipolar disorder is inherited by children of parents with the disorder more often than by children of unaffected parents (Andreasen et al., 1987; Rice et al., 1987).

However, the level of heritability and the degree to which the condition may reflect a biological vulnerability or merely a set of repeated, troubled familial interactions remains unknown. Kestenbaum (1982) speculated that when bipolar disorder occurs in children (a rare event) it may be useful in revealing "specific equivalent behaviors that are the precursors of the cyclothymic personality and manic-depressive states of young adulthood" (p. 248). Feinstein further postulated that the affective/limbic system in cases of manic-depression may possess a basic vulnerability leading to drastic, uncontrollable shifts in mood when it becomes overstimulated. If this is true, great benefit might derive from closer study of this condition in children.

As a final consideration, in addition to bipolar disorder and the other types of depression discussed so far, the DSM-III posited a third residual category of depression in adults termed *atypical depression.* In DSM-III-R, this category has been changed to *depressive disorder not otherwise specified.* In either case, the category pertains to individuals with depressive symptoms who cannot be diagnosed as having a major or other specific affective disorder or adjustment disorder.

James: A Year of Change and Loss

James is a $4\frac{1}{2}$-year-old boy who lives with his mother and his older brother. His parents separated a few months ago, following more than a year of loud verbal parental fights that were witnessed by James and his brother. James's father has expressed suicidal wishes and has been hospitalized for depression since the separation. James's mother reports that in the past James was always high-spirited, energetic, and could be difficult to control. During the past year, however, James's mother has noted that he is less energetic and often complains of being tired. She told of an incident when James ran into the street because he wanted to die after she yelled at him (he was not harmed). James's development has been normal except that speech was delayed until age 3. He also has a history of ear infections with intermittent hearing loss.

In school, James has sought out teachers to tell them that he is "stupid, dumb, and wants to die." He also has told them that he would kill himself by jumping off a roof or ingesting poisonous detergents. During class, James has trouble concentrating, and sometimes he loses control of himself. At the close of the school day, James often cries and screams that he does not want to go home. The school insisted that James be psychiatrically evaluated.

During assessment, James stated suicidal wishes. While playing, James and his brother—who was in for evaluation concurrently—were extremely aggressive and violent toward each other and toward the female therapist. James said that he was "angry" at his mother about her decision to divorce his father. It is noteworthy that, when James sees his father, his father asks about the mother's activities and blames her for all the problems leading to the divorce. James became noticeably distressed when the therapist asked him when he would see his father next. He said that he "worries about his father." James also alluded to his own feelings of sadness and despair and to his feelings of uncontrollability regarding the abandonment by his father, whom he rarely sees. Other elements of the mental status examination were developmentally appropriate.

The change in James from an energetic child who was difficult to control to an angry, hopeless, suicidal child occurred over more than 1 year, indicating that a dysthymia diagnosis is appropriate. James's feelings of abandonment and rejection may be predisposing risk factors to his condition, as might be the presence of depressive symptoms in his father. The degree of impairment in James's level of functioning, along with the inability of James, his mother, and his teacher to label a recognizable onset of James's transformation, indicate that his depressive symptoms are not in the context of a major depressive episode. James's symptoms are not part of any personality disorder.

Further assessment suggested that James's aggression and violence toward the female therapist are symptoms of his need for autonomy from his mother, and at other times his behavior suggested that he sought love and sought to boost his feelings of self-worth. The conclusion from assessment was that James suffers from dysthymia and that his mild, chronically depressed feelings, his fatigue, and his poor concentration can be remedied via individual therapy and weekly joint sessions with his brother and his brother's therapist.

Dysthymia.   The DSM-III-R delineates a second form of unipolar depression labeled *dysthymia* or *depressive neurosis* that is less intense than major depression. The essential features of this disorder were demonstrated by James, who was experiencing a chronically depressed mood and anhedonia that were not sufficiently intense to qualify as a major depressive episode. This mood may be continuous or intermittent with periods of normal functioning. If the periods of normal functioning last more than a few months, dysthymia cannot be diagnosed. Also, delusional episodes must not be present. During the depressive periods, at least two of the following six symptoms must be present:

(1) poor appetite or overeating

(2) insomnia or hypersomnia

(3) low energy or fatigue

(4) low self-esteem

(5) poor concentration or difficulty making decisions

(6) feelings of hopelessness. (DSM-III-R, pp. 232–233)

Seasonal Affective Disorder.   In differentially diagnosing depression, the clinician should always be alert to a possible seasonal pattern in the affected child. Seasonal affective disorder is characterized by recurrent fall and winter depressions that remit during the spring and summer (Rosenthal et al., 1986). While approximately 42% of adult patients who have seasonal affective disorder apparently experienced onset during childhood or adolescence, the symptoms are generally milder and not as clear-cut in childhood (Rosenthal & Rosenthal, 1984).

Children commonly experience the symptoms as being external in origin and fail to recognize the seasonal pattern.

Rosenthal and colleagues (1986) recommended that this condition be treated in adults and children by exposure to bright artificial light for 5 to 6 hours per day, although there is some indication that children may require less than this amount. Because it is easily treatable, the possibility of seasonal affective disorder should always be considered in children who have difficulties in school or at home that are most noticeable or prevalent in the fall-winter semester.

Depressive Disorder Not Otherwise Stated. In addition to major depression and dysthymia, the DSM-III-R posits this third, residual category of depression in adults. This category pertains to individuals with depressive symptoms who cannot be diagnosed as having a major or other specific affective disorder or adjustment disorder.

Depressive disorder not otherwise specified was labeled *atypical depression* in DSM-III. This term was originally used by West and Dally (1959) to identify a group of depressed patients who showed preferential response to the monoamine oxidase inhibitor iproniazid phosphate. Since that time, the term has been used widely and fairly indiscriminately, making precise definition difficult. For example, DSM-III-R uses this term to describe three different syndromes: major depression occurring with underlying schizophrenia, dysthymia with periods of normal mood lasting more than a few months, and any uncategorizable brief depressive episodes.

According to Davidson, Miller, Turnbull, and Sullivan (1982), other descriptions of atypical depression fall into two broad categories. The first is anxious depression (type A). Associated symptoms include anxiety, phobia, tension, and pain. The depression is mild, nonpsychotic, and rarely requires hospitalization. The second category of atypical depression describes a nonanxious form with atypical vegetative symptoms (type V). Associated symptoms include increases in weight and changes in appetite, libido, and sleep with mood lability.

Nondepressive Conditions in Children with Depressive Features

Joshua: Too Much Inconsistency

Joshua is a 5-year-old boy who lives with his mother, his father, and, until recently, his older sister. Joshua's father has been married four times. Joshua's mother is reportedly "narcissistic, moody, short-fused, unstable, inconsistent, and unable to separate from either of her children." Joshua's mother refused to nurse him and claimed that he would "wake her up at 2 A.M." When she went back to work 3 months after giving birth, Joshua was subjected to a succession of babysitters, one of whom set no limits and another who died. Both of Joshua's parents smile as they reprimand him. Joshua had a perfect birth, and his medical history consists of mild asthma and a sickle-cell trait. His developmental milestones were all reported to be normal.

Joshua's nursery school referred him for assessment 2 years ago primarily because he was aggressive to the extent that he required one-on-one supervision. Joshua would provoke and hit his classmates and use profanity. He would cry when limits of any sort were imposed on him, he could not articulate properly, and he referred to himself in the third person. Joshua's parents called him a "terror" who always wants his way immediately. He was described as a demanding, active and "uppity" child and had for the preceding 3 or 4 weeks begun to steal things (e.g, pencils, toys, blocks) from his classmates. He also liked to throw and bang his toys.

During assessment, Joshua, a good-looking, well-dressed child, exhibited constricted affect (denied sadness and fear) and extreme mood lability, changing quickly from laughter to tears and from friendliness to withdrawal. He denied having nightmares or self-destructive behaviors; his thought content, however, consisted primarily of "fires, wolves, broken ceilings, and children who have been abandoned or hurt." Joshua's fine motor skills were normal and his articulation was poor.

Joshua's behavior (namely, his hyperactivity, impulsiveness, use of profanity, reaction to limit-setting, and aggressiveness) implied that a diagnosis of attention deficit hyperactivity disorder was an appropriate one. This disorder is a common predisposing factor of dysthymia. In addition, Joshua's upbringing in a disorganized and rejecting environment made him more susceptible to dysthymia.

Major depression could be ruled out in this case; Joshua's long-lasting behavior was characteristic of a chronic mild depressive syndrome such as dysthymia rather than the acute changes that can be distinguished in a major depression. Oppositional defiant disorder also can be ruled out, for it is invalid if it occurs during the course of a dysthymic disorder. It is also clear that Joshua's mood swings were more severe than would be expected if they were merely developmentally appropriate fluctuations.

Thus a diagnosis of dysthymia was appropriate. It was recommended that Joshua have weekly therapy with the goal of increasing his frustration tolerance and helping to delay gratification. Both parents were to be seen occasionally, and Joshua's mother was referred to treatment as well.

Attention Deficit Disorder.   Fundamentally, there are six psychiatric diagnoses that are most often confused with major affective disorders in children and adolescents: attention deficit disorder, conduct disorder, anxiety disorders, eating disorders, substance abuse, and schizophrenia (Garfinkel, 1986). Attention deficit disorder enters into the differential diagnosis of depression because, according to DSM-III-R, it shares with depression the associated symptoms of increased psychomotor activity, difficulty in concentrating, mood lability, and occasional sleep disturbance. The primary area of risk lies in mistaking attention deficit disorder for dysthymia, due to the similarity of symptomatologies and the chronicity of both conditions, as can be seen in Joshua's case.

Conduct Disorder. Several researchers have found an association between major depression and conduct disorders in prepubertal and adolescent boys. Cytryn, McKnew, and Levy (1972) described antisocial behavior as a form of "masked depression," in which depression is acted out in the guise of delinquent behavior. Carlson and Cantwell's (1980) study of depressed children showed a high incidence of concurrent conduct disorders (32%), and Chiles, Miller, and Cox's (1980) study of admissions to a correctional facility (ages 13 to 15) found 23% of the cases to have major depressive disorder.

Puig-Antich (1982) studied 43 prepubertal boys admitted to a child depression clinic. He found that 37% of these patients met Research Diagnostic Criteria (RDC) (Spitzer et al., 1978) for conduct disorder. In the same period, none of the prepubertal girls met these criteria. Comparison of the boys who had conduct disorders with those who did not showed no significant differences in the clinical picture of the depression or in demographic variables such as socioeconomic status (SES), race, or age of admission to the clinic (average age 9 to 10 years). The types of behaviors that came under the heading of conduct disorders in this sample included chronic violation of rules at school and home (87% of the sample), fighting (75%), pathological lying (50%), stealing (44%), firesetting (31%), and truancy (31%). Behavior patterns were not significantly different between those with endogenous and those with nonendogenous depression, but the boys who had psychotic depressions showed a higher average number of antisocial acts.

In most of the cases (87%), the depression predated the conduct disorder, and when treated with antidepressant medication (Imipramine) the conduct disorders ceased in 11 out of 13 boys who showed antidepressive response. Puig-Antich's sample had histories of adverse conditions affecting their psychological well-being that were identifiable as risk factors for affective disorder. These included worse family situations than the group without concurrent conduct disorders and a greater incidence of psychiatric hospitalization. Of the 13 boys, 9 had been hospitalized because their antisocial and/or suicidal behavior had proved dangerous to themselves or to others.

In addressing the question as to whether the mixture of major depression with conduct disorder is a clinical entity fundamentally different from major depression, Puig-Antich concluded that the depression is the same whether a conduct disorder is superimposed or not. He further suggested that "the major depressive syndrome may play an important role as trigger for the emergence and persistence of conduct disorder patterns" (p. 125). If this hypothesis is correct, major depressive disorder may also be a risk factor for anxiety disorders, since there is equally strong evidence of the association of major depression with anxiety. Furthermore, as Marriage, Fine, Moretti, and Haley (1986) have noted, there are also implications for treatment of children with conduct disorder and depression. Such children or adolescents may respond well to antidepressant medication, with their troublesome behavior abating through alleviation of their depression.

Anxiety Disorders. Anxiety and depression frequently coexist in a manner that makes it difficult to assess which is the primary condition. Depression places the individual at risk for anxiety due to concern over his or her decreased ability to cope. Conversely, anxiety over the perceived reduced ability to cope can produce depression secondary to feelings of incompetence. Furthermore, there is strong evidence suggesting that these two conditions may be biochemically interrelated, since antidepressant medication (MAO inhibitors and tricyclics) also alleviate symptoms of panic disorder (Breier, Charney, & Heninger, 1985).

Adding to the difficulty in differentially diagnosing anxiety and depression is the fact that the symptoms of anxiety disorders are frequently difficult to distinguish from affective symptomatology (Hershberg, Carlson, Cantwell, & Strober, 1982). Symptoms common to depression and anxiety alike include dysphoric mood, sleep and weight disturbances, indecisiveness, agitation, and somatic complaints (Avant, 1984).

In a study of adolescent school refusers, Bernstein and Garfinkel (1986) found a high incidence of symptom overlap between affective and anxiety disorders. School refusal traditionally has been viewed as a function of separation anxiety (Eisenberg, 1958), but in a population with such a large number of risk factors associated with affective disorders, a high incidence of depression is a predictable outcome. Consequently, Bernstein and Garfinkel's findings that their sample showed a large degree of overlap between anxiety and affective disorder is not surprising.

These investigators examined a sample of 26 chronic school refusers aged 9 to 17 years (mean age 13 years, 7 months). Half of the sample were from single-parent families, and two thirds (69%) were from lower-class families according to Hollingshead and Redlich's (1957) scale of socioeconomic status. The investigators found that 54% of the sample had a family history of at least one immediate relative with alcoholism or drug dependency, 27% had family members with affective disorders, and 12% had a family history of anxiety disorders. Only 31% of the sample had no family history of alcoholism, drug dependency, affective disorders, or anxiety disorders.

Of the 26 children studied, 18 suffered from depression and 16 from anxiety, and 13, or half of the sample, had overlapping symptomatology of affective and anxiety disorders. Of these, two patients also had coexisting conduct disorders. The patients diagnosed as depressive suffered from dysphoria. The researchers found, as Sargent and Dally (1962) pointed out, that the symptoms of anxiety and depression were often difficult to separate and it was difficult to determine which was primary and which was secondary.

The overlap of depression and anxiety appeared to present a worse picture than anxiety alone but was not substantially different from depression alone. That is, the patients who had overlapping depression and anxiety had more severe symptoms than those who had only anxiety, but they were rated identical on most scales to the patients with depression alone. This concurs with Kovacs, Feinberg, Crouse-Novak, Paulauskas, and Finkelstein's (1984a) finding that the presence of concurrent anxiety disorders was not a factor affecting the course of major depressive disorder or dysthymic disorder in children, nor did it affect the risk for recurrence of major depression. However, it was found that major depression was a risk factor for exacerbating the effects of anxiety.

As a general guide for differential diagnosis, Roth, Mountjoy, and Caetano (1982), through exhaustive systematic investigations, have demonstrated that early morning awakening, psychomotor retardation, self-reproach, hopelessness, and depression are most indicative of major depression. Patients with anxiety states most often show marked tension, phobias, panic attacks, vasomotor instability, feelings of unreality, perceptual distortions, and paranoid and hypochondriacal ideation.

Schizophrenia.   As in the cases of anxiety, attention deficit disorder, and conduct disorder, differential diagnosis of depressed state in children must take into account the distinctive manifestations of schizophrenia. Several studies have cited a high rate of morbidity for depression among schizophrenic outpatients (Johnson & Rosenblatt, 1981). Epidemiological studies by Watt, Katz, and Sheperd (1983) showed a 40% incidence of depression over a 5-year period among schizophrenics.

Roy (1986) pointed out that depression can occur during any phase of schizophrenic illness—before, during, or after a schizophrenic episode. He reviewed studies citing a rate of attempted suicide among schizophrenics between 18% and 55%. Roy stated that a history of major depressive episodes was more common in a population of schizophrenics who had attempted suicide than among those who had not made suicide attempts. For purposes of treatment, it is useful to know that fewer attempts at suicide were made by schizophrenics while they were in a hospital setting, and Roy found correlations between risk factors for depression (e.g., social isolation, unemployment) and living situations that increased the risk of suicide for many chronic schizophrenics.

AGE-RELATED FORMS OF DEPRESSION

Adolescents

While it is useful to be aware of the many symptom overlaps that can confound an accurate diagnosis of depression in childhood, it is also of practical value to have some idea of the particular guise a depressive state is likely to have at a given stage of development. Unfortunately, much work remains to be done in this area. However, Kandel and Davies (1982) moved in this direction by performing an epidemiological study of 8,000 14- to 18-year-old teenagers in New York state.

The sample was randomly distributed with regard to sex, race, and SES, and data were collected from self-report questionnaires and parental questionnaires. The adolescents were not evaluated according to DSM-III criteria for depression. Instead, they were assessed more globally for depressive mood, a procedure that was likely to be more sensitive in detecting depression in this nonadult age group.

The two strongest demographic relationships found were between depression and sex and family income. Girls showed a substantially higher incidence of depressed mood than boys from age 13 onward. This sex difference was larger than that seen in adulthood. Furthermore, adolescents from families with incomes below $3,000 were found to be more depressed than any other group.

Other findings in this study indicated that self-report of depression was greater among adolescents than among their parents. The strongest association of all was between low self-esteem and depressed mood. Furthermore, peer orientation played a strong role in depressive affect. Teenagers who were delinquent and were oriented toward their peers and away from their parents were more depressed than those who were not delinquent or those with less peer involvement. However, those with little peer involvement were also found to be more depressed than those with positive peer interaction. In sum, teenagers who are isolated from either family or peers may be at greater risk for depression.

One other influence on depressive state was found, that of family decision-making patterns. Teenagers from families that were either highly authoritative or laissez-faire in management attitudes were shown to be more depressed than those from more democratic families. Thus, it seems likely that family functioning and closeness between parents and children (which helps forestall depression) are closely related.

The question of sex differences in depressed mood was examined with regard to the possibility that antisocial behavior in boys takes the place of depressed mood. When the questionnaires were assessed by adding the number of adolescents who were either delinquent *or* depressed, the difference in proportion between boys and girls disappeared. Delinquent behavior is assumed to be more socially acceptable among boys than girls, and girls were found more likely to be both depressed and delinquent than boys. Therefore, it appears that delinquent behavior in boys may indeed reflect depressed mood, since delinquent behavior more easily substitutes for depression in boys than in girls.

The appearance of delinquent behavior in association with depressed state is relevant to one of the few differences between depressed children and depressed adults noted in DSM-III-R: anger. According to the DSM-III-R schema, irritability/anger in children may be the diagnostic equivalent of sadness/depression in adults.

The association between depression and anger was perhaps first noted by Abraham (1927), who distinguished between grief and melancholia. Grief was viewed as a normal response to loss, whereas melancholia contained anger and hostility directed at the lost object. Whether the depressive state is induced by loss or by some other factor commonly seen in the history of depressed children (e.g., abuse), the component of anger may not be directed at the angering object but may be displaced onto less threatening elements of the environment, thus manifesting as conduct disorder.

Investigations are beginning to produce converging evidence of the significance of irritability as symptomatic of depression in children and adolescents. For example, Ryan and co-workers (1987) compared symptom frequency and severity in two sequentially referred samples of 95 children and 92 adolescents between 6 and 18 years of age. All children met unmodified RDC for major depressive disorder. All were medically healthy and were assessed with the Schedule for Affective Disorders and Schizophrenia for School Age Children, Present Episode.

These investigators found relatively little variation in RDC depressive state between childhood and adolescence. Of further significance was the preponderance of symptoms that are frequently recognized as depressive but are not formally a part of RDC or DSM-III-R depressive criteria (e.g., somatic complaints, social withdrawal). In addition, these researchers found irritability/anger to be prevalent in this age group to such a degree that they believe it is a valid criterion for diagnosing depression in children.

Another study in which anger emerged prominently was performed by Kashani and co-workers (1984) using 50 children aged 7 to 16 years whose parents had been diagnosed with an affective disorder (either unipolar or bipolar subtype). Of these children, 14% were found to be depressed according to DSM-III criteria as taken from the Diagnostic Interview for Children and Adolescents. The Diagnostic Interview for Parents of Children and Adolescents was also used to gather data.

Among these children, depression was the most common diagnosis. Furthermore, they were seen to be more abused and more destructive when angry than the nondepressed children. While the authors cautioned that their results were somewhat less than conclusive due to an overrepresentation of female patients and the small number of subjects, they felt that this study provides further evidence of the validity of considering anger to be part of the phenomenonology of the depressive disorder in middle to late childhood through adolescence.

Along these same lines, Carlson (1984) has postulated that there may be an alternate form of bipolar disorder, occurring primarily in children, which can be described more in terms of affective lability, irritability, and explosive behavior than by euphoria with irritability. These postulations, derived from a theoretical review of the literature and the results of direct research by such investigators as Ryan and co-workers (1987) and Kashani and colleagues (1984), lend strong support to the validity of the anger component in the diagnostic criteria for depression in children and adolescents. Rather than viewing the situation as one in which anger substitutes for depression, it seems that anger is a direct reflection of depressed mood.

Depression in 9-Year-Olds

The elusive nature of depression begins to be especially evident when prepubertal children are compared to adolescents. Kashani and Priesmayer (1983b), Kashani and Simonds (1979), and Kashani and colleagues (1983a), studying populations of 9-year-olds in Missouri and New Zealand, found no sex differences between depressed and nondepressed children of this age. In fact, during psychological testing, no behavioral differences were observed between 9-year-old boys who were normal and those who were later assessed as depressed. Futhermore, there were no significant differences between depressed and nondepressed children in IQ, verbal comprehension, reading, spelling, motor development, or SES. Like adolescents, however, depressed children did show higher levels of negative self-perceptions.

Among 9-year-olds, minor depression appeared to be more common than major depression. Most of the children with depression at age 9 had behavior problems for at least 2 years. However, there was an indication that behavior problems associated with depression at this age may not be of the attention-seeking type, since teacher responses to the Rutter Questionnaire did not distinguish between depressed and nondepressed children.

Jill: A Difficult Adjustment

Jill is a 3-year, 11-month-old girl who lives with her mother, her older brother, and her younger sister. Jill's father lived with them until she was $2\frac{1}{2}$ years of age, when he and her mother separated. Jill's parents are in the process of filing for a divorce. Jill was the product of an unplanned pregnancy, during which her mother had a liver infection. She also experienced hair loss, for which no physical cause could be found and which disappeared following delivery. Jill's mother describes her as having been a "happy baby," whose eating and sleeping habits were regular and whose developmental milestones were normal. Jill attends nursery school and was referred for evaluation by her nursery school teacher.

The teacher reported that Jill's behavior underwent a marked shift starting 2 months prior to assessment and became progressively worse. She described Jill as a cheerful child who was always cooperative in play and friendly with the other children. Within the last few months, however, Jill was frequently in a sad mood, bursting into tears in response to no, or slight, provocation (a child accidentally bumping into her during recess, or having to wait to use a toy). Jill's interaction with the other children changed, too; she would hit any child who disagreed with her or who interfered with her use of a toy. More recently, Jill's aggressive behavior toward the other children has intensified and become dangerous. For instance, Jill smashed a fellow student in the face with a teakettle with no apparent provocation. The teacher described Jill's mood at the time of the assault as "depressed." On another occasion, Jill hit the teacher and bit her when the teacher tried to speak to Jill about her inappropriate behavior. In response to these outbursts, the teacher urged that Jill's mother have her evaluated for any psychiatric disorder that might underlie her maladaptive behavior.

During the assessment, Jill appeared neat and her speech and language usage were developmentally appropriate. She displayed a full range of affect and betrayed no evidence of psychoses. All other elements of her mental status were also judged to be normal. Discussion with Jill's mother revealed that Jill had complained about her father's absence and recently had become sad when she heard his name. Jill has not seen her father since the separation, and she asks her mother frequently when she will "have her daddy again." The extent to which Jill's symptoms interfere with her social interactions at school and the degree to which her symptoms are excessive suggest that Jill is suffering from an adjustment disorder that was precipitated by the stressor of her father's departure from the home. Her presenting symptoms are of both emotional and misconduct nature, thereby qualifying her diagnosis as adjustment disorder with mixed disturbance of emotions and conduct. The fact that her symptoms appeared within 3 months of the proposed stressor adheres to the criteria for an adjustment disorder. Her symptoms do not seem to be part of some other condition not attributable to a mental disorder that are a focus of attention of treatment (V code) because in such conditions there is no marked impairment in social or occupational function, as seen in Jill's case, and Jill's reaction is not a normal or expectable response to the stressor experienced. Jill does not indicate symptomatology of any personality disorder, so her adjustment difficulty would not be labeled as related to such a diagnosis. Jill's difficulties would not be diagnosed as psychological factors affecting physical condition since she has indicated neither physical difficulties nor complaints.

A diagnosis of adjustment disorder with mixed disturbance of emotions and conduct has been assigned, to be reassessed if Jill's symptoms persist for more than the 6-month limit for problems termed adjustment disorders. The clinician has recommended that Jill be placed in a special classroom of limited size so that she will have individual attention and more structured limit-setting. Individual psychotherapy for Jill and parent/child group therapy for Jill's siblings and mother have also been recommended as components of the treatment plan.

Depression in Children 5 Years Old and Younger

As can be seen, depression in its recognized adult form rarely occurs in preschoolers, presumably due to their limited language and conceptualization skills. Nevertheless, symptoms of depression do clearly exist in members of this age group, as can be seen from Jill's case.

One study by Kashani and co-workers (1984) observed dysphoric mood among 3- to 5-year-olds (average age 4 years, 6 months) who were referred to a child developmental clinic. They found that dysphoric mood was associated with other depressive symptomatology more than any behavioral problem for which children were referred to the clinic.

Data were collected by interviews between the child and a child psychiatrist and between caregivers and a child psychiatrist. The parents of 17 children reported their children as having dysphoric mood, although only 7 of those children admitted to feeling sad. No children reported themselves as feeling sad whose parents did not make a similar observation.

The dysphoric children showed differences from the nondysphoric population in family constellation and history, emotional-behavior problems in school, and IQ. Data showed that 18% of the dysphoric children were living with both biological parents, as opposed to 45% of the children in the nondysphoric group. The dysphoric children's families had a higher incidence of drug abuse, mental illness, depression, and violent behavior. Of the total sample, 20% were referred to the clinic for behavior problems. In the remaining 80%, the dysphoric children showed a higher incidence of behavior problems than the non-dysphoric children. In another, more recent study, Kashani, Ray, and Carlson (1986) used four independent sources of information to evaluate depression and depressive symptoms in 100 preschoolers from the general population. The evaluation techniques included psychological testing of the children; semistructured interviews of the parents; checklist evaluations of the children by their parents; and formal teacher reports regarding the child's behavior, performance, and peer relations.

Kashani and colleagues found that a significant number of preschool children may exhibit sufficient depression to be of concern to teachers and parents although they fall short of being clinically depressed. Teachers appear to be more accurate in detecting the presence of depression than parents. Furthermore, anger or irritability, rather than sadness, appears to be the hallmark of depression in children of preschool age. Finally, environmental factors play an important role in the depressive picture at this age, since parents of children with depressive symptoms reported more stressful life events than did those with non-depressed children.

CONCLUSION

Since follow-up data regarding the outcomes of children who are clinically depressed are still scarce, the predictive validity of diagnoses in this age group remains basically unknown. However, the results of one longitudinal study on a cohort of 1,037 9-year-old children in the general population serve to demonstrate the importance of efforts at follow-up, since 1.8% of these children were observed to manifest major depression and 2.5% were seen to have a more minor depressive disorder (Kashani et al., 1983b).

This study found trends in childhood affective disorder that differed from those in adults. While these findings may not be definitive, they serve to provide perspective on the possible age-related differences in the depressive state. First, Kashani and colleagues found that minor depression was the most common type of depression in the children they studied, whereas in adults major depression is widely regarded as being the prevalent condition. The investigators speculated that this could mean that depression in children begins more commonly with minor types that later evolve into major depression. The authors also noted that while depression in adults is commonly reported to occur more frequently in women, the reverse appears to be true for children, since boys are more frequently cited as experiencing mood disorder. They also noted, however, that this may be due to an overrepresentation of male patients seen in a clinical setting.

In general, it seems safe to say that full-fledged adult depressive syndromes such as those described in DSM-III-R occur infrequently in preschoolers but may show a higher incidence as age increases. The very existence of depressive symptoms in young children is no longer in dispute, although the degree to which these symptoms may aggregate into syndromes is still a matter of conjecture.

However, there is no reason to suppose that a great deal more is understood about symptom agglomeration in adults than in children. For example, Coryell and Winokur (1984) have attempted to describe depression in adults according to a new system that utilizes certain observed patterns in symptom presentation. Specifically, they have postulated that there is an illness that tends to manifest as depression in females and alcoholism in males. These groups were separated on the basis of being early-onset females or late-onset males. The early-onset females had a significant family history of alcoholism and so were considered to be the prototype of "depression spectrum disease." The late-onset males, on the other hand, lacked family histories of alcoholism and so were thought to be prototypes of "pure depressive disease." While these categories may or may not eventually prove useful, the system of Coryell and Winokur serves to illustrate the fact that the nosology of depression in adults is in nearly as much flux as that in children—a situation that is not altogether negative since the best results will likely emerge with the use of a system that incorporates all age groups. This is more likely to happen if nosologies in both age categories are undergoing change simultaneously.

With regard to a possible dynamic in which early symptoms may aggregate into later syndromes, it may be instructive to discuss briefly the phenomenon of *double depression,* in which there is a concurrent diagnosis of major depression and dysthymic disorder. In a prospective study of 65 children between the ages of 8 and 13, Kovacs (1984a) found that 38% of the cases of major depression had an underlying dysthymia. Thus, it is possible that depressive symptoms in children aggregate first into a dysthymic condition and that this mood state later produces an overlay of major depression.

This mechanism would also provide support for Kashani's postulation that depression in children originates with minor forms that later evolve into more serious types. However, as Keller and Lavori (1984) have noted, there are few if any published data on a clinical population experiencing a dysthymic disorder that did not develop into a double depression. Thus, it is not possible to conclude definitively that the majority of dysthymias develop into major depression.

One phenomenon that might fuel the progression of less severe to more severe depressive states in children is the observed frequency with which low self-esteem is seen to be closely linked to depressive symptomatology in young children. Wallace, Cunningham, and Del Monte (1984) have observed that systematic increases in self-esteem occur throughout adolescence. It is possible that this natural and beneficial process could be inhibited by the feelings of worthlessness that accompany depressed mood. Thus, depression in childhood likely retards ego development, which in turn may further predispose the individual to a depressive outlook.

CHAPTER THIRTEEN

Anxiety Disorders and Their Differential Diagnosis

Nathaniel: Painfully Worried

Nathaniel is a 5-year-old boy who lives with his mother, his father, and his $1\frac{1}{2}$-year-old brother. Nathaniel was born a few years after his mother's first pregnancy ended in miscarriage, and he was breast-fed for 2 weeks. His mother was uncomfortable breast-feeding, and Nathaniel was quite difficult at feeding. He was switched to formula at 2 weeks of age, developed thrush, and became colicky. At 5 months, the pediatrician diagnosed Nathaniel as allergic to the formula. He began soybean formula, and the colic remitted within a few days. Nathaniel has no history of other medical difficulties. His parents describe Nathaniel's developmental milestones as within normal ranges except for walking. At the age of 17 months, Nathaniel was still not walking. He was taken to a doctor who recommended surgery. Nathaniel's parents rejected this suggestion and claim that Nathaniel was able to walk within a month.

Nathaniel's mother and father both say he was a very affectionate, cuddly child, who took delight in being the focus of attention. They assert that he was always smiling and happy, and that his vocabulary was extremely well developed at an early age. He enjoyed drawing, and was quite creative in any type of play. Nathaniel started preschool a year ago, at which time his parents noticed a change in him. They say that he began asking more questions about the possible outcomes of situations, at times exhausting them with inquiry. He became hesitant to go anywhere unless he had both an explanation of what to expect prior to the excursion and reassurance of the lack of danger. Difficulty getting Nathaniel to go to sleep at night began to develop, with various reasons given, including: "sudden fear of the dark" "marked tension and worry" about the next day's schedule; and extreme "sensitivity to noise," which prevents him from falling asleep.

Nathaniel's teacher began to express concern about him almost immediately after he started school. She says that he is not able to interact easily with peers and often seems to be off in his own world. During these periods of detachment, the teacher tries to make contact with Nathaniel. His responses, when she asks what he is thinking about, usually reveal that he is thinking about the details of some planned activity, about whether his earlier behavior is going to "get him into trouble," if he should have "behaved differently," how the other children feel about him, and so forth. He is slow to participate in activities, often saying that he cannot do them well. His teacher also notes that Nathaniel never seems able to relax, even during play and quiet times. The teacher feels that Nathaniel's tension is impeding his ability to benefit from school activities, and she has recommended assessment to determine the roots of Nathaniel's difficulties.

During the assessment interview, it was noted that Nathaniel is an extremely attractive boy of average physical size. He had little difficulty separating from his mother at the start of the interview, but his manner was extremely cautious. Speech and motor behavior were normal, as were other elements of mental status. Themes expressed in Nathaniel's speech included his parents' disapproval of him and fears of animals and ghosts.

Nathaniel was unusually startled and fearful when he heard a siren during the session; he needed reassurance that there was no "fire in the building." When asked to draw, Nathaniel resisted, saying that he was not good at drawing and that he could not do it right. After encouragement from the therapist, he drew a boy who was getting yelled at by his parents because he had touched their newspaper. Nathaniel seemed tense and anxious throughout the entire assessment; he related his fears of getting in trouble for future and past wrongdoings and stated that he feels "bad and jumpy" much of the time.

Nathaniel's excessive fear about past wrongdoings and future events, his inability to relax, his need for extensive reassurances, his worry that he is not good at tasks, and his self-consciousness about his perceived flaws suggest that he suffers from the debilitating effects of overanxious disorder. His relative ease at separating from his mother at the interview and the absence of difficulty in separating to go to school rule out the possibility that fear of separation is the precipitant, thus making a diagnosis of separation anxiety disorder inappropriate. The nature of Nathaniel's concerns regarding future and past events is not characteristic of tension inducers in children suffering from attention deficit hyperactivity disorder, so this too was ruled out. Furthermore, his concentration span seems unaffected. At this time, a diagnosis of adjustment disorder with anxious mood would also be inappropriate because Nathaniel's symptoms have persisted for more than 6 months. Nathaniel displays no symptoms of an associated psychotic or mood disorder.

Thus, a diagnosis of overanxious disorder has been assigned, and individual psychotherapy and further psychological testing have been recommended. Family therapy has also been suggested as a way to identify and develop functional alternatives to stressors.

INTRODUCTION

Freud (1894) was the first to describe a syndrome characterized by a central condition of anxious expectation such as that experienced by Nathaniel. However, Freud's anxiety neurosis encompassed both chronic anxiety and anxiety or panic attacks. Within this earliest nosologic system, anxiety neurosis was viewed as being a chronic form of generalized anxiety that could exist independently of, or concurrently with, anxiety attacks. Anxiety attacks were described as being severe feelings of apprehension and threat of impending doom that occurred in the absence of any mental or environmental stimulus.

For the most part, clinical diagnoses involving anxious states continue to be derived from Freud's description. There is little debate regarding the most severe form of anxious dysregulation, panic attacks. An attack of acute fear accompanied by physiological symptoms such as sweating and palpitations and occurring in the absence of an internal or external stimulus is clearly a pathological phenomenon. However, pathological levels of anxiety apart from panic attacks are extremely difficult to isolate and measure.

The major source of difficulty lies in the fact that anxiety and fears are psychological constituents normal to all human beings. As Puig-Antich and Rabinovich (1986) stated, "It is as if, in most cases, the affective picture is superimposed on a background of anxiety symptoms/disorder" (p. 143). Thus, it appears that anxiety, to one degree or another, accompanies almost every mood disorder. The problem then becomes one of determining whether the anxiety is the primary disorder, whether it is secondary to (caused by) the mood disorder, or whether it is merely the longstanding level of anxious arousal intrinsic to the individual's temperament and life experience.

Despite these possible sources of confusion, Puig-Antich (1982) has provided a compelling argument for the validity of differentiating the emotional disorders into *depressive* and *nondepressive* types. In a controlled family history study of prepubertal major depression, Puig-Antich and Rabinovich (1986) found that families with children diagnosed as having a nondepressed emotional disorder did not differ from either those with normal children or those with children with major depression. However, the families of nondepressed children did have a significantly lower risk of developing alcoholism than did families of children with major depression, and they were indistinguishable from families of normal children in terms of the alcoholism measure.

These and other findings have led Puig-Antich and Rabinovich (1986) to conclude that affective disorders in childhood possess a long-term stability that may exceed that seen in nondepressed emotional disorders. Furthermore, these authors have stated that "there is sufficient evidence to support the validity of separating the emotional disorders of childhood into the categories of depressed and nondepressed" (p. 140). While there may be good evidence supporting the existence of depressed and nondepressed emotional disorders, a nosology must still be developed that will provide the means of definitively diagnosing these states.

Specifically, the delineation of anxiety states other than those accompanying anxiety attacks is limited by the following factors:

1. The presence of anxiety in normal conscious states.
2. The presence of anxious symptoms in most psychiatric illnesses.
3. The necessity of relying upon subjective measures.
4. The wide variety of anxietal manifestations (e.g., verbal, cognitive, psychophysiological).

5. The existence of acute (phobic) and general anxiety states (Breier et al., 1985; Werry, 1986).

In general, attempts to arrive at different clinical categories of non-panic anxiety have begun with making a distinction between fear and anxiety. Fear is focused on a very real and specific object or situation (e.g., spider, school setting), while anxiety is viewed as an unpleasant and unjustified sense of apprehension. The delineation allows for a nosological system wherein panic attacks are distinguished from phobic state (a mixture of anxiety and fear that is persistent and of an intensity out of proportion to the stimulus), and phobic states are, in turn, segregated from generalized anxiety (anxiety neurosis without panic attacks).

While this system is useful to some degree, accurate clinical assessment is hampered by the fact that, as noted in DSM-III-R, anxiety and fear generate essentially identical cognitive and affective pictures such as apprehension and feelings of impending danger. Both produce similar physiological reactions as well (e.g., predominantly autonomic activity such as sweating or trembling). Furthermore, there are no provisions under this schema for further delineating states that might exist outside the conditions of anxiety attacks and phobias. Generalized anxious conditions are much more difficult to differentiate from one another.

Subcategories of anxiety states aside from anxiety attack and phobia thus far have failed to extend beyond such nebulous terminology as acute anxiety versus generalized anxiety states. In the former condition, the individual is overwhelmed and incapacitated for a short period of time by intense feelings of fear and dread; the latter state is a more pervasive apprehensive feeling that causes the individual to be constantly vigilant (Rapoport & Ismond, 1984).

Determining pathology within the latter category remains a difficult task. As Werry (1986) has pointed out, symptoms within generalized anxiety that might agglomerate into subcategories would have to be assessed in terms of a large number of variables, including (1) severity and disabling effect, (2) persistence, (3) age-appropriateness, (4) associated symptomatology, (5) unusualness or bizarreness, and (6) family or peer group norms.

As mentioned, one step toward identifying pathological states of general anxiety involves the attempt to segregate anxietal states from depressive states. The interrelatedness of these states is suggested by the fact that panic attacks can be treated successfully with antidepressant medications. In addition, the fact that these agents alleviate panic symptoms before reversing symptoms of generalized anxiety strongly suggests that panic anxiety is distinct from generalized anxiety (Breier et al., 1985). This finding provided the basis for the DSM-III-R distinction between panic anxiety and generalized anxiety, but the relationship between depression and anxiety has yet to be unraveled.

As will be noted shortly, the close juxtaposition of anxiety and depression is very noticeable in DSM-III-R because depression must be excluded in order to confirm many of the anxiety states described therein. For example, Kovacs, Feinberg, Crouse-Novak, Paulaskas & Finkelstein (1984a) reported that DSM-III criteria for anxiety disorder were met concomitantly by about 35% of those in their sample who were suffering from depression.

At present, the most precise formulation that can be made calls for recognizing the existence of a single, broadband, "internalizing" diagnostic dimension that includes symptoms indicative of anxiety, depression, and social withdrawal (Quay & LaGreca, 1986; Wolfson, Fields, & Rose, 1987). Attempts at reaching subclassifications of this broad spectrum have so far produced equivocal results despite the evidence suggesting that depressed and nondepressed disorders do exist.

In children, the problem of diagnosing affective states limited to anxiety is made even more difficult because of two main factors. First, the emotional discomfort and subjective feelings of distress that are the hallmarks of internalizing disorder are difficult for adults to recognize and evaluate in children. Second, behavioral manifestations of fear/anxiety become progressively more differentiated as development continues (Trad, 1987). Regarding the latter consideration, the development of cognition institutes a trend from concrete to abstract interpretations of environmental stimuli. This results in larger individual differences between children in what they regard as fearful.

In general, however, certain trends do emerge. It is useful to recognize that newborns tend to fear sudden and loud stimuli, heights, and lack of support (Bronson, 1972; Jersild & Holmes, 1935) and that this changes at around 12 months of age, when fear becomes attached to strangers and new objects in the environment (Bronson, 1972; Scarr & Salapatek, 1970). Furthermore, as Bowlby (1969) has discussed, 1-year-old infants begin to fear separation from their primary caregivers. As cognition progresses, preschool children develop fears of animals or imaginary creatures and fear of the dark, all of which decrease with increasing age (Bauer, 1976).

While these considerations complicate assessment, two relatively stable broadband spectra of behavior problems in children have been described. The first is commonly referred to as *internalizing* or personality problems (Wolfson et al., 1987). This category is analogous to the internalizing dimension described for adults with anxiety disorders and includes withdrawal, inhibition, and dissonances within the personality. The second dimension refers to *externalizing*, or behavior problems, including problems of conduct such as aggression and delinquency.

The following discussion of the diagnosis and consequences of anxiety in childhood will take into account the possible co-involvement of
depression and anxiety along the broadband internal/external (person-
ality/behavior) dimension. All of this will be considered within the context of age-specific developmental criteria.

In order to achieve as complete an overview as possible, all DSM-III-R
categories with associations to anxiety will be considered. Therefore,
anxiety disorders that are not strictly limited to children (social phobia,
simple phobia, panic disorder, obsessive-compulsive disorder, posttraumatic stress disorder, and atypical anxiety disorder) will be discussed
with regard to differential diagnosis in addition to the DSM-III-R anxiety disorders of childhood or adolescence (separation anxiety, avoidant
disorder of childhood or adolescence, and overanxious disorder).

DIFFERENTIAL DIAGNOSIS
OF CHILDHOOD ANXIETY STATES
ACCORDING TO DSM-III-R CRITERIA

Jason: Fearing Loss

Jason is a 2-year-old boy with no siblings who lives with his mother and
father. Until he was 7 months old—when his mother went back to work
once a week—Jason never had a babysitter. When he was 10 months old,
Jason's mother went to work full time and he was left at a babysitter's. After
5 months, Jason's mother decided she was not comfortable with the arrangement and found a sitter who could come to the family's home. She felt
uncomfortable again 5 months after the initiation of this new arrangement
and found a neighbor to babysit. This situation was satisfactory. However,
after about 8 months, the sitter's husband was transferred out of town and
Jason's mother was left, once again, in need of child care for Jason. Her
choice was to return to the first babysitter. Jason was cooperative, but he
did ask repeatedly for the previous babysitter, their neighbor.

With Jason's verbalized desire to return to the neighbor's house came
changes in his speech pattern (he repeated the final words of his statements
two or three times) and in his behavior. He was irritable and nasty. After
the new arrangement had been in effect for 2 weeks, Jason's paternal grandparents visited. For 1 week, Jason's father did not go to work and Jason did
not have to go to the babysitter's. Jason enjoyed a great deal of attention
from his grandparents during that week. The next week, Jason's father returned to work, and Jason resumed his schedule of going to the babysitter's
house without objection.

At the end of this second week, Jason's grandparents left and his mother
noticed that he was again becoming nasty and that he had started hitting.
Her reaction was to explain to Jason that, while she loved him, she did not

like his behavior. His behavior worsened, and he cried every morning when dropped off at the sitter's house. He began biting, throwing his toys, hitting, and stuttering. He started waking up during the night and running into his parents' room, telling them that there were monsters. Because these behaviors intensified, Jason's mother discontinued the babysitting and his father left his job to stay home and care for him.While in his father's care at home, Jason would look out the window for his mother, whom he feared was lost. When in her company, Jason clung to her, opting to be with her instead of playing by himself or with friends as he had done previously. Jason's stuttering never affected his pronunciation of "mommy," but had otherwise worsened along with his fears, which had recently become pervasive. His referral for psychiatric assessment followed observations that he was crying, biting, hitting, and stuttering; that he had sleeping difficulties and nightmares; and that he worried about his mother and was clinging to her.

During the initial assessment, both the child's mother and father were present. Jason played exclusively within close range of his mother, and she initiated play by giving toys to him. His facial expression betrayed fear and concern, and he did not maintain eye contact with the clinician. He interacted with neither his father nor the clinician. In play, he stuttered with nearly every word, but he displayed orientation, cooperation, and a good attention and concentration span. Other elements of the mental status examination were assessed as being within normal ranges. During the next session, which Jason attended with his mother, his mother told of Jason's questioning about where she had been during the day. He expressed fear and mentioned cars in connection with that fear. His mother's understanding was that Jason was telling her he wanted her to stay home. In the third, and final, session, Jason's mother reported that he enjoyed having her stay home more, but that his sleep was still disturbed. She would have to lie in bed with him to get him to fall asleep.

Initial evaluation of Jason's symptoms pointed to the diagnostic picture of separation anxiety disorder; he displayed all criteria associated with that diagnosis, including worry about harm to the attachment figure or the failure of the attachment figure to return (fear that his mother was lost); refusal to go to sleep unless the attachment figure is present; physical symptoms prior to separation (Jason experienced some constipation during the period when he resisted going to the babysitter); clinging to his mother; nightmares; and fantasies about monsters. Differential diagnosis against criteria for overanxious disorder was important because in overanxious disorder the anxiety is not focused on separation, as it is in separation anxiety disorder and as it was in Jason's case as well. Pervasive developmental disorder, major depression, and schizophrenia were also ruled out because Jason failed to exhibit characteristic symptoms of those disorders. Jason's anxieties could not be attributed to a condition of panic disorder with agoraphobia for the following reasons: Jason showed no evidence of panic attacks and his anxiety was focused on separation from his mother, not on fear of being in an unescapable situation, as it is in panic disorder with agoraphobia. Conduct disorder, although it often includes refusal to attend expected activities, was not an appropriate diagnosis for Jason because his resistance was in regard to separation and did not have oppositional or antisocial motives.

Thus, a diagnosis of separation anxiety disorder was made in which the patient was alternating between practicing separation and an inability to separate, an inconsistency due in part to the changing of caregivers. Weekly therapy was recommended for Jason and his parents together.

General Conventions

Jason illustrates another important aspect of anxiety, that is, anxiety generated as a result of fear of loss. Presumably, unlike Nathaniel's case, this anxietal state is associated with a specific cause and will abate with resolution of the child–mother relationship. For purposes of quickly and accurately delineating all the different states of anxiety postulated to exist according to DSM-III-R, the following general conventions will be adopted. The most empirically defensible scheme of anxiety to date places panic attacks at the most extreme level of pathology and intensity. Next in severity is phobic or acute anxiety state, which, in turn, is followed by generalized anxiety.

An anxiety or panic attack, occurring in the absence of an internal or external stimulus, comprises a special, well-delineated pathological category of anxiety. Threats to bodily or psychological integrity produce fears that generate acute or generalized anxious states. Varying degrees of anxiety can be experienced in response to a primary stimulus (e.g., a dog or a snake) or a secondary stimulus associated with loss of security (fear of being abandoned by a caregiver or of performing poorly on school academic and social tasks). In addition to these are the normal childhood fears of the dark and of strangers. It is also important to keep in mind that the intensity of anxiety feelings increases under conditions in which a number of these fears overlap.

Separation Anxiety Disorder

Benjamin (1963) has described a neurophysiologic maturation with noticeable EEG changes in infants at 3 to 4 weeks of age. This change appears to be related to the hooking up of input from the senses to the central nervous system. During this period, as Schecter (1978) has pointed out, the mother must function as a protective stimulus barrier, or mediator, to prevent the infant from becoming overwhelmed by potentially threatening and strange new stimuli. Variability in the adequacy of parenting at this time may account for later variability in the predisposition to anxiety.

Thus, anxiety on separating from the environment and from the caregiver is an emotion experienced by every infant, and these early anxious feelings may form the prototype for all such feelings (excluding panic attacks) in later life (Trad, 1986). That is, separation anxiety may well function as an organizer for related anxieties during later stages of development. For this reason, anxiety will be discussed in greater theoretical detail in a later section, along with other common manifestations of childhood anxiety such as school refusal and obsessive-compulsive disorder.

According to DSM-III-R, separation anxiety disorder is characterized by excessive anxiety concerning separation from persons to whom the child is attached. An "excessive" degree of anxiety is considered to be present if the child manifests at least three of the following nine signs or symptoms:

(1) unrealistic and persistent worry about possible harm befalling major attachment figures or fear that they will leave and not return

(2) unrealistic and persistent worry that an untoward calamitous event will separate the child from a major attachment figure, e.g., the child will be lost, kidnapped, killed, or be the victim of an accident

(3) persistent reluctance or refusal to go to school in order to stay with major attachment figures or at home

(4) persistent reluctance or refusal to go to sleep without being near a major attachment figure or to go to sleep away from home

(5) persistent avoidance of being alone, including "clinging" to and "shadowing" major attachment figures

(6) repeated nightmares involving the theme of separation

(7) complaints of physical symptoms, e.g., headaches, stomachaches, nausea, or vomiting, on many school days or on other occasions when anticipating separation from major attachment figures

(8) recurrent signs or complaints of excessive distress in anticipation of separation from home or major attachment figures, e.g., temper tantrums or crying, pleading with parents not to leave

(9) recurrent signs of complaints of excessive distress when separated from home or major attachment figures, e.g., wants to return home, needs to call parents when they are absent or when child is away from home). (DSM-III-R, pp. 60–61)

The disturbance must have been present for at least 2 weeks before a diagnosis of separation anxiety can be made. Furthermore, it must be determined that the disturbance did not occur exclusively during the course of a pervasive developmental disorder (PDD), schizophrenia, or any other psychotic disorder.

In differentiating separation anxiety from PDD (autism or pervasive developmental disorder not otherwise specified) or schizophrenia, the primary factor to keep in mind is the direct relation of the anxious state to the fear of separation from major attachment figures. As a look at the descriptive symptomatologies for PDD or schizophrenia will reveal, the anxious components of these disorders are generally less focused than those of separation anxiety.

In PDD's, among which autism is the only subtype recognized by DSM-III-R, there is a qualitative impairment in the development of reciprocal social interaction, in the development of verbal and nonverbal communication skills, and in the development of imaginative activity. In autism, the most severe and prototypic PDD, the child commonly displays imperviousness to the feelings of others and a marked lack of communication of any kind and is distressed over trivial changes in his or her environment.

The absence of delusions or hallucinations differentiates both PDD and separation anxiety from schizophrenic disorder, in which delusional content is abundant. Age of onset of schizophrenic disorder normally occurs during adolescence or early childhood. Both PDD and schizophrenia represent a greater degree of emotional-cognitive dysregulation than is evidenced in children with separation anxiety. As mentioned before, the anxious state seen in cases of separation anxiety is closely tied to need for proximity to the caregiver. Anxiety resulting from delusional fears in schizophrenics will be less tied to separation content. For example, complaints of sickness on school days may derive not from fear of being abandoned but from anxiety related to an inner voice telling the child that there is no air outside the house.

In cases of PDD, the child may cling to the caregiver or display panic symptoms, but these behaviors are less tied to the caregiver per se than to the anxiety that accompanies a more pervasive and severe inability to function effectively. Thus, the presence of asociality is often useful in segregating cases of PDD from separation anxiety. Furthermore, the ability to empathize is often much poorer in children with PDD than in those with separation anxiety. Empathic abilities are commonly highly developed in children with anxious attachments due to the fact that these children feel that they must lend their every effort to deciphering the ambivalent behavior of the caregiver. The ability to identify the mother's mood from moment to moment provides vital cues for coping in the face of inconsistent feedback.

Thus, in reaching a diagnosis of separation anxiety disorder, the clinician should focus concern on the caregiver, for the roots of this disorder lie in distorted attachment relationships. The child should be interviewed and assessed for any delusional or hallucinatory tendencies to rule out schizophrenia, and an inability to empathize may indicate the presence of PDD.

Avoidant Disorder of Childhood or Adolescence

The DSM-III-R classification of avoidant disorder calls for the following four basic components:

A. *Excessive shrinking from contact with unfamiliar people, for a period of six months or longer, sufficiently severe to interfere with social functioning in peer relationships.*

B. *Desire for social involvement with familiar people (family members and peers the person knows well), and generally warm and satisfying relations with family members and other familiar figures.*

C. *Age of at least $2\frac{1}{2}$ years.*

D. *The disturbance is not sufficiently pervasive and persistent to warrant the diagnosis of Avoidant Personality Disorder.* (pp. 62–63)

The most salient feature of this disorder is a fear of strangers so intense that it interferes with social functioning. Other aspects of functioning such as reality testing are only moderately impaired, and these may lead to slight depression. Temperament may be the most important factor to consider in terms of differentially diagnosing the anxious condition. A child who is "slow to warm up," who may be socially hesitant initially but eventually engages in age-appropriate peer interactions, should not be classified as avoidant (Rapoport & Ismond, 1984).

Overanxious Disorder

Children with overanxious disorder manifest restless behavior and seek approval as a result of generalized anxiety regarding aspects of their appearance or performance. According to DSM-III-R, four of the following seven persistent concerns must be present in order to confirm a diagnosis of overanxious disorder:

(1) excessive or unrealistic anxiety or worry about future events

(2) excessive or unrealistic concern about the appropriateness of past behavior

(3) excessive or unrealistic concern about competence in one or more areas, e.g., athletic, academic, social

(4) somatic complaints, such as headaches or stomachaches, for which no physical basis can be established

(5) marked self-consciousness

(6) excessive need for reassurance about a variety of concerns

(7) marked feelings of tension or inability to relax. (pp. 64–65)

If another Axis I disorder is present (e.g., separation anxiety disorder, phobic disorder, obsessive-compulsive disorder), the focus of these symptoms cannot be limited to it. For example, if separation anxiety is present, the symptoms cannot be exclusively related to anxiety about separation. Furthermore, the disturbance must not occur only during the course of a psychotic or mood disorder.

Overanxious disorder should not be diagnosed if symptoms have occurred exclusively during the course of a pervasive developmental disorder, schizophrenia, or any other psychotic disorder. If the individual is 18 years old or older, criteria for general anxiety disorder must not be met. Since the diagnosis of this disorder hinges largely on making an assessment as to the level of general anxiety, there are many alternative causes that must be ruled out. The characteristics of separation anxiety, PDD, and schizophrenia have already been described.

As mentioned in DSM-III-R, phobic disorder and obsessive-compulsive disorder, as well as others, can coexist with the overanxious condition. Phobic disorder is characterized by irrational fear of objects or of situations in which the individual may be subjected to scrutiny and be seen to behave in an embarrassing way. The fears are recognized by the individual as irrational, but are nonetheless uncontrollable. Obsessions are irrational thoughts that are viewed by the individual as senseless or repugnant and are experienced as invading his or her consciousness. Compulsions consist of ritualized behavior(s) directed at relieving tension by preventing the occurrence of some feared future event. The activity is either excessive or unrealistically connected to the "it" that it is intended to forestall. As with phobic disorder, the irrationality of the activity is recognized and felt as a source of distress. Overanxious disorder can be differentiated from phobia by the fact that phobia is driven by one or more specific objects or situations. Furthermore, overanxious disorder is set apart from both phobia and obsessive-compulsive disorder by the fact that individuals with either of the latter two conditions are aware of the irrationality of their actions and/or fears.

In differentiating overanxious disorder from major depression, it must be recognized that negative affect is identified by presence of dysphoric mood or loss of interest or pleasure in all usual activities. Characteristics of the dysphoria are sadness, hopelessness, and irritability. The mood disturbance must be prominent and persistent, but it need not be the most prominent symptom, and momentary shifts from one dysphoric mood to another (e.g., anxiety to depression to anger) should not occur. (For children under 6 years of age dysphoric mood may have to be inferred from a persistently sad expression.)

Furthermore, at least five of the following symptoms must have been present nearly every day for at least 2 weeks before major depression can be confirmed, and at least one of the symptoms must be either depressed mood or loss of interest or pleasure:

(1) *depressed mood (or can be irritable mood in children or adolescents) most of the day, nearly every day, as indicated either by subjective account or observation by others*

(2) *markedly diminished interest or pleasure in all, or almost all, activities most of the day, nearly every day (as indicated either by subjective account or observation by others of apathy most of the time)*

(3) *significant weight loss or weight gain when not dieting (e.g., more than 5% of body weight in a month), or decrease or increase in appetite nearly every day (in children, consider failure to make expected weight gains)*

(4) *insomnia or hypersomnia nearly every day*

(5) *psychomotor agitation or retardation nearly every day (observable by others, not merely subjective feelings of restlessness or being slowed down)*

(6) *fatigue or loss of energy nearly every day*

(7) *feelings of worthlessness or excessive or inappropriate guilt (which may be delusional) nearly every day (not merely self-reproach or guilt about being sick)*

(8) *diminished ability to think or concentrate, or indecisiveness, nearly every day (either by subjective account or as observed by others)*

(9) *recurrent thoughts of death (not just fear of dying), recurrent suicidal ideation without a specific plan, or a suicide attempt or a specific plan for committing suicide.* (DSM-III-R, pp. 222–223)

As can be seen from this symptomatic picture, anxiety stemming from depression can, at the grossest level, be differentiated from that deriving from overanxious disorder by the greater restlessness of the individual with overanxious disorder. The persistent, generalized worry exhibited by the overanxious person is likely to produce a greater level of vigilance than that seen in someone who feels that action may be futile. Furthermore, the emotional shifts of the overanxious person are usually more volatile than those evidenced by someone with major depression.

In differentiating overanxious disorder from separation anxiety, the primary consideration is the generalized anxiety relating to performance exhibited by the overanxious person versus the more focused anxiety regarding separation from the caregiver evidenced by the child with separation anxiety. Anxiety stemming from schizophrenia or PDD can be differentiated from that emanating from overanxious disorder by paying attention to the greater cognitive abilities of the child with overanxious disorder who, as an example, is likely to have a more developed empathic ability. Differentiating between the anxious state stem-

ming from avoidant disorder and anxiety deriving from the overanxious condition may be more difficult than separating it from the other
categories discussed thus far. Both conditions manifest a strong need
for support and approval. However, familial relations of the child with
avoidant disorder may be somewhat warmer than those of the overanxious individual.

In sum, the diagnosis of overanxious disorder is a demanding one
in which many alternatives must be ruled out. However, as operative
suggestions, the self-knowledge of the obsessive-compulsive individual
regarding the irrationality of his or her fears and actions; the decreased
emotional capability of the depressed individual; the strong focal
source of the anxiety of the child with separation anxiety (i.e., the caregiver); the lesser cognitive and empathic abilities of children with
schizophrenia or PDD; and the more felicitous familial relationships
seen in avoidant disorder may provide some means of detecting the
presence of overanxious disorder.

Phobia

Social Phobia. This disorder is characterized by a persistent irrational fear of, and compelling desire to avoid, a situation in which
the individual is exposed to possible scrutiny by others and fears that
he or she may act in a way that will be humiliating or embarrassing.
There is significant stress due to the disturbance, and the individual
recognizes that his or her fear is excessive or unreasonable. The phobic
reaction should not be due to another mental disorder such as major
depression or avoidant personality disorder.

Differential diagnosis of social phobia from major depression centers
around the pervasiveness of the negative affect and the lack of specific
anxiety-inducing stimuli in the latter condition. Social phobia can be
distinguished from avoidant personality disorder by the higher incidence of warm intrafamilial relationships and poor peer relationships
among members of the latter group.

Simple Phobia. Unlike social phobia, the phobic reaction in simple
phobia is not associated with possibly humiliating social situations.
Rather, the inciting stimulus is commonly an animal, heights, or close
spaces. As in cases of social phobia, the individual experiences distress
and the recognition that his or her fear is excessive or irrational. This
condition is not associated with another mental disorder such as schizophrenia, in which the phobic response may be elicited by a delusional
stimulus, or obsessive-compulsive disorder, in which the phobic stimulus is intrusive and linked to subconscious ideation.

Panic Disorder

A diagnosis of panic disorder requires either a minimum of four unexpected panic attacks over a period of 4 weeks, or one or more attacks
that have been followed by a period of at least a month of persistent
fear of having another attack. The attacks do not occur in response to
any recognizable or socially threatening stimulus, and they are marked
by onset of extreme feelings of terror and impending doom. At least
four of the following symptoms must develop during at least one of the
attacks: dyspnea; palpitations; chest pain; choking; dizziness; vertigo or
unsteady feelings; nausea or abdominal distress; derealization or depersonalization; parasthesias; hot and cold flashes; sweating; faintness;
trembling or shaking; or fear of dying, going crazy, or doing something
uncontrolled during an attack.

This disorder is usually associated with agoraphobia (fear of being in
places where uncontrolled behavior will be humiliating or where help
will not be forthcoming). Physical disorders and organic factors such
as amphetamine or caffeine intoxication must be ruled out, as must
schizophrenia. In the latter case, delusions, hallucinations, or marked
loosening of associations are the primary differentiating characteristics.

Obsessive-Compulsive Disorder

In this condition, the individual experiences either obsessions or compulsions. The latter are characterized by repetitive and seemingly pur-
poseful behaviors performed according to certain rules or in a stereotyped fashion. Although there is no realistic causal relationship
between the behavior and the event it is intended to forestall, some
measure of tension relief is obtained upon performance of the activity.
Furthermore, the individual is aware of the irrationality of his or her
fears and/or behavior. Obsessions are recurrent, persistent ideas,
thoughts, images, or impulses that are not experienced as being produced voluntarily. Rather, they are viewed as invading the consciousness, and since they are experienced as senseless or repugnant, attempts
are made to suppress them.

The obsessions or compulsions must be a significant source of distress
to the individual, interfering with social role or functioning. Symptoms
of this disorder cannot be attributable to schizophrenia, major depression, Tourette syndrome, or organic mental disorder.

As stated previously, obsessive-compulsive disorder can be differentiated from schizophrenia by the fact that individuals with the former
condition have an awareness of the irrationality of their thoughts and
actions. Individuals with major depression may exhibit psychomotor
agitation, but this is rarely ritualized to the degree seen in individuals
with obsessive-compulsive disorder.

Tourette syndrome, with an onset between the ages of 2 and 15, is characterized by recurrent, involuntary, repetitive, rapid, and purposeless motor movements affecting multiple muscle groups that can be suppressed for minutes to hours. Multiple vocal tics are also seen. Symptom intensity varies over minutes to hours and the condition must have been present for at least 1 year. This syndrome can be differentiated from obsessive-compulsive behavior relatively easily by the fact that the movements are random and not directed at alleviating tension. Essentially the same criterion can be applied to differentiating obsessive-compulsive disorder from organic mental disorders (e.g., delirium, dementia, amnestic syndrome, organic delusional syndrome, organic hallucinosis, organic affective syndrome, organic personality syndrome).

Posttraumatic Stress Disorder (PTSD)

This syndrome is the direct result of the occurrence of a stressor outside the range of normal human development that would evoke high levels of distress in almost anyone. Individuals with this disorder always reexperience the trauma, as evidenced by at least one of the following symptoms:

(1) recurrent and intrusive distressing recollections of the event (in young children, repetitive play in which themes or aspects of the trauma are expressed)

(2) recurrent distressing dreams of the event

(3) sudden acting or feeling as if the traumatic event were recurring (includes a sense of reliving the experience, illusions, hallucinations, and dissociative [flashback] episodes, even those that occur upon awakening or when intoxicated)

(4) intense psychological distress at exposure to events that symbolize or resemble an aspect of the traumatic event, including anniversaries of the trauma (DSM-III-R, pp. 250–251)

Responsiveness to, or involvement with, the outside world is significantly diminished following the trauma. This is demonstrated by at least one of the following (none of which were present prior to the trauma):

(1) efforts to avoid thoughts or feelings associated with the trauma

(2) efforts to avoid activities or situations that arouse recollections of the trauma

(3) inability to recall an important aspect of the trauma (psychogenic amnesia)

(4) markedly diminished interest in significant activities (in young children, loss of recently acquired developmental skills such as toilet training or language skills)

(5) *feeling of detachment or estrangement from others*

(6) *restricted range of affect, e.g., unable to have loving feelings*

(7) *sense of foreshortened future, e.g., does not expect to have a career, marriage, or children, or a long life* (DSM-III-R, pp. 250–251)

Finally, there are at least two of the following symptoms of persistent arousal that were not present prior to the traumatizing experience:

(1) *difficulty falling or staying asleep*

(2) *irritability or outbursts of anger*

(3) *difficulty concentrating*

(4) *hypervigilance*

(5) *exaggerated startle response*

(6) *physiologic reactivity upon exposure to events that symbolize or resemble an aspect of the traumatic event (e.g., a woman who was raped in an elevator breaks out in a sweat when entering any elevator)* (DSM-III-R, pp. 250–251)

There are very few controlled investigations into PTSD in children. However, it is clear that vulnerability to this disorder depends on a number of factors. Individuals not only vary in terms of their level of response to threat, they also vary in their ability to perceive danger and the degree to which they interpret a given situation to be dangerous.

While these dimensions of individual temperament undoubtedly play some role in determining the onset and course of PTSD, there is some evidence that they are secondary in importance to the nature and intensity of the trauma (Silverman, 1986). Moreover, in adults at least, it appears that personal and family backgrounds may not be good predictors of posttrauma psychopathology (Leopold & Dillon, 1963).

With regard to PTSD in children, Gleser, Grenn, and Winget (1981) examined the impact of the Buffalo Creek flood on families affected by it. All families were found to be adversely affected by the trauma. Parents exhibited increased cigarette and alcohol consumption as well as elevated use of prescription drugs in the years following the flood. It appeared that school-aged children were more severely affected than preschoolers and that the deficits in children over all were related to their parents' emotional destabilization and the disruption of home life.

In one of the few follow-up studies performed with children, Terr (1981) performed a nonblind, uncontrolled study on the population of children involved in the Chowchilla bus incident in 1976. These 26 children, aged 5 to 14 years, were kidnapped and buried in their school bus for 27 hours. They were evaluated after digging themselves out and each was found to suffer from posttraumatic emotional sequelae.

When evaluated, 4 to 5 years after the incident, each child was found to be experiencing PTSD. However, unlike adults, these children did not experience flashbacks, amnesia, or psychic numbing. Rather, they showed reenactment of the incident in their play and had difficulty recalling the occurrence of events during the incident in their proper order or time frame. The authors concluded from their investigation that children do not appear to be more flexible than adults in the aftermath of a powerful psychic trauma.

Given the fact that many children seen in psychiatric clinics come from extremely chaotic and/or abusive environments in which they are likely to be traumatized, it seems reasonable to suggest that the symptomatology for PTSD should be looked for in cases of suspected anxiety disorders. This is especially true since, as Silverman (1986) has suggested, exposure to severe trauma may actually recalibrate the entire emotional response system of the individual. Trauma may cause the neuroendocrine system to maintain an abnormally high level of vigilance while lowering the threshold of arousal. Thus, PTSD, to one degree or another, may lie at the root of many manifestations of anxiety symptoms, especially in children who are abused or who feel terrified and powerless for any other reason.

Atypical Anxiety Disorder

This is simply a catch-all category, intended for use when symptoms of anxiety do not appear to meet the criteria for any of the other specified anxiety disorders.

As should be clear from the foregoing discussion, the differential diagnosis of anxiety states can be a difficult task. The mere existence of a category such as atypical anxiety disorder is indicative of the confusion that still remains in assessing anxiety states. Nevertheless, three factors emerge that may be of general use when attempting to discover the etiology of an anxious state. First, it is important to screen for depression and to ensure that, if present, it is not the primary condition which in turn is producing secondary anxiety. Second, the anxious state should be assessed along an axis of specificity. That is, the clinician must attempt to determine whether the condition results from a focused source (e.g., separation anxiety, simple phobia, posttraumatic stress disorder) or is a more generalized phenomenon (e.g., obsessive-compulsive, avoidant disorder, overanxious disorder). Finally, it is important to consider all possibilities of pathophysiologic etiology.

Yvonne: Worry About the Future

Yvonne is a 5-year-old girl who has lived with her foster mother for the past 8 months. Yvonne's foster mother plans to adopt her. Yvonne is the second of four daughters born to her natural parents. Three of the daughters (including Yvonne) were removed from the care of their biological parents by the Children's Protection Services. When the agency first intervened 5 years ago, Yvonne was placed in the hospital for pneumonia, allegedly due to neglect. Strap marks were discovered on her older sister's back at this time. Yvonne was not removed from her home until age 2, when she was placed in emergency foster care. Since that time, she has been in various foster homes. Yvonne has reportedly become very attached to her current foster mother and, until 2 months ago, had been making "considerable intellectual gains." At this time, the court ordered supervised visits between Yvonne, her sisters, and her natural parents. As noted by the psychiatrist who supervises these meetings, Yvonne's natural mother is functioning at a borderline intellectual level. She has a history of being abused by her parents and her lovers. She is currently living with Yvonne's natural father, who is "usually unwashed, with a face mutilated by scars from knife fights." There is no information about Yvonne's birth or about her medical history, except that she had pneumonia and that she is severely farsighted.

Yvonne's foster mother reports that Yvonne demands constant attention and is very difficult, demanding, and intrusive. "She is nonstop wanting to know where I am and what I am doing." Yvonne also claims to have frequent stomachaches, for which a thorough medical examination found no source. Yvonne's day-care teacher also notes that Yvonne is very needy of adult attention; she attaches indiscriminately to strange adults and at times tries to follow them out of the room. In addition, Yvonne reportedly cries easily and gets into fights with her classmates. Both sources state that Yvonne's symptoms have worsened since she has begun visiting with her natural family.

During assessment, Yvonne was found to be overly friendly; she lacked timidity and any fear of strangers. She is a short, heavy-set child with a boyish appearance that is exaggerated by an unflattering haircut. Yvonne's gross motor movements appeared slightly immature; she had difficulty hopping and walking a straight line, but had no trouble alternating stairs. Her fine motor coordination was normal, as were her language capabilities. Yvonne's mood throughout the evaluation was happy, but she reported being sad when she thought about her parents having hurt her. Yvonne also reported being frightened when left alone. She denied having any hallucinations and did not exhibit any suicidal or self-destructive tendencies. During play, Yvonne chose the role of nurturer (by offering food) and was quite demanding, insisting that the examiner play games with her. Yvonne's performance during the session implied that she is of average intelligence. Her attention and concentration were both variable and her psychomotor activity was high. Yvonne was oriented and in touch with reality. Her behavior throughout the session was impulsive, and thus her judgment was impaired.

Yvonne's symptoms point to a diagnosis of overanxious disorder: She manifests an excessive worry about the future (fearing what will happen when she is left alone), and she has excessive need for reassurance and marked feelings of tension and somatic complaints without any physical basis. Yvonne has had these symptoms for more than 6 months, the minimum length of time necessary to make this diagnosis.

Differential diagnosis of separation anxiety disorder can be ruled out because Yvonne's anxiety is all-encompassing; it does not center only on situations involving separation. A diagnosis of attention deficit disorder can also be ruled out because, although a child with this disorder is usually tense and nervous, he or she is not unduly concerned about the future. Adjustment disorder with anxious mood is not an appropriate diagnosis for Yvonne because her symptoms have lasted longer than 6 months. It is also clear that Yvonne is not psychotic, for there was no "gross impairment of reality testing."

Thus, a diagnosis of overanxious disorder is appropriate in this case. Individual psychotherapy has been recommended to address Yvonne's fears, chronic neediness, and extreme anxiety about abandonment. Her foster mother has been advised to enter supportive parent counseling to help her deal with her child's particular needs.

COMMON MANIFESTATIONS OF CHILDHOOD ANXIETY

Fears of the Infant and Development of the Attachment Bond: Separation Disorder

As mentioned previously, separation anxiety may provide the template for all later forms of anxiety. As such, it is worthy of further discussion. Yvonne's case provides an excellent example of the great affective power of worry—the cognitive aspect of anxiety. It also illustrates the pervasiveness of the separation theme in anxiety states. The importance of being able to establish and maintain an attachment to the caregiver was graphically illustrated during World War II, when infants who were placed in residential nurseries or hospital wards displayed a predictable sequence of behaviors during their separations, namely, protest, despair, and, finally, hopeless detachment (Bowlby, 1969; Field, 1986). Defensive reactions directed at reducing anxiety from more minor separations include, but are not limited to, the following:

1. Physiological motor regression combined with avoidance of visual perceptions in order to kinesthetically restore the feeling of the mother's presence.
2. Attempts to master the environment by overcoming intervening obstacles in order to follow the mother.

3. Inhibition of activity to fend off anxiety arising from failed attempts at mastery. (Tennes & Lampl, 1969)

The dynamics underlying abnormally high levels of fear regarding separation from the caregiver depend on three factors: the innate fears common to all infants; the development of an anxious, ambivalent attachment bond with the caregiver; and the temperamental make-up of the infant. Bowlby (1973) has cogently argued that the infant is essentially "programmed" at birth to fear such things as loud noises, heights, loss of support, and looming objects.

Later, when cognitive development has progressed sufficiently to initiate the learning process, the infant grows to fear strangeness and being alone. Within this framework, objects that are feared may or may not be dangerous in fact. The caregiver plays a mediational role in determining the degree of fear felt in response to perceived environmental threat. An available and responsive caregiver aids the child in achieving a sense of security and trust that brings fear of potential threats into normative bounds. However, an unresponsive or undependable caregiver will generate the opposite effect, causing the child to experience exaggerated levels of fear in response to what are perceived to be threatening stimuli.

In Bowlby's view, the level of anxiety about loss and abandonment that continues to varying degrees over the course of a life is determined in large part by early experiences with the caregiver. In other words, the early natural need of the infant for protection and nurturance sets the tone for later emotional perception of security versus threat as mediated by the caregiver.

In the normal course of development, the infant begins to build a focused attachment to the caregiver, seeking protection from the caregiver and avoiding strangers. *Separation anxiety* describes the infant's dismay if the mother departs as well as the infant's worry about some anticipated absence. The same is true for children of preschool age (Blehar, 1974). Bloom-Feshbach and Blatt (1981) studied the adaptation to a nursery school of 20 3-year-olds and found that distress on separating from the caregiver each day was universal for the first 2 weeks and was present in many cases for the first 4 weeks. Separation distress continuing after the first month of school attendance was found to be correlated with social-emotional problems of the angry, defiant type. Thus, separation distress after 4 weeks might be one way of differentiating children with normal separation anxiety from those with more profound emotional difficulties, at least in those attending nursery schools.

Treatment of the Infant.   While separation anxiety is a normal phenomenon among all infants, the degree of anxiety experienced is determined by a number of factors including age (Stayton, Ainsworth, & Main, 1973), previous experience, the type of situation (Weintraub & Lewis, 1977), and, significantly, the quality of the attachment bond (Ainsworth, Blehar, Waters, & Wall, 1978).

Of these influences, perhaps the greatest is the quality of attachment between the infant and caregiver, and it must be realized that the infant makes a contribution to this bond by way of its innate reactivity to stress and other factors of temperament. Wolfson and co-workers (1987) have cited the work of Block and Block (1980), who defined two dimensions that can be used to measure the stable aspects of a child's adaptive ability and style. Ego-resiliency is defined as the degree to which a child can modulate impulses, desires, and feelings. Ego-control, on the other hand, is a measure of the ability of a child to contain or express impulses, feelings, and desires.

Block and Block (1980) suggested that, with regard to ego-control, children who exhibit brittle (nonresilient) overcontrol may be at risk for significant pathology. Brittle undercontrol, on the other hand, may be suggestive of a predisposition toward attention deficit or hyperactivity. In testing this hypothesis, Wolfson and colleagues (1987) studied 47 4- to 6-year-olds, 27 of whom were in therapeutic nursery programs and were diagnosed according to the DSM-III as having disturbances of emotion and mood. All cases of conduct disorder, attention deficit disorder, PDD, and psychoses were excluded from the study.

Contrary to the hypothesis, brittle undercontrollers were found to be at greatest risk for pathology, manifesting significantly higher scores on the externalizing dimension of the Child Behavior Profile and higher scores on aggression and depression scales. These children also scored higher on the activity dimension of temperament. Overall, the clinic children were less ego-resilient and temperamentally lower in adaptability and more negative in mood than the nonclinic controls. The temperamental characteristic of negative mood was the salient feature that distinguished the anxiety-disordered children from their normal peers. Wolfson and co-workers stated that this might have been due to concern over being separated from a parent. As Puig-Antich and Rabinovich (1986) have pointed out, this is a realistic concern since the overlap of depression and anxiety is very complex in cases of separation anxiety. Nevertheless, Wolfson and colleagues argued that it is more likely that constitutional factors interacting with early stress in members of the clinic group produced a lesser tolerance for negative emotions.

This reduced tolerance produces poor self-control, greater withdrawal and anxiety, and decreased flexibility. It is not difficult to see that a child with such a temperamental predisposition would place extra demands on the caregiver, who in turn might not be able to provide the full measure of responsiveness and security needed by such a child. It is indeed vital to consider temperament in the genesis of any anxious state in childhood.

School Refusal

The widely recognized phenomenon of refusal to go to school is another common manifestation of childhood anxiety and one that throws into high relief the various considerations that must be taken into account when diagnosing anxious conditions in children. School refusal is more properly looked at not as a diagnosis but as a syndrome of emotional distress that indicates an acute reaction to stress (Turner-Boutle, 1984). The fact that it is still a matter of question as to whether this disorder is a single syndrome presenting with a variety of symptoms or a number of syndromes with a common presenting symptomatology highlights the importance of determining the cause of the behavior. However, the task of discovering the etiology for this behavior is compli-cated by the fact that, as is so often the case with anxious disorders, children frequently present with a mixed anxious-depressed symptom-atology. For example, one study by Bernstein and Garfinkel (1986), in which 26 patients were referred from schools across the state and from two juvenile court systems, found that 69% of these early-adolescent chronic school refusers met DSM-III criteria for depression, 62% met the criteria for anxiety disorder, and 50% met the criteria for both dis-orders.

The first step in diagnosis is to determine whether it is the actual school setting that is the feared stimulus (as implied by "school phobia"), or whether the behavior derives from the desire to remain at home with the caregiver. In this way, for example, separation anxiety could present as school phobia. However, separation anxiety can be detected by the extreme difficulty encountered in separating the child from caregivers under any circumstances, school or otherwise. As another example, chil-dren with overanxious disorder might also refuse to go to school, but these children can be distinguished from those who are truly phobic toward school by the presence of global, persistent worrying (Werry, 1986).

To segregate other possible nonphobic causes of school refusal, it is helpful to refer to the origins of this condition. The original description by Broadwin (1932) was little more than a variant on truancy, a persist-ent form of nonattendance of school that subsequently came to be called *school phobia* by some investigators and *school refusal* by others (Hersov, 1985). The differentiation of school refusal from truancy is perhaps the first step to take in assessing a pattern of nonattendance.

According to Broadwin (1932), this phenomenon is distinguished from truancy by the fact that the parent knows where the child is at all times and the absence from school is consistent. Also, the absence is not comprehensible by either parents or the school. The child is happy and seemingly content at home but becomes extremely unhappy and fearful when forced to go to school, usually escaping to flee home as soon as an opportunity presents itself. Onset is sudden, and previous school performance has been at acceptable levels.

Broadwin's description is largely viable to this day. However, research has progressed since then to divulge that, when compared to truants, school refusers tend to come from smaller families at a higher level of income. Disciplining tends to be overanxious (Cooper, 1966). Furthermore, 20% of the mothers of children who refuse to go to school have a history of psychiatric disorder, usually affective (Berg, Butler, & Pritchard, 1974).

These results are in agreement with a later study by Last, Francis, Hersen, Kazdin, and Strauss (1987), who also found a significant incidence of psychiatric disorders among the mothers of children with school refusal. However, in their study, Last and co-workers used DSM-III (not DSM-III-R) criteria for separation anxiety disorder and phobic disorder of school to separate and compare school nonattenders. Their findings showed that the incidence of affective illness was four times greater in the mothers of children with DSM-III separation anxiety. Furthermore, separation anxiety appeared to be a more serious disturbance since 92% of the children with this diagnosis met criteria for at least one concomitant diagnosis, while the same was true for only 63% of the school phobia group.

Suggesting the feasibility of differential diagnosis, the study by Last and co-workers did find significant differences between the two groups of children with respect to the factors mentioned as well as symptoms and demographic characteristics. Children with separation anxiety were predominantly female and prepubertal and came from lower income families, while those with school phobia tended to be male and postpubertal and of higher socioeconomic backgrounds. These results are similar to those of Reeves, Werry, Elkind, and Zametkin (1987), who studied 105 children between the ages of 5 and 12 who had diagnoses of anxiety, attention deficit, conduct, or oppositional disorders. As in the findings of Last and colleagues, children with anxiety disorder were less predominantly male and had more anxious or disturbed parents.

These results notwithstanding, differential diagnosis of this condition can be an extended procedure. First, school refusal must be separated from truancy and nonattendance induced by a parent who keeps the child at home to work or for some other reason. Once truancy and voluntary withholding by a parent are ruled out, it must be determined whether the behavior is the result of separation anxiety, a phobia regarding something at school or the school setting as a whole, an aspect of depression, or a disorder related to psychosis or personality (Hersov, 1985).

Obsessive-Compulsive Disorder

Obsessive-compulsive disorder (OCD) has been generally thought to be rare in childhood (approximately 1% of child psychiatric inpatients), although it is receiving increasing attention (Rapoport, 1986). Compulsive ritualization of behaviors is a normal part of development, as evidenced by such prolonged childhood games as hopscotch and jacks. However, pathology can set in when the child experiences intensely repressed impulses from the unconscious.

In order to break into the conscious realm, the impulse becomes attached to an idea that has no logical connection to the impulse, causing the child to be puzzled as to why he or she has become obsessed with the idea. Since the content of the impulse is usually repugnant, the child may behave in a way opposite to that dictated by the impulse. Thus, the child may wash excessively as a futile means of counteracting the unconscious urge to make a mess (Karush, 1979).

There is still some debate as to whether or not OCD in children is actually an anxiety disorder. Berg, Zahn, Behar, and Rapoport (1986) tested the hypothesis that obsessive-compulsive symptoms develop to alleviate unacceptable feelings with 30 adolescent patients diagnosed as having severe or primary OCD.

After extensive interviewing and testing it was found that four patients also met the DSM-III criteria for overanxious disorder and one for separation anxiety disorder. Results testing the hypothesis were somewhat equivocal in that there were marked differences on autonomic arousal between sexes. Obsessive-compulsive boys were above normal on this measure compared to controls, whereas girls were lower than controls.

These results led Berg and co-workers to speculate that feelings of discomfort related to OCD in boys are more likely to be fears and anxiety, while girls may experience shame and guilt. As a final possibility, these investigators postulated that OCD may be more independent from anxiety or depressive disorders in childhood than in adulthood. It seems clear from this discussion that the dense cognitive-emotional content underlying OCD gives rise to feelings that have yet to be adequately delineated.

CONCLUSION

The predisposition to anxiety within a given individual depends on a number of factors about which little is known at the present time: factors of temperament and heredity, prenatal and early postnatal experiences, and the birth experience itself. Nevertheless, the DSM-III ambitiously attempts to define a great number of anxiety subcategories in children and adults at the risk of sacrificing reliability. Still, as Werry (1986) pointed out in his recent review of DSM-III criteria, the organization does allow for the arrangement of anxiety disorders along with age-specific guidelines. In this way, overanxious disorder is seen as being exaggerated elemental anxiety present at birth; avoidant reaction can be viewed as persistent stranger anxiety; separation anxiety may be separation fear; and phobia anxiety may be seen as specific conditioned anxiety. Under this scheme, for example, obsessive-compulsive disorder appears as a combination of escape-avoidant behavior in response to phobia-type anxiety experienced by an overanxious person.

However, much research regarding anxiety in children remains to be done. Little longitudinal research has been done on the organic course of children's fears and anxieties in nonclinical samples. For example, it is still an open question as to whether an anxiously attached infant develops into an insecure and fearful preschooler as Bowlby's (1973) work would predict. In addition, assessing anxiety in children is still problematic in that there is poor reliability among different scales and measures. Nevertheless, the DSM-III-R criteria as currently structured do provide a useful framework for interpreting the results of further investigations and making refinements.

CHAPTER FOURTEEN

Attention Deficit and Conduct Disorders and Their Differential Diagnosis

David: Energetic Inattention

David is a $4\frac{1}{2}$-year-old boy. He has been described as a curious explorer of his environment who particularly enjoys assembling and reassembling objects. He lives with his two younger brothers, aged 1 and 2, and with his parents. David fights frequently with his 2-year-old brother, especially when his brother wants to share or borrow his belongings. David usually settles these disputes with violent actions. When he was 3 years old, David's parents were separated for a 4-month period, during which David stayed with his mother at a shelter. David's father suffers from temporal lobe epilepsy, for which he has been hospitalized. David's mother described David as an extremely "passive" infant, whom she had to awaken to initiate or continue feeding. He sat up, began walking, and started talking within normal ranges. David's mother commented that David became "like a different kid" during his second year; her impression was that he was unusually distractible. For example, while standing in his playpen, David would suddenly become distracted by some stimulus and would then release his grip on the playpen bar and fall backward. His toilet training began after age 2 and took 11 months; he continued to wet at night until he was almost 4.

David was initially referred for evaluation after his nursery school teacher noticed that he acted as though the other children were not present. Psychological evaluation at that time concluded the following: bright-normal intelligence; severe articulation difficulties with expressive language deficits; attention deficit disorder without hyperactivity; and a lack of relatedness, described as "a peculiar quality of nonadaptivity." David's symptoms worsened over the months, with continued aggressiveness and unresponsiveness plus what his teacher described as an inability to "shift gears." Three different medications—Cylert, Imipramine, and Elavil—were prescribed by his pediatrician and a neurologist. The net result of drug therapy, as observed by David's teacher, mother, and the school psychologist, was ambiguous. A second psychological evaluation concluded that David suffered from depression secondary to attention deficit disorder.

Behavior characteristics that prompted referral for a third evaluation included the following: general aggressiveness; attempts to dominate the play situation; and exhibitions of extreme anger when others do not comply with his wishes. When enraged, David is likely to yell at or hit other children. Sometimes he loses interest in group play and wanders away to engage in solitary activities. David disrupts class by calling out. He has trouble staying in his seat and completing and organizing his schoolwork. His mother describes him as moody and demanding and tells of his temper tantrums, during which he will scream and cry uncontrollably for at least 20 minutes. She has also noticed that David cries easily when his feelings are hurt or when he feels frustrated. David may become deeply absorbed in an activity, but he cannot be redirected to other activities unless he becomes tired of the activity and elects to do something different. Other elements of the mental status examination were within normal ranges.

David's symptoms pointed to a diagnosis of attention deficit disorder with hyperactivity. His failure to complete and organize his schoolwork, his impulsiveness, and his inattention to the presence and needs of others are symptoms that are commonly found in attention deficit with hyperactivity. Specific developmental disorders such as developmental articulation disorder and developmental expressive language disorder are common associated diagnoses, and were considered in this case. It is not uncommon for children with attention deficit hyperactivity disorder to be functionally enuretic, as was David for a prolonged period after he completed toilet training. The possibility of David's having an associated diagnosis of epilepsy was also seriously considered, especially with his family history of epilepsy. He underwent neurological evaluation (including electroencephalographic examination), which yielded no positive findings, and the diagnosis of petit mal was ruled out.

Differential diagnosis against pervasive developmental disorder was kept in mind. This disorder was unlikely, however, because David does not manifest symptoms such as abnormalities of posture and motor behavior, abnormalities of mood, or odd responses to sensory input. A diagnosis of mental retardation was inappropriate because David's intellectual functioning deficits are not markedly subaverage and are most likely due to specific developmental deficits. A differential diagnosis of mood disorders was ruled out as well, on the basis of David's ability to maintain concentration and his psychomotor normalcy, conditions that would be disturbed in mood disorders. It was also determined that David's hyperactivity is not appropriate for his developmental stage and that his environment is not disorganized or chaotic enough to be responsible for causing his symptoms.

A recommendation for treatment will be made after completion of differential diagnoses of specific developmental disorders and epilepsy, so that all facets of David's difficulties and strengths can be incorporated into an effective improvement strategy.

INTRODUCTION

The association of hyperactivity with behavioral, social, and learning problems has been recognized for nearly a century. The early postulations of an organic etiology for this condition (e.g., organic brain syndrome, minimal brain dysfunction) may well prove true, but the fact is that what is unknown far outweighs what is known about hyperactivity and its associated phenomena. However, the ramifications of repeated episodes of frustration in task completion are becoming increasingly clearer. As David grew older, he began to cry and develop aggressive behaviors in response to frustrating tasks. The development of aggression is only one of many possible outcomes.

The most recent approach in attempting to unravel the relationships involved in attentional problems has been to perform research that focuses not on hyperactivity per se but on attention deficits that may, in one way or another, lead to hyperactive behavior and its concomitants. The diagnoses in DSM-III of attention deficit disorder, conduct disorder, and oppositional disorder were based on the postulation that a deficit in attentional ability may have causes and sequelae separate from those associated with conduct disorder or oppositional disorder.

DSM-III-R exerts further efforts in this direction, slightly changing the criteria for these disorders and grouping them under the new class of disruptive behavior disorders. In this new system, attention deficit disorder (ADD) without hyperactivity is essentially eliminated by renaming it as undifferentiated attention deficit disorder, observing that diagnoses of ADD without hyperactivity, according to DSM-III criteria, were hardly ever made. Attention deficit disorder with hyperactivity in DSM-III-R is now termed attention deficit hyperactivity disorder (ADHD). In turn, the new DSM-III-R criteria for ADHD have been modified so that no single feature is required. Rather, an index of behavioral items was selected in an attempt to better discriminate ADHD from conduct disorder (CD) and oppositional defiant disorder (ODD).

Despite these attempts at clarification, research continues to be published that contradicts the conclusion of DSM-III-R that diagnoses of ADD without hyperactivity are rarely made. The recent work by Lahey, Schaughency, Hynd, Carlson, and Nieves (1987) is a good example. Using a reliable assessment procedure, these investigators evaluated 41 clinic outpatients, 6 to 13 years of age, who were given a diagnosis of attention deficit disorder with hyperactivity (ADD/H) and 22 patients who were diagnosed as having attention deficit disorder without hyperactivity (ADD/WO).

In each case, the subject and at least one custodial parent (usually the mother) were interviewed separately. Decisions about the presence or absence of each DSM-III symptom were made by subjectively weighing and combining all information rather than employing a set algorithm. In addition to parent and child interviews, information was obtained by teacher interview and a range of teacher rating scales.

Lahey and co-workers found that ADD without hyperactivity can be diagnosed reliably, at least in a clinic-referred population. While a majority (68%) of the ADD/WO subjects received at least one additional diagnosis, nearly the same percentage (61%) of ADD/H subjects also had additional diagnoses. In general, children with ADD/H were found to be more impulsive and display a greater intensity and severity of CD than those with ADD/WO. On the other hand, children with ADD/WO were more sluggish in their cognitive processing and seemed more likely to show coexisting internalizing disorders. Just as children with ADD/WO were likely to show a preponderance of internalizing disorders, those with ADD/H more often displayed externalizing disorders.

Since research into the relationship between attention and hyperactivity and between the attention-hyperactivity axis and associated behavioral problems is still in the early stages, the attempt by DSM-III-R to separate ADD from CD and ODD is probably a fruitful one—at least in terms of guiding research efforts. While it is possible that a deficit in the capacity for sustained attention is a prime cause of hyperactive behavior and its associated symptomatology, it is very likely not the only cause, and it may in some instances be a secondary feature. For example, a deficit in learning ability could produce poor concentration due to poor comprehension. In this situation, the act of paying attention would be unrewarded. Thus, the child would begin to orient toward more rewarding stimuli—a process that could easily lead the adult observer to assess the child wrongly as being inherently distractible. Impulsivity could well become part of this picture if the child gradually learned to hurry through the unrewarding behavior of school tasks (Levine, Busch, & Aufseeser, 1982). In addition, the learned inattention (learned as a result of the learning disability), in combination with the learning disability itself, could well generate frustration, thereby facilitating aggressive behavior (Campbell & Werry, 1986; Levine et al., 1982).

The foregoing example, which is only one of many possible scenarios, serves to illustrate the difficulty in establishing which among the primary symptoms of ADD, CD, and ODD comes first in any given situation—hyperactivity, inattention, impulsivity, or aggression. It may be that the universality of the aggressive component provides the strongest reason for grouping these three disorders into one class—a possibility that is not directly acknowledged in DSM-III-R. In any case, as is reflected in the restructuring of DSM-III-R, it is important when discussing these disorders to be continually aware of the lack of specificity of the separate symptoms that comprise their structure.

An example of this lack of specificity was provided by Shapiro and Garfinkel (1986), who screened the entire population ($n = 315$) of children attending grades 2 through 6 at a Minnesota rural public school. Among this nonreferred population there were 153 girls and 162 boys. Mean age was 9 years, 10 months. Instruments were chosen with a view toward garnering data from as many varied sources as possible. Homeroom teachers completed the CTRS (Conners, 1969), while the students were given the Diagnostic Interview for Children and Adolescents (DICA) (Herjanic & Campbell, 1977). In addition, the children received a computerized attentional battery consisting of a continuous performing task, a progressive maze, and a group of tests assessing reading, arithmetic, and language achievement.

Using this extensive analysis, Shapiro and Garfinkel found that 7 (2.3%) of the children displayed inattention-overactivity, while 11 (3.6%) had significant indicators of aggression. However, 9 (3.0%) manifested problems in both areas. This represents 33% of the index group and clearly demonstrates the interdependence of symptoms commonly associated with the diagnoses of ADD and CD.

Much of the confusion lies in the fact that a good deal of the clinical symptomatology is far removed from the hypothesized causes of these conditions. It therefore seems likely that they will be definitively differentiated from each other (primarily ADD from CD) only when the specifics of brain function become more thoroughly understood.

Perhaps the most provocative finding to date regarding brain functions has been the observed relationship between hyperactivity and a reduced ability to receive incoming stimuli. Orris (1969) compared the performance of normal adolescents with undersocialized delinquents in a sustained attention task and found that the delinquent group performed significantly worse. In addition, the undersocialized group performed more activities directed at alleviating boredom (e.g., singing and talking to themselves) rather than attending to the task.

Others have duplicated the early results of Orris, leading to the general conclusion that the efficacy of amphetamine treatment for hyperactive children derives from the drug's ability to bring the mind "up to speed" so that the individual is able to experience normative levels of environmental stimulation (Skrzypek, 1969; Whitehill, DeMyer, & Scott, 1976). This forestalls the need to generate input through disruptive hyperactive behavior.

Another biological realm that promises to be of use in differentiating between different types of hyperactivity is that of family history. August and Stewart (1983) performed an intriguing study of 125 child psychiatric patients admitted over a period of 16 months with a diagnosis of hyperkinetic syndrome of childhood. They isolated two familial subgroups within this sample, those who had at least one natural parent with a diagnosis in the antisocial spectrum and those who had neither parent with such a diagnosis.

Grouping hyperactive children according to the psychiatric diagnosis of their parents proved useful. Those whose parents were in some way antisocial showed deviance on several dimensions of behavior and presented a clear picture of conduct disorder. Hyperactive children whose parents lacked any psychiatric diagnosis demonstrated more intellectual deficits but exhibited relatively few behavior problems beyond their problems with attention and impulsivity. Moreover, the siblings of these "pure hyperactives" tended to have similar developmental learning problems but a marked lack of conduct disturbances.

August and Stewart pointed out that their results run parallel to those of Stewart, DeBlois, and Cummings (1980), who found that the male offspring of parents with personality disorder and alcoholism frequently develop conduct disorders, while hyperactive boys without conduct disorder rarely come from parents with these conditions. Along these same lines, Biederman, Munir, and Knee (1987) found that the rate of major affective disorder was significantly higher (27%) in the immediate relatives of 22 children with attention deficit disorder than in the relatives of normal control subjects (6%). Furthermore, the children with attention deficit disorder were more likely to have coexisting affective disorders than were the normal controls (32% versus 0%).

The findings that some hyperactives do come from families with a negative history for psychiatric disorder points to a third, but not directly biologic, possible source of this behavior: the interaction of the child with his or her caregiver and/or family. Prior, Leonard, and Wood (1983) compared 20 preschool children diagnosed as hyperactive with 20 nonhyperactive matched controls. While the two groups were found to be significantly different, the greater behavior disturbance in the hyperactive children was found to be closely tied to issues of family temperament.

In their study, Prior and co-workers found that the tempermental characteristics of the hyperactive children clustered on the "difficult" side, suggesting that a difficult temperament might play a significant role in garnering a label of *difficult, unmanageable,* or *hyperactive* for a child. Prior and co-workers concluded that, rather than resorting to drug therapy, it might be more appropriate in many instances to devote attention to facilitating the interaction between the child and his or her mother.

In support of this contention are the findings of Hewitt and Jenkins (1946) and Lewis (1954), who reported that children with aggressive conduct disorder were frequently rejected by their parents when they were very young. Also, Cohen, Sullivan, Minde, Novak, and Keens (1983) found that mothers of kindergarten-age hyperactive children attempted to control their children's behavior more than the mothers of normal children by showing more disapproval and specifically telling the children what to do when confronted with problem-solving situations. The hyperactive children in this study demonstrated an exaggerated, anxious self-awareness in that they commented more frequently on their performance and requested more feedback than did controls. It is perhaps no small wonder that Varley (1984) reported that he has observed poor self-concept and feelings of isolation and loneliness in almost all children with ADD.

A recent study by Jacobvitz and Sroufe (1987) has substantiated the findings of Cohen and co-workers regarding the association of maternal intrusiveness with hyperactivity. Other aspects of child–caregiver interaction in association with hyperactivity were also examined in this prospective study of a large sample of infants who were considered to be at high risk for later caregiving problems since they came from low-income families.

Jacobvitz and Sroufe based their experiential measurements on the work of Douglas and Peters (1979), who hypothesized that ADHD is the result, at least in part, of the child's inability to adequately modulate or regulate his or her arousal level to meet situational demands. Jacobvitz and Sroufe measured three parenting variables that are conceptually linked to the infant's failure to adequately modulate its state of arousal: maternal intrusiveness during infancy and two later assessments of maternal behavior, one of seductive behavior and one of overstimulating behavior. Patterns of these maternal behaviors were assessed at 6 months, 2 years, and $3\frac{1}{2}$ years. During the first $2\frac{1}{2}$ years of life, the children were assessed repeatedly in terms of 38 early-childhood variables including neonatal behavioral assessments and ratings of activity level by parents and observers.

At the end of kindergarten, when the children were approximately 6 years old, their teachers completed the Achenbach Child Behavior Checklist for all 184 children in the study. This scale was administered to determine the presence or absence of hyperactive tendency. From this pool, 34 hyperactive children were chosen and compared to 34 matched, nonhyperactive children from the same pool. The two subsamples of children were compared regarding the early caregiving variables, child variables, additional characteristics of the mothers, and distractibility ratings taken at 42 months.

Like Cohen and colleagues (1983), Jacobvitz and Sroufe found that the caregivers of hyperactive children engaged in significantly more intrusive/interference behaviors with their infants than did the matched controls. Furthermore, mothers of the hyperactive children scored higher on the overstimulating care scale at 42 months. However, no correlation was found between seductive behavior on the part of the caregiver and later hyperactive behavior in the child, and only 1 of the 38 early-childhood measures (taken from newborn through 30 months) was found to correlate with later hyperactivity. It was discovered that hyperactive kindergartners had been significantly less motorically mature on the 7- to 10-day composited Brazelton factor—a result that needs replication since it is an isolated finding.

Jacobvitz and Sroufe concluded that since two of the three parenting measures (intrusiveness and interference) derived from a theory of arousal modulation were significantly related to hyperactive outcome, it is very likely that psychogenic antecedents for ADHD exist in many kindergarten children. Pending replication of their results, the authors have noted that overstimulating care may play a predominant role in some hyperactive children, while for others, organic factors such as motor coordination may be more important. Still others may have in their histories a combination of these and other factors.

One other factor that plays a significant role in the etiology of hyperactivity is the infant's temperament (Trad, 1987). The results of a study by Kagan and co-workers (1987) have given extra credence to the probable contributions of temperament as measured by reaction (inhibited/withdraw versus uninhibited/approach) to unfamiliar and cognitively challenging events.

In this longitudinal study, more than 400 children were screened in order to find groups of 60 consistently uninhibited and 60 consistently inhibited children. There was an equal number of boys and girls in each group, and children were selected at either 21 or 31 months of age. Signs of behavioral inhibition included long latencies before interacting with or immediate retreat from unfamiliar people or objects, proximity to the mother, and cessation of play or vocalization. Uninhibited children showed the opposite behaviors.

Kagan and associates found that the behaviors characterizing inhibited and uninhibited children were very stable across time, remaining essentially unchanged from early toddlerhood through the age of 5 and beyond. Given this stability in terms of inherent reaction to stress, a child who is inhibited and who, in addition, receives intrusive and/or interfering caregiving might be at especially great risk of developing ADHD.

While this possibility is of little predictive value since it would be difficult to assess every child and family for inhibited temperament and intrusive caregiving, there is some hope of prediction in a subgroup of children with certain minor physical anomalies. Waldrop, Bell, McLaughlin, and Halverson (1978) reported that neonates with relatively high numbers of anomalies drawn from the following list are likely to demonstrate short attention span, peer aggression, and impulsivity at age 3: head circumference out of normal range; more than one hair whorl; epicanthus; hypertelorism; malformed ears; low-set ears; asymmetrical ears; soft, pliable ears; no ear lobes; high-steepled palate; furrowed tongue; curved fifth finger; single palmar crease; wide gap between first and second toes; partial syndactalia of toes; and third toe longer than second toe.

Within a clinic population of 81 hyperactive boys, a subgroup with high anomaly scores had greater plasma dopamine-beta-hydroxylase (DBH) activity, earlier age of onset of hyperactivity, more fathers with histories of hyperactivity, and more mothers who reported bleeding during the first trimester as compared to a subgroup with low anomaly scores. Since the presence of these anomalies can be detected within 5 to 10 minutes in a newborn examination, they may prove useful in alerting parents and health care personnel to the possibility of later behavioral problems.

Waldrup and colleagues noted that these minor physical anomalies may be developmental abnormalities resulting from genetic transmission or from an insult during early pregnancy. It might be that the factors producing the deviation in early pregnancy could influence the occurrence of both the anomalies and some deviation in the development of the part of the central nervous system that is responsible for the hyperactive behavior.

The sum of these findings suggests that while the construct of attention deficit provides a way to conceptualize certain aspects of behavioral difficulties (particularly learning problems), the symptom complex characteristic of attention deficits is probably indicative of different phenomena in different individuals. To forestall confusion in the ensuing discussion, ADD in its pure form will be viewed as an essentially cognitive disorder involving defective arousal and attentional mechanisms, as suggested by Rosenthal and Allen (1978).

Furthermore, as suggested by August and Stewart (1983), it seems reasonable to hypothesize that attention deficit disorder and conduct disorder may exist along a continuum on which the former is a less severe form of the latter. This contention seems at the very least to be of heuristic value in light of their findings regarding the differences in hyperactive offspring of parents with psychiatric versus those with nonpsychiatric histories. While this hypothesis has by no means been proved, it remains a useful means of examining and relating the diverse symptomatologies in question.

DIFFERENTIAL DIAGNOSIS: ATTENTION-DEFICIT HYPERACTIVITY DISORDER (ADHD), CONDUCT DISORDER (CD), AND OPPOSITIONAL DEFIANT DISORDER (ODD)

Attention-Deficit Hyperactivity Disorder

There is still a general consensus that a deficit in attention during the school years is a primary source of developmental and behavioral dysfunction. Therefore, the proper diagnosis of this disorder, while it can be difficult, is of great clinical value (Palfrey, Levine, Walker, & Sullivan, 1985).

The DSM-III-R describes a child with ADHD as displaying signs of developmentally inappropriate inattention, impulsivity, and hyperactivity. The signs must be reported by adults in the child's environment, such as parents and teachers. Since the symptoms are typically variable, they might not be observed directly by the clinician.

When reports of teachers and parents conflict, primary consideration should be given to the teacher's reports because of their greater familiarity with age-appropriate norms. Symptoms typically worsen in situations that require self-application, as in the classroom. Signs of disorder may be absent when the child is in a new or one-to-one situation.

In an effort to improve the usefulness of DSM-III with regard to discriminating ADDH from CD and ODD, the DSM-III-R criteria comprise an index of symptoms of which no single feature is required. Specifically, the DSM-III-R diagnostic criteria for ADDH (renamed ADHD) require a disturbance lasting at least 6 months during which at least eight of the following behaviors are present:

(1) often fidgets with hands or feet or squirms in seat (in adolescents, may be limited to subjective feeling of restlessness)

(2) has difficulty remaining seated when required to do so

(3) is easily distracted by extraneous stimuli

(4) has difficulty awaiting turn in games or group situations

(5) often blurts out answers to questions before they have been completed

(6) has difficulty following through on instructions from others (not due to oppositional behavior or a failure of comprehension), e.g., fails to finish chores

(7) has difficulty sustaining attention in tasks or play activities

(8) often shifts from one uncompleted activity to another

(9) has difficulty playing quietly

(10) often talks excessively

(11) often interrupts or intrudes on others, e.g., butts into other children's games

(12) often does not seem to listen to what is being said to him or her

(13) often loses things necessary for tasks or activities at school or at home (e.g., toys, pencils, books, assignments)

(14) often engages in physically dangerous activities without considering possible consequences (not for the purpose of thrill-seeking), e.g., runs into street without looking (pp. 52–53)

Onset of ADHD must be prior to age 7, and the individual cannot meet the criteria for a pervasive developmental disorder (PDD). The characteristics of PDD will now be briefly enumerated for purposes of comparison. The reader is advised to refer to Chapter Nine for differentiating between the various symptoms associated not only with ADHD and PDD but also with other conditions that can present confounding symptomatic pictures.

DSM-III-R revises the pervasive developmental disorders so that autism is viewed as the most severe and prototypic—and the only recognized subtype—of PDD. Certain aspects of autism can resemble the behaviors noted in ADHD. For instance, these children may have in common the impairment of reciprocal social interaction as manifested in lack of awareness of the feelings of others, lack of play or presence of abnormal play, and impairment in the ability to make peer friendships. Furthermore, children with either disorder may exhibit markedly abnormal nonverbal communication and may have difficulty initiating or sustaining a conversation with others.

However, there are many behaviors demonstrated in autism that usually are not present in children with ADHD. Some of these may include lack of any means of communication, verbal or otherwise; abnormal seeking of comfort at times of distress; stereotyped body movements; persistent preoccupation with the parts of objects; and markedly restricted range of interests and preoccupation with one narrow interest.

In addition to autism, the clinician must be alert to the possible inducement of attentional lapses due to absence seizures (petite mal) that may not be recognizable. Absences may occur many times a day and cause attentional lapses lasting from 1 to 10 seconds. Subtle clonic limb movements and blinking at a rate of 3 times per second are also usually present, as are automatisms—simple, repetitive, and purposeless movements such as plucking distractedly at clothing. During an absence seizure, mental and physical activity are interrupted but muscle tone and bladder control are maintained. Following the seizure, there is no confusion, agitation, or sleepiness and the individual has no awareness of the incident (Kaufman, 1985).

In differentiating ADHD from symptoms generated by an affective affliction, changes in body weight and sad expression may be particularly helpful. In addition to PDD and affective disorders, mental retardation can produce symptoms that might be confounded with ADHD. However, except in infants, this condition is not overly difficult to detect since it includes significantly subaverage general intellectual functioning accompanied by concurrent deficits or impairments in age-appropriate adaptive behavior. The border between retarded and normal poses a more difficult diagnostic situation when ADHD is being considered.

When summing the various symptom complexes that can emanate from disorders other than ADHD, the DSM-III-R tactic of distinguishing a hyperactive disorder deriving from deficits in attention from CD and ODD seems at least semantically justifiable. Only ADHD contains symptoms under all three headings of inattention, impulsivity, and hyperactivity.

Conduct Disorder

The DSM-III subtypings of this disorder were streamlined in DSM-III-R to include only conduct disorder, solitary aggressive type, group type, and undifferentiated type. These revised DSM-III-R criteria comprise a single index of symptoms directed at improving the description of the disorder's manifestations in order to enhance the ease of diagnosis.

Youngsters with CD are often truant from school and may run away from home. Furthermore, physical aggression is common in all forms of CD, with afflicted children exhibiting such behavior as cruelty to animals or people and destruction of property, frequently by fire setting. Jacobson (1985), in a study of 104 child fire setters in London, concluded that children engaging in this behavior, while few in number, form a subgroup of severe conduct disorders. They are distinguished by a younger peak age (8 years), a higher male-to-female ratio, and more severe psychosocial disturbance. Supporting this notion are the results of Kelso and Stewart (1986). When they followed up 53 boys with aggressive conduct disorder, these investigators found that fire setting was a predictor for the persistence of CD.

Specifically, DSM-III-R criteria for conduct disorder are as follows:

A. *A disturbance of conduct lasting at least six months, during which at least three of the following have been present:*
   (1) has stolen without confrontation of a victim on more than one occasion (including forgery)
   (2) has run away from home overnight at least twice while living in parental or parental surrogate home (or once without returning)
   (3) often lies (other than to avoid physical or sexual abuse)
   (4) has deliberately engaged in fire-setting
   (5) is often truant from school (for older person, absent from work)
   (6) has broken into someone else's house, building, or car
   (7) has deliberately destroyed others' property (other than by fire-setting)
   (8) has been physically cruel to animals
   (9) has forced someone into sexual activity with him or her
   (10) has used a weapon in more than one fight
   (11) often initiates physical fights
   (12) has stolen with confrontation of a victim (e.g., mugging, purse-snatching, extortion, armed robbery)
   (13) has been physically cruel to people. (p. 55)

If the individual is 18 or older, he or she must not meet the criteria for antisocial personality disorder.

In the group type of CD, there is a predominance of conduct problems occurring within a social context with peers. The solitary aggressive type of CD is characterized by the predominance of aggressive physical behavior, usually toward both adults and peers, initiated by the person and not as a group activity. The undifferentiated type of CD is reserved for children or adolescents with CD containing a mixture of clinical features that cannot be classified as either solitary aggressive or group type.

Patrick: Focus on Defiance

Patrick is a 4-year-old boy who lives with both of his parents; he has no siblings. He began attending nursery school at the age of 1 year, 11 months, reportedly because his mother was overwhelmed by the job of taking care of Patrick and needed some relief from those responsibilities. Patrick's mother breastfed him, with supplemental bottle feeding to compensate for her inadequate supply of milk. She reports that it was physically painful to breastfeed, adding that Patrick would watch her while she fed him and she felt he had perhaps sensed her pain. Patrick's parents have reported no developmental abnormalities, although he does still occasionally wear a diaper to bed. Patrick has been extremely active since the time he started to walk.

A few months before initial evaluation, Patrick was ill with a fever in the 102- to 103-degree range, a rash, lethargy, and enuresis. Patrick's father was away on a business trip at the time of Patrick's illness. (According to his parents, Patrick is always more difficult while his father is away on his frequent business trips.) After staying home for 3 days because of his fever, Patrick returned to school, where he behaved destructively and was unresponsive to his teacher. Patrick's mother was called by the school and asked to pick him up. Patrick yelled and fought for 5 more minutes before his mother arrived to take him home. Following this illness and the ensuing difficulty at school, Patrick's parents took him to a medical doctor, who noted nothing unusual except for impetigo.

About a month later, Patrick ran into the street while his class was walking to the playground. The school responded by warning his parents of serious problems. The warning included a description of Patrick as an intelligent child who prefers to play alone and who has fast mood swings that are accompanied by impulsive and destructive behavior. It also stated that Patrick must have constant supervision because he is likely to engage in dangerous activities such as dumping sand on himself, banging heads with another child, putting objects into his mouth, or trying to climb out windows. His teacher commented that Patrick throws things, hits other children, and has particular difficulty at mealtime. For example, he might eat a napkin or stuff a large piece of food into his mouth without taking bites. She felt that he has difficulty coping with changes in routine. Patrick's mother added that he refuses to follow her directions and is often a behavioral problem at home. There have been similar complaints from camp counselors about his refusal to abide by rules and his misbehavior.

Soon after the school sent the report, Patrick's parents took him to a psychiatrist in the town where Patrick's uncle lives. That doctor reported that Patrick was attentive and friendly during the interview and felt that he might have symptoms indicating attention deficit disorder exacerbated by a recent viral illness. He referred Patrick for further treatment in his home town. At the interview at a major urban hospital, Patrick was polite and had no trouble separating from his mother. His coordination was fine, but he immediately complained that all the toys were "boring." Soon, however, he started to play with trucks and dinosaurs and exhibited particularly aggressive themes. Patrick was reluctant to stop this play when asked to draw, but eventually he agreed. He answered questions while drawing, except those about school or camp, and he refused to share personal stories. In a diagnostic play group, Patrick exhibited oral rage, poor socialization, and a lack of curiosity. In a family play group, Patrick's puppet character had difficulty relating to the other characters, except at one point where he pretended to be serving the other characters at a party. His parents scolded Patrick for "interfering" when he was disruptive during the post-family-play discussion in the clinician's office. In another play group, Patrick was very aggressive and was unresponsive to limit setting. Other elements of the mental status examination were within normal ranges. In discussion, Patrick seemed to have difficulty organizing and expressing his thoughts.

Evaluation of Patrick's presenting symptoms suggested that a diagnosis of oppositional defiant disorder would be appropriate, since he displays defiant and deliberately annoying behaviors but does not violate the rights of others in as severe a manner as would indicate a diagnosis of conduct disorder. Typical oppositional symptoms that Patrick manifests include the following: mood lability; temper outbursts; defiance of adults' requests; refusal to perform chores or other mandatory tasks; and the evidence of these behaviors within and outside of the home. The mental status examination revealed no indication of hallucinations or delusions, thus ruling out an associated diagnosis of a psychotic process. Patrick's behaviors and the evaluation did not indicate evidence of a depressive or bipolar disorder, so the oppositional behaviors were judged not to be related to associated diagnoses of dysthymia, a manic or hypomanic episode, or a major depressive episode.

The clinician recommended individual therapy for Patrick twice a week and family therapy with both parents every other week.

Oppositional Defiant Disorder

The DSM-III-R describes this disorder as containing a pattern of negativistic, hostile, and defiant behavior, lacking the violation of the basic rights of others that is seen in conduct disorder. Patrick fits this profile rather well. Children with ODD are often argumentative with adults, losing their tempers easily, swearing, and being readily annoyed by the behavior of others. Symptoms may not be present to a great extent in school but are almost invariably present in the home, where impairment of function is greatest.

DSM-III-R criteria for ODD are as follows:

A. *A disturbance of at least six months during which at least five of the following are present:*

(1) *often loses temper*

(2) *often argues with adults*

(3) *often actively defies or refuses adult requests or rules, e.g., refuses to do chores at home*

(4) *often deliberately does things that annoy other people, e.g., grabs other children's hats*

(5) *often blames others for his or her own mistakes*

(6) *is often touchy or easily annoyed by others*

(7) *is often angry and resentful*

(8) *is often spiteful or vindictive*

(9) *often swears or uses obscene language.* (pp. 57–58)

The individual must not meet the criteria for CD, and the behavior must not occur exclusively during the course of a psychotic disorder, dysthymia, or a major depressive, hypomanic, or manic episode. In achieving differential diagnosis, it is important to note that all of the features of ODD are likely to be present in CD. Therefore, CD preempts the diagnosis of ODD. Likewise, symptoms of ODD are often observed in the prodromal phase of a psychotic disorder, and a psychotic disorder therefore also preempts the ODD diagnosis. Similarly, when ODD symptoms are noted during the course of dysthymia, manic hypomanic, or major depressive episode, the additional diagnosis of ODD is not made.

Much has been written about the association of antisocial behavior and ADD. However, it is still not known whether this is an actual causal relationship or an association that arises due to some other factor associated with both conditions. The results of a recent prospective study by Wallander (1988) suggest that the latter may be the case. Wallander studied a cohort of 265 children between the ages of 10 and 13 years, using teacher ratings to assess them for attention problems. Their cumulative arrest frequency was obtained 8 years later.

While there was a weak correlation between early attentional problems and later antisocial behavior, this relationship was almost entirely obviated when variance due to IQ and maternal reports of paternal difficulty controlling alcohol intake was removed. Thus, it may be that antisocial behavior and deficits in attention tend to co-occur as a result of some other causative factor. In light of the previous discussion in this chapter, a good candidate for this common factor might be excessive or inappropriate aggressive behavior in the home on the part of one or both parents.

In light of the multiple diagnoses seen in ADD patients, Munir and co-workers (1987) have proposed that the presence or absence of a major DSM-III-R co-diagnosis might be a more useful means of defining or classifying this heterogenous disorder. In examining 22 ADD patients with psychiatric disorders, they found that the rates of conduct disorder, oppositional disorder, major affective disorders, non-Tourette tics, encopresis, and learning difficulties were significantly higher than the norm. The authors suggested that subgrouping ADD patients by means of epidemiological elaboration of these associations might lead to the identification of a more homogenous group of patients with common course, outcome, family history, and biological markers.

Support for this approach was given by Rescorla (1986), who noted that the best data on behavioral problems in preschoolers come from epidemiological surveys. He suggested a system that might prove useful as a first step toward the process proposed by Munir and associates. Rescorla noted that while factor analytic studies on preschoolers consistently report two major dimensions of behavior, externalizing and internalizing, very little research has been done that makes use of this behavioral split (externalizing behaviors are characterized by undercontrolled, acting out, and aggressive tendencies, while internalizing factors include overcontrolled, withdrawn, and anxious symptoms).

A powerful approach to the study of ADD and its related disorders could be initiated by an approach in which children are first assessed in terms of externalizing or internalizing traits and then further broken into subgroups according to the scheme of Munir and colleagues.

ATTENTION DEFICIT: A FUNCTION OF MANY FACTORS

Prospective Studies

The prevalence of behavior problems among preschool and school-age children is considerable. Chazan and Threlfall (1978) reported that 24% of a sample consisting of 725 children between the ages of 5 years and 5 years, 7 months showed some indication of behavioral disturbance. Follow-up studies have shown that a significant proportion of children with DSM-III ADD develop conduct disorder by adolescence, which may then lead to antisocial behavior in adulthood (Biederman et al., 1987). However, quantifying and categorizing ADD-derived behavior is difficult. As Campbell and Werry (1986) pointed out, the child becomes a matter of clinical concern only after an adult at home or in the school decides the child's behavior is problematic and then labels it hyperactive—a process that almost cannot help but confound the diagnosis of ADD and CD from the very beginning.

In their study involving a population of children referred for school-related problems, Levine and co-workers (1982) compared individuals having significant attention deficits with those who had other types of learning problems. These investigators pointed out that children with "primary" attention deficit not attended by any other disabilities would have average or better facility with language, age-appropriate memory ability, good conceptual capacity, and adequate visual-spatial orientation. Nevertheless, they would experience difficulty in exerting sustained selective attention and might have trouble modulating activity.

At the other extreme of this hypothetical clinical picture would be children who have no difficulty concentrating and regulating their activity but experience deficits in cognition (perceptual, language, or others). Levine and co-workers speculated that the primary attention deficit group would have greater difficulty with behavior and social adjustment. However, their data indicated that while these two groups may exist, mixed forms are far more common, and Levine and co-workers stressed that it is vital to understand that an attention deficit is likely to have more than one contributing factor as well as confounding sequelae.

If the probable multiple etiology of attention deficit is kept in mind, the results of prospective studies, though few, can yield maximum results. In a study by Campbell and co-workers (1986), 46 parent-referred problem 3-year-olds were compared to 22 matched normals. The investigators followed up 54 of the children at age 4, and 53 were assessed again at age 6.

Overall, children with the most severe symptoms tended to come from families with high levels of stress and disruption. Children who came from this family type, which was usually lower in social class, and who had mothers who were more directive and controlling, were more likely to be rated high on both hyperactivity and aggression at intake and at follow-up. Thus, Campbell and co-workers suggested that the ultimate effect of stress on children may be mediated through its effect on maternal tolerance and disciplinary factors.

Maternal behavior also emerged in the etiology of hyperactivity in 20 preschool children compared with a group of nonhyperactive children by Prior, Leonard, and Wood (1983). These investigators also stressed the child's temperament as a contributing factor to troubled mother–child interaction and emphasized the damage that could ensue from focusing solely on a difficult child as opposed to a difficult mother–child interaction.

Social ecology also was an important contributor to persistent attentional problems in a prospective study of 174 children by Palfrey and co-workers (1985). Children who exhibited early symptoms of attentional problems and continued to do so until school entry were more likely to have mothers with a high-school diploma or less. Furthermore, boys were found to comprise most of the group with persistent problems.

Donald: Aggression in the Service of Defiance

Donald is a 4-year-old boy who lives with his mother. He has seen his father only twice in his life; he was married to another woman at the time Donald's mother became pregnant with Donald and severed contact with Donald's mother until recently. Donald's mother reports that she became severely depressed after Donald's birth and tried to get his grandmother to help in caring for him. When help was refused, Donald's mother says she began to resent and feel oppressed by the infant's continual demands on her and subsequently neglected his care at times. When she began to ignore his needs, he became oppositional at feeding time, and, as a result of this, he would frequently vomit. Her reports of Donald's developmental milestones indicate no abnormalities. As Donald grew older, his behavior at home worsened, and his peer relationships at nursery school were also marred by his aggression.

The nursery school insisted on a psychiatric assessment of Donald, threatening to expel him otherwise. His nursery school teacher stated that Donald throws toys at other children, refuses to follow instructions that he understands, frequently initiates both verbal and physical fights with other children, and has attempted more than once to leave school during the day. A recent episode, which precipitated the school's insistence on Donald's evaluation, occurred when he stole money from a teacher's purse. He was caught in the act of stealing by the teacher, yet he denied his actions and blamed them on another child in the class. Donald's mother also reports that Donald steals from her. He refuses to do his chores at home and sometimes walks out of the yard, does not return for several hours, and then refuses to tell his mother where he has gone. A neighbor told Donald's mother that she had discovered Donald in her yard, poking her dog in the eyes with a branch. Donald's mother interpreted the neighbor's complaint as a lie motivated by the neighbor's dislike of her.

During assessment, Donald was friendly and likeable, although he did lie and was demanding at times. When he put his shoes on the furniture and threw toys in the therapist's office, his mother told him to stop, but her admonition had no effect. When asked to draw, Donald drew a picture of a man—whom he explained was a soldier—and several guns. He demonstrated a full range of appropriate affect. Other elements of his mental status were judged to be within normal limits. An interview with Donald's mother suggested that she may be suffering from a mixed personality disorder. Intelligence tests revealed that Donald's IQ is above average. His described behaviors fit the criteria for conduct disorder.

The direct assaults on others and violation of social rules suggest that Donald's condition is too pervasive to be diagnosed as oppositional defiant disorder. The presence of specific learning problems has not been noted, but Donald is not yet involved in structured language and arithmetic learning activities, so an associated diagnosis of specific developmental disorders might later be considered if Donald's academic performance does not meet his measured abilities. Donald does not exhibit symptoms of attention deficit hyperactivity disorder such as fidgeting and distractibility; therefore, this commonly associated diagnosis was ruled out.

In addition to his presenting symptoms, other factors in Donald's history strengthen the likelihood of the accuracy of a conduct disorder diagnosis. Often children who have this disorder are from homes where there is no father present or where the father is dependent on alcohol. It is also common for children who are rejected by their parents—as Donald was by his mother—to be diagnosed as having conduct disorder. Thus, the diagnosis of conduct disorder was assigned, and recommendation was made for placement in a therapeutic nursery where Donald would experience consistent limit setting. Recommendation was also made for further assessment of and treatment for Donald's mother.

The Role of Aggression

Hyperactivity and/or attention deficits are disproportionately represented in low-income families where high stress is prevalent, and the same is true for aggressive behavior (Parke & Slaby, 1983). This suggests that maternal and environmental suppression of the child's normative aggression and assertions of self might play a significant role in modulating the severity of the attention deficit and concomitant behavior. However, the fact that Donald comes from a middle-income home and his mother was not overly suppressive provides evidence that aggression can develop in response to frustration of any kind. In this case, Donald became aggressive in order to oppose his feelings of frustration and helplessness in the face of ambivalent maternal care.

Keeping in mind that aggression can develop in response to frustration of almost any kind and that deficits in attention rarely exist in isolation, it seems useful to speculate that the most severe forms of behavioral disruption occur when inattention and its frustrating concomitants (e.g., inability to learn, social isolation) are accompanied by a strong maternal and/or environmental suppression of the child's freedom to expand his or her sense of self. Using this construct, conduct disorder would be the result of inattention in the presence of strong suppression, while attention deficit disorder might represent a milder form in which inattention occurs in the relative absence of social stressors or is produced de novo from social stressors in the absence of organic causes.

While aggressive behavior (whether it be active or passive) is a component of conduct disorder, attention deficit disorder, and oppositional disorder alike, its expression takes on its severest manifestations in CD, is somewhat less severe in ADD, and is least severe in OD, where it is almost completely passive in nature. The legitimacy and heuristic value of focusing on the aggressive component of the attention deficit state seems clear and is further supported by the observed stabilities for both hyperactivity (Campbell, Breaux, Ewing, & Szumowski, 1984; Hechtman, 1985; Levy & Hobbes, 1982) and aggression (Olweus, 1979). Aggression is also deserving of increased attention due to the fact that there may be an underlying neural mechanism governing its expression, just as there are mechanisms governing attention and impulsivity (Trad, 1986). The existence of such a mechanism is suggested by the nature of the episodic dyscontrol syndrome, whose chief characteristic is aggressive and potentially very harmful behavior (Nunn, 1986a,b). While there are no epidemiological data regarding incidence in childhood, this disorder may represent a condition in which all other symptoms are secondary to the intermittent expression of violent aggressive urges. Thus, it seems likely that closer observation of the aggressive component can provide the key to further clarification of the disorders characterized by hyperactivity, inattention, and impulsivity.

It will also be important to further define the parameters of the development of acceptable behavior. Straker (1979b) suggested that investigations along this line should focus on what are generally thought to be the most important factors contributing to the development of normative behavior. These are an intact nervous system, "good enough mothering," adequate models for identification, and the opportunity to experience both instinctual gratification and frustration in such a way that frustration can be tolerated.

CONCLUSION

The lack of experimental data relating to attentional processes, particularly with regard to young children, is the prime contributor to the confusion that remains pertaining to attention deficit hyperactivity disorder, conduct disorder, and oppositional defiant disorder. It seems plausible to begin clarifying the various factors contributing to these disorders by directing research toward factoring out causes that produce increasing gradations of aggressive behavior throughout this behavioral spectrum. Thus, as August and Stewart (1983) have suggested, these disorders may eventually lie along a continuum as defined by the aggressive component, CD being the most severe, followed by ADD and finally OD.

Neurological research will also help to define the nature of these disorders. Quay (1986) proposed that the DSM-III undersocialized conduct disorder (Group CD, DSM-III-R) represents a situation in which there is an overactive reward system coupled with a subnormal behavioral inhibition system. This juxtaposition results in impulsive, disinhibited, reward-seeking behavior.

Quay postulated that there may be an underlying neurochemical mechanism responsible for this behavior in that norepinephrine (NA) is the primary neurotransmitter in the behavioral inhibition system and dopamine (DA) appears to be integral to the reward pathways. Quay pointed out that very low levels of dopamine-beta-hydroxylase (DBH), which converts DA to NA, may result in an excess of DA and a decreased amount of NA. Thus, subnormal levels of DBH may be responsible for an overenergized reward-seeking system and a disinhibited behavioral inhibition system. However, even if this system proves true, the question must still be answered as to whether the condition is primary or secondary to environmental influences.

Thus, it appears that attentional deficit may be a process, a disorder, or both; that is, it may be the result of other behavior and learning problems. As Levine and co-workers (1982) have stated,

> *Further research on the causes and management of attention deficits needs to take into account the possibility that this condition may be either a discrete neurologically based dysfunction or a phenomenon analogous to an inflammatory response. Just as the latter can accompany trauma, infection, autoimmunity, and other conditions, so attention deficits may appear as a nonspecific host response.* (p. 394)

There is good support for the notion of attention deficit as an "inflammatory" response to a wide array of environmental stressors. Sleator and Ullman (1981) and Hebben, Benjamin, and Milberg (1981) have demonstrated situation-specificity of the behavior of hyperactive children in one-on-one situations or during activities they enjoy. Thus, it may be more proper to consider nonorganic cases of attention deficit as an application deficit (Torgeson, 1977).

Observing this aspect of so-called "attention deficit," Prior and Sanson (1986) pointed to the need for further research into the development of attention. Knowledge about such issues as the relative rates of maturation of the visual, auditory, and other senses would be invaluable in assessing whether or not deficits related purely to attention are developmentally normal or truly pathologic.

In sum, it appears that the strategy adopted in DSM-III and DSM-III-R, which centers on the attentional component of ADHD, has met with mixed success. Werry, Reeves, and Elkind (1987) have suggested that the revision of DSM-III may have been premature, since insufficient time was allowed to generate enough research to test the hypotheses on which the diagnoses were based. In their extensive table of the symptoms attributed in different studies to the three conditions under consideration here, the most noticeable finding was the similarity of characteristics among all three diagnoses. It seems probable that this overlap will continue either until further research reveals the nature of the development and willful use of attention or until scrutiny of a different component in the symptomatic picture—such as aggression—yields more specific results.

CHAPTER FIFTEEN

Elimination Disorders and Their Differential Diagnosis

Sam: Profoundly Disordered Elimination

Sam is a 9-year, 7-month-old male. He has a 7-year-old brother with whom he has always gotten along. Their parents are currently going through divorce proceedings. Sam was the product of an unplanned pregnancy. His mother had two previous abortions and, although Sam's father wanted the pregnancy to be terminated, she refused to have a third abortion. Sam's mother reported that she had wanted a girl. Other than being a forceps delivery, Sam's birth was uncomplicated. His medical history is normal except for continued encopresis and enuresis. His mother stopped breastfeeding him after 3 months because Sam had frequent episodes of projectile vomiting. Sam's parents describe his developmental milestones as having been within normal ranges. Sam was never completely toilet trained, and his mother notes that from the time of the birth of her second child, when Sam was almost 3 years old, Sam exhibited behavior problems and fecal incontinence.

Sam was seen by a psychiatrist on two occasions prior to this evaluation. The first was at age 3, on the recommendation of his teachers at the Montessori school he attended. This recommendation was based on Sam's aggressive behavior toward other children: he would often tease them and fight with them. Counseling was discontinued after 2 years because of financial difficulties. However, seeing that Sam was still aggressive with other boys, his parents took him to another psychiatrist, who prescribed Mellaril. This resulted in weight gain but no change in behavior. Sam is still not fully capable of either bowel or bladder control, and he has recently begun to steal toys from other children.

During assessment, Sam, an attractive child, was open and friendly. He exhibited no discomfort when leaving his mother. Thought and affect were both observed to be normal, but fine motor coordination was slightly impaired. Sam took things from the office a number of times and, as a result, strict limits had to be set for him. His self-esteem was judged to be low, and he clearly expressed the belief that he was "bad" and his younger brother was "good." Intelligence tests revealed Sam to be of average to superior intelligence and functioning at a level beneath his full potential. Past medical examination had ruled out any physical cause for Sam's elimination abnormalities.

Sam's symptoms indicate that he has primary functional enureses, both diurnal and nocturnal, and primary functional encopresis. Commonly associated features such as sleepwalking and sleep terror disorder are not evident. Predisposing factors such as delayed toilet training and specific psychosocial stressors, namely the birth of a sibling and the impending divorce of his parents, were noted.

Sam's behavior, although aggressive and overactive, does not fit the necessary qualifications for a diagnosis of attention deficit hyperactivity disorder; he does not engage in physically dangerous activities or consistently lose things necessary for tasks at school or at home. He also does not blurt out answers to questions before they have been asked. Sam only meets three of the five criteria necessary for a diagnosis of oppositional defiant disorder: he actively defies his parents; behaves in a way that annoys others; and is often angry, resentful, and spiteful. A diagnosis of developmental coordination disorder is inappropriate because Sam's fine motor coordination is not impaired to the extent that it significantly interferes with his daily life or academic achievement.

Thus, the evaluation points to a diagnosis of primary functional encopresis and primary functional enuresis. Weekly individual therapy was recommended for Sam, along with family therapy and parent counseling once each week.

INTRODUCTION

The age by which children are expected to achieve voluntary control of their eliminative functions varies from society to society and within cultures as well. Nevertheless, as each individual grows there is a developmental trend toward control of these functions. Sensory development progresses in the direction of being able to make finer and finer distinctions between various internal as well as external stimuli (Mikkelsen, Brown, Minichiello, Millican, & Rapoport, 1982). However, as Sam has demonstrated, bodily functions can become disorganized in response to a disorganized, stressful environment, and they may be mobilized as a weapon in the fight for attention and control.

In the case of micturition, the first step in this progression is immediate evacuation in response to bladder distention during the first 6 months of life. During the next 2 years this response becomes progressively curtailed, probably due to the development of unconscious inhibition. In normative cases, the infant begins to comprehend and express a desire to void between 18 and 30 months. Ultimately, during sleep, afferent stimuli from the bladder will cause the child to awaken and go to the bathroom (Levine, Carey, Crocker, & Gross, 1983).

The ability to retain feces entails a somewhat more sophisticated series of physiologic interactions. The rectal response to distension can be difficult for a child to perceive and define, making it problematic for the clinician and child alike to obtain a clear impression of whether or not the child feels rectal fullness or is aware of passing a stool. Additionally, normal bowel function is a somewhat complicated mechanism in which the striated and internal anal sphincters interact in complementary fashion. The former muscle strongly contracts for up to 30 seconds in order to suppress a rectal contraction wave, while the internal sphincter is able to maintain steady tonic pressure to prevent leakage of fecal material between periods of rectal activity (Hersov, 1985).

Gesell, Ilg, and Ames (1974) have described voluntary defecation as being much more than a simple localized reaction. Rather, it is a complete neuromuscular response. As such, social learning interacts with maturational factors and this interaction results in fluctuations of bowel behavior that are dependent on elements of temperament, personality, growth rate, and habit formation.

Hersov (1985) profiled the normal fluctuations in elimination behavior, stating that by approximately 40 weeks, the infant is able to sit and react adaptively to toilet training. However, by 12 months, resistance again appears. At 15 months, when the child can stand, resistance lessens, irregularity declines, and some children may instinctively assume the "squat" position. Hersov pointed out that in terms of development the task is to establish a working balance between contraction and relaxation, which come under voluntary control separately.

Because of the variations in individual development and inter- and intrasocietal expectations, there is no universally accepted age at which a child is judged to be enuretic or encopretic. However, encopresis can generally be defined as the regular passage of formed or semiformed stools in the underwear or any other inappropriate place after 4 years of age (DSM-III-R, APA, 1987; Levine et al., 1983). Enuresis, according to Shaffer's (1985a) extensive review, may be thought to exist if wetting occurs in children age 4 years or older. The decision to make the cutoff point at 4 years was based on the results of many studies demonstrating that children who are still wetting at 4 years are different from those who are wetting at an earlier age because the probability of becoming dry in the following 12 months falls sharply after age 4. The DSM-III-R, however, requires that the child have a chronological age of at least 5 and a mental age of at least 4.

Encopresis and enuresis are often broken into two subtypes, primary and secondary. Again, the definitions of these subtypes vary somewhat. In general, children who have reached the age of 4 or 5 and have never learned control are considered to exhibit the primary condition, whereas those who have demonstrated control for a significant period of time and subsequently lapse may be regarded as having secondary encopresis or enuresis.

The diagnosis and treatment of either primary or secondary forms of elimination disorders make a vital contribution to the emotional poise and overall functionality of the child and the child's family. A great deal of confusion still exists as to whether disordered elimination is the cause of intrapsychic and intrafamilial discord or the reverse is true and it is emotional and environmental discord that lead to disordered elimination. Regardless of the issue of causality, treatment of elimination disorders frequently results in improved well-being of the child and family alike.

DIFFERENTIAL DIAGNOSIS OF ENCOPRESIS AND ENURESIS

Encopresis

Perhaps the most important part of diagnosing an elimination disorder of any kind is maintaining a nonjudgmental posture. The symptom of encopresis is likely the result of many interacting factors, and emotional disturbance is only rarely a primary cause (Levine et al., 1983). Only a small minority of encopretic children have an underlying primary behavioral and/or psychological disorder (Cavanaugh, 1983). Therefore, in the absence of clear evidence, it should never be assumed that an encopretic child is emotionally disturbed.

In cases where psychogenic encopresis is suspected, however, Johns (1985) noted that the encopresis in these instances usually follows a painful incident associated with the conscious suppression of the urge to defecate. Furthermore, Johns noted that children with a primary emotional disturbance may appear more passive than the norm, being uninvolved in their problem and showing little inclination to improve. They frequently display an isolation of affect, and when asked to simulate defecation they are able to demonstrate a normal external sphincter response without paradox.

Regarding the issue of what psychological disorders may be primary causes of encopresis, little is known definitively. As mentioned, children with attention deficit/hyperactivity may be prone to developing the constipation/encopretic syndrome. Young children exhibiting strident oppositional behavior may engage in acts of "encopretic revenge" against toilet training that was too harsh or began too early.

Organic causes of constipation that can lead to encopresis are anatomic, neurologic, endocrinologic, or metabolic. Children with encopresis generally appear well-nourished and healthy, but they may develop encopresis from drug use or insufficient exercise (Cavanaugh, 1983; Levine et al., 1983).

Cavanaugh (1983) recommended that a spinal cord disorder such as a tumor, trauma, infection, or malformation be excluded prior to making a diagnosis of encopresis. DSM-III-R requires exclusion of aganglionic megacolon. Endocrine and metabolic disorders such as hypothyroidism, hypokalemia, and porphyria must also be excluded, as must the rarer causes of constipation such as hypercalcemia, adrenocortical hyperplasia, renal acidosis, and diabetes insipidus. Anatomic lesions such as perianal fissures also can lead to stool withholding, and obstructions from such conditions as Hirschsprung's disease, anal stenosis, and intestinal mass lesions must be considered as well.

While relapses may occur during periods of stress, treatment of encopresis commonly results in alleviation of the condition and of secondary behavioral and emotional problems. The defecation process should be "demystified" for the child, and he or she should be made to realize that the stretched colon also has stretched nerves. This accounts for why the feces appear to just come out without warning (Levine et al., 1983). Frequently, the encopresis will respond to initially high doses of lubricants in combination with "demystification" counseling. Eventually, dosage can be decreased, and as normal anal stimuli are reestablished, a normal defecation pattern will resume (Johns, 1985).

Enuresis

As noted previously, approximately 30% of children with encopresis also have enuresis (Dejonge, 1973). Like encopresis, enuresis has many possible etiologies, ranging from adverse environmental circumstances and psychological disturbances to physiological mechanisms (Young & Young, 1985). Like children with encopresis, only a few with enuresis have an underlying primary behavioral or psychological disorder; thus it is inadvisable to assume psychiatric difficulties in the absence of clear evidence (Shaffer, 1985a). In some cases the enuresis may be secondary to the fecal impaction of the encopretic condition. When defecation does not occur daily, or is prolonged or painful, it can contribute to urological symptoms. Therefore, treatment of constipation with mineral oil, laxatives, and/or dietary manipulation may cause resolution of enuresis as well as encopresis in cases where the encopresis is responsible for reduced functional bladder volume (FBV).

A reduced FBV also may be the cause of or a contributor to enuresis in the absence of encopresis. Starfield (1967) found that the maximum volume eliminated after fluid load by enuretics in school clinics was one standard deviation below the mean for their age group. From these data, Shaffer (1985a) concluded that the bladders of many enuretic children do indeed function differently, causing them to feel the urge to urinate when the bladder is holding only relatively small amounts of urine. Unfortunately, the pathophysiology of reduced FBV remains unknown.

In order to differentiate between the various pathophysiological and potential environmental and psychological causes of enuresis, Maizels and Firlit (1986) stressed the importance of taking a complete history. To this end, they proposed that questions be grouped into eight categories; perinatal complications, complications in infancy, toilet training, micturition patterns, urinary infection, defecation pattern, perineal symptoms, and food sensitivities. Birth defects such as posterior urethral valves or ectopic ureter may also be at fault.

Maizels and Firlit pointed out that children with urinary frequency, urgency, and/or incontinence more often have histories of perinatal problems than do nonenuretic children. They suggested that this extra trauma may generate subclinical effects that lead to the maturational delay generally believed to be at the root of primary enuresis. The diagnostic lesson is that those who have had perinatal stresses are generally less likely to have a structural urological problem.

Another important aid in differential diagnosis of enuretic children is the voiding diary, covering an extended period and recording both volume and frequency of urination. Definition of the voiding pattern helps to differentiate symptoms that may appear to be related to voiding but are actually caused by rectal or genital problems. For example, dysuria may be relieved in some children by alleviating a fecal impaction. If the child is a female, the same relief may be achieved by treating vaginitis.

Toilet training is also an important issue in diagnosing enuresis. The history should include information such as whether or not the child has ever had daytime or nighttime urinary continence for at least a year. When was toilet training attempted, and when did the child achieve continence? As in the case of encopresis, it is possible in some instances that failure to gain continence is secondary to an oppositional mindset developed during toilet training that was too harsh or initiated too much in advance of muscular development.

Another issue that needs to be addressed when discussing the diagnosis of enuresis is that of sleep architecture. In the past it was believed that enuretic children slept more deeply than normals or that bed wetting was more likely to occur in normal children during delta sleep, while those who were psychiatrically disturbed most often urinated during REM. However, the consensus of opinion has now shifted against either of these hypotheses, indicating that while there may be sleep differences between enuretics and nonenuretics, these remain to be fully identified (Shaffer, 1985a; Young & Young, 1985).

Fortunately, once overt organic and psychological causes have been ruled out, enuresis can be treated effectively as long as the treatment includes a measure of patience. While tricyclic antidepressants are effective in controlling the condition, they are ineffective once therapy is discontinued. The bell-and-pad method, which has undergone continuous refinement in terms of ease of use and efficiency, has been found to be 75% effective, with the average relapse rate being 41% (Doleys, 1977). Subsequent retraining in those who relapse usually proves effective (Goel, Thomson, Gibb, & McAinsh, 1984)

PREVALENCE AND ETIOLOGY
OF ELIMINATION DISORDERS

Enuresis

Prevalence.   As mentioned, the manifestations and course of the elimination process are closely tied to developmental events, since both enuresis and encopresis are commonly considered self-limiting, rarely being a problem once adulthood is reached (McGuire & Savastano, 1984). Enuresis has been described since the beginning of recorded history. Since primary nocturnal enuresis is far more common than daytime, or diurnal, enuresis, most estimates concern the former variety.

Dejonge (1973) reported an incidence of 1% in children between the ages of 7 and 12. In a study drawn from the child population of the Isle of Wight, Rutter, Yule, and Graham (1973) found that prevalence of enuresis varied according to the criterion of frequency of wetting. Of the 7-year-old boys in the study, 15% were found to wet less than once a week; however, only 7% wet more frequently. The DSM-III-R claims a 7% rate of enuresis in boys at age 5 and 3% for girls of the same age. At age 10, the rate drops to 3% for males and 2% for females, and by age 18 enuresis exists in only 1% of males and is essentially nonexistent in females.

An important aspect of enuresis is the probability of relapse after a period of dryness. This is most likely to occur around ages 5 to 6 and happens more often in boys than girls. Oppel, Harper, and Rider (1968) have reported that up to one fourth of children who have been continent for 6 months or longer will begin wetting again.

Etiology.   Before discussing possible etiologies underlying enuresis, it is necessary to be aware of the developmental trends during the normal course of acquiring control. In his comprehensive review, Shaffer (1985a) noted that girls usually become continent at a younger age than boys. However, the incidence of enuresis for both males and females is roughly the same between ages 4 and 6. The ratio of boy to girl enuretics increases after age 7 until, by age 11, boys are twice as likely to be enuretic as girls. Shaffer pointed out that this is partially attributable to the fact that males are twice as likely as females to develop secondary enuresis. Additionally, boys have a slower rate of spontaneous acquisition of continence.

One of the primary factors entering into the assessment of possible etiologies for enuresis is the fact that this condition frequently runs in families. In a study by Kaffman and Elizur (1977), 67% of enuretic children reared partially away from their parents on a kibbutz were found to have enuretic siblings. This compared with only 22% of dry kibbutz children. Twin studies by Bakwin (1973) also revealed high genetic concordance. For example, in the study by Bakwin, enuresis was seen to be significantly greater in monozygotic than dizygotic twins (68% versus 36%).

Beyond this apparent genetic association, the specific mechanism of which has yet to be defined, the next strongest causal factor appears to be socioeconomic/environmental. A number of studies (e.g., Essen & Peckmam, 1976; Levine et al., 1983) have found enuresis to be more prevalent in children of low social class living in disadvantaged circumstances. Institutionalized children also show higher rates.

It is often assumed that enuresis, whether among socially disadvantaged children or those more fortunate, is a result of another psychiatric disorder or premature or harsh toilet training procedures. However, these relationships, if they exist, are elusive. Shaffer (1985) reported no differences in the rates of psychiatric disorder between children with and without family histories of enuresis, and Mikkelson and Rapoport (1980) found no difference in treatment response either to Imipramine or to the bell and pad between enuretics who were psychiatrically disturbed and those who were not. Furthermore, removal of the symptom of enuresis has rarely been seen to result in the emergence of other symptoms (Levine et al., 1983a). In the realm of personality traits, however, there are some suggestive data showing that three types of personality may be more prone to develop enuresis at 4 years of age: children who are highly dependent, children who resist change, and those who are hyperactive (Kaufman & Elizur, 1977).

As with possible psychiatric etiology, it is also not possible to definitively ascertain the causal role of toilet training procedures. Brazelton (1962, in Levine et al., 1983a) asserted that early toilet training is a prime contributor to enuresis. However, Kaffman and Elizur (1977), in a carefully controlled longitudinal study, found that toilet training was more effective when started between 12 and 15 months than when it was begun after 20 months of age.

Nevertheless, it seems probable that toilet training technique does play some mediational role in the development of elimination problems. Undue harshness on the part of the caregiver may easily create unwanted effects. However, it is difficult to know whether the harsher approach has been elicited by a difficult child.

The child's temperament undoubtedly plays a role in learning the elimination process just as it plays a role in learning any new task. In Levine and co-workers' (1983a) analysis of the National Health Examination Survey data, enuretic children between the ages of 6 and 11 were more frequently noted by their parents to be "high strung" and to "lose their tempers easily." This association held across all social classes.

Furthermore, both male and female enuretic adolescents between 12 and 15 years of age were more likely to describe themselves as being tense, having difficulty sleeping, and having bad dreams. Again, it was not possible to determine causality from these data. That is, it was not clear whether temperament played a primary causal role or whether increased tension due to enuresis over time was manifested as temperamental instability. Mikkelsen and co-workers (1980, in Shaffer, 1985a) attempted to explore the relationship between enuresis and neurological status and found that while there appears to be no difference in prevalence of neurological soft signs between controls and enuretics in males between the ages of 5 and 13, psychiatrically disturbed enuretics did have significantly higher neurological soft sign scores than enuretics who had no psychiatric symptoms.

In addition to these findings, both Rapoport and co-workers (1980) and Shaffer, Gardner, and Hedge (1984) have found that disturbed enuretics show more developmental and biological abnormalities than do nondisturbed enuretics. These findings led Shaffer (1985a) to speculate that the association between psychiatric disorder and enuresis may be linked to some other, as yet unknown, common factor. One candidate for a common factor might be self-image or locus of control. Moffatt, Kato, and Pless (1987) measured improvements in self-concept following treatment for nocturnal enuresis. While changes in self-image were greatest in those who had the largest reductions in wetting frequency, these changes were not statistically significant. However, the authors noted a movement toward a more external locus of control in children who failed to become dry after conditioning.

In sum, given the close tie between wetting and developmental progress, a conservative description of the etiology of enuresis would entail the recognition of the relationship between the higher prevalence of enuresis in boys and the slower maturation of boys compared to girls. Further, the higher prevalence among the lower classes may be at least partly attributable to more coercive means of toilet training, particularly at ages that are premature in terms of the child's level of physical development. As to whether psychological or environmental factors are primary in causing enuresis, it is likely that both may be the case, depending on the individual and the circumstances.

Robert: A Defiant Child

Robert is a 4-year-old boy who lives with his mother and his maternal grandparents in their home. Also living in the house are his 2-year-old brother Joe and his mother's three sisters. When he was 2 years old, after his parents' separation, Robert moved with his mother and his brother into his grandparents' home. The separation followed several months of loud fights, which Robert occasionally interrupted to plead for them to stop. Before entering nursery school at age 3, Robert had babysitters intermittently when his mother went to work. Robert's mother asserts that Robert had no difficulties with these separations, except during a 2-week period immediately following his parents' separation.

Robert's development of motor coordination and language were without abnormality, and his mother initiated toilet training at the age of 18 months, which was 1 week before his brother Joe's birth. After Joe's birth, Robert refused to sit on the potty and insisted that he wanted to wear diapers again. Following the pediatrician's advice, his mother complied. When Robert was 3, his mother began toilet training again. Robert required a diaper at night, but not during the day. His pattern of elimination consisted of using the toilet only to urinate and waiting until he was diapered to have a bowel movement. Usually, he would move his bowels soon after diapering, which was most often right after dinner. This pattern prevailed for 3 months, until Robert entered nursery school.

Robert's mother sent him to nursery school without a diaper until November, at which time the school requested diapering because Robert habitually soiled himself during the day. When Robert was sent to school with a diaper, he would be changed into pants in the afternoon, after he moved his bowels. Other children at the school teased Robert, calling him "Stinky" or "Baby." Robert responded by screaming at the children. Robert and his brother no longer attend the nursery school because their mother and the school staff had several incidents of conflict.

Robert was referred for psychiatric assessment after his pediatrician could find no physical cause for Robert's primary encopresis. At the time of evaluation, Robert, age 4, still required nighttime diapering and would move his bowels only when diapered. His mother reported that Robert had verbalized a fear of falling into the toilet for the past 6 months. She also expressed frustration and anger about Robert's lack of toilet training and tried a few strategies to encourage his fecal continence. First, she promised Robert that he could sleep in a bed instead of a crib if he would use the toilet; this did not have the desired effect because Robert enjoyed sleeping in his crib. Other strategies included telling Robert that he could not go to school or could not have a certain toy unless he used the toilet. Robert would promise compliance in these instances and invariably break his promise. Another attempt was made to encourage his continence by not changing Robert's diaper immediately, with the idea that sitting in a dirty diaper for a long time would prompt him to use the toilet. This, too, was unsuccessful, in part because his grandmother would almost always change him in response to his complaints soon after soiling.

During the assessment interview, Robert's appearance and behavior were normal. His mood seemed anxious, as demonstrated through play involving battles in which he was solely responsible for devastating the enemy's forces. Robert's vocabulary was found to be very rich, and he was described as having an active, vivid imagination. Robert refused to hop on one foot during the interview, giving the excuse that such an activity was for older boys to do. When asked to draw, he drew something other than what he was shown, even though it was clear that he had understood the request. He seemed strong-willed; his mother added that he was "stubborn." Other elements of the mental status examination were assessed as being within normal ranges.

Robert's behavior during the interview and his case history are indicative of functional encopresis with oppositional defiant disorder; his parents' divorce is a relevant stressor. Several factors that are commonly associated with a diagnosis of functional encopresis are present in Robert's case. His mother's inconsistency in toilet training him, his brother's birth, the stress of his parents' separation and the related relocation, and his entry into school can all be viewed as predisposing factors. The accompanying diagnosis of oppositional defiant disorder is based on Robert's demonstrated refusal to comply with adults' requests. Review of the case suggests that Robert has not resolved the losses he experienced a few years ago, namely, the loss of his father through parental separation and the loss of his mother's full attention with the birth of his brother. In reaction, Robert manifests a desire to be treated like an infant, perhaps due to anxiety about being independent and more autonomous. His protracted struggle over toilet training may be his method of controlling an otherwise unpredictable and chaotic environment.

Encopresis

Prevalence. Any child 4 years of age or older who involuntarily passes stools on a regular basis qualifies for the diagnosis of encopresis (Cavanaugh, 1983; DSM-III-R, APA, 1967). However, Robert's case demonstrates that like enuresis, encopresis can be used as a means of defiance, although in the case of encopresis the defiance is more often unconscious. In a study of 8,863 7-year-old children, Bellman (1966), using a parent questionnaire, found that the frequency of encopresis in children between 7 and 8 years of age was 1.5% in boys, with a boy-to-girl prevalence ratio of 3.4 to 1. Other studies have produced ratios as high as 6 to 1, with boys being significantly more prone to this condition (Levine, 1975).

In addition to these epidemiologic figures, encopretic cases comprise from 10 to 25% of referrals to pediatric gastroenterology practices (Johns, 1985; Taitz, Wales, Urwin, & Molnar, 1986). Furthermore, it is estimated that 30% of encopretic children are also enuretic (Silverman et al., 1983, in Johns, 1985).

Etiology. Lack of control over defecation is extremely dehumanizing and damaging to self-esteem. Parents, siblings, (and in the past many psychotherapists) frequently interpret soiling as an aggressive act and blame the innocent child for the serious curtailment in family activities that results from his or her condition. Because of shame, these children are usually unaware that others in the community have the same problem.

In the majority of cases, encopresis is the end result of a process in which severe, chronic constipation leads to involuntary overflow due to fecal impaction (Cavanaugh, 1983; Johns, 1985; Levine, 1975). Once constipation has become chronic, the child is at risk of becoming trapped in a pain-fear cycle in which painful defecation leads to increased efforts at retaining stools. Eventually, sensory feedback from the bowel becomes impaired and the rectal wall stretches and loses its ability to forcefully contract (Cavanaugh, 1983).

Levine, Carey, Crocker, and Gross (1983) identified three stages of vulnerability in the pathogenesis of encopresis. Noting that encopresis is the end stage of a multifactorial process, Levine used a developmental scheme in which stage I, "Early Experience and Constitutional Predisposition," covers the events of the first 2 years of life; stage II, "Training and Early Autonomy," encompasses ages 3 to 5; and stage III, "Extramural Function," pertains to the early school years.

During the first stage, in the first 2 years of life, consistent and calm management of bowel function will keep problems to a minimum. Some children have a history of "early colonic inertia," which may be an endogenous tendency toward poor intestinal motility. Others have a congenital anomaly, such as imperforate anus, for which they have had surgery. Although the surgery may have been entirely successful, undue anxiety may continue to be centered around bowel movements. Food intolerance can also lead to constipation and the encopretic cycle of pain and fear.

When there is a constitutional predisposition to encopresis, the problem can be exacerbated by parental overreaction in terms of either reward or punishment. Furthermore, if an abundance of suppositories or other direct anal manipulations are employed, the child is at risk of becoming anally fixated and may actually begin to manipulate parental behavior by means of his or her bowel performance. This is one situation in which oppositional behavior, secondary to intrusive coercion, may develop and generalize to situations other than the bathroom.

During stage II, between the ages of 3 and 5, the child begins to explore the issues of autonomy and independence. Children who were vulnerable to the encopretic dynamic during stage I are at highest risk for developing new factors that will generate negative associations with the toilet during stage II. For example, these children may dread the bathroom environment as a harbinger of pain, discomfort, and embarrassment. Anxiety regarding toilets is common in such children, and they may even fear that the toilet is capable of flushing them away or that it is a place where they may be bitten from "down below." Also

during this stage, conflict between parental control and the child's burgeoning need for autonomy may trigger latent bowel dysfunction.

During stage III, early in elementary school, the child with previous
encopretic tendencies is subjected to new stresses, not the least of which
is the public school bathroom. The lack of doors on toilets or the inability to void at the same time as at home may well cause the child to
restrict bowel behavior. If the decision is made to withhold going to the
bathroom until after school, the urge may be gone by the time the child
gets home and normal defecation is thus deranged.

In addition to feeling trauma from strange bathrooms, the child may
overindulge in foods such as milk or chocolate during the early childhood years—elements that certainly do not aid intestinal motility.
Another possible contributing factor to encopresis at this age, and one
that brings us to the issue of differential diagnosis, is that of *hyperactivity.*
A child who is impulsive and task-impersistent frequently fails to complete an act, a tendency that may extend in some instances to the act of
defecation. Munir and co-workers (1987) performed a controlled study
of 22 children with attention deficit disorder (ADD) and 20 normal controls and found significantly higher rates of encopresis in the children
with ADD. Also more frequent in children with ADD were learning disorders, conduct and oppositional disorders, major affective disorders,
and non-Tourette tics.

While causal relationships are difficult to isolate, predisposing factors
may be less so. One interesting study by Rappoport, Landman, Fenton,
and Levine (1986) investigated the relationship between locus of control and treatment outcome in 50 encopretic children between the ages
of 9 and 12 years. Those who improved significantly were found to have
a more internal locus of control and showed better compliance than
the children with a predominantly external locus of control.

CONCLUSION

The early view that enuresis is symptomatic of underlying emotional
distress has largely been negated by the recognition that there are actually very few emotional differences between enuretic and nonenuretic
children. Studies are lacking, but it appears that the clinical picture
of encopresis is less benign, although not drastically so. The observed
association of encopresis and ADD and the considerable individual and
family upheaval that accompanies this condition are cause for clinical
concern.

The results reported by Rappoport and co-workers (1986) and Moffatt and co-workers (1987), investigating issues of self-image and locus of control, suggest that enuretic or encopretic children with at least

minimally positive self-image and a predominantly internal locus of control are most likely to respond well to treatment. Perhaps the psychiatric issue of most long-range importance in elimination disorders is the progressive feeling of loss of control. If protracted, this feeling could make the child resistant to treatment and render him or her vulnerable to depression.

These issues aside, it is vital for clinicians not to underestimate the potential degree of trauma associated with both enuresis and encopresis. Treatment for both conditions is generally effective despite the fact that, as yet, relatively few predictors of treatment success have been found.

CHAPTER SIXTEEN

Sleep Disorders and Their Differential Diagnosis

Mark: Eruptions of Unconscious Fears

Mark is a 4-year, 7-month-old boy who lives with his 9-year-old sister and their parents. Mark was cared for by a housekeeper from birth until he was age 4. For 3 weeks after the housekeeper left, Mark's behavior was markedly aggressive and very demanding of others' attention. Mark's mother had a normal pregnancy, and there were no birth complications. She describes him as having been a "happy, easy, fair-tempered baby." Mark began walking at a developmentally appropriate age, but he was difficult to toilet train. He occasionally wets his bed. Mark's medical history is normal.

Mark's mother decided to divorce his father 6 months prior to Mark's presenting illness. One month after this decision was made, Mark, his mother, and his sister moved in with his maternal grandparents. Mark's parents report that since he, his mother, and his sister moved back in with his father 3 weeks after they left, Mark has become aggressive both at home and in school. Mark has also refused to attend school numerous times and is clingy and dependent. He has reportedly begun to wake up in the middle of the night screaming and crying. Mark's parents state that, although they try to comfort him, he seems almost oblivious to their presence. "He just calls out for help against crocodiles or monsters and then, after a few minutes, lies back down and falls asleep." Mark's mother states that he does not seem to remember his awakenings in the morning.

During assessment, Mark, a cute, well-dressed boy, alternated between clinging to his parents and exploring the room. His play was loud and aggressive (he broke crayons and yelled on the phone). Mark exhibited some difficulty when his parents left the room; once, he ran out to get some more toys from his mother. His affect was labile, shifting from anger to sadness. Mark had no evidence of perceptual disorders; he was fully oriented and denied suicidal and homicidal ideations.

Mark's nocturnal symptoms point toward a diagnosis of sleep terror disorder. He has recurrent episodes of abrupt awakening that begin with a panicky scream. He is relatively unresponsive to his parents' efforts to calm him during these episodes.

A diagnosis of dream anxiety disorder can be ruled out; Mark's episodes of agitation are more severe than would be expected with this diagnosis. Moreover, children with this disorder usually remember their dreams.

Mark's dreams also should not be confused with hypnagogic hallucinations, which occur during the transition between wakefulness and sleep. The possibility of seizure disorder has not been ruled out; however, Mark's EEG, measured during one of the nighttime awakenings, was within normal limits.

Mark's diurnal behavior meets the criteria for a diagnosis of adjustment disorder. He is reacting to an identifiable psychosocial stressor (his parents' impending separation) that occurred less than 2 months prior to the onset of his symptoms. Mark's reaction to the stressor has led to an impairment in functioning in school, and his maladaptive behavior has not lasted more than 6 months.

If Mark's maladaptive behavior was a condition not attributable to a mental disorder (i.e., phase of life problem), his social functioning would not be affected. With a diagnosis of psychological factors affecting physical conditions, the predominant symptom is an actual physical condition or disorder, and this is not the case with Mark.

Thus, Mark was diagnosed as having sleep terror disorder and adjustment disorder. Individual psychotherapy, parental counseling, and couples treatment were recommended.

INTRODUCTION

Mark's nocturnal terrors in response to separation stress are probably nothing new in child development. In fact, the impact of sleep quality and quantity on health and disease has been recognized since the time of Hippocrates. However, refinement of these relationships had to await the development of the means to measure electrical activity, not only of the brain but of other organ systems as well. Therefore, the importance of sleep physiology in clinical medicine was not recognized until the 1950's.

In the 1930's, Loomis, Harvey, and Hobart (1937) measured human brain-sleep potential and reported major changes in electrical activity in comparison with readings in the waking state. Their work was seminal to the later efforts of Aserinsky and Kleitman (1953) and Dement and Kleitman (1957), who discovered the two fundamental types of central nervous system activity during sleep, the rapid eye movement (REM) and non-REM states. Both of these types of sleep recur cyclically, and each is controlled by different neurophysiological and biological regulators.

Two developments resulted from this discovery. The association of REM sleep with dreaming touched off renewed interest in the biological basis of mental illness. Additionally, the study of disordered sleep was triggered by the observed association of certain respiratory changes with the sleeping state.

Orr (1985) noted that the definition of sleep in terms of certain physiological changes, which are neither evident in the waking state nor predictable from any parameters of waking physiology, established the legitimacy of sleep as an area of science and medicine. As Orr put it, "The human organism is now understood to be a center of sleep and waking physiology" (p. 1155).

Perturbations in sleep architecture can take many forms, all of which can have a negative effect on waking performance. In normal functioning, the REM state is characterized by rapid eye movements in which the eyes move in synchrony as though looking at something. These eye movements occur in association with dreaming and a low-amplitude, fast-frequency encephalographic pattern. Peripheral muscle activity is inhibited, so that in normal individuals dreams do not give rise to motor activity. There is also some irregularity and acceleration of cardiac and respiratory activity (Levine et al., 1983).

In contrast, the non-REM state exhibits an EEG that is characterized by slow-frequency, high-voltage wave forms. In general, body movements are infrequent, being limited to gross changes in position. Resting muscle activity is tonic, and cardiac and respiratory rates are slow and regular.

The normative functioning of sleep physiology is almost totally reliant on a regular sleep schedule in which the individual obtains enough sleep to fulfill his or her particular need for sleep. While the amount of sleep needed by each person varies greatly, the body requires a certain percentage (approximately 20%) of REM sleep each night (Long, 1987). If a significant amount of REM time is lost during one night, there will be a "REM rebound" the next night in order to restore the body's quota for REM. In the infant, however, this dynamic is slightly different. Rather than rebounding the next night, the infant tends to show tenacity for the ongoing sleep state, striving to return to it immediately following the disturbance.

As yet, there is no satisfactory explanation for why we need REM sleep, or even why we sleep at all. However, there is speculation that REM sleep serves as a mechanism of CNS autostimulation, which is particularly important during uterine development and immediate postpartum life. The highly active REM state might serve as an important source of stimulation in the absence of environmental input, enhancing the development and organization of the brain (Anders & Weinstein, 1972).

Very little more is known about the function of sleep in infants or about the developmental parameters of sleep. In general, it is known that patterns of REM activation and non-REM inhibition do occur in fetuses. However, these are not yet linked to a clear diurnal rhythm. Sleep architecture continues to evolve from birth through adolescence. Levine and co-workers (1983) have outlined the basic dynamic changes in both REM and non-REM sleep over the course of time.

REM sleep evolves in a direction from more to less. Newborns spend 8 to 9 hours in REM sleep per night, while adolescents and adults require only 1 to 2 hours. In the first year, the newborn progresses from going from waking to REM to going from waking to non-REM. Periodicity of the REM state also occurs. At birth, REM periods recur every 50 to 60 minutes, while the adult REM cycle has a periodicity of 90 to 100 minutes. Finally, there is a change in the temporal organization of REM and non-REM states. At birth, the REM period is equally long in the beginning and at the end of sleep. However, by 6 weeks of age, the diurnal pattern is apparent in that there are short periods of REM in the early night followed by longer periods during the morning hours.

Maturation of the non-REM state is characterized by the evolution of four electroencephalographically identifiable states. The stage 1 non-REM pattern is denoted by fast, low-amplitude activity similar to waking and REM patterns. Stage 2 contains "sleep spindles" and K complexes against a background of low-voltage firing. In stages 3 and 4, there are increased proportions of slow, high-voltage, synchronous delta waves. As puberty progresses, the proportionate amount of stages 3 and 4 decreases. In preadolescence there may be a second or third period of stages 3 and 4 non-REM, while these stages are largely confined to early night in adolescence and adulthood.

In the newborn, the sleep pattern tends to be erratic, since sleep is broken every 20 minutes to 6 hours. These wakings probably occur because there are inherent sleep-wake and rest-activity cycling patterns in the newborn. Also, hunger alerts the child, causing awakening, and there is as yet no diurnal rhythm allowing the consolidation of sleep into a single period during the night (Ferber, 1985). However, after 6 months of age, sleep is largely consolidated during the night in normal infants.

Thus, when diagnosing sleep problems, at least in newborns, the primary difficulty is in discerning the point at which perturbations in sleep should be considered a problem instead of an annoyance. This is made even more difficult by the fact that newborns, children, and adolescents alike rarely complain of sleep difficulties themselves—any more than they complain of emotional, behavioral, or learning problems (Simeon, 1987). Nevertheless, investigators and clinicians alike stress the importance of making an effort at early intervention in cases where sleep problems exist. Disordered sleep may not only give rise to long-lasting family destabilization, it may also be negatively associated with longevity and cardiac function (Bidder, Gray, Howells, & Eaton, 1986; Long, 1987).

DIFFERENTIAL DIAGNOSES OF SLEEP DISORDERS

Fundamental Categories of Sleep Disturbance

Roffwarg (1979), in attempting to standardize the nosology of clinical sleep disorders, has developed four major categories: (1) the hypersomnias, which are characterized by excessive time spent in sleep or somnolence; (2) insomnias, in which there is difficulty initiating and maintaining sleep; (3) parasomnias, characterized by dysfunctional occurrences associated with sleep such as nightmares and sleepwalking; and (4) phase lag syndromes, in which there are aberrations in the sleep-wake schedule.

The DSM-III-R utilizes these basic differentiations but groups all the sleep disorders under only two general headings, the dyssomnias and the parasomnias. The dyssomnias are segregated into primary and secondary insomnias, hypersomnia, and three types of sleep-wake schedule disorders: advanced or delayed, disorganized, or frequently changing. The parasomnias include dream anxiety disorder, sleep terror disorder, sleepwalking disorder, and parasomnias not otherwise specified, such as nocturnal myoclonus (leg jerks).

As stated previously, children over 6 months of age in general should not exhibit sleep disturbances as a consequence of maturational mechanisms. Thus, disturbed sleep after 6 months should stimulate a search for interfering factors. Perhaps the most prevalent of these factors are associated with the lack of recognition on the part of the parents that even children learn to fall asleep in certain ways and with certain associations (e.g., a stuffed animal) (Ferber, 1985). Thus, if the infant or child is subjected to inconsistent sleep cues, or if he or she fails to associate crib or bedroom with sleep, erratic sleeping patterns may develop— patterns that usually resolve quickly when the offending intervening factors are corrected.

Another common etiology for erratic sleep stems from the caregiver's complaint that the child awakens at night. These wakenings are normal, and the child, if left alone, will usually fall back to sleep. However, if the child goes to sleep in a room other than the bedroom and is then taken into the bedroom while asleep, he or she will likely be frightened on waking in a different place and therefore experience difficulty in going back to sleep.

Prevalences of Various Sleep Disorders

It is estimated that nearly half of all Americans over the age of 15 experience difficulty sleeping at some point in their lives (Walsh, Sugerman, & Chambers, 1986), and 22 million Americans have a chronic complaint about their sleep (Orr, 1985). Furthermore, sleep problems are the primary complaint of parents who bring their children to a pediatrician or other clinician (Edgil, Wood, & Smith, 1985).

Waking at night and irregularity of the sleep pattern are problems that continue to plague parents and health practitioners in 25 to 50% of infants (Levine et al., 1983). However, the etiologies, aside from the obvious possibilities just discussed, remain obscure, being related to temperament, maturation, and environmental factors. Bixler, Kaies, and Soldatos (1979) surveyed medical practitioners and found insomnia to be reported in 5.1% of pediatric referrals while hypersomnia occurred in 1.3%. The frequency of nightmares was the greatest, occurring in 7.4% of all patients. The frequency of parasomnias ranged from 1.2 to 7.8%.

Diagnostic Considerations

General Guidelines. Leaving aside the issue of incidence for the moment, the first step in determining the existence and nature of a sleep disturbance is to take a full history. Information as to when the problem began, the details of the sleep pattern, and measures taken to resolve the problem are necessary. The past need for sleep should be assessed, and characteristics of the parent should also be noted. Is the mother nervous or does she seem depressed? Is this her first child?

Aside from paying attention to the characteristics of the mother that might influence the sleep behavior of her child, it is also useful to find out the reason why she is seeking help at this particular juncture. It is beneficial to inquire about any changes in the household routine, where the child sleeps, whether or not the child attends a playgroup, and who the caregiver is during the day (Valman, 1987).

Behavioral observations of the child in the presence and absence of the mother are also a potential source of valuable information. If the child quiets on seeing the parents walk into the room and is not overly troubled in their absence, a complaint of insomnia is more likely to be unrelated to separation stress. Thus, the clinician can begin to look for a lack of ritual at bedtime, unnecessary response to the child's nightwaking, or a physical cause such as sleep apnea. In addition, the evaluation of sleep disorders requires assessment of daytime sleepiness, behavioral functioning while awake, and the organization of nighttime sleep (i.e., observation of 24-hour diurnal organization and biorhythmic function) (Levine et al., 1983).

While physical examination of infants and young children commonly provides little information regarding sleep complaints, the clinician must have sufficient working knowledge of the uses and capabilities of the sleep clinic in cases where such evaluation is warranted. Orr (1985) reported that most evaluations of infants in sleep clinics pertain to the possible existence of a sleep-related breathing disorder. These cases commonly occur in infants during the first 6 months of life who have had a significant clinical episode of apnea.

Applicability of DSM-III-R Nosology to Childhood Sleep Disorders. DSM-III-R does not differentiate between disorders of sleep in adults and children. This is justifiable because the essential features of most types of sleep disturbances are the same for both groups. However, it is important for the clinician to know that the parasomnias are represented in childhood more frequently than the dyssomnias described in DSM-III-R.

Broughton (1968), Anders and Guilleminault, (1976), Roffwarg (1979), and Levine and co-workers (1983) have identified a group of four sleep disorders that share common features and occur more often in the preschool and school-age years. Night terrors (DSM-III-R sleep terror disorder), sleepwalking (sleepwalking disorder), sleeptalking (parasomnia not otherwise specified), and primary nocturnal enuresis (considered by DSM-III-R to be a parasomnia but listed under disorders usually first evident in infancy, childhood, or adolescence) all occur at a particular point in the sleep cycle. They usually appear after a prolonged stage 3 or 4 non-REM period, just prior to a transition to the REM state. These disorders also tend to appear between 70 and 120 minutes after sleep onset; all can occur in the same child; a family history for the disorder is usually positive; males outnumber females by a ratio of 4 to 1; and there is retrograde amnesia regarding the episodes.

In general, sleep terror disorder (night terrors, pavor nocturnis) occurs frequently, but irregularly, primarily in preschool children. The most important differentiation to make is between sleep terror disorder and dream anxiety disorder (nightmare disorder). The most salient differential feature between the two is that nightmares are recalled, whereas an episode of sleep terror is not. In the case of sleep terror, the child sits suddenly upright and screams. The episode rarely lasts longer than 5 minutes and is not remembered in the morning.

Sleepwalking disorder and sleeptalking tend to substitute for sleep terror during the school-age years. Movements and speech are rambling and unfocused. Usually the conditions resolve spontaneously, but when they persist, or when speech or sleepwalking are directed, a psychological disorder may be suspected.

While the parasomnias are more common in childhood than the DSM-III-R dyssomnias (insomnia, hypersomnia, sleep-wake schedule disorder), they do nevertheless occur. It is important to make two determinations when diagnosing these conditions in infants and children. First, transient insomnia due to temporary anxiety and impaired parent-child relations should be differentiated from the chronic condition (Pearce, Akamine, Kapuniai, & Crowell, 1986). Second, when the condition has lasted more than a month, it is important to differentiate the inability to sustain a continuous long period of sleep from a disturbance in the diurnal regulation in sleep. That is, the child may be sleeping uninterruptedly for a long period, but the period does not occur at a time that is convenient for the parents. In such cases, the child may awaken and remain awake late at night, but has nevertheless rested adequately. Thus, the sleep-wake schedule disorder (delayed sleep phase syndrome) may be mistaken for insomnia.

When insomnia is actually present, it may be the result of an internal physiological dysregulation or it may be associated with sleep apnea, in which case there may be a complaint of hypersomnia during the daytime, which is actually symptomatic of and secondary to the insomnia condition. An important indicator of childhood-onset insomnia is its frequent association with other symptoms of childhood pathology, such as attention deficit hyperactivity disorder (Pearce et al., 1986).

DEVELOPMENTAL CONSIDERATIONS IN THE ETIOLOGY OF SLEEP DISORDERS IN INFANTS AND CHILDREN

It may be significant that the highest percentage of childhood sleep disorders found by Bixler was attributed to nightmares. Simonds and Parraga (1982) found that while 93.5% of the children and adolescents in a normal population slept soundly, the disturbances that did occur were usually associated with anxiety. These investigators found that the most common complaints were restlessness, fear of the dark, need for a security object or bedtime ritual, and talking during sleep. Fears regarding going to sleep were reported in 6.7%, and nightmares occurred at least once a week in 9.7%.

Anna Freud has noted that the human infant may be the only infant among mammals who sleeps alone, without contacting the skin or feeling the warmth of another creature. Given the data of Simonds and Paraga, its seems likely that, at least in young children, disordered sleep may be associated with separation trauma—perhaps in this instance the fear is of being separated from consciousness (and hence from a sense of control). This is especially likely to be a contributing factor if the child is customarily allowed to go to sleep in one place and wakes up alone in another.

In older children, around the ages of 8 to 11 years, there may be a confusion between sleep and death. Since the death concept matures around this time, incomplete understanding can produce faulty associations with loss of consciousness. Connell and Sturgess (1987) reported six case studies in which six children in middle childhood developed sleep phobia. After close observation, the investigators found that these children showed a predisposition to separation anxiety as a result of early separation trauma. Furthermore, their reactions were triggered by the recent death of someone important to them. All six also showed a tendency to equate death with sleep.

The cases reported by Connell and Sturgess serve to highlight the importance of clarifying developmental and social factors when evaluating sleep disturbances in children. Since sleep seems vulnerable to an anxious state, the problem may lie in current parental difficulties or in changed interactional patterns among family members. Furthermore, if the child receives inadequate nurturing during the day, he or she may demand increased attention, negative or positive, during the night (Ferber, 1985).

It is also important to recognize that sleep disturbances are likely to occur during the attempt to achieve developmental milestones such as toilet training or separation due to school attendance. Inadequate coping with these challenges may result in the prolongation of sleep problems—a process that further diminishes the child's coping capacity.

Studies by Edgil and co-workers (1985), Kataria, Swanson, and Trevarthan (1987), and Clarkson, Williams, and Silva (1986) are not only indicative of the developmental issues related to sleep discussed so far, but also shed additional light on symptomatologies associated with different developmental levels. Edgil and co-workers (1985), noting that sleep problems are the primary behavioral complaint motivating parents to seek treatment of their children, selected 40 mother-child pairs from a private pediatric practice according to the following criteria: children were between 9 and 48 months of age and had no developmental delays or current physical illnesses. The mean age of the children was 20.9 months.

The children were assessed with the Denver Prescreening Developmental Questionnaire, while the parents responded to an interview that was developed by the investigators to determine such variables as parental age and educational level, employment status, number and ages of siblings, and primary caregiver during daytime hours. Prenatal, perinatal, and neonatal histories were also obtained.

It is interesting that the most commonly cited maternal goal for an infant's behavior was that he or she sleep through the night. This goal was followed in popularity by getting the child to go to sleep easily and to obtain adequate night- and daytime sleep. Since these were children who had no disease or developmental delays, it seems likely that problems in sleeping, if any, were associated with the lack of ritual or sleep-associated stimuli already mentioned—factors that are fairly easy to correct.

Another interesting finding, and one that has significant implications for research efforts in the field, was that being a firstborn increased the likelihood of sleep problems. As Edgil and colleagues have noted, it seems likely that mothers who have had more than one child tend to define sleep behavior more realistically.

Noting that nightwaking appears to decline in prevalence in school-age children and that bedtime struggle appears to increase in frequency between the ages of 3 and 4, Kataria and colleagues (1987) undertook a study to map the persistence of these and other sleep disturbances in young children. In this longitudinal study, 60 normal children between the ages of 15 months and 4 years (mean age 26.4 months), selected randomly from medical school and private pediatric practices, were followed for 3 years.

Sleep questionnaires were completed by mail, telephone, and personal interviews at the beginning and the end of the study. A sleep disturbance was defined as nightwaking or bedtime struggle that occurred 3 or more nights out of the week and was present for at least a month at the time of the interview. Nightwaking was defined as being present if crying and demand for parental attention occurred. Bedtime struggle, in turn, was defined as occurring if the child took more than an hour to settle after being expected to go to sleep.

The results of this study again highlighted the importance of anxiety in the etiology of sleep disorders. Among the 23 children who were found to have disturbed sleep, the most common stress factor was unaccustomed maternal absence. This was reported in 7 of the sleep-disturbed children and in none of the 37 children without sleep problems. Also in line with other studies were the prevalences of sleep disorders found. Nightwaking was experienced by 22%, bedtime struggle by 13%, and both nightwaking and bedtime struggle by 7%.

Perhaps most significant, however, was the finding that the sleep disturbance persisted over 3 years in 8.4% of the sleep-disturbed group. This suggests that in the absence of treatment, sleep problems may be tenacious, being the result of stress and ongoing negative family dynamics. In light of their findings the authors stressed the importance of early intervention.

In combination with the results of Kataria and colleagues, a longitudinal study by Clarkson and colleagues (1986) may shed additional light on the developmental trends and stability of sleep disorders in children, since an older population of children was used (5 to 9 years). Noting that nightwaking recently has been reported to decline from 50% of preschool children to 20% at age 12, and that bedtime struggle increased from 8% at age 2 to 40% at age 10, these investigators sought to define the characteristics of sleep disorders in middle childhood.

Nearly 1,000 children were followed from ages 5 through 9. Information regarding sleep was collected from the parents when the children were age 5, 7, and 9 years. Children were also interviewed directly at age 9. Mothers were asked to estimate the total time the child spent in bed and the total time asleep and were asked if there had been any sleep problems on the night prior to the interview.

Overall, sleep time was found to decrease with age, as reported widely in other studies, although the variability at each age highlighted the importance of using a flexible approach when evaluating an individual child's sleep requirement. Sleep problems decreased over time as well, although there was low agreement among parents, teachers, and children in terms of day- and nighttime behaviors—an occurrence common in developmental studies. Only 0.3% of the total sample experienced a problem that persisted over the entire period.

This low persistence of sleep problems in middle childhood led the authors to conclude that these problems are infrequent, are inconsistently reported by parents and children, and do not identify a psychologically disturbed group of children.

Thus, the results of Kataria and Clarkson and their co-workers suggest that the trend of decreasing prevalence of sleep problems from ages 1 to 5 years continues into middle childhood. Clarkson and colleagues pointed out that it would interesting to discover when the frequency of sleep disorders begins to rise again toward its adult level and what developmental factors are responsible.

PSYCHOLOGICAL PHENOMENA ASSOCIATED WITH MATURATIONAL STAGES OF SLEEP ARCHITECTURE

Psychopathology and Temporally Associated Sleep Stages

Much work remains to be done on correlating development of sleep architecture with emotional/psychological disturbances. Much of the difficulty lies in the fact that the development of sleep in the newborn is still poorly understood. Anders and Weinstein (1972) delineated a general scheme in which the first year of life is most commonly troubled by failure to sleep through the night. They cited studies showing that 70% of babies settle by age 3 months and 83% do so by 6 months. It is generally believed that failure to settle is related to the process of CNS maturation, since insult to the CNS (e.g., anoxia) frequently results in delayed settling (Preston, 1945).

During the second year of life, as already noted, sleep disturbances are characterized by anxiety. During this period, however, the possibility first arises for neurotic conflict. With psychological and cognitive components being added to the physiological sleep requirement, the child clings to consciousness, fearing severance from the waking world. Thus, presleep rituals become important sources of reassurance. In some cases, the rituals may have their roots in more deepseated conflicts, in which case the excessively practiced rituals are in effect the early precursors of psychopathology. According to Anders and Weinstein, the third to fifth years of life are almost always marred to some degree by some form of sleep difficulty (e.g., slow to fall asleep, nightwaking, nightmares, fears of ghosts and wild animals, inability to sleep alone or in the dark). Most of these difficulties are transient, but if one or more persists for a long time, it may be an indicator of burgeoning psychopathology stemming from conflicts developed perhaps as early as the second year of life.

Attempts to further refine the temporal association between different types of psychological disturbance and level of sleep maturation have only begun to yield results. That this is a difficult task at best is demonstrated by the fact that all-night studies of psychotic children, while few in number, have failed to show any major differences in sleep pattern in these children compared to controls (Simeon, 1987). Studies with autistic children, however, have revealed maturational defects related in particular to REM sleep differentiation and vestibular function (Ornitz, 1978).

The picture is further obfuscated by the failure to associate changes in sleep architecture with psychopathological symptoms such as depression. Puig-Antich and co-workers (1983b) performed a 3-night polysomnographic study of 54 prepubertal children rigorously assessed by research diagnostic criteria to have major depressive disorder. Two groups of nondepressed controls were used for comparison. One group ($n = 25$) was comprised of children with emotional disorders, the other ($n = 11$) was comprised of normal children with no psychiatric condition.

After comprehensive polysomnographic assessment, it was found that the children with major depression showed none of the well-established EEG sleep characteristics of adults having the same disorder (i.e., shortened latency of onset of REM after falling asleep; increased REM density; decreased delta sleep; lessened sleep efficiency; and abnormal temporal distribution of REM over the course of the night).

In explaining their results, the investigators ruled out the possibility that children and adult depressives have basically different disorders, maintaining instead that the lack of sleep findings in depressed children stems from maturational factors that modify the expression of depressive illness. If this hypothesis is accurate, the sleep disturbances noted in depressed adults would be due not only to depression but also to an interaction between depressive illness and age.

Continuity of Sleep Disturbances

If sleep characteristics are ever to be used effectively as an aid in diagnosing psychiatric disorder, it seems evident that the effects of maturational phases will have to be taken into account. In reaching this goal, it will be helpful to define which types of sleep disturbances occur over the full course of maturation and which ones are limited to certain age ranges.

In this regard, Simonds and Parraga (1982) comprehensively studied sleep disorders and behavior in a rural population of school-age children (5 to 20 years old) using maternal reports. They found that nightmares, although they decrease in frequency with age, affect children of all ages. Also frequent but declining with age were occurrences of sleeptalking (the most prevalent sleep phenomenon), sleepwalking, bruxism, and bedwetting. The only two disorders found to remain relatively constant over time in terms of frequency were narcolepsy and primary hypersomnia. The fact that most of these behaviors occurred more prevalently in younger children demonstrates a maturational phenomenon at work.

Several investigators have sought to discover whether unsettled sleep during the preschool years is at all predictive of later sleep disturbances and/or psychological difficulties or is merely an artifact of CNS maturational stages. It does appear that early sleep disturbances may not be strictly the result of CNS development. Salzarulo and Chevalier (1983) investigated sleep difficulties in 218 children between 2 and 15 years of age and found a clear relation between early sleep–waking rhythm disturbances and later sleep problems. Thus, it may be that there is an extra element of internal conflict in some children with sleeping difficulties that emerge over and above normal maturational changes.

Discovering whether or not this is the case in a given child is still a very difficult task—one that may not ultimately prove worthwhile since other investigators have found that early sleep disturbances are not predictive of later sleep difficulty, even in children who are psychosocially burdened (Klackenberg, 1982). It may indeed prove to be the case that maturational changes make sleep disorders ineffective as a means of diagnosing childhood disorders, since other studies show little if any correlation between early sleeping problems and behavioral difficulties (e.g., Clarkson, Williams, & Silva, 1986).

CONCLUSION

Perhaps the most important consideration in diagnosing disorders of sleep in childhood is the contribution of the parents to the apparent pathology. It is crucial to discover the bedtime habits and rituals to which the child is or is not exposed in order to rule out parental contributions to the child's sleep behavior. Children should associate sleep with the bedroom and be introduced to bedtime rituals such as a warm bath prior to going to bed. Security is the key that enables a child to openly express his or her in-built need for sleep. In the second year of life especially, security concerns of the toddler become paramount.

In the vast majority of cases, behavioral therapy to "reset" the diurnal clock or build associations of items or rituals with sleep prove to be very effective. Drug treatment is almost never justified in young children with sleep disorders.

In the future, the study of sleep disorders in children may yield valuable information about other psychiatric conditions. The well-noted association of depression with increased or decreased sleep has led many to speculate that insomnia or hypersomnia may be markers for depression. If this association could be ascertained in young children, many questions about mood disorders in early and later life might be answered.

CHAPTER SEVENTEEN

Eating Disorders and Their Differential Diagnosis

David: Mysterious Eating Habits

David is a 3-year, 8-month-old boy who lives with his parents and his 1-year-old brother. David is the product of a normal pregnancy; however, due to prolonged labor, an emergency cesarian section had to be performed. David's medical history is significant for a fall at 1 year of age that resulted in a large subcutaneous hematoma but no loss of consciousness. David has reached his developmental milestones within normal age limits with the exception of speech and language development. His language has been significantly delayed since age 2. He rarely speaks and usually uses only disconnected words. However, he is capable of constructing two- to three-word sentences.

David was referred for assessment after undergoing a speech/language and hearing evaluation when he was enrolled in a language-oriented preschool program. He was administered the Stanford-Binet Intelligence Test to discover which class he should be placed in. David's IQ was found to be in the low-normal range (70–75). At this time an audiologist assessed David's hearing to be normal. He was also given a neurological examination 6 months prior to assessment, which resulted in no remarkable findings. David was tested for lead poisoning as well, because since age 2 he has been ingesting numerous nonnutritive substances. David's parents and nursery school teachers noted that he will chew on his clothing and his shoes and eat sand. It was also reported that David has trouble socializing with his peers. Although he is never physically abusive to other children, he does attempt to scare them with animal noises.

David was brought to the assessment office by his mother. He refused to separate from her during the first interview, but at the second testing session he separated easily. David appeared his stated age, but was inattentive and distractible to a greater extent than is expected for children his age. David fidgeted constantly and attempted to eat facial tissue, a pencil, and crayons at different times throughout the session. Fine motor and gross motor movement were assessed to be normal. David exhibited good comprehension skills; however, he rarely spoke. When he did speak it was mostly in the form of nonsense syllables and single words. Affect was constricted, but full range. Mood ranged from happy to tearful. David's concentration and attention spans were judged to be poor. His insight was assessed as fair, as was his judgment.

Based on David's repeated eating of nonnutritive substances (e.g., sand, clothing) since age 2, he was diagnosed as having pica. Although other disorders, namely schizophrenia and autism, may also present this symptom, David meets none of the other criteria for these disorders. His affect is not flat or inappropriate as it would be in schizophrenia, nor is there any evidence (either reported or observed) of delusions or hallucinations. Furthermore, David's socialization difficulties are not severe enough to warrant a diagnosis of autism.

David's socialization problems may, however, be an associated feature of his Axis II diagnosis: developmental expressive language disorder. David shows evidence of the essential feature of this disorder: marked impairment in the development of expressive language. As was exhibited by his results on the Stanford-Binet Intelligence Test, this impairment is not due to mental retardation. Further testing resulted in the finding that neither hearing impairment nor a neurological disorder is present. The fact that David's comprehension skills were judged to be normal rules out a diagnosis of elective mutism. David also does not meet the criteria for a pervasive developmental disorder, in which expressive language impairment may be present. Although acquired aphasia has criteria similar to those of developmental expressive language disorder, the former is usually accompanied by seizures, EEG abnormalities, or "hard" neurologic signs, none of which was found in the results of David's neurological examination.

Thus David was diagnosed as having pica and developmental expressive language disorder. The clinician recommended that he continue in his language-oriented preschool program and begin weekly individual therapy to address his eating disorder. Plans were also made for David to enter group therapy to help him socialize more effectively.

INTRODUCTION

As a subclass of disorders, the DSM-III-R conservatively defines eating disorders as being characterized by gross disturbances in eating behavior. As can be seen from David's case, these disturbances rarely occur in the absence of psychiatric stressors. Eating disorders include anorexia nervosa, bulimia nervosa, pica, and rumination disorder of infancy. Obesity is not included due to its apparent lack of association with any specific psychological factors in the etiology or course of any given case of obesity. However, it can be indicated by noting psychological factors affecting physical condition.

Eating disorders, when defined more broadly as the *misuse of eating in an attempt to solve or mask conflicts of living,* comprise a category of childhood disturbance that is more important in making clinical diagnoses than might first be apparent upon reviewing DSM-III-R (Bruch, 1973). The major significance of disturbed eating behavior derives from the fact that the social patterns of interaction between the child and mother develop and become entrenched during the first few weeks of life, when the nature of these interactions are largely related to feeding (Levine, Carey, Crocker, & Gross, 1983). Therefore, an eating disturbance can provide the clinician with a strong indication that there is something amiss within the child's psychosocial matrix (Satter, 1986; Trad, 1986, 1988).

Adding to the clinical importance of early feeding patterns is the fact that eating behavior is particularly vulnerable to distortion because the state of hunger carries with it aspects of both an innate drive and a learned experience. Bruch (1981) illustrated its complexity by pointing out that hunger can refer either to the physiological state of nutritional depletion or extreme food deprivation or to prolonged starvation. It can also be taken to mean a recurrent psychological experience defined by an unpleasant, compelling sensation that is felt in the prolonged absence of food and that also gives rise to urgent searching behavior, and even fighting, in an attempt to assuage it. Language derived from this human experience provides yet another common way of viewing hunger. When we are moderately hungry or when we desire a particular food, we often describe this condition as an *appetite*.

Theorists such as Bruch (1981) and Levine and colleagues (1983), by making the necessary attempt to speak of *hunger awareness,* rather than the more labile term, *hunger,* have recognized the fact that two forms of behavior have to be differentiated from each other from the time of birth: behavior that is initiated within the individual and that which occurs in response to external stimuli. Normal development requires the presence of "sufficient appropriate responses to clues originating in the child, in addition to stimulation from the environment" (Bruch, 1981, p. 214).

It is not difficult to envision how this system can go awry within the context of early feeding interactions. If the caregiver offers food in a way that is in synchrony with the infant's internal signals for nutritional intake, the child will come to recognize internal clues of hunger. That is, hunger awareness will evolve. However, if food is offered on a schedule inappropriate to the child's internal needs, whether due to neglect or to the fact that the mother responds solely to her own needs and perceptions in the matter of feeding, the infant may become confused. The infant may then fail to differentiate between hunger and satiation and may not be able to discriminate either of these feelings from some other, unrelated source of comfort or discomfort.

The ready manner in which interactional problems in the infant-mother dyad can become incorporated into eating behavior is exacerbated by the fact that infant health is judged almost solely in terms of growth measurement, which in turn depends on nutritional intake. The focus on growth and eating by the lay and medical community facilitates the evolution of a nearly obsessive preoccupation with the infant's eating (Bruette, 1984). This provides a fertile context for maternal overconcern, which may cause a mother to overwhelm the infant's internal hunger cues.

Given the ease with which disturbances in eating behavior can arise, as a result of both aberrant intrafamilial interactions and social overconcern, it is clear that eating provides a sensitive barometer of emotional state. Frequently, disturbances in eating are the first indicator of less obvious but primary psychosocial problems. This is an important clinical fact to recognize when encountering an eating-disordered child for the first time. When a parent presents a child with an eating complaint, it remains for the clinician to differentiate between such possibilities as aberrant feeding patterns due to maternal insensitivity or misconceptions, depression, food intolerance or allergy, a specific nutritional deficiency, or accidental ingestion.

DIFFERENTIAL DIAGNOSIS OF EATING DISORDERS

Disorders First Manifesting in Adolescence: Anorexia Nervosa and Bulimia Nervosa

Neither anorexia nor bulimia becomes apparent before adolescence or early adulthood, but it is widely agreed that these conditions are related by way of having similar etiological roots in infancy and childhood. The child is deprived of the opportunity to develop an accurate inward awareness of hunger when feeding times and circumstances do not proceed according to his or her internal needs but are dictated by the mother's feelings.

A discussion of the family characteristics of patients who severely restrict their food intake will follow. However, before describing these conditions it is important to know that awareness of hunger is rarely the only source of distortion in the perception of internal state in children who will grow to develop anorexia or bulimia nervosa. Other feeling states are usually mislabeled as well (Bruch, 1981). For example, these children may be told repeatedly that they "must" be cold, tired, happy, and so forth at times when these labels do not apply to how they actually feel. This maternal tendency toward global lack of touch with the infant's internal state can be invoked to explain the potentially dire effects of both anorexia and bulimia nervosa.

Both anorexia and bulimia occur much more frequently in females than males, and both are characterized by the adoption of extreme measures to control body size and weight. Anorexia nervosa is the more severe of the two conditions in terms of current functioning and later outcome, being characterized according to the DSM-III-R by four major features:

A. *Refusal to maintain body weight over a minimal normal weight for age and height, e.g., weight loss leading to maintenance of body weight 15% below that expected; or failure to make expected weight gain during period of growth, leading to body weight 15% below that expected.*

B. *Intense fear of gaining weight or becoming fat, even though underweight.*

C. *Disturbance in the way in which one's body weight, size, or shape is experienced, e.g., the person claims to "feel fat" even when emaciated, believes that one area of the body is "too fat" even when obviously underweight.*

D. *In females, absence of at least three consecutive menstrual cycles when otherwise expected to occur (primary or secondary amenorrhea). (A woman is considered to have amenorrhea if her periods occur only following hormone, e.g., estrogen, administration.) (p. 67)*

Weight loss is most commonly achieved by reduction in total food intake, often in conjunction with arduous exercise regimens. Many of these individuals have concurrent diagnoses of bulimia nervosa since they are unable to exert continuous control over their intention to restrict food intake and so compensate by binging and then inducing vomiting.

Bulimia nervosa is characterized, as is anorexia, by an overconcern with body size and shape. In addition to dieting, bulimics make repeated attempts to control what they perceive as negative physical traits by vomiting or the use of diuretics and/or cathartics. Because they also engage in alternate episodes of binge eating and fasting, these individuals frequently exhibit weight fluctuations. Some may be slightly underweight, while others may be overweight. Depressed mood is commonly observed, and these people are often diagnosed as having psychoactive substance abuse or dependence, most commonly also involving sedatives, amphetamines, cocaine, or alcohol.

The specific DSM-III-R criteria for bulimia nervosa are:

A. *Recurrent episodes of binge eating (rapid consumption of a large amount of food in a discrete period of time).*

B. *A feeling of lack of control over eating behavior during the eating binges.*

C. *The person regularly engages in either self-induced vomiting, use of laxatives or diuretics, strict dieting or fasting, or vigorous exercise in order to prevent weight gain.*

D. *A minimum average of two binge eating episodes a week for at least three months.*

E. *Persistent overconcern with body shape and weight. (pp. 68–69)*

Disorders First Manifesting in Infancy and Childhood

Pica. Like anorexia nervosa and bulimia nervosa, children exhibiting pica—the persistent eating of a nonnutritive substance for at least 1 month (DSM-III-R)—are often subjected to an increased level of psychosocial stress, although of a different and usually less severe variety.

Singhi, Singhi, and Adwani (1981) studied 50 children with iron deficiency anemia with pica and compared them to 50 other children who were also iron deficient but who exhibited no tendency toward pica. The children were matched for age, sex, socioeconomic class, and degree of anemia.

It was found that the children in the pica group had significantly greater stress scores than children in the control group. Specifically, the factors associated with pica were maternal deprivation, caregiving by someone other than the mother, parental separation, parental attitude of neglect, joint family, child beating, too little mother-child interaction, and too little father-child interaction. In another study by Singhi and Singhi (1982), low socioeconomic status was significantly related to the occurrence of pica.

The implication of these studies was that the psychosocial setting of children with pica should be evaluated and treatment should include an attempt to alleviate stress (Singhi & Singhi, 1983). This idea gains some support from a report in which pica was seen to occur in rats subjected to stress (Burchfield, Elich, & Noods, 1977).

Similar but somewhat different results were obtained from another study using a population of Indian children (Tamer, Warey, Swarnkar, & Tamer, 1986). Most of the children were between 1 and 3 years of age, with an average age of 2.3 years. Unlike the children in Singhi and Singhi's (1983) study, pica was unrelated to family type. However, 9% of the parents engaged in pica as children, as did 37% of the mothers during their pregnancies.

Pica may not appear very often as a solitary problem. In one study of 180 children with pica by Singhi and Singhi (1982a), 57% were found to have associated behavior problems. The most common of these was temper tantrum (33%), followed by bruxism (18%), breath holding (11.4%), and thumb sucking (11.4%).

The results of these studies are indicative of the confusion that still exists with regard to the etiology of pica. First of all, geophagia, the eating of earth, has been noted to occur throughout the world in association with religious beliefs or with the purpose of providing a full feeling to supplement poor diet (McLaughlin, 1987). This has been noted in areas ranging from rural Mississippi to the inhabitants of tropical forests. Furthermore, the Greeks and Arabs of ancient times ate clay to relieve nausea and vomiting (Laufer, 1930). Thus, there appears to be a certain component of normative social behavior associated with pica that makes its diagnosis somewhat tricky.

This aspect of pica is enhanced by the fact that the eating of nonfood substances appears, in some instances, to be associated with a strong urge to maintain internal homeostasis, as in the case of consuming iron-containing items to relieve iron deficiency. Unfortunately, investigations into the hypothesis that pica is a physiological-need-based behavior have been equivocal to date (Chen et al., 1985; Singhi & Singhi, 1982a).

Regardless of the lack of evidence about the degree of internal need association in pica, the choice of the item is usually highly specific. Choices may include ice, clay or soil, grass, leaves, starch, plaster, paint chips, string, paper, cigarettes, buttons, and insects. The child may begin eating these items between the ages of 12 and 24 months or even earlier (DSM-III-R). According to Sayetta (1986), several groups have been identified as being at particular risk for developing pica. The foremost factor is low socioeconomic status, which implies that hunger may predispose to pica. Other groups include those with high nutritional demands (e.g., infants, young children, pregnant women, and nursing mothers); brain-damaged, epileptic, mentally retarded, and psychotic individuals; blacks in the United States; and Middle Eastern populations with diets marginal in phytates and fiber.

Although pica frequently remits with time, it may be risky to wait for spontaneous resolution of this condition since a number of medical complications can occur. Among these complications are persistent vomiting, bowel obstruction, gut perforation, chronic constipation, iron deficiency, hypercalcemia, lead intoxication, obesity, parasitic worm and enteropathogen infections from earth or pet food, growth disorders, and hypogonadism (McLaughlin, 1987; Newton, Stack, Blair, & Keel, 1981). For children with suspected pica, it is important to obtain a comprehensive medical evaluation and institute management of any associated behavioral and emotional problems.

When diagnosing pica, the DSM-III-R stipulates that the child must not meet the criteria for autistic disorder, schizophrenia, or Kleine-Levin syndrome. It is also important to be aware of the fact that children also ingest foreign, sometimes poisonous, substances independent of pica. These incidents occur with less frequency than the eating of non-nutritive substances in children with pica. However, they are not necessarily "accidents" attributable to the random intersection of the child's oral explorations, the availability of toxic agents, and lapses in the attention of caregivers.

Bithoney, Snyder, and Michalek (1985) pointed out that psychosocial stress appears to be a factor in the lives of children with histories of such ingestions, since the families of these children show a generally higher prevalence of family problems. As in pica, ingestion of poisonous substances is likely related to a combination of family stress, maternal stress, and developmental factors. Thus, it may be advisable for the clinician to view poisonous ingestions initially as a subclass of pica, meriting the same attention to familial interactions and stress.

Rumination.   As defined in DSM-III-R, rumination disorder of infancy is characterized by:

A. *Repeated regurgitation, without nausea or associated gastrointestinal illness, for at least one month following a period of normal functioning.*
B. *Weight loss or failure to make expected weight gain.* (p. 70)

Furthermore, the infant may either eject the food from the mouth or rechew and swallow it. Often, sucking noises are made with the tongue, and the infant gives a clear impression that considerable satisfaction is associated with the rumination activity.

The aspect of pleasure associated with rumination has attracted a good deal of theoretical attention. As Chatoor, Dickson, and Einhorn (1984) pointed out in their excellent review, two basic theories of rumination have evolved in this regard. Within the psychodynamic approach, it is believed that rumination develops as a somatic means to alleviate tension. Basically, the infant feels fearful about maintaining an investment in a love object and so turns inward for satisfaction and safety (Trad, 1986).

Those who favor the behavioral approach believe that rumination is a learned behavior, being negatively reinforced in certain children when it assists them in avoiding situations that are more aversive than those associated with the rumination itself. Chatoor and colleagues have favored a somewhat different approach in which organic, psychodynamic, and behavioral theories are integrated to explain a given condition of rumination. An example of the usefulness of this approach is the case in which some anatomical problem such as hiatal hernia leads to vomiting in the infant. At some point the infant may learn to initiate vomiting, turning it into rumination in an attempt at self-regulation.

The aspect of self-regulation may prove central to the etiology of rumination, since this behavior was observed to decrease in a dose-dependent manner in a woman with lifelong postprandial rumination after administration of paregoric, an opiate agonist (Chatoor et al., 1984). In turn, naloxone, an opiate antagonist, blocked that effect of paregoric. While the evidence was not conclusive, Chatoor and colleagues pointed out that this finding suggests that opiate receptor insensitivity or a reduction in endorphinergic transmission might be involved in the pathophysiology of rumination. They further pointed out that this hypothesis gains support from experimental evidence showing that endorphins may play a mediating role in attachment bonds. Maintenance of bonds is associated with the presence of endorphins, while separation is not. Thus, the frequent observance of poor or disrupted attachment to the caregiver in babies who ruminate may provide a basis for postulating that rumination occurs in an attempt to reestablish a disrupted endorphinergic system.

In short, Chatoor and colleagues postulated that when the infant is unable to obtain loving attention or tension relief via the caregiver, rumination occurs as a way to achieve self-stimulation or tension relief. Since rumination, once established, can develop into a very resistant habit disorder, the clinician is well advised to attempt readjustment of the family interaction patterns once a medical etiology has been ruled out.

Food Allergy and Food Intolerance. All children, indeed individuals of every age, express dislikes and preferences for certain foods. It is important to be able to distinguish between an attitude about food due to allergy, intolerance, or taste and one that derives from psychological sources alone. The degree of tolerance shown by parents toward individual taste is an indicator of the degree of control they impose on the child's need for independence and autonomy. As noted previously, when parents are noticeably concerned about eating behavior and food dislikes, food itself is less likely to be the problem than parental overcontrol (Levine et al., 1983).

When differentiating between food aversion due to allergy or intolerance and that due to familial conflict, it is important to keep in mind that knowledge regarding the immune response system of healthy newborns and infants and the mechanisms protecting them from harmful immune responses is still very limited. However, the clinician should in no way condone the practice of a mother who severely restricts the diet of her child, believing erroneously that food allergy is the cause of some problem behavior (e.g., hyperactivity).

Food intolerance and allergy during childhood are indicated by a number of associated symptoms including vomiting, diarrhea, failure to thrive, abdominal pain, eczema, wheezing, urticaria and other rashes, mood alteration, flatulence, abdominal distention, migraine, epilepsy, and enuresis (Bruette, 1984). The presence of true allergy to or intolerance of a food is best established by repeatedly exposing the child to the food in question (food challenge) and obtaining reproducible effects on exposure and withdrawal.

Obesity. Although the DSM-III-R considers obesity to be primarily a physical disorder, Bruch (1981) noted that the development of obesity in an infant or child can be an expression of underlying emotional problems. Bruch drew attention to the fact that anorexia nervosa and developmental obesity can derive from the same source: the misuse of the eating function to solve problems of living that seem otherwise unsolvable. In both conditions there is an intense preoccupation with food and weight, which reflects an enormous concern with social approval— a vulnerability that reflects underlying emotional and personality problems.

The very development of obesity in a child is often an indicator of these other developmental disturbances and, in adolescent children, the clinician has cause to become suspicious if an obese teenager is noticeably inactive. This conspicuous inactivity is very often the result of an overanxious mother who perceives danger in everything her child does outside of her direct control (Bruch, 1981).

According to Bruch, rapid increases in weight that are associated with other psychodevelopmental problems may occur at times of emotional distress. These weight gains may then be counteracted (usually unsuccessfully) with frantic attempts to reduce. When the individual's inner sense of emptiness and despair is met with overeating, the consequent frantic attempts to lose weight may lead to depression or acute disturbances such as schizophrenia in those who pursue dieting with total determination. Those who fail to stay with dieting give up and resume overeating, not only regaining the previously lost weight but usually overshooting the previous weight level.

Woolston (1983) noted that obesity of infancy and early childhood represents a final common pathway resulting from the interaction of many different factors such as genetic make-up, parental experience, familial and cultural practices, emotional dimensions, and activity level. Before diagnosing obesity with attendant emotional disturbance, the clinician must rule out hypothyroidism, hypercortisolism, Froelich's syndrome, Laurence-Moon-Biedl syndrome, Prader-Willi syndrome, and disorders of glycogenesis (Woolston, 1983). Woolston further noted that children who are obese for genetic reasons are commonly short, being at less than the 5th percentile in height, and show delayed bone age. Children with so-called simple obesity, on the other hand, are nearly always above the 50th percentile and have normal or advanced bone age. The diagnosis and treatment of obesity in infants is made even more important due to the fact that obese infants more commonly become obese adolescents and adults than do nonobese infants.

CHARACTERISTICS OF FAMILIES WITH EATING-DISORDERED CHILDREN

Adolescence

If the definitions of anorexia nervosa and bulimia nervosa are examined, the issue of control becomes immediately apparent. Individuals with these disorders are excessively consumed with the need for control. Furthermore, all efforts at control are directed inward, literally toward the shape of the self. These facets of anorectic and bulimic behavior have led investigators such as Satter (1986) and Bruch (1981) to attempt to isolate early dynamics within the family that could potentially lead to such excesses of inward-directed control.

Working independently, these investigators have arrived at many of the same conclusions. Most of the investigation into the family characteristics and dynamics of families with eating-disordered children has been done in relation to anorexia nervosa. This is partly due to the fact that anorexia is a more severe condition and partly because many family therapists have asserted that anorexia nervosa is a valid diagnosis pertaining to a certain type of family (e. g., Minuchin, Rosman, & Baker, 1978).

Satter and Bruch both called attention to the fact that anorexia nervosa occurs very frequently in individuals who are described as being "perfect children." The early feeding histories of these children are conspicuous in that they are so remarkably free of trouble. In other words, the child is reported as having eaten exactly what was offered, without fussing. Tellingly, many mothers describe how they reliably "anticipated" the needs of their children and never permitted them to "feel hungry."

What circumstances within the family, then, lead to this kind of treatment of the infant? Satter and Bruch concurred that, while the families of anorectics do not appear on the surface to be disturbed, there is a definite unacknowledged, underlying tension between the mother and father that is extended to the children as well. These families are often characterized by overprotection, enmeshment, and rigidity (Minuchin et al., 1975, 1978). Overprotection leads to an excess of parental control and reduces the child's opportunity to take risks and develop autonomy. Furthermore, since the members of the family tend to isolate themselves, becoming overinvolved with one another, a rigidity of atmosphere develops in which the need for social and physical growth is suppressed in the service of keeping the family in a static state.

In addition, Bruch noted that anorexia nervosa develops most often in families of the upper-middle and upper classes. The parents in these families commonly place great importance on attaining success, and the intense pressure for achievement, combined with the deficits in autonomy and inner awareness, very likely gives rise to a situation in which the adolescent sees in his or her own body the only possibility of achieving control and some sense of selfhood. If this desperate attempt at control fails, the intensity of feelings and the level of confusion about the difference between internal needs and those imposed from the outside may cause schizophrenic levels of disorganization. Thus, when presented with a patient who is in conflict with the family overeating patterns, it is extremely important for the clinician to be sensitive to the potential dangers that may evolve later.

Infancy

Dahl and Sundelin (1986) and Dahl, Eklund, and Sundelin (1986), in their study of 50 infants between 3 and 12 months of age who were reported to a child health care facility for some form of eating problem, found that eating problems were fairly common during the first year of life and particularly so during the early period after birth. These children also became temporarily difficult to feed following change of food or external stress such as an acute infection. While these were transient effects, they were times of vulnerability during which problems that may have developed between infant and mother became exacerbated. Thus, clinicians should take care to assure that eating difficulties during times of stress do not turn into long-term problems.

Dahl and Sundelin found three main categories of eating problems. More than half the infants (28) refused to eat, 9 showed colic, and 8 were referred for vomiting. The problems often began at an early age and persisted for a long time (mean age at onset 4.3 months; mean duration 4.5 months). The investigators estimated that the prevalence of eating problems as defined in their group was 1.4 per 100 infants between the ages of 3 and 12 months (Dahl & Sundelin, 1986).

In a follow-up of the same children, Dahl and co-workers (1986) found four main maternal factors that were associated with eating problems in infants: (1) a mother's feeding problems during her own infancy; (2) breastfeeding problems experienced by the mother; (3) great anxiety experienced by the mother during her pregnancy and; (4) psychosomatic complaints in the mother, possibly indicating overstress as a result of the pregnancy. Although these indications of maternal disturbance hardly exhaust the possibilities, they do serve to demonstrate the importance of the maternal role in the genesis of feeding problems, especially since the mothers in this study typically demonstrated negative mood and irritability about feeding their children.

CONCLUSION

In distinguishing between an eating disorder and a simpler eating problem or disturbance, the clinician must make an assessment of the resistance to change and the level of affective arousal. It is important to keep in mind that eating attitudes and behaviors, both good and bad, quickly become entrenched and are comprised of experiences accumulated from the individual, the family, and the society at large. However, an eating disorder will likely exist in families where there is an extreme level of parental control imbued with intense feelings that may or may not be immediately apparent.

The ideal situation is one in which the mother and infant develop a mutually rewarding interaction that results in a sense of competence for both. This entails the evolution of a feeding interaction in which timing, pacing, and tolerance of frustration are mutually agreeable. A timely cue for clinical intervention is provided when feeding ceases to be a pleasurable experience for mother and infant. Sensitive responding at this point on the part of the clinician has the potential to forestall tension and unhappiness in the short run and prevent the development of overt pathology over the long term.

CHAPTER EIGHTEEN

Tics and Stereotypy/Habit Disorders and Their Differential Diagnosis

Jack: Classic Symptoms and No Fault of His Own

Jack is a 5-year, 1-month-old boy who lives with his maternal grandfather and his grandfather's girlfriend. Jack was the product of an uneventful full-term pregnancy, and his birth was normal. Jack reached all his developmental milestones within the appropriate age ranges. He was toilet trained by age 2, but still has occasional accidents. Jack's biological parents are both alcoholics who come from families of alcohol and drug abusers. Jack was witness to violence, fighting, screaming, and yelling between his parents. Both parents abused him physically and emotionally. Jack's maternal grandfather is an alcoholic who attended Alcoholics Anonymous and claims to have been sober for the past 2 years. He has been Jack's legal guardian for approximately 1 year.

Jack has a long history of behavioral problems such as explosive outbursts, biting others, slamming doors, and cursing. Since age 4, Jack has exhibited a variety of tics; he periodically makes grunting noises and clears his throat. He also curses for no apparent reason. These tics have changed over time, beginning with reports of involuntary twitches in his face and excessive, repetitive eye blinking.

Throughout the assessment, Jack was restless and anxious. He was neatly dressed and well-groomed and appeared much younger than his stated age. When he was asked about hallucinations, he was very vague, first claiming to have experienced them, then denying their presence and refusing to elaborate. His mood was normal and his affect was appropriate. Gross motor coordination was intact; however, it was noted that Jack had mild difficulty performing activities requiring fine motor skills (i.e., tying shoelaces). Jack expressed suicidal ideations ("Sometimes I feel I want to die"). He expressed homicidal ideations as well (to "beat or kill someone"); however Jack has never attempted aggressive acts on anyone. He feels he is "too small" and "not strong enough" to do so. Jack also reported that he sees himself as "bad, ugly, and very weak," indicative of poor self-confidence. Intelligence testing proved Jack to be capable of functioning in the high-average range. His short-term memory (concentration) appeared weak, and his judgment was affected by quick, impulsive, and nonreflective responses. Although Jack has been reported to have a short attention span, he was able to establish a rapport with the examiner on a one-to-one level. Jack's speech is quite rapid and his sentences are choppy ("I gonna die." " I fall apart." "I am bad." "I'm kidding.") and interspersed with grunts and yelps. In addition, during the assessment he perpetually touched things (e.g., a corner of the desk, his shoe, a Lego block), but when this was pointed out he claimed not to have been aware of his actions.

Jack's symptoms indicate that a diagnosis of Tourette syndrome is appropriate. He has exhibited both multiple motor tics (eye blinking, touching, facial twitches) and vocal tics (grunts, throat clearing, yelps) for well over 1 year. The anatomic location, the severity, and number of the tics have changed since they first began to appear.

The symptoms present in Tourette syndrome may be found in other disorders, and so differential diagnoses must be made. As a part of Jack's physical examination, a urine analysis for toxicology was performed. The results enabled the clinician to rule out the possibility of ingestion of any psychoactive substance (e.g., amphetamine) as well as a diagnosis of organic mental disorder induced by psychoactive substances.

Jack also underwent a neurological examination which revealed soft neurological signs and nonspecific EEG abnormalities. These symptoms constitute an associated feature of Tourette syndrome according to some sources. (Some 50% of patients with Tourette syndrome show soft neurological signs and 13 to 15% of patients with Tourette syndrome exhibit minor EEG abnormalities.) Stereotypy/habit disorder, unlike Tourette syndrome, consists of apparently intentional behaviors that are often rhythmic. As shown during assessment, Jack's continued touching of objects (a motor tic) was entirely unintentional and without pattern. A diagnosis of obsessive-compulsive disorder may be ruled out on this basis as well, for compulsions differ from tics in that the former are intentional behaviors and the latter are involuntary. Finally, a diagnosis of schizophrenia may be ruled out: Although schizophrenia may present with abnormal motor movements, it does not involve vocalizations like the grunts, yelps, and words of Tourette syndrome.

Thus, a diagnosis of Tourette syndrome was assigned, and it was recommended that Jack enter individual treatment once weekly to help him overcome his feelings of inferiority and to aid in reducing his symptoms of Tourette syndrome.

INTRODUCTION

Analysis of tic disorders and habit disorders requires more than an integration of neurologic and psychiatric perspectives. Since these disorders first appear in childhood or adolescence, the clinician must also take *developmental* factors into account (Trad, 1986, 1988). Tics, which occur in Tourette syndrome, chronic motor or vocal disorder, transient tic disorder, and stereotypy/habit disorder (DSM-III-R), are rapid, repetitive, aimless, and, with the exception of stereotypy/habit disorder, involuntary movements of functionally related muscle groups (Cohen et al., 1987; Matthews, Leibowitz, & Matthews, 1983; Williams, Pleak, & Hanesian, 1987).

From a developmental perspective, regardless of the specific subclass of tic disorder, tics in children are characteristically transient in nature, a fact that makes assessment of their incidence and clinical significance extremely difficult. One estimate is that tics appear in 1 to 5% of the population (Azrin & Nunn, 1977). The individual may be aware of the particular mannerism, but tics usually occur automatically and unconsciously (Goldenson, 1970). Other features of tics in general are that they rarely, if ever, occur during sleep; they appear to be most common between 8 and 12 years of age, with an onset between 5 to 7 years; and they occur approximately three times more often in males than in females (Matthews et al., 1983). Spontaneous recovery from tics has been reported to be at least 50% after 2 to 15 years' duration (Corbett, Matthews, Connell, & Shapiro, 1969).

Whether tics occur within the context of the tic disorders as delineated in DSM-III-R (Tourette syndrome, chronic motor or vocal tic disorder, and transient tic disorder) or within the context of stereotypy/habit disorder (e.g., nail biting, hair pulling, head banging, etc.), the psychiatric sequelae of tics can be quite severe. Shaffer (1985b) has demonstrated that children with brain injury—which is very probable in the case of most tics—experience a greater rate of psychiatric impairment than do children with comparable degrees of non-CNS physical disabilities.

This is probably attributable to the fact that children afflicted with a CNS-associated handicap have more to cope with than the deficit in self-esteem that attends all handicapping conditions. The clinician must take into account the fact that there is a potential direct neurophysiological impact on the emotional, cognitive, and behavioral capacities in individuals with CNS dysfunction. In addition to the possibilities of reactive anxious and depressed states, children with tic or habit disorders are at risk of becoming overdependent on parental or adult care—an occurrence that can lead to exhibiting psychosomatic complaints to maintain adult concern (Williams et al., 1987). Finally, children with sufficiently severe tics may be excluded from social activities, thereby contributing to developmental lags—a risk that already exists in many of these children since tics also frequently occur in association with hyperactivity and deficits in attention.

For all these reasons, early diagnosis and, if possible, control of tics by dopamine-blocking agents are essential if the individual is to be spared many years of suffering and ridicule. Adults in whom the diagnosis has not been made sometimes seek seclusion and take jobs in which they work alone. While early intervention may forestall these events, detection is often difficult because individuals with Tourette syndrome may become proficient at controlling their tics in public until they can go to a private place to let go.

DIFFERENTIAL DIAGNOSIS: TICS AND THE TOURETTE SYNDROME

Features and Diagnostic Criteria of Tourette Syndrome

Tourette syndrome (TS) is the most debilitating of the tic disorders, and it provides a good example of the way neuropsychiatric disorders of childhood are the result of interaction between genetic, behavioral, and environmental factors. In fact, many investigators view Tourette syndrome as a model of childhood onset of neuropsychiatric disorders (Cohen et al., 1987; Williams, Pleak, & Hanesian, 1987). This view of TS as a paradigm for all CNS-related psychiatric disorders stems from the fact that the expression of symptoms varies with age in a way that may parallel the development of the CNS, as symptoms vary in severity with fluctuations in environmental stress (Cohen et al., 1987). There appears to be a significant degree of genetic transmission of vulnerability to TS (Williams et al., 1987).

The DSM-III-R implicitly concurs with the view of Tourette syndrome as something of a model for childhood neuropsychiatric disorders in that it makes note of the existence of data indicating that TS and chronic motor or vocal tic disorder may represent different symptomatic expressions of the same underlying disorder. Therefore, close attention to the signs and features of Tourette syndrome will provide a sound basis for identifying not only Tourette, but other disorders associated with tics.

Before presenting the definition and associated features of Tourette syndrome, it is first necessary to explain more fully the nature and manifestations of tics. As noted in DSM-III-R and elsewhere (e.g., Cohen et al., 1987), tics can be motor or vocal, simple or complex. A simple motor tic is a fast, darting, repetitive, and directionless contraction of an involved muscle group. Some examples of simple motor tics are facial grimacing, eye blinking, neck jerking, shoulder shrugging, and finger jerks. Simple vocal or phonic tics consist of linguistically meaningless noises and sounds such as grunting, sniffing, throat clearing, coughing, barking, or hissing.

Complex motor tics are characteristically slower, more organized and more functional than the simple variety. They can involve any type of motion and can manifest as facial gestures; grooming behaviors; touching, hitting, or biting one's self; smelling an object; clapping; kicking; hopping; throwing; or dystonic posturing. It is vital to note that complex motor tics, in addition to having more components than simple tics, are often ritualistic and carry a component of compulsion with them so that, for example, the repeated performing of an act such as picking up a chair to find out "just the right spot" for it can provide a measure of tension release.

Complex vocal tics erupt suddenly and unpredictably and are comprised of inappropriate words or phrases such as "Ha ha!" "Oops!" or "Uh Uh!". Also, words or phrases may be uttered out of context; unintentional, socially unacceptable outbursts or outright obscenities may erupt (coprolalia); or the person may repeat his or her own sounds or words (palilalia). Echolalia might also occur, as might echokinesis (imitation of the movements of someone who is being observed).

Simple or complex motor or vocal tics are neurologically expressed and irresistible in the same manner that actions of an individual with obsessive-compulsive disorder are psychologically experienced, but they can usually be suppressed for a variable length of time (as is also true of the action in OCD). Furthermore, the severity of all forms of tics can be increased by environmental stress and may become decreased by absorption in a project such as reading a book or sewing.

Tourette syndrome thus represents a kind of worst-case scenario in terms of tic pathology, one that can contain all of the various types of tics described above. Therefore, it is useful to conceptualize tic phenomena along a continuum from simple tics to full-blown Tourette symptomatology. The essential features of Tourette syndrome are both motor and vocal tics. According to DSM-III-R criteria, an individual with TS has multiple motor tics and at least one vocal tic:

A. *Both multiple motor and one or more vocal tics have been present at some time during the illness, although not necessarily concurrently.*

B. *The tics occur many times a day (usually in bouts), nearly every day or intermittently throughout a period of more than one year.*

C. *The anatomic location, number, frequency, complexity, and severity of the tics change over time.*

D. *Onset before age 21.*

E. *Occurrence not exclusively during Psychoactive Substance Intoxication or known central nervous system disease, such as Huntington's chorea and postviral encephalitis.* (p. 80)

Either type of tic can occur at different times during the illness, and they can also occur simultaneously. There are two features of the way tics appear that complicate diagnosis of Tourette syndrome. The tics may appear several times daily, nearly every day or intermittently throughout a period of more than 1 year. The tics in TS are also variable in that their number, anatomic location, complexity, and severity can change over time.

In TS the tics occur in bouts and may involve the head and other parts of the body. Coprolalia is present in up to a third of cases, and complex motor tics such as touching, squatting, deep knee bends, retracing of steps, and twirling while walking are also frequently present.

The first symptoms to appear in approximately half the cases are bouts of a single tic. Commonly, the first tic to appear is eye blinking, but squatting, tongue protrusion, sniffing, hopping, throat clearing, stuttering, and coprolalia can also occur initially. In other cases the disorder begins with multiple symptoms, which may include any of the tics mentioned thus far as well as various noises such as barks, grunts, screams, yelps, or snorts.

The median age of onset of Tourette syndrome is given as 7 years in DSM-III-R, and it may occur as early as 1 year of age. In the majority of cases onset occurs prior to age 14. The course of the disorder is lifelong in the vast majority of cases, although periods of remission may occur lasting from weeks to years. Severity and frequency of symptoms may abate in some instances during adolescence and adulthood, and the symptoms also may become less varied over time in these individuals.

There is some degree of familial transmission of Tourette syndrome, since all tic disorders occur more frequently in first-degree biological relatives of people with TS than among the general population.

In terms of differential diagnosis of Tourette syndrome, it is first necessary to differentially diagnose tics in general. They should be distinguished from other movement disturbances such as choreiform (dancing, random, irregular, and nonrepetitive movements); dystonic (slow, twisting movements occurring between periods of prolonged muscular tension); athetoid (slow, irregular, writhing most frequently in the fingers and toes but often in the face and neck); myclonic (brief bursts of sharp muscle contractions that may affect parts of muscles or muscle groups in nonsynergistic manner); hemifacial spasm (irregular, repetitive, unilateral jerks of facial muscles); synkinesis (movements of the corner of the mouth when the person intends to close the eye or vice versa); and dyskinesias (e.g., tardive dyskinesia—oral-buccal-lingual masticatory movements of the face and choreoathetoid movements of the limbs.

Second to be eliminated in the differential diagnosis of Tourette syndrome are stereotyped movements such as head banging, rocking, or repetitive hand movements that are intentional and often rhythmic in nature. Also, compulsions resulting from obsessive-compulsive disorder must be differentiated from tics by way of their intentional nature, although, as will be discussed shortly, many individuals with TS report compulsive-like feelings associated with their tics. Finally, Tourette syndrome must be differentiated from amphetamine intoxication and numerous other neurological disorders such as stroke, Lesch-Nyhan syndrome, Wilson's disease, Sydenham's chorea, Huntington's chorea, and multiple sclerosis. Organic mental disorders and schizophrenia may also present with abnormal motor movements, but these and other conditions can be distinguished from TS by a careful history, appropriate laboratory tests, and observation since there is no other disorder that mimics the full symptomatology of TS.

Stereotypy/Habit Disorder

Habit disorders such as thumb sucking, hair pulling, head banging, body rocking, teeth grinding, and skin picking, while they are phenotypically similar, actually appear to be less related to the symptomatology of Tourette syndrome than do the behaviors seen in OCD or autism/PDD. This stems largely from the fact that these behaviors are distinguishable from tics in that they are voluntary and nonspasmodic (Matthews et al., 1983).

The DSM-III-R cites three criteria necessary for making a diagnosis of stereotypy/habit disorder. First, the behavior must be intentional, repetitive, and nonfunctional (e.g., shaking or waving hands; biting nails; mouthing objects; swallowing air; noncommunicative, repetitive vocalizations; breath holding; face slapping; hand biting; hyperventilation). Second, the disturbance must either cause physical injury to the child or markedly interfere with normal activities. Finally, PDD and tic disorders must be ruled out. Another aspect of stereotyped behaviors that aids in differential diagnosis, aside from their presumably voluntary nature, is their frequent association with mental retardation.

Transient Tic Disorder

The diagnostic criteria for transient tic disorder and for chronic motor or vocal tic disorder are as follows:

Transient Tic Disorder

A. *Single or multiple motor and/or vocal tics.*

B. *The tics occur many times a day, nearly every day for at least two weeks, but for no longer than twelve consecutive months.*

C. *No history of Tourette's Disorder or Chronic Motor or Vocal Tic Disorder.*

D. *Onset before age 21.*

E. *Occurrence not exclusively during Psychoactive Substance Intoxication or known central nervous system disease, such as Huntington's chorea and postviral encephalitis.* (DSM-III-R, p. 82)

Chronic Motor or Vocal Tic Disorder

A. *Either motor or vocal tics, but not both, have been present at some time during the illness.*

B. *The tics occur many times a day, nearly every day, or intermittently throughout a period of more than one year.*

C. *Onset before age 21.*

D. *Occurrence not exclusively during Psychoactive Substance Intoxication or known central nervous system disease, such as Huntington's chorea and postviral encephalitis.* (DSM-III-R, p. 81)

It is apparent that these disorders represent less severe subsets of the symptomatology seen with Tourette syndrome. When compared to those with TS, children with transient tic disorder characteristically have milder symptoms that may not require pharmacological treatment and interfere minimally with schoolwork and social interaction. The clinician should be aware, however, that the symptoms of transient tic disorder may in some cases become chronic and more severe, evolving into Tourette syndrome.

The most common tic in this disorder is eye blinking or some other facial tic. There may be just one or a number of tics of either the motor or vocal variety. In cases where there are a number of tics they may occur simultaneously, sequentially, or randomly. The primary distinguishing characteristic in differentiating this disorder from Tourette syndrome and chronic motor or vocal tic disorder is the fact that the latter conditions last for at least one year.

Chronic Motor or Vocal Tic Disorder

It is also a relatively simple matter to distinguish this disorder from the other two tic disorders because Tourette syndrome involves not one but both kinds of tics, whereas in transient tic disorder the disturbance is always less than a year in duration. In comparison to those seen in Tourette syndrome, the tics in chronic motor or vocal tic disorder are much less severe. Functional impairment is also much lower.

PREVALENCE AND ASSOCIATED FEATURES OF TOURETTE SYNDROME

Prevalence

Reports of the prevalence of Tourette syndrome vary widely. In fact, the highest reported estimate is 160 times greater than the lowest (Burd, Kerbeshian, Wikenheiser, & Fisher, 1986). However, Caine (1985) noted that, as with all relatively rare disorders, TS may be significantly under-reported, since prevalence is usually estimated on the basis of number of cases diagnosed within a certain population.

Noting that the prevalence rate of Tourette syndrome has been generally estimated to be between 1 and 5 in 10,000, Burd and co-workers (1986) performed a study oriented toward obtaining a more accurate figure based on data from a geographically and demographically defined population of normal school-age children. These investigators used DSM-III criteria and drew from the North Dakota population of 140,580 school-age children, finding a TS prevalence rate of 5.2 per 10,000. This figure broke down into 1.0 per 10,000 for girls and 9.3 per 10,000 for boys. Thus, the male/female ratio for this population was

9.3 to 1, which is considerably higher for boys than the data used in DSM-III-R.

Associated Features

In their study, Burd and co-workers noted the possibility that children with Tourette syndrome, due to school and parent referral, may be more likely to come to the attention of physicians than adults with this syndrome. They therefore suggest that prevalence studies should be based on populations of children alone in order to obtain a more reliable idea of the prevalence of TS.

The reason for referral of children with this disorder is not limited to the incapacities associated with it. However, the fact that specific learning disabilities, such as attention deficit disorder (ADD), are often found along with tic complexes further increases the chances of referral for assessment and treatment. Children with TS commonly show impulsiveness, frustration intolerance, subnormal ability to concentrate, hyperactivity, and obsessions and compulsions. Cohen and colleagues (1987) estimated that 50 to 60% of children with TS who are referred to clinics in major medical centers may also satisfy diagnostic criteria for ADD (inattentiveness and impulsivity) and hyperactivity. In many cases, these characteristics may develop prior to the onset of TS.

When symptoms of ADD occur it is very important to withhold stimulant medication until a thorough screening for tic symptoms is made. If this screening is not done, a child in whom the symptoms of ADD are precursors of tics may suffer an earlier onset of the tics due to exacerbation from the medication. Furthermore, the tics may never emerge in some children without aggravation from medication for ADD (Lowe, Cohen, Detlor, Kremenitzer, & Shaywitz, 1982). Thus, a strong family history of Tourette syndrome argues strongly against the institution of stimulant therapy for alleviation of hyperactive symptoms. Furthermore, if a child on such medication begins to develop tics, therapy should be discontinued immediately.

Another interesting feature of Tourette syndrome is that it is frequently associated with obsessive-compulsive symptoms (Grad, Pelcovitz, Olson, Matthews, & Grad, 1987). Recent research has indicated that obsessive-compulsive disorder (OCD) is far more common in patients with TS than in the general population. In fact, one study reported that obsessive-compulsive behavior is the most frequent associated behavior seen in patients with this disorder (Nee et al., 1980).

While the observed association between Tourette syndrome and OCD needs further elucidation, it does serve to call into question the usual description of tics as being "involuntary." Some children and adults do experience their tics as coming unbidden, but many others report antecedent, evanescent sensory signals or urges that might suggest participation by sensory systems and/or motor pathways (Cohen et al., 1987). These urges are experienced as an increasing tension and anxiety with regard to one area of the body. As in cases of OCD, the tension builds unbearably until the individual paroxysmally discharges it by performing a certain action (or tic).

One possible indication of the nature of the relationship between TS and OCD may be derived from neurochemical studies in which it has been found that clonidine not only attenuates the frequency and severity of tics but also partially relieves the compulsive feelings of individuals with Tourette syndrome (Cohen, Detlor, Young, & Shaywitz, 1980). While these findings and others implicate dopaminergic involvement, the full mechanism remains to be described. In any event, the clinician should be aware of the compulsive component of TS and of the possible presence of this disorder in children diagnosed with OCD.

In addition, Pauls and Leckman (1986), noting the numerous reports of increased obsessive-compulsive disorder among patients with Tourette syndrome, performed a genetic study of 30 nuclear families identified through 27 index cases of TS. They found evidence to support the hypothesis that OCD is etiologically related to TS and chronic tics. Thus, it is possible that chronic tics and OCD are alternative phenotypic expressions of the diathesis of Tourette syndrome.

Like OCD, there are many aspects of autistic-like behavior that appear to be related to Tourette syndrome. In particular, the stereotypic movements, vocal expostulations, and echolalia seen in autism may confound the diagnosis of TS. Further compounding the difficulty is the fact that tics and stereotypies can occur in the same individual. However, the observation that stereotypic behaviors and tics, as well as compulsions, all respond favorably to clonidine is evidence of dopamine involvement along the whole spectrum of disorders associated with tics and/or atypical movements (Jeste, Karson, & Wyatt, 1984). As to the specifics of clonidine action in these disorders, little is known for certain. Leckman, Detlor, and Cohen (1983) noted that the observation that clonidine is effective in only 50 to 60% of patients argues against an underlying deficit in noradrenergic systems in TS. Rather, it appears that central noradrenergic mechanisms become involved at some later point in the development of the condition.

Further supporting the notion of Tourette syndrome as a paradigm for these disorders are the findings of Burd and co-workers (1986), who studied 59 patients whose early history indicated infantile autism or other pervasive developmental disorders (PDD). Of the patients studied, 12 later developed TS, and these scored significantly higher on IQ measures and measures of receptive and expressive language. Based on these findings, Burd and co-workers hypothesized that development of symptoms of Tourette syndrome following the onset of PDD may be a marker of more favorable developmental outcome. Furthermore, children with PDD who also meet the criteria for Tourette syndrome may comprise a distinct subgroup of children with PDD.

Vivian: Example of an Unconscious Internal Circuit

Vivian is a 3-year, 10-month-old girl who lives with her two younger siblings and their parents. A year ago, Vivian's maternal grandmother lived with the family for 3 months; however, she left to live with her son and died 3 months later of pneumonia. Vivian was born of a normal, full-term pregnancy, and there were no complications. All her developmental milestones were reportedly normal; however, she was bottle-fed until age 5 because she "watched her younger sister using the bottle and wanted to do the same." Vivian is described by her father as being a "daydreamer," and her pediatrician reports her to be a "quiet, passive child." Vivian's medical history is unremarkable. Her parents report that when she was approximately 3 years of age, she began twirling her hair while she was sucking her thumbs. She would then pull out the knots she created. This behavior stopped spontaneously after about 6 months. Vivian began playing with her hair again 2 months ago, but it was not until 1 month later that her mother noticed that she was pulling out her hair from both her scalp and her eyebrows in an approximation of the balding pattern of her father. During her hair-pulling episodes, Vivian has been described as "staring." Vivian is reportedly an excellent student. She has friends and gets along relatively well with her siblings. Her mother reports only that Vivian bites her nails, picks her cuticles, and tends to be more testy with her than with her husband.

Vivian, a cute Hispanic girl, was cooperative throughout assessment. She sat quietly unless asked a direct question. Vivian's hair had been arranged so as to make her bald patches less obvious. At times, she would fidget anxiously with her fingers or a piece of string. Her range of affect was full, and her mood was reserved. Vivian did not exhibit gross thought disorganization. She denied both suicidal and homicidal ideation. Her attention and concentration were unimpaired, and her insight and judgment were deemed fair.

Vivian's symptoms point to a diagnosis of trichotillomania; she has recurrently failed to resist impulses to pull out her hair, and this has resulted in a noticeable hair loss. This hair pulling has no association with a preexisting inflammation of the skin, and it is not a response to a delusion or a hallucination. However, the lack of information regarding Vivian's feelings immediately prior to and following her hair-pulling episodes necessitates differential diagnoses.

Although Vivian is "often touchy," a diagnosis of oppositional defiant disorder is easily ruled out because she has no other criteria necessary for this diagnosis. A diagnosis of dysthymia can also be ruled out primarily because Vivian is not reported to be depressed in any way, nor does she claim to be sad. In addition, Vivian's appetite is normal, as is her sleeping pattern, and her concentration is intact. A diagnosis of stereotypy/habit disorder seems appropriate, for Vivian engages in an "intentional, repetitive, nonfunctional behavior." However, this diagnosis is made only when a disturbance causes physical injury to the child or markedly interferes with normal activities. Obsessive-compulsive disorder is an appropriate diagnosis for Vivian because her hair-pulling behavior has no seeming purpose, nor does she claim to do it in order to prevent or produce some future event or situation. Extensive neurological examination has ruled out the possibility of petit mal seizures. This finding is supported by Vivian's awareness of her maladaptive behavior and lack of postepisode drowsiness.

Thus, a diagnosis of trichotillomania has been assigned, with a recommendation to assess family functioning (i.e., clarify secrecies and conflict resolution) and to engage Vivian in individual treatment.

CONCLUSION

The results of recent research suggesting that children with CNS-related disorders are more vulnerable to the development of psychiatric illness provides a compelling reason to detect and treat tic disorders. This task is made complicated by the fact that the symptoms in tic disorders characteristically wax and wane over time and are responsive to fluctuations in environmental stress. One factor that makes differential diagnosis somewhat easier is the recognized genetic transmission of vulnerability to tic disorders. A family history of tic disorder can be instrumental in making the discrimination between a true tic disorder and some other condition with aberrant movements such as stereotypy/habit disorder.

The heuristic aspect of the analogies associated with Tourette syndrome also should not be overlooked. The fact that some individuals with this disorder experience an inner tension that can only be discharged with the performance of a certain action is highly suggestive of an underlying CNS mechanism, probably dopamine-related, uniting tic disturbances and obsessive-compulsive disorder. The potential heuristic value of Tourette syndrome is further indicated by the hostile, aggressive nature of the complex vocal tics (coprolalia) when they are present. Apparently, when this occurs, there is disinhibition of aggressive urges. Further understanding of the neurobiochemical mechanism underlying this phenomenon could prove beneficial in the understanding and treatment of hyperactivity and conduct disorders.

CHAPTER NINETEEN

Somatoform Disorders and Their Differential Diagnosis

Stacy: Frozen in Defiance

Stacy is a 4-year, 3-month-old girl who lives with her younger brother, older sister, and their parents. Stacy was born of an uneventful pregnancy and, with the exception of a prolonged labor, birth was normal as well. Stacy reached all developmental milestones within the appropriate age ranges. Her medical history is unremarkable. Stacy is, according to her family, "the most important person in the house." She admits to being her father's favorite child and is not above exclaiming to either her siblings or her mother "Daddy loves me the best." Stacy's father is a salesman and must frequently go on business trips. When he is away, reports Stacy's mother, Stacy is "unmanageable and disrespectful. She alternates between staring at the mirror and gluing her eyes to the television, and she won't listen to anyone." Stacy's father admits to being "a trifle indulgent" with his daughter, but claims that it is only because she "always seems to need reassurance that we love her." According to Stacy's nursery school teachers, she has always been an average student; however, she has been described by many as being "immature." Stacy "rarely waits to be called on and merely calls out whenever she so desires." Reports from both her school and her family show that Stacy is prone to throwing temper tantrums in order to get her way.

Stacy's parents brought her in for evaluation because, for 2 months, her right arm had been "stuck." Her head was tilted to the point that it nearly touched her right shoulder, and her arm was outstretched at a 45-degree angle from her shoulder. Stacy claimed to be incapable of moving either her arm or her neck. This "paralysis" began, according to both Stacy and her mother, on the evening after Stacy's father had left on one of his business trips. Stacy and her mother had got into a fight that culminated with Stacy's mother shouting, "If you continue acting like this, I'm going to send you to your grandmother's house." A few hours after this argument, Stacy reportedly reached for the telephone and from then on was "paralyzed." Stacy's parents had taken her to numerous physicians and neurologists, none of whom could find any explanation for her so-called paralysis. One physician reported that when he attempted to bend Stacy's arm, her elbow became hyperextended, and when he tried to flex her arm, he encountered resistance as well; this resistance is inconsistent with actual paralysis. What Stacy's parents found most odd was that, in contrast to Stacy's usual behavior (which tended to be "overly emotional and exaggerated"), she seemed relatively unconcerned with her lack of mobility. Her parents also reported that Stacy moved freely in her sleep, but she denied any assertion of this capability.

Throughout the examination Stacy openly expressed her willingness to "do anything to help the examiner." Stacy appeared her stated age and was dressed quite fashionably. During the entire interview her arm remained extended. Her right fist was clenched tightly, and her head was tilted onto her right shoulder. In order to make eye contact with the examiner, Stacy had to move her entire body; this was done slowly and deliberately as if she were in pain; however, she denied any discomfort. Stacy's affect was judged to be normal. Thought content revealed a preoccupation with physical attractiveness and a fear of being disliked and then abandoned. Her speech and language capabilities were age appropriate. Stacy exhibited neither suicidal nor homicidal ideations. She was well oriented, and both attention and concentration were assessed to be normal. Stacy's judgment was impaired by her tendency toward impulsive decision making.

Due to her apparent paralysis, reports from her parents, and the psychological evaluation, Stacy was diagnosed as having conversion disorder. She exhibited a loss in functioning suggestive of actual paralysis; however, after appropriate investigation (both physical and neurological), this could not be explained by a known physical or neurological disorder. Stacy was reportedly unaware of producing her condition and, after careful deliberation, it was decided that the threat of being sent out of her home exacerbated Stacy's fear of abandonment, thereby initiating her symptoms. This temporal relationship between a psychosocial stressor (argument with mother) that is related to a psychological need (to be liked) and initiation of a symptom (paralysis) is a criterion for a diagnosis of conversion disorder. Furthermore, Stacy was not conscious of producing her "paralysis," and this too is a requirement of conversion disorder.

Differential diagnosis of a physical disorder (such as multiple sclerosis) was ruled out by both the absence of any significant finding in a thorough physical examination and the fact that Stacy's "paralysis" was inconsistent with the anatomical distribution of the nervous system. If Stacy's symptoms were indicative of an undiagnosed physical disorder, there would be no evidence that they served a psychological purpose. Although other disorders, namely, somatization disorder and schizophrenia, may have conversion symptoms, Stacy did not meet the criteria for either of the two disorders. Differential diagnosis of hypochondriasis was made because there was no actual loss of body functioning. The fact that Stacy's symptoms were unintentionally produced ruled out both a diagnosis of factitious disorder with physical symptoms and a diagnosis of malingering.

Stacy's constant demands for reassurance (as reported by her father), her concern with physical attractiveness (as expressed in the evaluation), her frequent temper tantrums, and her lack of tolerance for waiting (as noted by her teachers) pointed to a diagnosis of histrionic personality traits. This is a frequent predisposing factor of conversion disorders. Although with dependent personality traits the individuals are excessively dependent on others for praise, they are without the exaggerated emotional features of histrionic personality disorder. A diagnosis of narcissistic personality disorder was also ruled out on the basis that Stacy lacked the preoccupation with a grandiose sense of self and intense envy.

Thus a dual diagnosis of histrionic personality traits and conversion disorder was made. Twice-weekly individual therapy was recommended for Stacy and once-weekly counseling for her parents.

INTRODUCTION

The DSM-III-R defines somatoform disorders as a group of conditions whose principal features are physical symptoms suggesting physical disorder for which there are no recognizable organic findings—a definition that seems to apply to Stacy well enough. These symptoms, in the absence of physical findings, are then considered to be linked causally to psychological factors or conflicts. The nature of the symptoms in somatoform disorders is different from those seen in malingering or factitious disorder because the symptom production is not intentional. Although the symptoms in this class of disorders are physical in nature, the specific pathophysiology underlying their development cannot be determined by existing laboratory or medical examination techniques. Therefore, the pathophysiological processes involved must be conceptualized by means of psychogenic constructs (Trad, 1988).

Within DSM-III-R nosology, several factors can account for the development of this type of symptomatology. In *body dysmorphic disorder* there is preoccupation with some imagined defect in appearance in a normal-appearing person. *Conversion disorder* describes a psychological development leading to alteration or loss of physical functioning to a degree that suggests a physical disorder. *Hypochondriasis* is a psychological reaction formation producing irrational fears or beliefs about having one or more diseases. Finally, *somatoform pain disorder* is characterized by preoccupation with pain unattributable to any other mental or physical disorder. A somatoform disorder is a usually chronic disorder beginning early in life in which there are recurrent and multiple somatic complaints of many years' duration.

Ford (1983) viewed the concept of somatization as a "process in which the body is used for psychological purposes or personal gain" (p. 1). Ford envisioned the psychological uses of somatization as being threefold:

1. Displacement of unpleasant emotions into a physical symptom, as when a child becomes preoccupied with bowel dysfunction in lieu of feeling an underlying depression.
2. Use of the symptom as a symbolic means of communicating an idea or an emotion, such as when hysterical paraplegia develops in order to communicate helplessness.
3. The alleviation of guilt through suffering, an example of which would be the development of a pain syndrome following the death of an ambivalently regarded person.

In terms of the second function of somatization, personal gain, Ford delineated four fundamental possibilities:

1. Ability to manipulate relationships (e.g., I can't visit you because I'm ill).

2. Obtaining release from duties and responsibilities such as consciously or unconsciously feigning illness or disability in order to avoid going to work.

3. Financial gain, such as when disability payments are made following a false "whiplash" injury.

4. Seeking attention or sympathy from another person, as when concern and worry are aroused in response to self-induced skin lesions.

In effect, Nelson (1983) took Ford's broad purposes of the somatization process and grouped them into two types of psychosomatic illness: conversion (hysterical) reactions and psychophysiologic disorders. Conversion reactions are characterized by sudden onset and are usually traceable to a precipitating environmental event. These types of reactions most commonly are manifested through the voluntary musculature or sense organs (e.g., hysterical blindness). Psychophysiologic disorders are more difficult to define in terms of onset and may involve different organ systems in response to chronic anxiety (e.g., eczema, bronchial asthma, ulcerative colitis, peptic ulcer).

From these brief descriptions it can be seen that the interplay of various psychological factors and/or conflicts can result in a wide variety of bodily effects, real or imagined. Understanding of these variations in unexplained somatic symptoms is hampered by the fact that in many cases (e.g., body dysmorphia, somatization disorder, and undifferentiated somatoform disorder) there is still little or no genetic or other information about predisposing factors.

However, information is beginning to emerge regarding the type of psychosomatic symptom that is likely to occur in relation to a given psychiatric condition. Goldberg, Regier, McInerny, Pless, and Roghmann (1979) stated that among children with mental health problems referred to pediatricians, complaints regarding the gastrointestinal tract are the most common. This led Wasserman, Whitington, and Rivara (1988) to evaluate 18 girls and 13 boys between 6 and 16 years of age who were referred to a pediatric gastroenterology clinic for recurrent abdominal pain. They found that gastrointestinal complaints occurred most often in anxious, internalizing children who had experienced traumatizing events and who came from families whose members had a history of abdominal complaints.

On a more specific level, Livingston, Taylor, and Crawford (1988) evaluated 95 psychiatrically hospitalized children 6 to 12 years of age and found that abdominal pain and palpitations were significantly associated with separation anxiety disorder and psychosis. To a lesser degree, children diagnosed with major depression also evidenced gastrointestinal complaints. Pseudoneurological problems, on the other hand, were found to be more common in children who also reported psychotic symptoms. Many more studies like this and the one by Wasserman and co-workers are needed in order to reach greater specificity regarding somatic complaints and their relation to psychiatric stressors.

In trying to unravel the pathogenesis of psychosomatic or somatoform illness, Kenny, Bergey, and Young-Hyman (1983) have emphasized the importance of abandoning the dualistic notion of mind-body separation. These investigators have suggested that somatoform complaints be placed on a continuum ranging from those that are largely psychological in etiology to those that are largely physiological in nature with a smaller psychological component. Graham (1985) has supported this idea, noting that while the physical and psychological components of any given clinical problem should be taken into account, their relative importance will vary considerably in terms of etiology and treatment. Graham has proposed a system wherein common medical conditions of childhood might be ranked according to the degree of contribution made by psychological involvements. In ascending order of importance of psychologic contributions, Graham has listed these conditions as follows: congenital malformations, cancers, metabolic disorders, infections, epilepsy, failures of growth, bronchial asthma, enuresis/encopresis, accidents, and emotional/behavioral disorders.

This chapter takes a nondualistic viewpoint to examine the nature of somatoform disorders and suggests that trauma and stress play a major role in the pathogenesis of these disorders. In other words, stress and/or trauma may trigger not only distinctive behavioral disorders but distinctive physiological vulnerabilities as well. These vulnerabilities may then become transduced into a certain type of somatoform complaint depending on the individual's specific biological make-up, psychological system, and previous experience. Support for this contention is gained from studies showing that severe stress significantly affects not only psychological functioning but physiological functioning as well (e.g., down regulation of the immuno-response system) (Trad, 1988).

By inference, this argument also impinges on what the DSM-III-R refers to as "psychological factors affecting physical conditions." Under this rubric, investigators have focused on environmental stimuli that are temporally related to the initiation or exacerbation of a physical condition and to physical disorders with either demonstrable organic pathology, such as rheumatoid arthritis, or a known pathophysiological process (e.g., migraine headaches or vomiting).

DIFFERENTIAL DIAGNOSIS
OF SOMATOFORM DISORDERS

Body Dysmorphic Disorder

The DSM-III describes seven ways in which the body is observed to be used for psychological or personal gain, along with a catch-all category, somatoform disorder not otherwise specified, that is intended to cover any other ways that might be encountered. The first of these, body dysmorphic disorder, is characterized by a preoccupation with some imagined defect in appearance in a normal-appearing person. In some cases there might actually be a slight physical anomaly, but the person's interpretation of its severity is grossly exaggerated. In order to be diagnosed as body dysmorphic, the preoccupation cannot be of delusional intensity, as in delusional disorder, somatic type, and its occurrence cannot be exclusively during the course of anorexia nervosa or transsexualism. Differential diagnosis from adolescent concerns about body image revolves around the greater intensity of concern in those who are dysmorphic, and the exaggeration of defects seen in major depression, avoidant personality disorder, and social phobia are only symptoms and not the primary disturbance.

Conversion Disorder

The predominant feature of this condition is an alteration or loss of physical functioning that suggests a physical disorder but, as in Stacy's case, is an expression of a psychological conflict or need. As Stacy also serves to illustrate, patients may exhibit a relative lack of concern about what appears to be a very serious problem. For a diagnosis of this disorder to be reached, the person must not be conscious of the symptom production; the symptom cannot be a culturally sanctioned response pattern and cannot be explained by a physical disorder; and it cannot be limited to pain or to a disturbance in sexual functioning. Thus, malingering is differentiated from conversion disorder by the intentionality of the symptom production in the former disorder. Furthermore, it is important not to make this diagnosis in cases where there is disease such as asthma or irritable colon, in which psychological factors play a role but there is still organic involvement.

Hypochondriasis

In this disorder there is preoccupation with the fear of having, or the belief that one has, a serious disease. For this diagnosis to be made, the supposed symptoms cannot be those of panic attacks. The fear must persist even in the face of medical reassurance to the contrary regarding the disease, and this disturbance must have existed for at least 6 months. Furthermore, the fear cannot be of delusional intensity. The most important and sometimes difficult differentiation to make in this disorder is between hypochondria and true organic disease.

Somatization Disorder

The essential features of this manifestation of using the body in the service of psychological or personal gain are recurrent and multiple somatic complaints of several years duration for which medical attention has been sought but for which no organic cause has ever been found. Several classes of symptoms can potentially be employed in this disorder, involving problems with the gastrointestinal tract or the cardiopulmonary and neurologic systems, sexual troubles, and problems of the female reproductive tract. In order to make this diagnosis there must be a history of many physical complaints or a belief that the person is sickly beginning before age 30 and persisting for many years. Furthermore, the symptoms cannot have occurred only during a panic attack, and they must have caused the person to take medication. As in hypochondriasis, it is of great importance to rule out true physical disorders in somatization disorder.

Somatoform Pain Disorder

In this condition, the principal feature is preoccupation with pain in the absence of physical findings that might account for the pain or its intensity. For this diagnosis to be made, the preoccupation with pain must have existed for at least 6 months. Also, appropriate evaluation must uncover no organic pathology, or, when there is related organic pathology, the complaint of pain or the resulting impairment must be grossly in excess of what would be expected from the physical findings. It is important to differentiate individuals with this disorder from those who have histrionic personality traits. Furthermore, in malingering, the symptoms are intentionally produced in pursuit of a goal that is obviously recognizable, a condition that does not pertain in somatoform pain disorder.

Undifferentiated Somatoform Disorder

This category is intended to describe clinical pictures that do not meet the full symptom criteria of somatization disorder. In this condition there is usually either a single symptom such as difficulty in swallowing or, as is more commonly the case, an array of multiple complaints such as fatigue, loss of appetite, and gastrointestinal problems.

EMPLOYING A PSYCHOLOGICAL PERSPECTIVE FOR THE UNDERSTANDING OF SOMATOFORM DISORDERS

Necessity of the Psychological Viewpoint

A model of psychosocial medicine is crucially important in revealing the mechanisms underlying all forms of somatoform disorders and complaints. Knapp (1980) has argued for the validity of the psychosocial context as applied to medicine by compiling a wide range of data that strongly implicates psychological factors as catalysts in a variety of organic diseases. For example, Knapp has noted that great progress has been made in comprehending the relationship between central nervous system phenomena and peripheral body processes as mediated by neuroendocrine transmitters and their receptors. Along these lines, Weiner (1977) has identified six psychosocial or psychosomatic diseases involving the operation of a neuroendocrine component at some level: hypertension, bronchial asthma, peptic ulcer, thyrotoxicosis, rheumatoid arthritis, and ulcerative colitis.

The most powerful implication of this line of research is that virtually all organic diseases have etiologic components deriving from both biological constitution and level of psychological adaptation. To further explore the relationship between these two major contributors to disease, Knapp recommended the use of Molina's (1983) biopsychological model.

The Biopsychological Model

Molina (1983) noted that the principal advantage of a biopsychological approach stems from the fact that it provides a view of disease as a multidynamic process, one that originates from the interaction between biological, psychological, and sociocultural factors. This view is more in line with reality, since normal living organisms are not stagnant but exist in constant flux, striving to adapt to a continuous line of environmental challenges. Thus, it is most accurate to view physiological disorder not as an isolated entity that occurs apart from those life forces, but rather a process born in a cauldron of multiple interactions.

The central dynamic underlying Molina's biopsychological model is that of increasing or decreasing vulnerability. For example, psychological vulnerability grows with the number of personally experienced roadblocks to coping or development. In addition, genetic factors are likely to play a role in the evolution of psychological vulnerability. It has now been established that a number of conditions are associated with strong familial predispositions (i.e., a number of metabolic, endocrine, and cardiovascular conditions as well as some psychiatric disorders such as mood disorders, schizophrenia, and panic attacks). Interacting with a genetically determined temperament or constitution, developmental problems such as a childhood relationship with an overly intrusive caregiver can give rise in adulthood to psychological vulnerability when a person is faced with circumstances requiring individuality and autonomy.

Along these lines, Molina noted that cultural and societal factors associated with developmental problems can combine to predispose an individual to be more or less socially vulnerable to certain circumstances. For example, homosexuals may be more exposed to social discrimination than heterosexuals. By extension, the property of being male or female or being the first or last child in a family, when combined with cultural norms, will make an individual more or less susceptible to various types of stressors.

Other deterrents to normal development can also be seen as contributing to overall vulnerability in the individual. For example, information about such factors as prenatal, perinatal, childhood, and adult accidents that have an impact on biological development can affect both psychological and biological vulnerability. An example of such factors might be exposure to teratogenic drugs in the prenatal period leading to congenital malformation that would negatively affect the infant's later psychological and social development. Thus, in assessing biological vulnerability, the clinician should try to determine whether or not the individual suffered a biological accident that left psychological sequelae in its aftermath. Sequelae of biological and psychological developmental vicissitudes might include poor frustration tolerance, learned helplessness, low self-esteem, limited capacity for trusting others, and fear of intimacy (Trad, 1986, 1987).

Finally, but certainly of great importance, is another precipitating factor that interacts with the individual's internal vulnerabilities and increases susceptibility to illness: stress. Stress that causes an alteration in biological or psychological equipoise or a major change in social environment can result in the disruption of at least one of these adaptive systems. Furthermore, since these systems are coexistent, disruption of even one will threaten the stability of the entire person. Thus, when studying a given disorder, the clinician should take into account the individual's overall state of vulnerability. This requires an analysis of the biological, psychological, and social systems of the individual as well as an index of current life stresses. Following such an analysis, the dynamics of the disorder will be better understood, and this will facilitate the development of an effective treatment plan (Trad, 1987).

Emilio: Coping . . . Barely

Emilio is a 3-year, 7-month-old boy who lives with his father and his mother. His parents are currently experiencing a significant degree of marital discord. According to the mother's psychotherapist, there is "a lot of tension and verbal fighting" in the home. There has been some discussion of a legal separation.

Emilio was born of a full-term, planned pregnancy. His birth was normal, and both Emilio and his mother were released from the hospital after 3 days. Emilio was breastfed for $3\frac{1}{2}$ months until, his mother reports, "my milk ran out and I was exhausted." Both Emilio's mother and his father had previous marriages. His mother is currently unemployed, and his father owns a saloon. Although Emilio's past medical history includes no abnormalities, for the past 8 months, he has been complaining of "very bad tummyaches" almost daily. Emilio's developmental milestones were all reached within normal age expectations.

The recommendation that Emilio be assessed came from his mother's psychotherapist. Emilio's parents have both expressed extreme frustration with their son vis-à-vis his strong-mindedness and constant complaints of gastrointestinal discomfort. According to Emilio's mother, he is very "stubborn and defiant and sometimes drives me crazy. We took him to six doctors and they didn't find anything wrong with him. I don't know what to do with him anymore."

Assessment included both Emilio and his parents. All were found to be alert and oriented. Emilio's parents fought during most of the session and devalued each other constantly. In response to their verbal abuse, Emilio told his parents to "shut up." He often placed his hand over their mouths or covered his ears with his hands as if he did not want to hear his parents' voices. Toward the middle of the interview, Emilio claimed he had a "tummyache," but when he came back from the bathroom with his mother, "nothing happened." The pace and volume of Emilio's speech was judged to be normal. His play behavior consisted of erecting and knocking down buildings with Lego blocks and, to her annoyance, shooting his mother and the evaluator with the space gun. When she asked him to stop shooting, Emilio refused and began to swear at her. Emilio exhibited no evidence of psychotic, suicidal, or homicidal symptoms. He denied the presence of either hallucinations or delusions. Emilio's cognition was judged to be intact, as were his memory skills. Emilio's affects were full range and appropriate. Both fine and gross motor movements were judged to be normal. Following the psychological assessment, Emilio underwent a full physical examination. No abnormalities were found on either of the two evaluations.

Emilio's symptoms point to a diagnosis of undifferentiated somatoform disorder. He has complained of gastrointestinal discomfort for which appropriate evaluation uncovered no organic pathology or pathophysiologic mechanism. His complaints have persisted for more than the 6 months required to make this diagnosis.

However, differential diagnosis must be made: somatoform pain disorder requires a "preoccupation" with pain, which Emilio does not manifest. In somatization disorder there is the requirement of a minimum number of characteristic symptoms of several years' duration; Emilio's symptoms have only been present for 8 months. This time frame also rules out the possibility of adjustment disorder with physical complaints, for which the required duration of symptoms is less than 6 months. Since there is no evidence of any "physical condition," psychological factors affecting physical condition can be ruled out as well. Finally, Emilio's disorder is not malingering, because his symptoms are not intentionally produced in pursuit of an obviously recognizable goal, which is necessary for this diagnosis to be made.

A diagnosis of oppositional defiant disorder was also made based on Emilio's defiance of his parents' requests, his use of obscene language, his angry and touchy demeanor, and his insistence on doing things that annoy others. Although these symptoms are also observed in conduct disorder, Emilio does not violate the rights of others, a criterion inherent in this diagnosis. Emilio's symptoms do not match any of the criteria necessary for a diagnosis of attention deficit disorder with hyperactivity. No evidence of psychotic symptoms were found during assessment; thus, a psychotic disorder was ruled out. Additionally, Emilio's mood and affect were both judged to be normal and appropriate, so a mood disorder was ruled out as well.

Thus, the diagnosis of undifferentiated somatoform disorder and oppositional defiant disorder was made. The clinician recommended that evaluation be continued for the parents alone, Emilio alone, and the family together. Once-weekly therapy for Emilio and once-weekly family therapy were recommended.

MEDIATION OF STRESS: COPING STYLE

It is evident from Emilio's case and others like it that stress can lead to somatic complaints in situations in which the individual fails to cope with internal dissonances or dissonances between the self and the external environment. Rutter (1979) noted that most forms of psychosocial stress do not constitute a short-term, single stimulus. Rather, they are a complex set of shifting conditions with their own histories and futures attached. Coping provides the child with the psychosocial tools needed to fend off the debilitating effects of stressors, allowing the child to continue coping at an optimum level. Many factors should be taken into account when determining whether a child possesses an adequate coping style (and thus protection from somatoform complaints), among them socioeconomic status, age, sex, family constellation, temperament, cognitive and affective regulatory capacities, and consistency of parental relationships.

Rutter's concept implicitly includes the idea that the child's developmental status will strongly affect coping ability. Garmezy and Masten (1986) have noted that this element and the others just mentioned, in addition to being *predictors* of competence, are also *moderators* of competence.

The theories and data generated by Rutter's many studies have produced a useful body of information that can be integrated into the purvue of a physical examination. For example, it is vitally important to find out whether or not the child is being exposed to any of the specific stressors Rutter has mentioned: imminent hospitalizations, recent birth of a sibling, and parental divorce. Likewise, stressors that might be less obvious should also be searched for (e.g., marital discord, family financial problems, school pressures). After assessing the child along these lines, the clinician can proceed to assessment of coping capacity. This phase of the evaluation should include integration of developmental factors such as the child's age, developmental stage, type of temperament, attachment status, and level of self-esteem.

With regard to assessment, Minuchin and co-workers (1975) attempted to isolate the factors responsible for childhood psychosocial disorders. They distinguished between two forms of symptomatology: primary psychosocial disorders and secondary psychosocial disorders. In the former category, a physiological disorder was already present (frequently a metabolic disorder such as diabetes or an allergic diathesis as exists in asthma). The psychosocial element in the primary form lies in the emotional exacerbation of already existing symptoms.

In secondary psychosocial disorders, there is no predisposing physical disorder in evidence. In these cases, the psychosocial element lies in the transformation of emotional conflicts into somatic symptoms. Occasionally, these symptoms can escalate into severe illness such as anorexia nervosa. An interesting and useful finding that emerged during the course of the investigation by Minuchin and co-workers was that both types of psychosocial illness were seen to be associated with a particular type of family organization typified by enmeshment, overprotectiveness, rigidity, and lack of mechanisms for conflict resolution.

Minuchin and co-workers found that interventions modifying the familial orientation of the psychosocially ill patient facilitated remission more successfully than did interventions that were focused only on the patient. Overall, the notion of a *psychosomatogenic family* helps to isolate problem areas within the child's primary life context—an approach that circumvents a good deal of the necessary initial exploration for areas amenable to intervention. In other words, information about family organization and functioning as it pertains to possible psychosocial problems can be used in prophylactic treatment strategies.

Along these same lines, it might be advantageous to examine the work of Anthony (1986), who summarized theories about the response of children to severe stress. Anthony first called attention to a model of self-induced pathology in which individuals are likely to develop helpless or hopeless responses in relation to their psychological or constitutional vulnerabilities. This theory was originally advanced by Schmale (1972) and implies that psychosocial factors are prime triggers in episodes of physiological illness.

Anthony postulated a second model based on Rutter's theory of individual differences in vulnerability to stress-induced disorders. This model centers around the fact that disturbing events in a child's life may be perceived as being uncontrollable, and feelings stemming from this perception extend to the child's relative ability to maintain an internal locus of control in times of extreme stress.

A third model has also been developed in relation to factors predisposing to physical illness. This model is derived from research into physiological and psychological responses to stressful stimuli. It assumes that individuals differ in vulnerability in terms of their suppression of awareness of threatening stimuli. Alternatively, an individual might be hyperalert to these stressful situations. The implication is that those who are either hyperalert to problems or too strongly suppress awareness of stressful situations may be at increased risk for physical disease.

PHYSIOLOGICAL AND PSYCHOLOGICAL RAMIFICATIONS OF STRESS

Physiological Sequelae

Prior to discussing the psychological ramifications of stress in children exposed to traumatic events, it will be advantageous to summarize the general effects of stress on physiological functioning. Research results regarding the effects of stress in children are limited to date, primarily because measurement has been limited largely to noninvasive techniques such as measurement of heart rate. However, the newly developed technique of analyzing hormones in free-flowing saliva promises to correct this situation (Gunnar, 1987). Despite the paucity of data on relationships between hormones and stress, Rice (1987) performed research on the various interactions that lead the brain to translate the effects of emotional or stressful stimuli into various physical manifestations. Rice hypothesized that the brain reacts to a stimulus that has an emotional charge with output via the autonomic nervous system and hypothalamo-pituitary-adrenal axis that mobilizes the natural defenses of the body.

These responses are represented in a heightened state of arousal, which includes increased cardiac output, higher blood pressure, and increased rate of arterial plaque formation. When confronted with situations of extreme stress, however, the body may not be equipped to respond optimally. In such cases, individuals resort to more primitive coping strategies such as denial, withdrawal, or resistance.

Coddington (1972), who investigated the overall effects of life events in the development of disease processes in young children, noted that as children expand their social sphere they also increase their risk of exposure to more dramatic positive and negative life events. Thus, at each stage of development the child must readjust to the new stresses encountered. For example, the first such milestone is when the child enters school. A later adjustment is needed with the onset of puberty. In general, Coddington reported that health is especially dependent on the child's ability to maintain a balance between the internal milieu and the external environment. Thus, the ability to combat disease, according to Coddington, depends upon the child's skill at adapting to the progressively stressful changes in the surrounding environment.

Psychological Sequelae

Terr (1979, 1981, 1983) performed a series of studies involving the children of the Chowchilla school bus kidnapping that are valuable for understanding the intimate interplay between physical and psychological factors. In 1976, a bus carrying 23 children attending summer school was hijacked by three men. The children were forced into a van, which was then buried in a deserted section of the road. The children remained buried for 16 hours before two of the older boys dug an escape route.

Terr first studied these children 5 to 13 months after the event and found that they had not only posttraumatic stress syndrome but also clusters of symptoms relating to the trauma. These included persistent nightmares and acute anxiety that surfaced even during normal daily activities. Terr reported personality changes, fear of the future, and reenactment of the events.

Terr also found that repetitive phenomena occurred during the recovery period. Some children reported dreaming of their own death, while others displayed peculiar behaviors, including fantasies that first occurred during the kidnapping. Of the children involved, 14 almost obsessively played and replayed the kidnapping experience with their friends. When questioned, many of these children said that they felt they could be kidnapped again. Although most of the children came from stable and secure backgrounds, their parents noted that they no longer seemed able to fully "trust the world."

In 1983, Terr conducted a follow-up study of the kidnapped children and reported some disturbing results. Among other things, Terr found that the posttraumatic effects of the event remained the same or had actually intensified. Also prevalent were denial, a sense of a foreshortened future, nightmares, and an obsessive desire to reenact the event through fantasy play. In addition, many of the children felt mortified and shamed by the event.

Family problems began to develop during this later period as well (e.g., deaths of children or parents, alcoholism, divorce), and symptom severity was found to be significantly correlated with the degree of family problems. Children from multiproblem families, isolated families, or families with recent problems tended to show the severest clinical manifestations. Also, children who had previous physical or emotional problems demonstrated a more intense type of posttraumatic stress.

Handford and colleagues (1986) also studied children subjected to a stressful environmental event, the Three Mile Island nuclear accident. There were 92 families in the sample, with a total of 164 children who lived within a 30–mile radius of the reactor. These were narrowed to 35 households with one child each (mean age 13.2 years).

While the accident resulted in no physical damage to individuals, children and parents felt that they had to cope with the possibility that long-term radiation exposure might seriously curtail their lives and activities. The parents showed increased levels of anxiety, hostility, and paranoid ideation following the incident—responses that receded after $1\frac{1}{2}$ years. The children, however, showed repercussions of anxiety that persisted and even increased over time. Additionally, the children reported stronger and more symptomatic responses than the parents. Their reactions to the accident were affected by the consistency of the mood and reactions of their parents. This study was similar to Terr's studies of the Chowchilla incident because both showed that trauma can exert persistent effects on the perceptions of children and that the responses of children to stressful events may be more pronounced than those of the adults in their families.

Because both the Chowchilla and Three Mile Island incidents involved the imposition of trauma on the children and their families independent of any actions on their part, these situations suggested conditions of learned helplessness. In other words, the children were subjected to seemingly random events in an uncontrollable and indifferent universe. Just as children experiencing learned helplessness manifest cognitive and affective deficits, so did these childhood victims of posttraumatic stress show disturbances in perceptual and cognitive capacities.

A study of 1,000 preschoolers in child development clinics by Kashani and Carlson (1987) might reveal a mechanism whereby such stresses are transduced into somatic complaints. Of the 1,000 children studied, only 9 were found to meet DSM-III criteria for depression. However, all 9 demonstrated somatic complaints. Thus, it might be that severe stress produces somatic symptomatology mediated by powerful dysphoric mood states such as depression or anxiety. Of course this hypothesis needs substantiation.

More generally, misperceptions and cognitive distortions can cause the child to lose sleep or develop eating disorders, which heightens vulnerability not only to organic disease but also to accidental injury. Also, the child may become oblivious to his or her own symptomatology and therefore fail to comply with medication or other therapy. Parents may exacerbate this situation by underestimating the impact of stress once their child has been diagnosed as not having any physical reason for the symptomatology.

In such a case the clinician's task is manifold. Initially, the child should be examined directly for signs of injury or organic disorder directly attributable to a stressful event. The possibility and operational mechanism of posttraumatic syndrome should also be assessed. Parents should be interviewed to discern their level of coping with their child's stress. Thorough analysis of the child's trauma followed, if possible, by catharsis of the trauma is the most effective means of forestalling or softening the aftermath of stress.

Sociocultural Sequelae

Somatoform illness represents a significant health problem, in terms of both its incidence of occurrence and its nonspecific, difficult-to-diagnose symptomatology. Ford (1983) estimated that (excluding psychiatric treatment) the cost of all medical care in the United States to persons with no organic illness is $20 billion, 10% of gross health expenditures. It is difficult to tell what proportion of this figure is apportioned to children with psychosomatic illness. However, Werry (1986) has estimated the incidence of somatoform disorders in children to be about 5%.

Data are also lacking as to the prevalence of specific disorders in children and what predisposing factors there might be to these various disorders. Nevertheless, in Ford's (1983) comprehensive review of somatoform disorders in children, a common history of disturbed childhood was found. This history resolved into two types. The first is characterized by inconsistency stemming from a chaotic, overstimulating environment. Children from this background typically develop Briquet's syndrome, factitious disorder, or Manchausen syndrome.

The second type of factor predisposing children to the somatoform process is characterized by stability without warmth. Parents of these children are frequently described as hypochondriacal themselves, and one is often more dominant than the other. Children from these homes typically develop hypochondria and nonspecific pain complaints. While these classifications may be of some diagnostic and heuristic utility, it is clear that further refinement of the pathogenesis of somatoform disorders is needed.

CONCLUSION

The mechanisms underlying the transduction of stress to somatic complaints with ill-defined organic origins are still largely unknown. However, there seems little doubt that such transductions do take place in individuals with poor coping abilities or in those, such as the children involved in the Chowchilla incident, whose coping mechanisms are overwhelmed.

In testing for the possible involvement of stress in a given somatic complaint it is useful to apply Coddington's technique of taking into account the continual expansion of the child's social and overall environmental sphere. For example, if a child is being subjected to a stressful family life (e.g., divorce) at the time of a developmental milestone such as entering school or beginning puberty, his or her coping mechanisms may be at least temporarily overcome and psychosomatic complaints may be the result. The particular somatoform disorder to evolve may be inferred from variables such as temperament, past experience, family dynamics, and genetic predisposition to certain kinds of malaise such as respiratory difficulties.

CHAPTER TWENTY

Gender Identity Disorders and Their Differential Diagnosis

Bradley: Losing More Than a Father

Bradley is a 5-year-old boy who lives with his mother and his older brother. Bradley's father was a traveling actor who spent time at home only sporadically and for short stays; he died 4 months prior to initiation of Bradley's treatment. Bradley's mother stated that developmental milestones were without abnormality. Toilet training included bowel continence at age 3 with urinary continence achieved at $3\frac{1}{2}$ years. Bradley's mother returned to work full time 8 weeks after his birth, and Bradley was taken care of by a nurse. Bradley was cared for by a different woman from age 18 months to 2 years, when the family moved to a different geographic area. At age 3, Bradley entered nursery school without separation difficulty. When he was 4, his family moved back to the East and he entered a day-care center.

Bradley's mother indicated that the father's death affected the family significantly in many ways. For his part, Bradley has indicated that he "puts those feelings [about his father's death] in a file cabinet in my head." Thus, it is difficult to assess how Bradley has been affected by the loss of his father, who was rarely present before his death. Bradley's mother sought evaluation of Bradley because he sometimes wears her clothes; he started doing so at age 2. In nursery school, Bradley always opts for stereotypically female roles in play; for example, he chooses to be the bride. At age 5, Bradley asked his mother "if it was possible to have an operation that could change a boy into a girl." Bradley has told his mother that he "wishes he were a girl." All of Bradley's friends are girls, with the exception of one older male friend whom he sees only once or twice a month. Bradley and his older brother fight frequently, and his brother teases Bradley, saying that he is "effeminate."

During assessment, Bradley was dressed in appropriate male clothing and evidenced no motor or speech abnormalities except that his speech was particularly clearly pronounced for a boy his age. He uses his hands a great deal when he speaks, and his manner is, to a degree, affected. He seems happy, and the content and form of thought revealed during assessment were not indicative of any psychoses. Intelligence tests and observation showed that he is unusually bright, with an IQ in the superior range. Bradley spoke of bad dreams he has in which robbers break into his house; these dreams interfere significantly with his sleep. Other elements of the mental status examination were within normal ranges. Interestingly, Bradley did not mention concern over his gender identity, even though he has told his mother of such troubling thoughts. He spoke about his hobbies, which include designing clothes for his dolls and doing needlework.

Bradley's comments during the assessment interview and his mother's description point toward a diagnosis of gender identity disorder of childhood without related dysphoria or serious interpersonal deficits. His preference for stereotypically female activities, his cross-dressing behavior, his assumption of female roles in play, the predominance of friendships with girls, and poor relationships with same-sex peers (his brother) are all factors of Bradley's persona that may be present in a diagnosed case of gender identity disorder of childhood. The teasing often suffered by children with this disorder usually becomes evident and problematic, possibly leading to depression and anxiety, about the age of 8, so Bradley has not yet been subjected to ridicule by others—except his brother, with whom Bradley also fights about typical sibling issues.

Bradley's behavior would not be classified as merely not fitting cultural gender stereotypes because female activities are dominant and he has expressed a desire to be a girl. Physical examination revealed no abnormalities, so an associated abnormality of the genitals was not labeled. Recommendation was made for individual exploratory therapy three times a week with a male therapist. Therapy and counseling were also recommended for Bradley's mother.

INTRODUCTION

Among the many life forms in existence, confusion about gender identity occurs in the human species alone. Sexuality may be the most fundamental defining characteristic across all species, but along with the faculties of consciousness and reason comes the potential for error, even in the most basic matters of nature. However, for Bradley and for other male children whose association with their fathers is vestigial, the term *error* may not be appropriate. To make an error there must first be a choice, and establishing a sexual identity in the absence of a same-sex parent hardly provides a choice.

Green (1980) defined psychosexual development as the ontogeny of sexual identity. As such, it consists of three components. The first is the awareness that one belongs to one of two categories of human beings, male or female. Beyond this first fundamental perception is a second component of psychosexual development, gender role of masculine and feminine behaviors. The third facet is comprised of the direction of erotic and romantic interests, the preference of one sex over the other for sexual partnering. The evolution of these three psychosexual components is governed in turn by three other factors: genetic contributions, parental and societal shaping of boy-like and girl-like behaviors, and the child's spontaneous learning of appropriate sex behaviors by means of imitation (Maccoby & Jacklin, 1974).

While gender cross-identification does occur in children, the momentum of evolution with regard to sexual reproduction is so great that it occurs only rarely. There is clear evidence that gender typing is an inherent facet of the make-up of every individual. Many differences have been observed between male and female newborns. For example, females have a stronger adverse reaction to stimulation with a jet of air and exhibit greater distress when a blanket is abruptly removed (Bell & Costello, 1964).

These and other differential responses of males and females are likely due to prenatal hormonal influences. As an example, male rats castrated shortly after birth show significantly more feminine behavior than those castrated at a later time, and testosterone administered to newborn female rats largely eradicates female responses and produces predominantly male behaviors such as aggression (Harris & Levine, 1962). Of course, it still is not possible to say how much correlation there is between findings in animals and humans. However, there is a good deal of correlation between the biological substrates of man and other mammals, and there have been reports indicating that contributions from sex hormones are far from insignificant to development of sexual identity in human beings.

For example, Green (1980) cited the early work of Money, Hampson, & Hampson, 1955) with girls in whom hyperadrenalism had caused masculinization of the external genitalia. If these girls were properly diagnosed and reared as females they became heterosexual, although they did exhibit "tomboyishness." According to Green, citing results in monkeys, this argues in favor of comparable prenatal hormonal effects in man and animals. For example, it is known that female monkeys who are exposed to a male hormone before birth are significantly more masculine in behavior than controls. However, exposure to the same hormone after birth fails to affect behavior, although it does masculinize the body.

Of course there are contributions to gender identity from sources other than hormones. Rekers (1979) delineated these contributors as "chromosomal status, fetal gonadal and hormonal development, maternal hormones, brain dimorphism, and genital dimorphism" (p. 373).

While the composite of all these factors is of considerable importance and conceivably could predispose certain individuals to gender confusion, the early experience of the individual is no less crucial. The biological imperative of sexual identity alone is not sufficient to shape the sexual identity of the child. In fact, variables relating to social learning traditionally have been regarded as the prime contributors to disturbances in gender identity (Meyer-Bahlburg, 1977).

In the absence of social and biological pathology, children simply learn the physical and social discriminative factors separating the sexes and come to understand their own sexuality. However, this simple-sounding process is largely dependent on the normative development of cognition. Kohlberg (1966) has approached sex typing as a cognitive process, taking the position that gender identity is primarily a mental image formed by the child and is limited by the child's ability to conceptualize and understand the physical world. Children in Piaget's preoperative stage of thinking (roughly ages 2 to 6) are unable to conceive of gender as a permanent, unchangeable attribute and therefore believe that gender can be changed.

The mechanism of gender identity formation is thus centered around the emotional and social factors that contribute to the child's ability and willingness to perceive and accept his or her own gender. First and foremost among these are the developmental changes between child and parents, that is, separation-individuation.

A smooth evolution of the awareness of separateness will allow for optimal role modeling. Troubled separations are more likely to produce problems. The character of the male or female parent also plays a pivotal part in sex role adoption, as does the nature of the relationship between the parents. Last, but by no means least, the biological sex of the child strongly affects acquisition of gender identity. Males have significantly more difficulty in establishing and maintaining their sexual status and autonomy, as evidenced by the fact that gender identity disorders occur far more frequently in males than females. However, it may be that identity disorders are noticed less frequently in girls because "tomboyishness" is considered an acceptable trait.

Therefore, prior to discussing factors relating to the differential diagnosis of the various gender identity disorders presented in DSM-III-R, it seems advisable to briefly discuss the influences underlying gender identity formation for boys and girls. Knowledge of the origins and mechanisms underlying the acquisition of gender awareness will help in properly distinguishing between the various possible deviations in sexual orientation.

DIFFERENTIAL DIAGNOSIS OF GENDER IDENTITY DISORDERS

In describing the various gender identity disorders, the DSM-III-R stipulates that gender identity is the private experience of gender role, while gender role is the public expression of gender identity. Gender identity disturbances can be mild, as in the case of an individual who experiences some but not extensive discomfort and a sense of inappropriateness in being male or female. When the disturbance is severe, the person has the strong sense that he or she actually belongs to the opposite sex. In most cases the onset of gender identity disorders can be traced back to childhood.

Gender Identity Disorder of Childhood

Both males and females with this relatively rare disorder experience persistent and intense distress about their assigned gender far beyond nonconformity to stereotypic sex role behavior. Individuals with this disorder either have a strong desire to be of the opposite sex or actively insist that in fact they *are* of the opposite sex. Girls in particular tend to show few if any signs of psychopathology. However, some girls and especially boys may show serious signs of disturbance (e.g., social withdrawal, separation anxiety, depression). Most cases of this disorder begin to develop before the age of 4 (in the midst of the separation-individuation struggle). While the ratio is unknown, many more males than females develop this condition, conceivably because of the difficulties inherent for boys in disidentifiying with the mother, as discussed by Greenson (1968).

DSM-III-R diagnostic criteria for gender identity disorder of childhood are as follows:

For Females:

A. *Persistent and intense distress about being a girl, and a stated desire to be a boy (not merely a desire for any perceived cultural advantages from being a boy), or insistence that she is a boy.*

B. *Either (1) or (2):*

    (1) *persistent marked aversion to normative feminine clothing and insistence on wearing stereotypical masculine clothing, e.g., boys' underwear and other accessories*

    (2) *persistent repudiation of female anatomic structures, as evidenced by at least one of the following:*

        (a) *an assertion that she has, or will grow, a penis*

        (b) *rejection of urinating in a sitting position*

        (c) *assertion that she does not want to grow breasts or menstruate*

C. *The girl has not yet reached puberty.*

For Males:

A. *Persistent and intense distress about being a boy and an intense desire to be a girl, or more rarely, insistence that he is a girl.*

B. *Either (1) or (2):*

    (1) *preoccupation with female stereotypical activities, as shown by a preference for either cross-dressing or simulating female attire, or by an intense desire to participate in the games and pastimes of girls and rejection of male stereotypical toys, games, and activities.*

    (2) *persistent repudiation of male anatomic structures, as indicated by at least one of the following repeated assertions:*

        (a) *that he will grow up to become a woman (not merely in role)*

        (b) *that his penis or testes are disgusting or will disappear*

        (c) *that it would be better not to have a penis or testes*

C. *The boy has not yet reached puberty.* (pp. 73–74)

In reaching a differential diagnosis of this disorder, close attention should be paid to family structure (e.g., one or two parents) and parental interactions in order to detect seductive practices such as age-inappropriate sleeping with the mother or father, lax bathroom behavior among family members, and the like.

Children whose behavior simply does not fit the cultural norms of masculinity or femininity should not be given this diagnosis in the absence of the full syndrome. Physical abnormalities of the sex organs are usually not associated with this disorder, but when present they should be noted on Axis III.

Transsexualism

This disorder is chiefly identifiable by the presence of persistent discomfort and a sense of inappropriateness about one's assigned gender in an individual who has reached puberty. The diagnosis is not made if the disturbance is limited to brief periods of stress. There is always the wish to live as a member of the opposite sex. The estimated prevalence of this disorder is considered to be 1 per 30,000 for males and 1 per 100,000 for females.

Generally uncomfortable wearing the clothes of their assigned sex, these individuals dress in clothes of the other sex and frequently engage in activities culturally associated with the other sex. They often find their genitals repugnant, leading them to request sex reassignment by hormonal and surgical means.

Their behavior, dress, and mannerisms become those of the other sex to one degree or another. Along with this disorder there is usually a coexisting moderate or severe personality disturbance, and anxiety and depression are frequently experienced. While cases of spontaneous remission have been noted, this condition is usually chronic.

DSM-III-R diagnostic criteria for transsexualism are as follows:

A. *Persistent discomfort and sense of inappropriateness about one's assigned sex.*

B. *Persistent preoccupation for at least two years with getting rid of one's primary and secondary sex characteristics and acquiring the sex characteristics of the other sex.*

C. *The person has reached puberty.* (p. 76)

Differential diagnosis of this condition requires the perception that it possibly had its roots in gender disorder of childhood and continued into puberty. Extensive femininity in a boy or masculinity in a girl during childhood increases the likelihood of transsexualism. Some individuals may experience the desire to belong to the other sex and be rid of their own genitals in times of stress. In such cases, since the wish has not been present consistently for 2 years, the diagnosis of gender identity disorder not otherwise specified should be considered.

Delusions of belonging to the other sex may be present in schizophrenia, but this potentially confounding factor is rare. Cross dressing may also exist in both transvestic fetishism and gender identity disorder of adolescence or adulthood, nontranssexual type. However, unless these disorders evolve into transsexualism, the wish to be rid of one's genitals is absent.

Gender Identity Disorder of Adolescence or Adulthood, Nontranssexual Type (GIDAANT)

As with the other conditions discussed, this disorder is characterized by a persistent discomfort and sense of inappropriateness about one's assigned sex. However, the persistent cross dressing may be in fantasy or reality, and GIDAANT differs from transvestic fetishism in that the cross dressing is not for the purpose of sexual excitement. It is different from transsexualism in that there is no persistent preoccupation for at least 2 years with transforming the primary and secondary sex characteristics into those of the other sex. Anxiety and depression commonly coexist with GIDAANT but may be relieved by cross dressing. In most cases, the clinical picture of gender identity disorder of childhood was present prior to puberty. It is believed that GIDAANT is more common than transsexualism, but the ratio is unknown.

The DSM-III-R diagnostic criteria for GIDAANT are as follows:

A. *Persistent or recurrent discomfort and sense of inappropriateness about one's assigned sex.*

B. *Persistent or recurrent cross-dressing in the role of the other sex, either in fantasy or actuality, but not for the purpose of sexual excitement (as in Transvestic Fetishism).*

C. *No persistent preoccupation (for at least two years) with getting rid of one's primary and secondary sex characteristics and acquiring the sex characteristics of the other sex (as in Transsexualism).*

D. *The person has reached puberty.* (p. 77)

The differential diagnosis of GIDAANT from transvestic fetishism and transsexualism has been discussed. In rare instances, a person with GIDAANT may develop transsexualism, in which case the diagnosis of GIDAANT is changed accordingly.

Both transsexualism and GIDAANT are subdivided according to the history of sexual orientation (i.e., asexual, homosexual, or heterosexual). These conditions, regardless of the particular sexual orientation, appear to be outgrowths of an initial childhood difficulty in achieving gender identity due primarily to problems in separation-individuation for which the parents bear the major responsibility (although elements of temperament should not be ignored). However, not all children who experience gender identification difficulties grow to be transsexuals or have GIDAANT. More prospective research is needed to discover the differences between children who do and do not develop adult gender disorders after being exposed to detrimental conditions of separation-individuation.

INDICATORS OF CROSS-GENDER IDENTIFICATION IN CHILDREN

Males

Experiments in cross-gender behavior, effeminacy in boys and tomboy-ishness in girls, is not unusual in childhood, being generally regarded as a passing phase (Bakwin, 1968). However, persistent disturbances in gender identity in boys is revealed in such behavior as cross dressing, feminine mannerisms and speech content, artificially high voice, use of women's cosmetics, avoidance of masculine-type activities, preference for female playmates, and assumption of the female role in play (Green, Fuller, & Rutley, 1972). However, the ratio of masculine to feminine play and any compulsive element in cross-sex play are more important determinants than isolated cases of cross-sex-role behavior (Rekers, 1981).

There is evidence suggesting that normal boys exhibit predominantly masculine preferences in toys and activities by the age of 3 or 4 (Rekers, Amaro-Plotkin, & Low, 1977; Rekers & Yates, 1976). Deviant activities occur at least this early and perhaps earlier (Bakwin, 1968).

Females

There is far less literature delineating specific masculine behaviors in young girls that are predictive of later gender pathology than there is for males. This is likely due to the fact that gender deviance is noted more frequently in males. While it is likely that the incidence of sexual disorders is in fact greater in males than females (see next section), Green (1980) pointed out that there are a number of factors that tend to focus attention preferentially on males. Males remain as the most valued sex in our society, and by extrapolation, masculine behavior is the most favored. Therefore, masculine behavior is more frequently rewarded within the hierarchy of the child subculture—a preference that extends to some degree to the behavior of girls. However, feminine behavior in boys is highly proscribed and immediately noticed. Since cross-gender behavior in young girls results in little intra- or interpersonal conflict, these children are seen in the clinic much more rarely.

The relatively intense focus on male behaviors by the populace at large places an extra tension on boys in terms of the appropriateness of their behavior—a tension that contributes in part to the probability that the male role in childhood is more rigid than the female role. Archer (1984) demonstrated this greater rigidity, as well as pointing to other differential factors in development between the sexes, by using a unique array of four related dimensions: rigidity, complexity, consistency, and continuity.

By *rigidity*, or *flexibility*, is meant the extent to which opposite-gender activities are avoided. Archer cited numerous studies such as those by Greif (1979); Lever (1976); Hargreaves, Stoll, Farnworth, and Morgan (1981); and Gold and Berger (1978) to demonstrate that males have less opportunity than girls for experimentation in terms of sexual identity along three dimensions: (1) the actions in which children engage; (2) children's perceptions of gender-appropriate activities; and (3) adults' reactions to gender-appropriate and cross-gender behavior.

In terms of *complexity* or *simplicity*, descriptive of the elaborateness of the content of the gender role, boys have a tendency to construct relatively simplified, incomplete images of their role due to the influence of incomplete role models, models in the media and elsewhere that tend to overstress such factors as physical strength and athletic skills.

Consistency refers to the extent to which there are conflicting requirements for the male or female role. Here, too, males may be subject to a higher level of confusion. Males receive conflicting information about traits that are expected of them. As men they are expected to be aggressive and strong; as boys they must be well-behaved and study hard. In addition, toughness in childhood and adolescence must give way to occupational status in adulthood.

Finally, with regard to *continuity* and *discontinuity* of the sexual role, Archer cited the discussion by Katz (1979) in which the disparity between childhood and adolescent gender roles is greater for females than for males. Katz argued that with the onset of adolescence, the girl begins to follow a more rigid set of rules than previously, rules oriented toward restricting their sexual accessibility. Boys, on the other hand, tend to exhibit a widening interest and begin to explore the more varied possibilities of the adult male role. It is almost as though, in this final stage, the rigidity and confusion of the male role is "fixed" by the reinforcement inherent in the reward of expanded possibilities. That is, there is little incentive, after adolescence begins, for the male to reexamine his gender assumptions.

While Archer's argument points to the relatively greater incidence of gender confusion in males, deviant behavior does occur at an early age in females. Like effeminate males, masculine girls strongly resist wearing female clothing, preferring boys' clothes and haircuts. Feminine activities such as housework are often resented, and they do not like to play with dolls, choosing instead the paraphernalia of boy's games. Like effeminate males, masculine females prefer the company of the opposite sex (Bakwin, 1968).

When weighing the importance of specific male-like activities in girls, Tauber (1979) pointed out that it is important to realize that girls are consistently more likely to play with male-associated toys than are boys to play with feminine-type toys. Thus, the play of girls encompasses a larger repertoire of behaviors than that of boys.

Stability of Childhood Indicators of Sex-Role Deviance

The majority of studies relating to the reliability of childhood indicators in predicting later homosexual or transsexual behavior have been retrospective. There are several possible sources of error associated with this research technique, the first of which is distorted memory. Rekers, Mead, Rosen, and Brigham (1983) pointed out that an adult who remembers his father as weak and effeminate may be citing his current impressions about his father during childhood rather than the actual traits present at the time.

It is also difficult, if not impossible, to assess from retrospective data the proportion of children who experienced the same conditions of childhood and yet did not manifest gender confusion as adults. Furthermore, the majority of early studies focused on homosexuals who were psychologically distressed, leading to possible confounding with other psychiatric conditions. More recent retrospective research efforts have introduced a possible sampling bias in that many of these studies used samples from homosexual organizations and communities, members of whom may be untypically vocal and less socially isolated than the norm.

Despite these limitations, results of retrospective studies are largely concordant. The results of a study by Whitam (1977) are typical. Questionnaires were administered to 206 male homosexuals and 78 male heterosexuals. The questionnaire dealt with what were considered to be six primary childhood indicators of later adult homosexuality. These included interest in dolls, cross dressing, preference of company of girls rather than boys in childhood games, preference for company of older women rather than older men, being regarded as a sissy by other boys, and sexual interest in other boys rather than girls in sex play.

The strongest indicators of later homosexuality were playing with cross-sexed toys, cross dressing, preference for female activities, and being regarded by other boys as a sissy. Preferring the company of older women appeared to be the weakest predictor of later sexual deviance. This study is suggestive of the results obtained in many others (e.g., Green, 1974) indicating that the majority of effeminate boys are very likely to have an atypical sexual identity as adults.

While the results of retrospective studies such as the one by Whitam are of some clinical value, prospective studies produce far more powerful findings. Fortunately, longitudinal studies are now being done with greater frequency. Green (1980) evaluated two groups of males (subjects and controls) in terms of indicators of gender identity, first in boyhood and later in adulthood.

One group ($n = 66$) came from families who were clinically or self-referred and contained boys with considerable cross-gender behavior. The other group ($n = 56$) was composed of demographically matched, paid volunteers. On initial evaluation, the age range of the boys was $3\frac{1}{2}$ to 11 years (average age, $7\frac{1}{2}$ years). Reevaluation for sexual orientation at least into early adolescence was performed on two thirds of each group. Of the 44 individuals who previously had shown extensive cross-gender behavior, 30 were found to be homosexually or bisexually oriented. This contrasted greatly with members of the control group, of whom none showed evidence of gender deviance.

These results agree with those of many retrospective studies, furthering the belief that boyhood nonerotic behaviors are closely correlated with erotic behaviors in adulthood. Green further emphasized the strength of this relationship by citing another study by Whitam (1980) in which homosexuals in three different cultures (Brazil, Guatemala, and the United States) more often recalled a preference for playing with girls' toys, engaging in girls' games, and cross dressing, as well as being regarded by other males as a sissy.

SEPARATION-INDIVIDUATION AND THE DEVELOPMENT OF GENDER IDENTITY

Gender Acquisition as a Learned Process

Genetic factors alone do not account for the very strong stability between early gender deviance and later sexual orientation. Diamond (1965) pointed to the fact that while there is ample evidence to support the contention of behaviorally fixed sexuality in animals from birth, this is definitely not the case in man.

Among the vertebrates, man is alone in this flexibility: *While gender is not modifiable by experience, gender role certainly is.* That is, regardless of whether or not an individual's sexual identity is consonant with his or her true sex, the individual rarely has difficulty perceiving which behaviors are appropriate for each gender. This is most graphically illustrated by the findings of Money and co-workers (1955), who worked with individuals who had anomalous external sex organs. The most reliable prognosticator of later gender identification and role in these hermaphrodites was their sex assignment and rearing. Chromosomal sex, gonadal sex, hormonal sex, accessory internal reproductive morphology, and ambiguous morphology of the external sex organs were far less potent predictors of sex role outcome.

The results of a study by Rekers, Crandall, Rosen, and Bentler (1979) also demonstrated the validity of looking to social learning variables as the prime contributors to sexual identity disturbances. In this study, 12 boys from 4 years, 10 months to 13 years, 6 months of age were independently diagnosed as having gender disturbances by three different clinical psychologists. These subjects then received a medical evaluation including history, physical examination, chromosome analysis, and sex chromatin studies. All the boys were found to be genetically and physically normal, with the exception of one who had an undescended testicle.

Differential Effects of Parental Influence on Boys and Girls

Before attempting to describe some of the social dynamics that can give rise to gender confusion, it is advisable to keep in mind the dynamics of optimal sexual maturation. Kohlberg (1966) stated the situation most succinctly. Gender identity is achieved when the child can label self and others, while gender role depicts the actual sexual behavior. Ideally, the two are congruent. When they are not, a gender disorder exists.

As children grow, they not only need to identify with their parents but must separate from them as well. Litin, Giffen, and Johnson (1956) suggested that dissonance along the identity role axis can be traced to adaptations of the ego while separating in the presence of abnormal parental influences.

Litin and co-workers have identified the following four familial factors contributing to gender confusion in children:

1) The child has suffered during its development the confusion and dissatisfaction that result from its parents' poorly integrated marriage. 2) One parent has been consciously or unconsciously seducing the child; usually the other parent has unwittingly colluded with the seduction (seduction is the process whereby the parent consciously or unconsciously imposes upon the young child an adult form of ambivalent sexuality which is totally inappropriate to the child's age). 3) The seduction may or may not be followed by genital frustration. 4) Concomitantly, the parent subtly defines a pattern of unusual sexual behavior. This behavior may be genital, or it may be pregenital and perverse. The child regards it as partially condoned and acceptable and therefore carries out the act. It may feel very little guilt and shame. (1956, p. 39)

Clearly, for both boys and girls, a wholesome and encouraging family atmosphere is the best environment in which to evolve a sense of sexual identity. However, in the presence of one or more of the family circumstances listed by Litin and colleagues, girls appear to emerge unscathed more frequently than boys, since more boys than girls suffer gender identity problems.

Greenson (1968) astutely pointed out that this may be attributable to an extra dimension of separation-individuation that the male must achieve but the female is spared. He called attention to the fact that, in terms of psychoanalytic theory, the female child must work through two conflictual areas on the way to achieving sexual identity. She must shift her primary erogenous focus from her clitoris to her vagina, and she must disengage from her mother as the primary love object and turn to her father and to other men.

While male children may be spared these steps, the female child is spared the vicissitudes of "disidentifying" with a parent of the opposite sex. That is, the girl's identification with her mother is not a hindrance to establishing her femininity, while to the boy it *is* a hindrance. The boy, too, strongly identifies with his mother but must break away and search elsewhere for a role model. He must develop a new identification with his father. This is problematic and difficult because it entails renouncing the pleasure and security of the primal association with the mother and trying to reestablish those feelings with the usually less emotionally accessible father.

Greenson pointed out that there are two primary contributors to the outcome of the boy's attempts at reintegrating his identity with his father. First, it is important for the mother to allow and even encourage her son in this endeavor. A second important determining factor is the motives offered by the father to his son for identifying with him. If the mother refuses to relinquish her bond with her son and if the father is a relatively passive, joyless person, the boy will have little chance and less reason to break away in favor of the father.

Because the boy, compared to the girl, is faced with this relatively greater leap in terms of gender identity, Greenson has postulated that "men are far more uncertain about their maleness than women are about their femaleness . . . women's certainty about their gender identity and men's insecurity about theirs are rooted in early identification with the mother" (p. 370). This observation seems borne out by the behavior of fathers with their children in a study by Jacklin, DiPietro, and Maccoby (1984) on sex-typing pressure in child/parent interactions. Fathers in this study tended to exaggerate the sex-typed nature of play with both sons and daughters, perhaps revealing a basic uncertainty in themselves with regard to this issue. Of course it is also possible that the exaggeration of sex-typed playing was due to the father's greater involvement in cognitive versus emotional concerns.

Greenson's argument blends nicely with the facts that gender disorders are far more frequent in males than females and that boys with gender difficulties frequently come from homes where the father is either absent or psychologically distant from other family members (Bakwin, 1968; Litin et al., 1956; Rekers et al., 1983). This argument also meshes with that of Socarides (1980), who further endorsed the importance of separation-individuation in the genesis of homosexuality. Noting that the entire process of acquiring a differentiated sexual identity depends on the child's ability to identify with the parent of the same sex, if difficulty in achieving this identity arises in the rapprochement subphase of separation-individuation, homosexuality is the likely result. As Socarides stated, "Homosexuality serves to repress a pivotal nuclear conflict: the urge to regress to a preoedipal fixation in which there was a desire to reinstate the primitive mother-child unity" (p. 334). In the upcoming discussion of differential diagnosis of specific childhood gender identity disorders, it will be beneficial to keep in mind the etiologies postulated by Greenson and Socarides as well as the familial factors previously cited by Litin and co-workers. Additionally, referral to Table 2–1 on page 32 will assist in keeping in mind the various conditions that may confound diagnosis of gender disorders.

CONCLUSION

The fact that some children outgrow their gender handicap lends hope to efforts directed toward treatment and prevention. Litin and co-workers (1956) have urged an approach of collaborative therapy in which the child and parent or parents are counseled simultaneously. In this way it is possible to answer such questions as why one particular child of all those in the family was chosen to be the recipient of parental sanction or seduction; why a specific kind of sexual behavior may have been permitted; and how the parent's need for this kind of unconscious gratification is communicated to the child.

Rekers (1981) also has advocated interviewing the parents both separately and together for the purposes mentioned above as well as to discover the child's role identifications, level of understanding of all aspects of sexuality, and history of any behaviors such as cross dressing that may reach pathologic proportions. Interviews with parents and children are also important therapeutically, since most children with sexual disorders cannot be identified on the basis of physical abnormalities.

Another important point has been highlighted by Fagot and Leinbach (1985), who pointed out that most of the research on sex role acquisition has been performed on children who were 3 years of age or older, possibly reflecting Freud's emphasis on this period as crucial in psychosexual identification. Since Fagot and Leinbach (1985) found that boys and girls react differently to the responses they elicit from other people by 25 months of age, it seems advisable to recommend that research into sex role development be expanded to include earlier age groups.

As research progresses it is beneficial to realize, as Green (1985) has pointed out, that a balance now currently exists in sexual research between the old school, which emphasized the importance of biological contributions to psychosexual development, and the newer school of social learning, which emphasizes the importance of the events occurring in the first 5 years of life. This balance is a favorable position from which to perform further studies.

CHAPTER TWENTY-ONE

Childhood Suicide and Suicide-Like Behavior and Their Differential Diagnosis

Alex: A Pervasive Wish to Jump Out of a Window

Alex is a 4-year-old boy who lives with his mother. His parents are separated, and his father visits sporadically, without prior notice. Before his parents separated, Alex witnessed many fights between them, which often involved his father's physically and emotionally abusing his mother. Alex's father once set fire to a family photo album and left ashes scattered in the living room. Alex's mother reports that Alex became fascinated with fire around the time that his father left the household. He acted out this attraction to fire by trying to set his clothing, his toys, and a mattress afire. She commented that when Alex was involved in fire setting or watching, he seemed hypnotized. Following incidents in which she intervened in Alex's fire setting, his mother would calm him down either by lying with him in her bed and stroking his hair or by exercising with him in her bedroom.

Alex was referred for psychiatric evaluation after a nursery school teacher reported that Alex was prone to profane verbal outbursts with patricidal wishes and that he failed to socialize well with the other children. During the course of therapy, Alex revealed destructive fantasies in addition to fire setting; he burned himself and announced a desire to jump from the office window. During these episodes he was unresponsive to the therapist; he continued to announce his intention to jump out of the window while running toward the window and smashing against it. This and the patient's talk of stabbing himself in the abdomen indicated to the therapist the presence of suicidal tendencies.

There are several approaches for evaluating these suicidal behaviors. First, the therapist must take into account that, for a young child, the notion of the finality of suicide is not understood; thus, the child's self-destructive behaviors are not actually understood by the child as permanent. Reasons for suicidal behavior in Alex's case could originate from various sources. A classic explanation would likely assert that Alex's wish to destroy himself was based in the fear that his father would discover his overly enmeshed relationship with his mother. Also, by harming himself, Alex could force his parents to reunite, which could restore the possibility of a male role model who would mediate Alex's libidinous energies that were directed toward his mother. Another explanation of Alex's suicidal behavior stems from the idea that people who are repeatedly subject to circumstances that are out of their control will attribute to themselves helplessness and inability to control their environments. Self-destruction, in this case, would provide a means for Alex to act out in a way that would ostensibly indicate his control over environmental factors. One more possibility is that a child suffering from low self-esteem might attempt to relieve himself of unendurable depression through a self-destructive escape.

Recognizing the various motivational possibilities, the therapist chose to move cognitively with the child, step by step, to help him achieve an understanding of the irreversibility of the outcomes of self-destructive behaviors. The therapist did this by questioning Alex about the consequences of acting out his fantasies in the real world. Gradually, Alex's cognitive abilities broadened, and he was able to understand the finality of damaging behaviors. The next step was to help Alex understand how he was feeling when he wanted to jump out the window and to model appropriate alternate behaviors. This was accomplished through play therapy, using a doll that Alex threw from the window when he had the urge to jump, and review of tapes of play interactions. Through watching tapes of the sessions, Alex learned to recognize the emotions connected to his self-destructive wishes. This, in conjunction with the transference relationship, facilitated his modeling of more adaptive behaviors. The transference relationship provided Alex with a means to reflect his sense of self and thus impart fuel for the development of his self-esteem.

INTRODUCTION

Despite the difficulties inherent in developing behaviors directed at self-preservation, very few young children, as in the case just cited, engage in suicidal behavior, and fewer still succeed in carrying the act to completion. As an example, according to one estimate, children between the ages of 10 and 14 comprised of 8.5% of the total population in 1978 but accounted for only 0.55% of all suicides for that year (Shaffer & Fisher, 1981). Nevertheless, suicidal behavior increases rapidly as age progresses, and it is relatively common among children and adolescents referred for psychiatric treatment (Schaffer, 1986). In general, it is estimated that suicidal behavior is the reason given for referral in at least 8 to 10% of children who are clinic patients (Mattsson, Seese, & Hawkins, 1969; Leese, 1969).

While these statistics are somewhat illuminating, they must be viewed with caution because the number of cases reported in children is subject to a number of limitations—all of which inhibit the reporting, study, and treatment of suicidal behavior (McGuire, 1983). Perhaps the single largest contributor to the obfuscation of childhood suicidal issues is the prevailing but incorrect notion that children cannot have conscious intentions to kill themselves. This simply is not the case, yet it is a fact that the United States Office of National Vital Statistics does not have a category of suicide for cause of death in children under age 10 years.

One of the reasons for the dearth of information regarding childhood suicidal behavior stems from the problem of definition. Many assume that children under age 10 are unable to understand the finality of death and therefore contend that completed suicide cannot be considered a cause of death in children under this age. However, it is the goal of achieving death that defines the act of suicide. As long as the child has some type of death concept, it is immaterial whether he or she believes death to be reversible or fails to recognize its universality or non-functionality.

Adopting this rational approach to the definition of suicide is helpful, but the problem of defining suicidal behavior in childhood remains. In order to gauge the suicidal child's concerns about death, one must first be aware of age-appropriate reactions to the dawning awareness of the existence and nature of death. Rosenthal and Rosenthal (1984) have documented the appearance of suicidal tendencies in children as young as $2\frac{1}{2}$ to 3 years.

Thus, as Pfeffer (1985) and Shaffer (1986) pointed out, it appears that self-destructive behavior can be expressed at any level of development. Accordingly, the inclusion of primary developmental processes such as separation-individuation and the development of empathy is essential in attempting to understand childhood suicidal behavior. Of the many factors available for study that influence development, those of temperament, loss, family instability, parental psychopathology, and concurrent mood disorders appear to have the most relevance for the etiology of suicide.

Pfeffer (1985a,b; 1986b) grouped these factors into four mutually interactive categories: early developmental experiences, ego functioning, interpersonal relationships, and affects. Under normal circumstances, these are in dynamic equilibrium. However, when stress along one or more axes builds to intolerable levels, ego functioning is overwhelmed and the child enters the spectrum of suicidal behavior at one of any number of stages, which Pfeffer described as moving from suicidal ideas to suicidal threats, suicidal actions, and finally suicide.

Examining the mutually interactive components that contribute to suicidal behavior seems to be the most appropriate approach. Not only are definitional issues simplified and a plausible mechanism of suicidal behavior presented, but this factorial approach allows the clinician to assess the individual contributions of the different factors in a given child.

As an additional support for the contention that suicide results, ultimately, from an overwhelmed ego, Pfeffer provided a plausible end point of this mechanism: the nearly universally reported phenomenon of psychotic constriction. In adults, this constriction is manifested by the evaporation of awareness of possible pain, the feelings of others, and all other consequences of the act accompanied by a pure concentration on achieving the means to end life. Pfeffer plausibly suggested that in children this constriction of awareness can be seen in such acts as repetitive pill taking, swimming out as far as possible in order to drown, running out into traffic, and jumping from a high place.

The ensuing discussion focuses on the major internal and environmental factors contributing to the various degrees of ego dysfunction that lead to suicidal behavior. It is important to keep in mind throughout that ego disorganization drastic enough to result in psychotic constriction is rare in children under age 15, but that risk increases with age and a good portion of the children referred for psychiatric treatment do exhibit some form of suicidal ideation or behavior in response to what is perceived as an overload of stress (Shaffer, 1982, 1986; Carlson, Asarnow, & Orbach, 1987).

INTERNAL PREDICTORS OR RISK FACTORS FOR SUICIDAL BEHAVIOR

Sex

The preeminent factor in the occurrence of suicidal behavior is male sex. In the United States and most Western countries, the ratio of male to female completed suicides is three to one (Schneidman, 1976). The opposite ratio holds for the number of women and men who attempt, but do not complete, suicide; that is, three times more women perform uncompleted suicide attempts than men. Also, males tend to use more violent means of suicide than females (Rosenthal, 1981).

It may be tempting to say that regardless of whether the higher rate of suicide among males is attributable to social isolation, hormone-related differences in aggressive tendencies, or any number of other possible causes, the clinician should be particularly sensitive to suicide-related statements in young boys. However, caution should be exercised at this time in acting on a generalization.

There are arguments such as the one by Suter (1976) indicating that the socialization process of young girls and women, implicitly dictating a passive role, causes them to develop in a direction opposite to personal mastery. This gives rise to feelings of incompetence and rage that could merge under stress to produce suicidal behavior—behavior that succeeds less frequently in its intent than in males because women tend to have less difficulty in asking for help (consciously or unconsciously) than do males, who also may fear the shame of a failed attempt.

These and other arguments that highlight the differential significance of developmental and social issues demonstrate the need for more careful assessment in the compilation of statistics on suicide. In children, it may indeed be that young girls actually attempt suicide more often than young boys but succeed less often in completing it. If so, since any attempt at suicide is to be forestalled, it may be judicious for clinicians to pay close attention to suicidal ideations from children of either sex but to consider completed suicide in boys as more probable.

Temperament

There has been little research performed specifically on the relationship between temperament and suicidal behavior in children. However, some temperamental theorists such as Plomin (1982) have hypothesized that impulsivity is one of four stable, inheritable dimensions of temperament playing a significant and lasting role in social interactions. Masters (1972) theorized that the roots of impulse control may be traceable to very early contingency experiences. Masters postulated that children who are particularly impulsive experience numerous episodes of noncontingency that cumulatively produce a failure to learn behavioral restraint.

While Masters's theory undoubtedly has some merit, most investigators have treated impulsiveness as a function of emotional and cognitive development. The ability to control impulses is frequently viewed as being associated with other aspects of development that are believed to be impaired in suicidal children (e.g., self-object representation).

Rothbart and Derryberry (1981, 1982) postulated that self-regulation is a temperamental variable that develops in step with neuroanatomy and biochemistry in the first years of life. They maintained that self-regulation plays an important role in coordinating attention and response in the developing infant. Along these lines, Vaughn, Kopp, and Krakow (1984) observed the ability to inherit response to a desirable stimulus in children as young as 18 months. However, they also found that the majority of children could not sustain this ability over time or across tasks. The consistency of the control improved only upon maturation of the child. Among the very young, relatively minor levels of stress may evoke impulsive behavior. If, in addition, the child has failed to achieve the ego strengthening that derives from successful separation from the caregiver, the level of self-control may be so poor that even self-destructive urges cannot be restrained.

Unfortunately, past and current research has failed to provide evidence with which to evaluate this theory. While many researchers have found high levels of impulsiveness among suicidal children (Brent, 1987; Cohen-Sandler, Berman, & King, 1982; Williams, Sale, & Wignall, 1977), there has been a paucity of developmentally oriented research directed at determining the trigger role of impulsiveness in children who engage in suicidal behavior. Differences in definitions and methodologies also make cross-study comparisons unreliable.

For example, in one study of latency-age children who had attempted suicide, Pfeffer, Conte, Plutchnik, and Jerrett (1979) found high levels of impulsivity, but they found no differences in impulsive behavior levels between suicidal and nonsuicidal children in a later study (Pfeffer,

1986b). In a study by Rosenthal and Rosenthal (1984), preschoolers were found to have a high degree of impulsivity. In this study, half the pre-schoolers exhibited both impulsivity and hyperactivity. However, it was not possible to isolate neurological or temperamental contributions from other factors such as family stress.

Pfeffer (1986a) suggested that while temperament undoubtedly fac-tors into suicidal behavior, there may be a dynamic within the suicidal behavior of children that causes observers to give impulsivity an inap-propriately high value. According to Pfeffer, a suicidal episode occurs as a result of an unstable equilibrium between forces that promote self-preservation and those that do not. It is an abrupt shift in the balance that produces what may appear to be an impulsive suicidal act. This would explain, as well, why suicidal episodes in children are transient and difficult to predict.

Empathic Development

The development of empathy has important implications for suicidal behavior in the young—particularly in the very young. During the first year of life, the infant's empathic responses are global, and, if repeat-edly exposed to the distress of another, especially the mother, the infant runs the risk of incorporating this distress (i.e., depression) as though it were its own. Certainly, in later stages of development, this process could predispose the child to hopelessness and make him or her prone to suicidal ideation and behavior.

After the first year, normal empathic development works to shield children from environmental distress as well as to sensitize them to it. Young children's growing representational abilities allow them to dis-tinguish stress rising within themselves from that emanating from oth-ers. However, under conditions of extreme stress, an individual may regress back to the less differentiated empathic responses of infancy in which another's distress may be confused with one's own. In fact, this may constitute a dynamic of the suicide pact in adolescents.

Furthermore, when empathy is regressed or underdeveloped, another dynamic pertaining to suicidal behavior begins to evolve. It has been widely observed that prosocial behavior is highly correlated with the empathic response to emotional or physical harm suffered by another. That is, children learn to control their aggressive tendencies through their empathic understanding of the distress of others. If this control fails to evolve adequately due to a deficit in empathic development, a child will likely be shunned by his or her peers and will become iso-lated—a condition that, if extreme, is intolerable and may well predis-pose the alienated child to suicidal recourse.

EXTERNAL/ENVIRONMENTAL RISK FACTORS FOR SUICIDAL BEHAVIOR

Loss

While the largely internal factors of empathy, impulsivity, and temperament are significant for suicidal behavior in children, stresses generated by demands of the external environment can overpower the child's will to survive. Perhaps primary among such stresses is the experience of loss and bereavement.

Freud originally put forth the relationship of object loss to depression and suicide in "Mourning and Melancholia" (1915). In 1982, Bowlby alerted the psychological community to the relationship of early loss to adult psychiatric disorders, including that of suicide.

Extensive research since then has supported the notion of loss as a critical risk factor in suicide. The history of suicidal children often reveals a past that includes one or more losses (Adam, 1982; Birtchnell, 1972; Bunch, 1971; Hill, 1969; Tennant, Bebbington, & Hurry, 1980). As an example, Goldney (1981) found that parental loss or separation was much more common in the histories of children who had attempted suicide than in controls. In a study by Kosky (1983), half the children exhibiting suicidal behavior had been confronted with a significant loss through death. This compared to only a quarter of the nonsuicidal children in the study who had experienced such a loss. Interestingly, most of the losses experienced by the suicidal group had occurred in the 12 months prior to the suicide attempt.

Husain and Vandiver (1984) postulated that loss creates a greater risk for suicide than any other factor. While loss may occur as a result of death, prolonged hospitalization, parental separation or divorce, or abandonment are also experienced as loss equivalents. Husain and Vandiver noted that children typically respond to such loss as though it were desertion. This provokes guilt, aggression, and anger, all of which may combine to produce suicidal behavior.

As is true for the proper development of empathy leading to prosocial behavior, the development of the ability to cope with loss of a loved one requires a sufficiently stable and differentiated self-object representation. When a child loses a valued object, he or she feels not only the loss of the object but the loss of self that was resident in the object.

In pathological cases, the boundaries between self and object are blurred, so that the child might attempt suicide as a means of reuniting the self and the object. Alternatively, death may be seen as a means of punishing the lost object, since self-directed aggression appears to be synonymous with aggression against the frustrating behavior of the inadequately externalized lost object. By destroying the self, the child may believe he or she is destroying an intolerable external reality.

Family Instability

Vying with loss for primacy among the risk factors for childhood suicide is family instability. More recent research has suggested that greater emphasis should be placed on chronic family stress and instability as the most significant risk factor predisposing to childhood suicidal behavior. Any factor, whether it be marital instability and separation/divorce or death of a loved one, that causes persistently drastic disruption in contingencies may be at least equally responsible for generating suicidal behavior in children. As discussed previously, noncontingency produces negative affect in the very young, and this affect, if extreme, may form the basis of a bridge between depression and suicide.

In keeping with this "bridge" hypothesis, it may be the instability surrounding a loss, rather than the loss itself, that determines outcome. As an example, it may be the family strife preceding marital dissolution rather than the dissolution itself that promotes suicidal ideation or behavior. In this context, divorce would serve as an index of long-term family instability instead of an abrupt loss acting as a stimulus for suicide.

Following this line of reasoning, the ability of a family to respond positively to a child's need for nurturance after loss governs the outcome as much as the loss itself. In support of this idea, Zeligs (1967) found family attitudes and responses to loss to be pivotal in shaping the child's response to death. Warm, caring relationships appear to ease the child's pain, whereas children from chaotic homes experience much difficulty in adjusting.

In the case of a disorganized home, it is often unclear whether it was the loss or the family strife that precipitated a child's suicide. Adam (1982), in his extensive investigations of the impact of death on children, proposed the concept of "poor outcome" loss to indicate that family discord plays an important negative role in a child's attempt to integrate loss. On the other hand, Adam also pointed out that in cases where prolonged illness or marital discord have dominated the home for a long time, death or divorce can become a positive environmental reorganizer.

These qualifications of the effect of loss on suicidal behavior are important in avoiding single-cause explanations for suicide. The search must be widened to include numerous factors that shape an individual's adaptive capacities. This is consistent with the tenets of developmental psychology emphasizing multiple adaptive mechanisms, and it is well indicated by a number of studies dealing with the backgrounds of suicidal children.

For example, as a single factor, recent stress did not distinguish hospitalized latency-age suicidal children from their nonsuicidal counterparts in a study by Pfeffer and co-workers (1979). Nor did early loss alone appear to influence the suicidal behavior in a study of 76 hospitalized children between the ages of 5 and 14 studied by Cohen-Sandler, Berman, and King (1982). These children were divided into three groups—suicidal, depressed, and psychiatrically impaired but nondepressed (controls).

Cohen-Sandler and colleagues (1982) found that during infancy and preschool years, when important attachments are formed, psychiatric controls experienced more separation than the suicidal and depressed groups combined. Although throughout their lives suicidal children had sustained more family life disruptions through separation, divorce, and remarriage, they typically remained in the home, intensely involved with family members, where they were exposed to the full impact of the turmoil. Thus, suicide for these children became a vehicle for retaliation against events and people they felt they could not control. These observations led Cohen-Sandler and co-workers to conclude that the life history of a child predicted suicidal behavior better than any particular symptomatology.

In league with this hypothesis are findings of many other studies that indicate the importance of the family milieu. In Adam's (1982) literature review of retrospective comparisons of family stability in suicidal and nonsuicidal homes before loss, approximately half of the nonsuicidal homes were rated as stable, in contrast to less than 10% of the suicidal homes. The nonsuicidal homes succeeded in eventually restoring preloss levels of stability while the loss appeared to have had a more permanent effect on the suicidal homes. Thus, chronic familial maladaptation to loss may contribute more than the loss alone to suicidal behavior in the young.

Most attempts to examine the family environment as a source of risk for suicide have isolated variables that affect attachment and self-object representation. The impact of these variables on other suicide-related aspects of development, such as impulse control, remains largely unexplored. However, in tracing the antecedents of self-regulation, Kopp (1982) noted that lack of maternal warmth may diminish compliance among the very young. She also suggested a possible relationship between divorce and a child's level of control. Furthermore, abuse and the experience of unalloyed aggression may transmit a model of poor impulse control to a child. In conclusion, it is vital to recognize the correlation between loss and family stability or instability underlying suicidal behavior in childhood.

Attachment

The pivotal role of loss and disruptive family life in generating child-hood suicidal behavior derives from the attachment bond between infant and caregiver, since models of attachment also strongly focus the dynamics of reaction to loss. The degree to which the infant is successful in achieving need fulfillment through the caregiver serves as a paradigm for future attempts at controlling the environment. If this early attempt at mastery fails (i.e., if high levels of noncontingency occur), the child is at risk of developing depression, which may shade all other attempts to cope and could predispose the child to suicidal behavior in the presence of extreme stress.

Suggestive of the role of poor or insecure attachment in suicidal children is the fact that these children are routinely described as emotionally isolated (Adam, 1982; Paulson, 1974). Furthermore, many of the patterns of pathological responses to separation, such as anger and protest, can be seen in much of the self-destructive activity of these children.

Children who feel angry about a perceived desertion may try to retain an idealized image of their loved ones and therefore must convert their anger toward these individuals into self-hatred, holding themselves to blame. This is clearly a mechanism whereby self-destructive behavior can then become manifest (Housain & Vandiver, 1984; Toolan, 1962). Miller (1971) reported that idealization of lost attachment figures is common among suicidal children.

Along these same lines, the attempt to deny or overcome (i.e., protest) the effects of separation may take the form of an attempt to reunite with the lost attachment figure. Therefore, fantasies of effecting a reunion with a lost family member may underlie a bereaved child's attempt to take his or her own life. This is especially so when the child has not yet made the transition from attachment to separation. In this case, in the face of parental death, the emergent reunion fantasies will postpone the development of self-object relationships—a factor that might facilitate performance of the suicidal act.

Attachment theory also provides a means of interpreting the hopelessness and helplessness so commonly reported among suicidal children (Ackerly, 1967; McIntire, Angle, & Schlicht, 1977; Weissman & Worden, 1972). These expressions of despair might well reflect the consequences of these children's continued failure to master their environment through their mothers. Beck, Steer, Kovacs, & Garrison (1985) argued that hopelessness constitutes an important link between depression and suicide.

Expressions of helplessness and hopelessness may form the foundation of a response in which a child perceives himself or herself as being unable to control an intolerable environment. Beck and colleagues hypothesized that reactions against this learned helplessness, rooted in the disordered attachment bond, might underlie suicidal behavior. In other words, suicide might represent the last resort for building contingency, providing the final hope that one's actions will result in a predictable, albeit annihilating, outcome.

In Adam's (1982) review of the literature on attachment and suicide, the histories of suicidal children show extreme insecurity in almost all relationships in their lives. Furthermore, the failure to form stable attachments, leading to extreme social isolation, appears to be a major factor in the etiology of suicide in children.

From the issues briefly reviewed here, it appears that factors of family stress and disordered attachment are inextricably linked. It seems unlikely that secure attachments between child and caregiver will be represented to any significant degree in families with high levels of discord, and it appears even more unlikely that members of such families will be able to establish the equilibrium following loss that a child so desperately needs in order to continue proper development. Children from disturbed homes who suffer loss are therefore at high risk for suicide.

TRENDS IN RISK FACTORS
FOR CHILDHOOD SUICIDE

It is clear from the foregoing discussion that additive stresses interacting at varying levels of coping ability appear to be the forces determining the balance of the urge to survive. Attachment, self-object representation, empathic development, coping with loss, gender and temperament all interact to facilitate or forestall suicidal behavior.

Rosenthal and Rosenthal (1984), in comparing 16 suicidal preschoolers between $2\frac{1}{2}$ and 5 years of age with 16 behaviorally disordered children matched by age, sex, race, and parental marital and socioeconomic status, found four categories describing the culmination of the various stresses in the lives of the suicidal children: *self-punishment* (six children); *escape* (three children); *reunion with the central nurturer* (four children); and *rectification of an unbearable life situation* (three children). Along these same lines, Friedman and Corn (1985), in their case report of a boy who attempted suicide at age 7 and was followed up at age $12\frac{1}{2}$, found that the suicide attempt was directed at achieving several ends, some of which contradicted each other. This boy's first hope was that his act would bring his parents back together, but he simultaneously wished to wreak revenge on his parents for separating. Finally, by suicide, he hoped to repair his self-image by comparing himself to his favorite hero, Superman, who jumped from windows—the means this boy used in his suicide attempt. While these observations are useful, further research is needed to discover the final common pathway(s) of these influences in either direction.

In reviewing the literature, Cohen-Sandler and co-workers (1982) found that the factors most consistently associated with suicide in children were family disorganization, conflict, or a broken home. Calling attention to the work of Stanley and Barter (1970), Cohen-Sandler and colleagues (1982) observed that when suicidal children are compared to nonsuicidal controls, it becomes apparent that this variable is not as important when it stands alone as when parental loss occurs before age 12 and when the loss is part of a progression toward increasing isolation.

The insubstantiality of individual stresses in the etiology of suicidal behavior in children is illustrated in a study by Shafii, Carrigan, Whittinghill, and Derrick (1985), who used the technique of psychological autopsy to evaluate 20 children and adolescents between the ages of 12 and 19 years who had committed suicide. They found no significant differences between a matched-pair control group and the experimental group for the variables of broken home, overcrowded family or large number of children, parental dependency on drugs or alcohol, demanding parents, poor academic performance, being behind age-appropriate grade level, or being a school dropout. However, differences were found in that the suicidal children had significantly *more exposure to suicide* and demonstrated greater suicidal ideation, threats, and attempts and frequent use of drugs or alcohol.

Cohen-Sandler and colleagues pointed out another distinction that is lacking in the literature: the discrimination between suicidal and nonsuicidal depressed children. While discriminating between these two groups may be difficult, such a discrimination, if successful, would provide useful information about those aspects of depression that are conducive to suicide. Accordingly, Cohen-Sandler and co-workers studied 76 children between 5 and 14 years of age who were discharged from an inpatient psychiatric unit. Stringent operational criteria were employed to separate the children into three groups: suicidal, depressed, or psychiatric nondepressed (controls).

The investigators did in fact find significant differences between suicidal and depressed nonsuicidal children. While 65% of the suicidal children were also diagnosed as depressed, only 28% of the depressed children engaged in suicidal behavior. Furthermore, suicidal children experienced greater and increasing amounts of life stress as they matured, especially during the year prior to their admission. Perhaps of even greater significance is the fact that particular types of stress were found to be more predictive for suicidal behavior—among them, loss. From the time the suicidal children entered school to the period just prior to their admission, they had experienced a disproportionate number of losses of all kinds. Counter to what has been reported in the literature, however, these children tended to remain in the parental home, remaining intensely involved with family members and peers. It can be assumed that these individuals were also grieving and/or depressed, and the cumulative atmosphere of sadness might have negatively affected the young children's coping ability.

Another significant finding from this study was that of the 100 symptoms evaluated, only 2 specifically characterized the suicidal group: (1) these children had depressed affect and (2) they engaged in threatening other people. These qualities were also found in the study by Shafii, Carrigan, Whittinghill, and Derrick (1985), who found that a large proportion of the suicidal children in their retrospective study had exhibited destructive behavior toward others.

Cohen-Sandler and colleagues pointed out that these findings suggest a common denominator: aggression that is readily expressed both inwardly and outwardly as intense rage directed toward the self and others. One possible predictor of imminent suicidal behavior may be the presence of aggression or rage that is directed globally toward the external and internal world.

Thus, over all, it appears that children who experience a disproportionate number of losses as part of an ongoing process of isolation before the age of 12, who remain in the home, and who demonstrate globally directed rage may be at highest risk for suicide.

CONCLUSION

Developing an adequate base for self-preservation is perhaps the single most important element of personality. Khantzian and Mack (1983, in Pfeffer, 1986b) theorized that the following six different functions must be developed in order to achieve it:

1. Enough positive self-esteem so that the individual feels that he or she is worth protecting.
2. The ability to anticipate risky situations.
3. The ability to control impulses.
4. Pleasure in mastering situations of risk.
5. Enough knowledge about the environment and oneself to make survival possible.
6. The ability to choose others who will enhance one's protection and not jeopardize one's existence.

If Khantzian and Mack are correct, there seems to be ample room for failure in developing the means of survival. Yet this process cannot be defeated without severe and sustained assault from the environment. The assault can occur on any of a number of levels, as is evidenced by the fact that few, if any, studies have provided data suggesting that suicidal children are a distinct diagnostic group in which a characteristic dynamic or predictable antecedents can be found.

One dynamic does seem clear, however. The chances for suicide increase with age and with previous attempts. Suicide appears to be related, at least in some cases, to the existence of suicidal thoughts or behavior in the family or in peers. Thus, suicide may be a "language" of sorts among a given subgroup of individuals—a language of desperation using the concept of suicide in the hope of attaining a restructured, more bearable existence. In these cases, at least, the clinician can hear and respond to the call.

However, as Rosenthal and Rosenthal (1983) pointed out, the clinician cannot depend on caretakers in chaotic families to provide diagnostically valuable information. In addition to probing past and present family functioning and the number and kind of stresses the child has been heir to, the clinician must also explore the child's internal emotional and cognitive approach to his or her actions. In many instances, risk for suicide will be confirmed by interviewing the child.

Part IV

Specific Risk Factors During the Preschool Years

CHAPTER TWENTY-TWO

Child Abuse and Neglect

Kevin: Reacting to Abuse

Kevin is a 2-year, 2-month-old boy who lives in a foster home where his 4-year-old brother also resides. He has a 1-year-old brother who lives in a different foster home. Kevin lived with his mother and his father, who were never married, until Child Protective Services placed him and his brothers into foster care about 4 months ago. Kevin's mother is 19 years old and is one of 11 illegitimate children, 9 of whom are females with illegitimate children of their own. Neither Kevin's mother nor any of her sisters are educated beyond the 10th grade, and his mother appears to have borderline intellectual functioning.

Kevin's father, who is not the father of either of his brothers, was expelled from school in the 11th grade after assaulting a teacher. He also has a drug and alcohol abuse problem (although he denies current abuse of alcohol, stating that he drinks only about one case of beer per week), and he has been arrested three times on burglary and weapons charges. Kevin's father's past includes several clear instances of antisocial behavior including a report that he killed, cooked, and ate a cat at the age of 2 or 3 and his statement that he cut off a dog's head when he was 13 because he thought it was a rat. Kevin's father has two brothers who have both been treated for psychiatric disorders. His grandfather abandoned the family when Kevin's father was very young, and his grandmother is described by both of Kevin's parents as being "crazy." Kevin's parents describe Kevin as being just like his father. Kevin's mother and father live together with Kevin's 16-year-old aunt. Kevin was carried to term in an uncomplicated pregnancy during which his mother received no medical care, and he reportedly has no medical problems.

Kevin and his brothers were placed in foster care following an incident in which the police were called by a neighbor in response to a loud family argument. The police enlisted the aid of Child Protective Services after arriving at the family apartment to find Kevin and his brothers in an alley outside the home. The youngest child had frostbite from exposure to the cold winter temperatures. Child Protective Services' interviews yielded information about the care situation, including the fact that Kevin's mother basically ignored Kevin and the youngest boy in favor of the oldest child. Kevin, according to his mother and father, enjoyed taking baths and was allowed to run his own bath water and bathe unsupervised. Kevin and the other children also had easy access to kitchen knives. Kevin's parents reported that Kevin threw his baby brother onto the floor and sat on him, smiling all the while. They added that he twice tried to stab his father with kitchen knives, and that he once stabbed his older brother with a fork and drew blood. At the time of Child Protective Services' intervention, Kevin communicated only through grunts and he would take off his clothes and then refuse to get dressed. Kevin's parents did not initiate toilet training. The parent-child relationship was characterized by the parents' making fun of the children. The parents are thought to be unreliable.

Immediately following his placement in a foster home, Kevin bit other children and strangled and killed a pet bird. Kevin's behavior became steadily less aggressive and his communication skills improved with development of language use as he adjusted to the consistent gratification of his needs in the foster home. Kevin's evaluation was concomitant with his removal from his parents' home and placement in foster care.

At the initial assessment, it was determined that Kevin's aggressive behavior and failure to develop mature language abilities likely resulted from his chaotic environment, in which adaptive cognitive stimulus was absent. It was recommended that he be evaluated to ensure that his language and behavioral problems could be resolved. Kevin's reaction to separation from his father was depressive in nature, and his response to reuniting was joyous. Separation from his mother precipitated no emotional response in Kevin, indicating the absence of a secure attachment and perhaps also suggestive of her abusive, negligent care. Since residing in foster care, Kevin's aggressive behaviors and language problems have declined steadily to virtual nonexistence, and toilet training has been accomplished. Kevin reveals no signs of psychoses at present, and all other elements of mental status have also been judged to be normal for a boy of Kevin's developmental level.

Formulation suggests that Kevin's difficulties may not have been accurately reported by his parents, who may have merely been projecting their own destructive and aggressive fantasies. His living in an environment that was unsafe (he had access to knives and was left in potentially dangerous situations by himself) is also a probable contributor to his maladaptive behavior. The delay in language development could have been due to long periods of stress and to the lack of adaptive interactions, especially with his mother, during which he could learn to model his speech. Constant teasing, opposition, and neglect were clearly apparent under his parents' (lack of) supervision. Because remarkable improvement and fine adjustment have been noted since foster placement, the nature of Kevin's difficulties can be characterized as situational rather than as the result of an internalized psychiatric disorder. Recommendation was made for Kevin's retention in current foster care with minimal, if any, supervised contact with his parents.

INTRODUCTION

The emergence of child abuse as a defined sociopathological phenomenon has occurred largely within the past decade. Identification of cases like Kevin's has happened not only as a result of a possible increase in the incidence of this phenomenon but also because of a long-delayed recognition of its existence. Social proscriptions regarding making judgments about child-rearing practices are strong and can be overcome only with great difficulty. In its most extreme form, the principle of family autonomy can be traced to Roman law, in which the father was given total authority over the life and death of his children (Miller,

Dawson, Dix, & Parnas, 1976). In terms of formal law, this situation changed little until the 19th century, when adequate parental care was at last considered to be enforceable (Garrison, 1987).

At its most extreme, abuse can lead to death of the child. The National Center on Child Abuse and Neglect has reported the most conservative statistics, finding that between 2,000 and 4,000 deaths resulted from abuse in 1978. In their nationwide survey of hospitals treating abused children, Kempe and Kempe (1978) reported that over 25% (85) of the 302 cases studied suffered brain damage and 33% of the children died. A study by Hampton and Newberger (1985), however, found that although 34% of the injuries in their study were serious, less than 0.5% resulted in death. Furthermore, the American Humane Association (1985) has estimated that major physical injury existed in only 3.2% of the abused child population of 1983.

Regardless of the exact figures, the focus of major concern to the clinician and to society should lie in the fact that it is the young child who must endure the largest share of severe maltreatment. In 1983 nearly two thirds of the reported cases of major, or major with minor, physical injuries were inflicted upon children from birth to 5 years of age (AHA, 1985). Furthermore, nearly half the cases of deprivation occurred within this age group.

Children younger than 5 years of age are the most poorly equipped to handle stress. Abusive treatment easily interferes with attachment to the mother and the development of cognition and self-concept. Such interference can produce lifelong deficits in coping ability. These deficits may later contribute to producing frustration, which, combined with the adult's own experience as an abused child, leads the individual to direct violent urges against the next generation (Trad, 1987, 1988).

The cyclicity of abusive behavior within the family, in combination with the fact that the birth to 5-year age group is also the population at highest risk for hospitalization-induced depression, only compounds the difficulty of treating these children and highlights the necessity of determining the roots of abusive behavior among parents (Trad, 1986). This is especially true in light of the fact that child abuse and neglect within the general population appear to be increasing. Estimates have risen from 711,000 cases in 1979 to 1.5 million in 1983 (AHA, 1985).

While the need is urgent, a disciplined approach to treatment is essential. Strategies to combat or counteract child abuse must begin with an adequate clinical definition of the phenomenon. Primary among difficulties inherent in defining abuse are other forms of abuse that do not actually culminate in violence. For example, threats are not only difficult to define but are nearly impossible to document as well. Nevertheless, Gelles and Straus (1979) considered that threats of abuse are in fact a powerful form of emotional abuse that can intimidate and terrorize the child. Aber and Zigler (1981) concurred, stating that threats of violence can have consequences as harrowing to the young child as the actual abuse itself. Furthermore, Herrenkohl, Herrenkohl, and Egalf (1983a) and Herrenkohl, Herrenkohl, and Toedter (1983b) have reported a high incidence of emotional cruelty over a 10-year period in the case records of welfare families cited for physical abuse or neglect.

Other important factors that relate to abusive behavior but complicate its definition are the so-called "sins of omission"—emotional and physical neglect. Unlike physical neglect, which is apparent from the witholding of food, shelter, clothing, and so forth, emotional neglect is more difficult to recognize and quantify. However, like the threat of abuse, emotional neglect (depriving the child of interaction with a responsive and stimulating caregiver who is aware of the infant's developmental abilities and need for nurturance) can have a profound negative impact on development. While estimates of the incidence of emotional neglect are difficult to make, Morse, Sahler, and Friedman (1970) cited studies that indicate matching rates for traumas related to physical abuse and gross parental negligence. Holter and Friedman (1968) found that in a survey of children under 6 years of age seen for injuries at a general hospital, 10% displayed injuries suggestive of physical abuse and an additional 10% showed traumas that were probably related to neglect.

Aside from the definitionally ephemeral but nevertheless potent threats of abuse and the various forms of neglect, the definition of this phenomenon has undergone some degree of refinement, reflecting the development of research in the field. One of the earliest definitions, the "battered child syndrome," presents the situation of a young child who has suffered serious physical abuse at the hands of a parent or caregiver (Kempe, Silverman, & Steele, 1962). Except for modifications in degree, this definition is still largely operational.

Parke and Collmar (1975) defined abuse as "behavior that results in injury of another individual," and added the element of intentionality to the actions of the caregiver. Thus, a child is abused if he or she "receives nonaccidental physical injury as a result of acts (or omissions) on the part of his parents or guardians that violate the community standards concerning the treatment of children" (p. 513). In addition to this definition, Green (1983) stipulated that the physical abuse must occur repeatedly within the context of a pathological parent-child and family relationship. Taken together, these definitions convey some idea of the nature of child abuse. What is most important to realize is that the direct application of these definitions to the specific situation usually provides an operational means of identifying the phenomenon (Trad, 1987).

The fact that at least some attributes of child abuse are readily perceptible makes the search for its causes a hopeful one. All parents have to respect the fact that their child is smaller and so must be treated with restraint in physical and emotional terms. Very young children are also inherently frustrating to some degree because of their limited ability to communicate. A third factor all parents must cope with stems from the extra financial burden that is automatically imposed on any family with the addition of a child. Nevertheless, certain individuals react to these universal stresses with violence toward the child while others do not.

In searching for the reasons, it should first be considered that abuse can arise from any one or a combination of three interacting social levels. This ecological approach assesses the parent's risk for developing abusive behaviors toward his or her child by studying the parent's environment and how it may or may not predispose the adult to engage in abusive behavior.

Bronfenbrenner (1977), who originated the ecological context or model, posited that the three environmental levels on which people perform are (1) the microsystem within one's household; (2) the exosystem within the whole of society; and (3) the macrosystem existing amid the predominant cultural morals. Thus, an individual's microsystem and exosystem, both personal and interpersonal, are given definition and context by the macrosystem.

In addition, the ecological model incorporates the property of bidirectionality between parent and child as a possible contributor to abuse. That is, the characteristics of the child are considered as well as the psychiatric and social interactional patterns of the parent. When confronted with a temperamentally difficult child, certain parents may be more prone to abusive behavior than they would be if the child were of an easier nature.

As Belsky (1980) demonstrated, the ecological model unites the parent, the parent-infant dyad, the infant, and the world at large, with all its encompassing cultural values, into one system that defines the parent's whole environment and his or her risk of developing abusive behavior patterns. In other words, the parent under stress from the environment (exosystem) may become abusive within the family environment (microsystem) if he or she meets with no opposition from the culture's child-rearing attitudes (the macrosystem).

The ecological approach seems essential if the effects of various life stresses are to be weighed, counterweighed, and compared in an attempt to determine the root causes of abusive behavior. This approach seems the most promising for determining the outcomes of abusive behavior as well, since maltreatment during the highly formative period of early childhood is likely to have intricate long-term consequences as well as more immediate and overt effects (Trad, 1987, 1988).

PARENTAL STRESS AND CHILD ABUSE

The Insufficiency of the Psychiatric Model

As a means of exploring the nature of child abuse, the strength of the ecological approach becomes apparent almost immediately if it is compared to constructs in which psychopathology is viewed as the sole cause. As an example, Gelles (1973) gave a compelling explanation of the way in which the psychopathological model can be used to explain child abuse via the parent's relationship with the child, while at the same time illustrating the narrowness of this approach.

Abusive parents may have a *transference psychosis,* in which they perceive the child as a persecuting adult, believing that the child feels guilty when in reality it is their own guilt they are experiencing. This transference leads to the perception of the child as being the psychotic portion of the parent, which the parent wants to destroy. Thus, the child is projected as being the cause for the parent's hostile urges.

Another psychiatric scenario that has received some attention is the case of parents who turn to their children for the *nurturance and protection* they themselves lacked as infants (Morris & Gould, 1963). Morris and Gould described this as a parent-child role reversal, in which the parents look to their children to meet their own unfulfilled dependency needs.

Leonard, Rhymes, and Solnit (1966), in a study of nonorganic failure to thrive (NOFT) infants, postulated that pregnancy often reawakens a mother's need for nurturance, which must be fulfilled in order for the mother to succeed in her role as a new mother. However, when the mother's need is unfulfilled, as in the case of an unwanted pregnancy, the new mother often fails to thrive as a mother. Such a caregiver, when confronted with raising a child who fails to thrive, may interpret her child's behavior as an indication of her failure as a mother.

Thus, the mother and infant become mired in a *destructive pattern of mutually unmet dependency needs.* Childhood depression and suicide have both been shown to originate within the sustained feelings of insecurity and helplessness found in impaired caregiver-infant dyads (Adam, 1982; Morris & Gould, 1963; Pfeffer, Conte, & Plutchnik, 1980; Pfeffer et al., 1979, 1982; Trad, 1986, 1987).

While the foregoing situations are psychiatrically plausible, Gelles pointed to the insufficiency of such explanations in accounting for all cases of child abuse. It is highly doubtful that, as the psychiatric model would have it, there is only a single causal variable (a mental disease) accounting for the phenomenon. Such a postulation is also inconsistent with the fact that not all child abusers are psychiatrically ill.

According to Paulson, Schwemer, and Bendel (1976), who conducted a comparative study of abusive and nonabusive parents for degree of psychopathology, approximately one tenth of the parents of abused children have been diagnosed with a classifiable psychiatric illness. Abusive parents were observed to display higher levels than controls when rated on the Psychopathic Deviate and Hypomania Scales.

Smith, Hanson, and Noble (1973) noted "abnormal personalities" among almost half (46%) and psychopathology among a third of abusive fathers when evaluated on the Eysenck Personality Inventory and the General Health Questionnaire. During the interview, nearly half of the mothers were described as neurotic, with symptoms of depression, anxiety, or a combination of the two. On the other hand, Spinetta and Rigler (1972) came to a different conclusion, finding little in the literature to suggest a high incidence of general psychiatric illness among parents of abused children.

Depression

Of the psychological variables that have been suggested as being associated with child abuse, depression is perhaps the most pervasive. Kaplan, Peleovitz, Salzinger, and Ganeles (1983) compared mothers of 76 abused children who had been reported to the New York State Department of Social Services with 38 control mothers. The results revealed an incidence of clinical depression among the mothers of abused children that was nearly four times that seen in the controls (51% versus 13%). Furthermore, 24% of the fathers of abused children showed depression as compared to only 16% of the controls.

In a study conducted by Susman, Trickett, Iannotti, Hollenbeck, and Zahn-Waxler (1985), a direct correlation was found between depression and abusiveness based on findings of similarities in child-rearing practices among the mothers of both the abused and control groups. Administering the Block Child-Rearing Practices Report to several groups (current major depressives, current minor depressives, abusers, and controls), Susman and co-workers found that the current major depressives paralleled the abusive mothers in 38% of the 21 child-rearing variables they examined. The two groups mirrored each other most closely on factors indicating affect expression and development of autonomy. The abusive parents differed from the control group in showing higher rates of alcoholism, drug abuse, antisocial personality, and labile personality.

Typologies

Employing the sort of studies just described, a number of psychiatric researchers have sought to identify traits within the parent in an attempt to construct a profile of characteristics predisposing to child abuse. The majority of researchers agree that abusive parents often lack the ability to control their aggressive feelings. One of the first investigators to evolve a typology of abusive parents, Merrill (1962) built a classification based on three fundamental categories: (1) *chronic hostility and aggression;* (2) *rigidity, compulsiveness, and unreasonableness; and* (3) *passivity and dependence.* Lack of empathy (Melnick & Hurley, 1969; Steele, 1983); impulsivity, hypersensitivity, and quickness to react (Bousha & Twentyman, 1984); self-centeredness (Melnick & Hurley, 1969); and avoidance of social interaction, fear of authority, feelings of guilt, and low self-esteem (Helfer, McKinney, & Kempe, 1976; Main & Goldwyn, 1984) have also been noted as traits prevalent in parents who are child abusers.

Stress of Low Income

As Gelles (1973) and others (e.g., Bland & Orn, 1986) have pointed out, while these psychiatrically derived traits may be of some use, their origins remain obscure in many instances. A large part of the problem derives from the fact that the psychiatric approach to child abuse fails to account for possible social causes of stress. Independent of any psychopathology that may be present, the single most important environmental stress contributing to child abuse appears to be low income. Being poor in an affluent society quickly and strongly produces frustration that can easily generate aggressive impulses.

While child abuse is by no means restricted to members of low-income families, the preponderance of cases do occur in this setting (Schneider-Rosen & Cicchetti, 1984). Gil (1971) found that *nearly half* of the fathers of abused children were unemployed during the year prior to exhibiting abusive behavior. At the time of the actual event, 12% were unemployed.

In a study of parent-child interactions in abusive and nonabusive families, Herrenkohl, Herrenkohl, Toedter, and Yanushefski (1984) actually found strong correlations between the relative warmth of family interactions and the level of income. In studying parent-child interactions in 259 families, Herrenkohl and co-workers found that the higher the income level the more positive and the less negative and hostile both parents and children were. Furthermore, parents at higher-income levels were found to be more task supportive of their children. Overall verbal interaction was higher as well in higher-income families. Lower-income families exhibited less child-centeredness, mutual acceptance, stimulation, and enjoyment and more parent-centered behavior and mutual rejection than families of higher income. There was also a greater prevalence of coercion as a control technique among the poverty group.

Effect of the Child's Status in the Family

Just as low income may predispose otherwise nonpathologic adults to engage in abusive behavior, the child's relative family status has the potential to generate stress that could increase parental vulnerability to abusive behavior. According to the Massachusetts Society for the Prevention of Cruelty to Children, half of the reported abuse cases involved premarital conception (Zalba, 1971). Bennie and Sclare (1969) found that many abused children were the product of unwanted pregnancies and that the abused child is likely to be the youngest child, indicating the possibility that the most recent birth may sometimes tip the scale against the parents' ability to cope (Trad, 1987).

Effect of Being Subjected to Abuse as a Child

While the stress of poverty, due to either low wages, unemployment, or a surfeit of children, is very real, it falls into the same category as the delineation of personality traits predisposing to abusive behavior— both must be studied together and in the broader social context before their relationship to child abuse can be assessed. Furthermore, specific parental, child, and environmental factors that mediate between stress and the quality of child care need to be outlined (Egeland et al., 1980).

One of these mediational factors is the manner in which the parent exhibiting abusive behavior was raised. Investigators agree that individuals who have experienced violence and abuse as children are more likely to become child abusers than those who did not experience such abuse as young children (Byrd, 1979; Cicchetti & Rizley, 1981; Curtis, 1963; Fontana, 1985; Main & Goldwyn, 1984).

A number of investigators have pointed to cognitive impairments in the parent as a prime source of risk for beginning or continuing abusive behavior. Low levels of intelligence and lack of awareness concerning a child's developing needs are two of many cognitive impairments cited by this group (see discussion of self-concept development and dysregulated bonds) (Cameron, Johnson, & Campos, 1966; Fisher, 1958; Holter & Friedman, 1968; Kempe et al., 1962; Simpson, 1967, 1968).

Furthermore, Main and Goldwyn (1984) demonstrated that mothers who have been rejected as children generally tend to display myriad cognitive deficits such as distorted views of their childhoods, failure to remember specific events, idealization of a neglecting parent, and incoherent discussion of their current attachment bond.

The number of studies supporting the contention that mothers who were emotionally or physically abused by their own mothers tend to abuse and reject their own offspring has led many investigators to examine the attachment bond between abusive caregivers and their infants. Crittenden (1985), after having observed social networks of abusive and neglecting mothers, contended that a person's own early attachment relationship with his or her parents infuses all of that person's familial and extrafamilial relationships. Thus, a parent lacking a stable and engaging set of attachment feelings is likely to establish the same flawed relationship with his or her own child.

Dysregulation of the Attachment Bond: Perturbations Contributing to the Propagation of Abusive Behaviors

Schneider-Rosen and Cicchetti (1984) pointed out that study of the development of the attachment relationship between infant and primary caregiver during the second year of life is very useful for examining the cognitive achievements underlying consolidation of attachment to the caregiver. Observation of the growth of this bond also provides a base from which to study the later effects of this relationship on affective and cognitive development.

Schneider-Rosen and Cicchetti hypothesized that infants in an abusive environment will be insecurely rather than securely attached. Since consolidation of the attachment bond marks the beginning of the differentiation between the self and the environment, a secure attachment promotes mastery. Insecure attachment, on the other hand, retards approach and mastery, providing a limited potential for exploring the environment due to insecure feelings about leaving the caregiver. Presumably, infants who have been abused will have experienced negative feedback from the caregiver that produces an insecure attachment.

To test this hypothesis, Schneider-Rosen and Cicchetti reasoned that the advanced exploration of the environment by securely attached infants should allow them to differentiate from the environment and recognize themselves earlier than insecurely attached infants. They studied 37 subjects from low-income families. Of these, 18 infants from 18 to 20 months of age had been maltreated, while the other 19 acted as controls. The quality of the attachment bonds of these infants was tested by the strange-situation procedure (Ainsworth & Wittig, 1969).

In agreement with attachment theory, the maltreated infants had a significantly greater number of insecure attachments when compared to nonabused children. The hypothesis of earlier self-recognition by the nonabused children was also supported. Maltreated infants were developmentally delayed in their affective responses to their images in a mirror under conditions of the standard mirror-and-rouge paradigm.

These results provide evidence of impairment in the development of self-concept in children who are maltreated. When such children mature and begin having children of their own, their lack of self-development can impose barriers to the formation of secure attachments with their own children. Their deficits in self-esteem can also make them vulnerable to stress due to diminished coping ability (Trad, 1986, 1987).

Galambos and Dixon (1984), in their study of adolescent abuse and the development of personal sense of control, obtained results suggesting that the cognitive deficit noted above may also influence the locus of control in adolescence. Specifically, these investigators noted that victims of severe physical and emotional abuse often display low self-esteem, high anxiety, lack of empathy, aggressive behavior, and suicidal tendencies. People with such feelings typically exhibit an external locus of control. Therefore, Galambos and Dixon hypothesized that the nature of the relationship between locus of control and experience of abuse may depend on the duration of the abuse. That is, the longer the maltreatment the more profound the feelings of worthlessness. If true, this finding would support the contention that vulnerability to stress produced by deficits in self-concept have their origins in insecure attachment bonding.

In their study, Galambos and Dixon did find a gradation between length of exposure to abuse and locus of control. Adolescents who experienced abusive behavior throughout childhood tended to be more externally oriented than adolescents abused for a shorter time. Thus, perturbations in the attachment bond may lead to insecure attachments, producing deficits in self-esteem that go on to produce vulnerability to stress (Trad, 1986, 1987). This vulnerability not only places the adult who was abused as a child at risk of performing abusive behaviors but tends to be replicated through attachment bonds and passed to the next generation.

The enormous impact of the quality of the attachment bond has been demonstrated recently in a prospective study by Troy and Sroufe (1987), who followed the development of victimization patterns in 38 children from a low-income urban setting. The term *victimization* was defined as a relationship characterized by a sustained pattern of exploitation and manipulation. The victimizer achieves this goal via control of resources (dominance, verbal hostility, and/or physical aggression).

The investigators' purpose was to see whether or not specific types of attachment (secure, anxious-avoidant, and anxious-resistant) were associated with the evolution of roles as victimizers, victims, or neither. Anxiously attached children were hypothesized to be more likely to engage in aggressive/manipulative or submissive behavior. Securely attached children were hypothesized to be sure enough of themselves that they entered into neither a victimizer nor a victimized role.

Children with differing types of attachment bond histories were assigned to dyads (play pairs) in order to assess the nature of their interactions. A total of 14 dyads were used in all. All possible combinations of attachment history were used in this study.

The results were dramatically in agreement with the initial hypotheses. The presence of a child with an avoidant attachment history was associated with victimization in five of seven pairs in which at least one child had an avoidant history. In counterpoint, none of the seven pairs without an avoidant child exhibited victimization. The authors pointed out that, specifically, victimization occurs in dyads containing a child with an insecure attachment history (either avoidant or resistant).

It was found that all victimizers had an avoidant attachment history and all victims were anxiously attached. In other words, victimization occurred in every case in which one member of the play pair had a history of avoidant attachment and the other had also been anxiously attached. Further adding to the strength of these findings were observations stemming from a pair of girls, both of whom had avoidant attachment histories. In this play pair, the direction of victimization switched back and forth several times during the course of the relationship.

Thus, it appears that *the victim has an active role in sustaining a pattern of victimization.* Furthermore, it seems feasible to identify victimization as a unique, maladaptive interactional pattern incorporating elements of aggression that could persevere into adulthood, and predispose the victim to abusive behavior not only toward children but toward others in the environment as well. This dynamic appears to be related to insecure attachments. The avoidant attachments give rise to victimizing behavior, while resistant attachments tend to produce an individual prone to being victimized.

The Differential Effects of Stress on Parents

Egeland and co-workers (1980) compared the effects of stress on mothers who provided adequate versus inadequate care and found that while environmental stress is an important etiological contributor to child abuse, it is still essential to determine why some mothers react to stress with violence and others do not. One reason may be the lack of self-esteem already noted.

Egeland and colleagues sought to discover additional reasons by examining variables that differentiated high-stress mothers who mistreat their children from high-stress mothers who do not. Employing a life event scale as well as measures of various personality traits such as aggression, succorance, impulsivity, and so forth, these researchers prospectively studied 367 primiparous women at risk for abusing their children.

The Cochrane and Robertson Life Events Inventory was administered to each mother 12 months after the birth of her infant, and a new scoring system was used to differentiate between mothers who were abusers and those who were not. Again, this study showed the importance of mother-child interactions since the patterns that most differentiated between the two groups were mother-infant interactions during feeding and play, changing life events, and babies' nonoptimal functioning.

High-stress mothers who were abusers scored higher on the aggression and dependence scale and lower on the succorance and social desirability scales. These mothers were easily frustrated and quick to respond to their frustrations in an aggressive, hostile fashion. High-stress mothers who did not resort to abuse, on the other hand, received more support from family members and friends and were better at feeling support.

In terms of cognitive development, it is interesting to note that the nonabusive mothers were more able to recognize the intent of their children's aggressive impulses and to mediate their reactions accordingly. This finding supports the hypothesis that mothers who were themselves abused lack fully developed empathic abilities perhaps related to self-concept deficits incurred from infancy.

Alcohol Use

One aspect of the differential effects of stress on caregivers may be the degree of alcohol use. Although Orme and Rimmer's review of the literature on alcoholism and abuse revealed no causal relationship uniting the two behaviors, many researchers have noted similarities between the personality profiles and psychiatric histories of alcoholics and child abusers. Feelings of powerlessness, ineffectiveness, and worthlessness have been ascribed to both populations, suggesting that those with alcohol dependency may be more at risk for abusive behavior than those who are not alcoholics. This may be especially true in light of the disinhibitory effects of alcohol.

Of particular interest is Hindeman's (1977) study in which he found that it was not uncommon for alcoholics to have a history of child abuse. In a questionnaire administered to 178 patients in treatment in the United States and Australia for drug and alcohol addiction, Kroll, Stock, and James (1985) found that alcoholics who had been abused as children had significantly greater levels of aggression than nonabused alcoholics. This aggression was directed both at others and at themselves in the form of domestic violence, violence against authority, and serious suicidal attempts. The abused alcoholics also tended to display more depressive symptomatology than those who were not abused.

While it has not been proved, it is possible that anxiety produced by early deficits in coping due to being abused contributes to the use of alcohol in adults who were abused. If this is true, the factors influencing whether or not a given adult turns to alcohol abuse would again follow an ecological paradigm in which genetic predisposition, family practices, and social mores interact to produce the end behavior.

ABUSE AND THE CHILD'S REACTIVITY TO STRESS (TEMPERAMENT)

Patterns of Stress Evolving from Character Traits

Thus far the discussion has focused on the parent's contextual contributions to the evolution of abusive behavior. The effects of the infant's genetic predisposition remain to be examined. The contributions of the infant's temperament to mother-infant interactions is not trivial. Defined as constitutionally based individual differences in reactivity and self-regulation, individual differences in temperament have been theoretically and empirically linked to resilience to stress, adaptivity of coping styles, and quality of parent-child relationships (Rothbart, 1986; Windle et al., 1986).

In the study by Egeland and co-workers (1980), it was noted that high-stress mothers who did not abuse their children tended to have infants who were more responsive to their mothers and who initiated more social interaction. Possibly, these babies were easier to care for and more rewarding to the mothers. As Egeland and co-workers postulated, when a highly anxious mother must cope with very stressful life events, the extra stress involved in attending to the needs of a less responsive infant may well increase the likelihood of abusive behavior.

Chess (1970) presented an excellent overview of the various ways in which vulnerability associated with traits of temperament can contribute to the development of behavior disorders. Defining temperament as the behavioral style of the infant—the how of his or her behavior, not the what (content) or the why (motivation)—Chess found a number of attributes and patterns of temperament that were more likely than others to predispose the child to damaging interactions with the environment.

Activity Level. Temperament in itself can neither cause nor prevent a behavior disorder, but certain possibly damaging characteristics should be watched for. Among these is activity level, defined as the motor portion of a child's functioning and the diurnal amount of active and inactive periods. As a rule, children with high levels of activity are more difficult to manage than more sedate children. Furthermore, demands for restraint that are too far beyond the child's ability to satisfy may lead to his or her being labeled "bad." If punishment for this seemingly intentional disobedience ensues, the child may conclude that all attempts to please are futile. This could lead to habitually disobedient behavior.

Rhythmicity. Defined as the regularity and predictability of hunger-feeding patterns, elimination, and the sleep-wake cycle, this variable may have high-risk consequences during infancy. As a general observation, irregularity is likely to be problematic in the clock-watching cultures of the West. Irregular sleeping patterns may interfere with the working schedules of the parents. Even the child with very regular patterns may encounter trouble due to the inability of the parents to make changes in their schedules.

Approach or Withdrawal. This is a key component of temperament that reflects the way in which an infant responds to a new stimulus. Some individuals move readily into new circumstances while others do not. The child who initially withdraws from entering into play may be pressured to do so. He or she may also come to be labeled as a "negative" person, and the behavior may be viewed as obstinacy or a desire to thwart the parents' wishes.

Adaptability. This variable refers to the speed and ease with which behavior can be modified as a response to changes in the environment. Children who require repeated exposures to adapt to a novel situation may come to withdraw even more if not given sufficient opportunity to adapt to each situation. A bright but slow-to-adapt child may be mislabeled by teachers as someone who is slow to learn.

Quality of Mood. The amount of pleasant, happy behavior exhibited by a child strongly influences the reaction of surrounding people. If the predominating mood is negative and the child tends to react to stress with whining and fussing, the likelihood of dissonant interactions with parents is greatly increased.

Intensity of Reaction. This dimension measures the energy level of response to a situation, whether it is neutral, positive, or negative. A predominantly intense child exhibits an "all or nothing" response, and if this response tends to be generally negative, the child may come to be judged as anxious or hostile. A child with mild reactions, on the other hand, might come to be viewed incorrectly as unresponsive or apathetic.

Distractibility. Children differ in the degree to which extraneous environmental stimulation interferes with ongoing behavior. Task completion may be difficult for children who are easily distracted, especially if this trait is accompanied by nonpersistence. While high distractibility can be problematic once the child attains school age, it can also be advantageous by contributing to a high degree of alertness and awareness.

Attention Span and Persistence. Taken together, these variables measure the length of time spent pursuing a particular activity as well as the degree to which the activity is continued in the face of obstacles. A child with a short attention span and little persistence will tend to give up too easily when confronted with the first signs of failure. This clearly inhibits the development of adequate coping behavior. However, a high degree of persistence is no guarantee of success, since children with this characteristic may persist in tasks that are not approved of by teachers, parents, or peers.

Trait Clusters

Chess (1970) pointed out that none of these characteristics of temperament occurs in isolation. Rather, they are interrelated to comprise three primary types of character: the easy child, the difficult child, and the child who is "slow to warm up."

Easy children are at least risk for developing behavior disorders. These children are largely regular, mostly positive in mood, readily adaptable, have low or mild intensity levels of their responses, and are affirmative in their approach to new situations. As infants, they quickly establish regular eating and sleeping cycles, and they quickly adapt to changes in school routine when they grow older.

Nevertheless, there are pitfalls attached to even this kind of character. A sharp difference in parental and extrafamilial standards in school may be overwhelming if the child finds himself or herself suddenly the target of criticism, punishment, or ridicule. As a defense, such a child may remain the same at home but withdraw or become aggressive while at school.

In counterpoint to easy children, difficult children typically have irregular biological functions, predominantly negative responses to new situations and stimuli, and a high degree of negative mood. They may respond to frustration with tantrums and tend to make special demands on their parents for unusually consistent or tolerant handling. These children have the greatest risk of developing behavior disorders. Chess pointed out that 70% of the children with this trait cluster in the New York Longitudinal Study developed behavior problems.

Slow-to-warm-up children display a mix of negative, though mildly intense, initial responses to new situations. They adapt only gradually after repeated exposure to new situations. Pressure for quick adapta-

tion tends to intensify the urge to withdraw, which may bring on a negative child-environment interaction.

Chess emphasized that temperament alone cannot produce a behavior disorder any more than vulnerability inevitably does in the individual. Nevertheless, certain constellations of temperamental traits appear
to be more frequently associated with behavior disorders. These include
the following:

> *a combination of irregularity, nonadaptability, withdrawal responses, and predominantly*
> *negative mood of high intensity; 2) a combination of withdrawal and negative responses*
> *with low intensity to new situations, followed by slow adaptability; 3) excessive persistence;*
> *4) excessive distractibility; 5) markedly high or low activity level.* (1970, p. 130)

Differences in Character Between Survivors
and Nonsurvivors of Abuse

It is informative to compare the temperament clusters cited by Chess
with those uncovered in a 14-year prospective study by Zimrin (1986).
Zimrin studied 28 children known to have been abused between the
ages of $3\frac{1}{2}$ and 5 years. These children were followed up 14 years later.
Those who had managed to survive their childhood trauma to become
well-adjusted individuals were compared to those who showed high degrees of psychosocial pathology.

Zimrin found three basic differences between survivors and nonsurvivors of abuse. First, survivors tended to express activity rather than
passivity and regression. Second, survivors evaluated their personal resources in a positive light, as opposed to the negative self-evaluations
of the nonsurvivors. Finally, survivors had a significant relationship
with an external figure other than the parents, whereas no such relationship existed in the nonsurvivor group.

It is impossible to draw definite conclusions regarding the contributions of temperament to the differences seen between survivors and
nonsurvivors, but certain of the variables cited by Chess for difficult
versus easy temperament do suggest themselves. Easy children, like the
survivors in Zimrin's study, if they are energetic and quick to approach
new situations, are more likely to seek the help of an adult outside the
parental relationship. On the other hand, the high degree of negative
mood expressed by difficult children may correlate with the negative
self-evaluations of the nonsurvivors.

On a global level, it is not difficult to infer a general correlation between the five difficult temperament clusters cited by Chess and the
characteristics of Zimrin's nonsurvivors that differentiated them from
the survivors. Thus, it appears that clinical attention to a child's temper-

ament will be of great value in any psychiatric evaluation, particularly so in cases of suspected abuse.

THE CONCOMITANTS OF CHILD ABUSE

Depression

Abused and/or neglected children are at particularly high risk for developing depression (Trad, 1986, 1987). In one representative investigation, Kazdin, Moser, Colbus, and Bell (1985) studied the relationship between physical abuse and depressive symptoms in 79 children between the ages of 6 and 13 who were referred for psychiatric treatment. None of the children showed evidence of neurological impairment, uncontrolled seizures, or dementia and none were receiving psychotropic medication. Median age was 10.4 years.

All diagnoses were based on DSM-III criteria, with symptom description obtained from direct child and parent interviews immediately prior to admission as well as following hospitalization. Two staff members completed independent diagnoses for each child.

Abuse was defined as "physical injury inflicted by a parent, guardian, or other adult responsible for the care of the child." The level of severity of abuse was assessed using physical signs, explanations about the appearance of these signs, and the pattern of the injuries, their explanations, and their treatment. Cases of neglect and sexual abuse were omitted from the study.

The principal finding of this study was that these physically abused psychiatric inpatient children demonstrated higher levels of depression and hopelessness and lower self-esteem in comparison with nonabused patients. It was interesting that the severity of the depressive symptoms varied with the history of abuse. For example, children who had been abused in the past but were currently not being abused had less severe depressive symptoms compared to children who were being abused in the present. However, it cannot be stated as yet that the negative effects of abuse on depressive symptoms diminish with time.

Another observation was that the effects of past abuse fail to diminish if abuse continues into the current time frame. The children with both past and current abuse exhibited the most severe signs of depression, hopelessness, and low self-esteem. Kazdin and colleagues suggested the possibility that the history of abuse retains its impact on the child and supplements the effects of current abuse. However, they noted that those with past and current abuse may be prone to experiencing more frequent and severe abuse over all.

This last postulation has an interesting correlate suggesting that there may be some similarity between the suffering of abusive events and the experience of events leading to posttraumatic stress syndrome (PTSD). Individuals vary in their ability to perceive dangerous stimuli. While an experience that proves devastating to one person may not so severely affect another, there is an implicit assumption in the psychiatric literature that there is a stress level that will do great harm to almost anyone (Silverman, 1986).

In light of recent research by Pynoos and colleagues (1987), it seems plausible at least to suggest that child abuse may in some cases engender reactions similar to PTSD. Studying 159 school-age children following a sniper attack in their school yard, these investigators found systematic self-reports of PTSD symptoms. Like the severity of depression in the study by Kazdin and colleagues, the type and number of PTSD symptoms increased as exposure to the trauma increased.

Over and above the risks for depression and/or PTSD, the abused child also experiences inconsistent and extreme levels of parental noncontingency. The child who in one instance may be commended for wanting to explore the environment may on another occasion be abused for engaging in similar behavior. As a result, the child may withdraw from the environment in order to protect the self. Ultimately, this could produce learned helplessness. Since the child cannot know who is ultimately responsible for the abuse—himself or herself, the caregiver, or simply a random universe—active participation in life may hardly seem worthwhile.

In addition to the depression induced by abuse, these children are prone to experience depression even when they are hospitalized for treatment of their injuries. As Spitz and Wolf (1946) and Bowlby (1944) have documented, children in institutional settings, particularly those between the ages of 6 months and 4 years (which is also typically the period of highest abuse), are highly susceptible to onset of depression. Hospitalization subjects the abused child, or any child, to insecure attachment, lack of parental support due to anxiety and guilt of the parent, and fear of abandonment (Kashani, Barbero, & Bolander, 1981; Mason, 1965).

Compounding the ill effects of hospitalization is the fact that an abused child returning from the hospital is at greater risk for further abuse and neglect, since hospitalization only aggravates the conditions that produce abuse in the first place, namely, behavioral difficulties (Ferguson, 1979; Prugh, 1983); depression (Pilowsky, Bassett, Begg, & Thomas, 1982; Reichelderfer & Rockland, 1963); insecure attachments (Bowlby, 1951; Ferguson, 1979); impaired ability to form relationships (Bowlby, 1944, 1951); and stress in the home (Prugh, Staub, Sands, Kirschbaum, & Lenihan, 1953).

Cognitive Deficits

Abused and depressed children with an external locus of control may become abusive themselves, transferring the abusive behavior forced on them out to the world in general (George & Main, 1979). This only reinforces their isolation from the world and exacerbates depressive behaviors. On the other hand, children with an internal locus of control, believing that they are the cause of their caregivers' abusive behavior, may direct their aggressive feelings not externally at the world but inward toward themselves, placing themselves at risk for suicidal behaviors (Husain & Vandiver, 1984; Kosky, 1983; Monane, Liechter, & Lewis, 1984).

In addition to cognitive deficits regarding locus of control, abused children have been shown to experience developmental delays affecting nearly every aspect of their functional abilities (Elmer & Gregg, 1967; Kempe & Kempe, 1978; Martin & Beezley, 1977). The development of motor skills is particularly sensitive to the ill effects of abuse. Children who are abused for practicing their developing motor skills such as walking, grabbing, and generally exploring the environment will be pressured to arrest the use of such skills. Language disorders such as delayed speech development and problems in articulation have also been noted (Elmer & Gregg, 1967; Green, 1983; Kempe & Kempe, 1978; Trad, 1988).

While the literature is replete with these associations and many others relating to learning disabilities, the causal relationships involved remain to be delineated. It may be that child abuse causes learning disability through any of a number of mechanisms ranging from sufficiently severe brain damage to the generation of pathological levels of anxiety. However, it may also be that an innate learning problem generates parent-child friction, which predisposes certain adults to act abusively. In their excellent review of the literature, Caplan and Dinardo (1986) concluded that at the present time there is no conclusive evidence to support the contention that abused children are more likely than non-abused children to have learning disabilities or that learning disabled children are more likely than children without learning disabilities to be abused.

Violence

The preponderance of violent behavior exhibited by abused children illustrates the severity of the experience of being abused. George & Main (1979) studied 20 children from disadvantaged circumstances. Of these, 10 had been physically abused and 10 were matched controls. Results indicated that the abused children were more prone to kick, hit, or slap than their equally disadvantaged but unabused peers. In addition, 70% of the maltreated children, compared to only 20% of the controls, displayed violent behavior or posed threats of violence toward their caregivers. Furthermore, the abused children, when confronted with distress among their normal peers, often displayed signs of anger, fear, or physical abuse.

Monane and co-workers (1984) studied the histories of abused and nonabused hospitalized psychiatric patients aged 3 to 17 years and found that violence is also prevalent among older abused children. While only 46% of the nonmaltreated patients behaved violently, 72% of those who were maltreated expressed acts of extreme violence. However, violent behavior in these children may not be exclusively learned behavior, since there is a strong possibility that many of these children may be brain damaged or impulse disordered.

The violence found among abused children corresponds to that of Zahn-Waxler, Cummings, McKnew, and Radke-Yarrow's (1984) study of the children of affectively ill parents. Abusive parents have themselves been found to exhibit depressed behavior. Thus, it is not unlikely that the children of abused and depressed parents will act like other children of depressed parents.

Like the violent behaviors seen among the children of the affectively ill, the abused children's violence may represent, in some cases, an inability to allay the empathic distress they feel for the emotional states of their parents. Therefore, while under normal circumstances prosocial behavior would become the normal means of venting empathic distress, those who have been maltreated, lacking a model of empathic response, may alleviate their distress in aberrant ways. Some possibilities include dulled emotional responsiveness or, again, aggressive behavior and violence. It is important to note also that many abused children have a severely restricted empathic ability, which may lead to blunting of affect and inappropriate or paradoxical emotionality. Thus, the overall effects of abuse encompass developmental distortions of all kinds—depression, production of future psychopathology, violence, and most inimicably, the likelihood of later becoming abusive as a parent (Trad, 1987, 1988).

CONCLUSION

The severe concomitants of child abuse, in combination with its ingrained cyclicity from generation to generation, make its detection and treatment the highest priority. It is possible that *this phenomenon accounts for a much greater portion of adult psychopathology than is presently recognized.* Interacting with the child's temperament, even the most caring of parents probably unknowingly inflict some psychic damage on their children from time to time. Because of the sensitive formative period of early childhood, even modest punishments can take on dire significance in later life. In cases where abuse is overt and severe, the fallout affects far more than the child in the present and the future. The ensuing behaviors of aggression/violence, depression, and suicide negatively affect all who come to care for such a person.

In looking for treatment recommendations, it seems reasonable to take some lessons from the children in Zimrin's (1986) study of children who survived early abusive treatment to become well-adjusted adults. First, as Zimrin pointed out, it would be beneficial to increase the means of family support to abused children. Since the survivors studied usually only needed one sympathetic advisor, this may not be as difficult as it might seem at first glance. The sincerity and stability of the relationship appear to be more important than the quantitative aspects of support.

Second, treatment should include strategies to strengthen the child's confidence in his or her inner resources. Coping behavior is centrally influenced by confident self-image, an area in which these children are extremely lacking. For instance, it might be useful to isolate performances at school and analyze them with the child, not in the light of the parent, but in the light of objective reality, with differential diagnostic attention given to developmental cognitive, as well as social, deficits.

Finally, coping behavior should be reinforced as much as possible. The child should be encouraged to engage in even the smallest of coping behaviors and then taught to see the positive effects of his or her actions. If carried out thoroughly, this process can have a snowball effect in which the child begins to engage in coping for his or her own gratification. Otherwise, abused children may well regress and accept their fate.

CHAPTER TWENTY-THREE

Separation Reactions to Day Care, Divorce, and Death

Tomas: Fearful Reactions

Tomas is a cheerful, active, affectionate, easygoing 5-year-old boy with many friends. His general development and his adjustment to school entry were without incident, and he enjoys drawing and listening to music. Tomas's only separations from his parents were when his two younger brothers were born. Both times he stayed with his maternal grandparents. A few months after Tomas started school, his parents separated for a 3-month period. During the separation period, Tomas began to order his mother around and provoke fights with one of his brothers. At school, Tomas became difficult; he would not listen or pay attention, and he would claim to not know how to do something even though he had been taught how to do it. For a few weeks prior to evaluation, Tomas had frequent temper tantrums and daydreamed often while at school.

When Tomas's father returned to the home, Tomas's behavior resumed its pre-separation character. However, after the first week, Tomas's mother noted that his maladaptive behavior seemed to be building up. Tomas started to interrogate and direct his mother as he had done when his father was absent. Tomas's mother responded to his directives inconsistently and remarked that whatever she said, her husband condemned her. Tomas started bossing his younger brothers around, too. His mother expressed a feeling of lack of control over her own children and her own life. When Tomas arrived for evaluation, his performance at school was weakening and he had recently destroyed some family photographs.

During the assessment interviews, Tomas was cooperative; he displayed normal attention and concentration spans and used normal, coherent speech. Thought, behavior, and affect were all observed to be normal. Tomas's thought content included references to fear of a "shark with sharp teeth," which he drew, and to the consequences of misbehaving, which included "going to jail." Developmentally, Tomas was assessed to be average; elements of the mental status examination were judged to be within age-appropriate normal ranges.

The temporary separation of Tomas's parents is an identifiable stressor in this case, which he reacted to with maladaptive behaviors within 3 months of its onset. Tomas's reaction included emotional features (i.e., anxiety about his father deserting the family), even after his father had returned home, and fear, as expressed in the assessment interview. Tomas's reaction was also characterized by conduct disturbance, including violation of family rules, for example, his telling his mother what she was allowed to do, his overseeing her actions as would a parent, and his initiation of fights with his brother. These observations led to an initial diagnostic impression of adjustment disorder with mixed disturbance of emotions and conduct.

Differential diagnosis of conditions not attributable to a mental disorder that are a focus of attention or treatment was ruled out because Tomas's reaction was in excess of normal and expectable adjustment and because his school functioning was showing signs of impairment. (In conditions not attributable to a mental disorder there would not be such impairment.) A personality disorder diagnosis was inappropriate as well, since Tomas's maladaptive reaction to the stressor was not within the context of his overall past development. Recommendation was made for sibling group therapy once a week plus family meetings every other week to help Tomas overcome his adjustment disorder with mixed disturbance of emotions and conduct.

INTRODUCTION

The individual's ability to handle separations during the course of life is inextricably linked to the etiologies of both mental health and psychopathology. There is first the awareness of being separate from the caregiver, driven by the onset of consciousness of the self. Later, as Tomas is painfully learning, separations from peers, parents, and possibly mates must be dealt with. Finally, the individual must come to terms with death—the separation from life itself.

The original template for learning to master separation is of course the *attachment bond,* the establishment and later modification of the early relationship between mother and infant (Trad, 1986, 1987, 1988). If the bond is secure, the child will respond organically to the pull of the mother's safety and the push of the opposing urge to explore the unknown environment. Eventually a balance will be struck between security and curiosity, and, optimally, the child will grow to feel secure away from his or her mother and come to devote most time to exploration and mastery.

It has long been believed that when this developmental process is interrupted, either by the loss of one or both parents or by sudden, prolonged separations such as beginning nursery school, the potential for the development of pathology may be greatly increased. In fact, parental loss has received the most attention in terms of being a risk factor for the later development of such conditions as depression, sociopathy, neuroses, and even schizophrenia (e.g., Barry & Lindemann, 1960; Brown & Epps, 1966; Brown & Harris, 1978; Granville-Grossman, 1966).

Perhaps because none of these studies has yielded definitive results (Tennant et al., 1980), many have argued that, at least in infants under 6 months of age, trauma from separation or loss cannot occur. In support of this contention, Kagan (1980, 1984) has theorized that interactions with the environment cannot have an effect over the long term except by *being registered through the aegis of cognition.* This is one plausible explanation for why the analyses of the long-term effects of early experiences have yielded few reliable data.

In opposition to such logical explanations is the fact that strong reactions to separation in young infants such as anaclitic depression have been well documented. Bowlby (1960) has been the principal proponent of the view that the responses of young infants to prolonged separation from the caregiver are very similar to those exhibited by adults who experience a loss. At first, infants exhibit a strong protest against the separation. This is followed, after varying periods of time, by despair. Finally, withdrawal and apathy set in to such an extent that the infant is indifferent if reunited with the caregiver.

The elements of this issue are revealed in the argument as to whether or not infants can experience bereavement. Freud (1926) stated that

> *Mourning occurs under the influence of reality-testing: for the latter function demands categorically from the bereaved person that he should separate himself from the object, since it no longer exists. Mourning is entrusted with the task of carrying out this retreat from the object in all those situations in which it was the recipient of a high degree of cathexis.* (p. 172)

This process is carried out by a mechanism in which "each single one of the memories and expectations in which the libido is bound to the object is brought and hypercathected, and detachment of the libido is accomplished in respect of it" (Freud, 1917, p. 245). When mourning is defined in this way, it hardly seems plausible to assume that infants are capable of the sustained stress and sophisticated understanding of object relations required to mourn.

Observations of the mourning process within a developmental framework also quickly reveal different dynamics in the coping strategies of children and adults once the events beyond the initial phases of protest, despair, and withdrawal are examined. Many researchers such as Shambaugh (1961) have noted children's use of primitive defensive mechanisms against loss. In his report of a 7-year-old boy whose mother had died, Shambaugh noted, among other reactions, denial, regression, and upheaval in object relationships over a period of more than a year. Shambaugh noted that "three factors, at least, separate a young child subject to an important loss from a bereaved adult: his real state of dependence on adults, his not yet fully incorporated superego, and his relatively undeveloped ego" (1961, p. 521). The limitations brought about by these factors were apparent as early as 1937, when Deutsch (1937), after examining instances of the absence of grief in four cases of adults who had experienced parental death in childhood or adolescence, concluded that the child's ego puts in operation self-protective mechanisms in order to bear the strain.

Thus, as Miller (1971) observed, the reaction to loss in children seems to have a precise but different purpose from that of adults. Rather than learning gradually to disassociate from the lost person, the child "[strives to] avoid the acceptance of reality and emotional meaning of the death and maintains in some internal form the relationship that has been ended in external reality" (p. 701).

These observations have also been supported by such investigators as Wolfenstein (1966), who retrospectively reported her psychoanalytic work with adults who experienced the loss of a parent in childhood or adolescence. The cases of adult pathological grieving seemed to have their roots in unresolved or unevolved childhood mechanisms against the loss. A defensive splitting of the ego can occur and persist, one in which the superficial acknowledgment of the parent's death remains isolated from wishes or expectations that the dead person will return. Thus, the reality testing remains impaired and the emotional pain goes unresolved.

In speculating on the mechanisms by which reality testing can continue to be impaired, Buchsbaum (1987) emphasized the importance of variability in memory. Memories of the parent are vital to the bereaved child because they cushion the loss, allowing the child to retain a portion of the internal consistency needed to continue the narcissistic self-nurturance inherent in normal development. Buchsbaum agreed with Pollock's (1978) approach, believing that mourning is possible in childhood, but it must be defined in terms of the particular child's affective, defensive, and cognitive capabilities. As Buchsbaum pointed out, one of the most important determinants of children's ability to cope with a loss depends on the as yet unanswered question of whether early memories retain the features characteristic of the age at the time of loss or whether they are progressively incorporated into age-appropriate schemas.

Although it is not conclusive or entirely illuminating, preliminary evidence from a 10-year prospective study by Wallerstein (1984) has shed some light on the relationship between memory and early loss. This study drew on a population of 131 children between $2\frac{1}{2}$ and 6 years of age who came from 60 divorcing families. Of these, 30 children were evaluated in the period following divorce and were then interviewed along with 40 of their parents 10 years after the event.

Few children retained conscious memories of the intact family or even of the period of marital rupture. However, for a significant portion (30%), the divorce itself (i.e., the fact that there was a major upheaval resulting in permanent change, regardless of whether or not the specifics were retained in conscious memory) remained as a central aspect of their lives. Economic deprivation was a major theme, as was the tendency to envision (imagine) the loss of what would have been a happier, more nurturing life. Many still had fantasies of reconciliation.

Indicative of the importance of developmental variables, particularly that of cognition, was the finding that the younger children in this study showed significantly less trauma in association with the divorce than did the older children. Wallerstein has noted that this is somewhat surprising in light of the fact that it was the younger children who showed the greater distress at the actual time of the break-up. As will be discussed later, results such as these suggest that divorce per se may not be the direct cause of poor social outcome in children. Rather, it may be that other factors such as punishment techniques or familial discord prior to the divorce are more directly responsible.

Given the problem of definition, the ambiguity of the data, and the inherent differences between the developmental and adult contexts, it seems wise to focus attention less on the issue of whether children and adults experience grief in a similar or dissimilar way and more on the sequelae of childhood defensive techniques against loss. Indeed, as early as 1963, Bowlby acknowledged that a significant number of the characteristics of "one or another variant of pathological mourning in adults are found to be almost the rule in the ordinary mourning responses of young children" (p. 521).

In studying the consequences of loss in infancy and childhood with a view toward specific defense mechanisms, developmental factors such as age, sex, extent of loss, and many others move into the foreground. In order to further enhance understanding, these factors will be discussed in relation to three levels of loss or separation—peer separation, loss of a parent through divorce, and loss of a parent through death.

PHENOMENA RELATED TO SCHOOL SEPARATION FROM PEERS AND CAREGIVERS

Social Importance

An examination of the dynamics and consequences of the less dramatic trauma of separation from peers (as opposed to caregivers) can provide a background for studying the sequelae of the increasingly severe shocks of partial separation from a parent via divorce and total loss due to death. While the developmental impact of child care outside the home has always attracted attention, it is doing so at an ever-increasing rate at present, since one out of every two children in the United States is currently receiving some form of this care (Phillips, McCartney, & Scarr, 1987).

Among the many factors related to child rearing in nursery-type facilities, the effect on prosocial behaviors has generated the greatest concern and the greatest research effort. Again, this interest is likely to increase, since it is projected that by 1990 75% of all mothers will work and there will be 10.5 million children in need of day care (Schindler,

Moely, & Frank, 1987; Urban Institute, 1980). In general, studies to date have claimed that in comparison with children reared at home those with day-care experience demonstrate more effective peer interaction, better communication, more advanced levels of play and perspective taking, more confidence in social interactions, enhanced cooperative behavior, and better task orientation (Clarke-Stewart, 1984; Cochran, 1977; O'Connell & Farran, 1982; Ramey, MacPhee, & Yeates, 1982; Rubenstein & Howes, 1979; Trad, 1987, 1988). On the other hand, children with day-care experience have been reported to be more likely to exhibit aggressive behavior (physical and verbal), be less cooperative with adults, and display negative affect (Haskins, 1985; Ramey, Dorval, & Baker-Ward, 1981; Rubenstein, Howes, & Boyle, 1981; Schwarz, Krolick, & Strickland, 1973; Schwarz, Strickland, & Krolick, 1974).

There are several plausible explanations for these findings, none of which has been proved as yet. Schwarz and co-workers (1974) wisely pointed out that in many studies it is impossible to ascribe the observed effects strictly to the day-care setting. The differences may well have appeared as a result of sampling bias. Nevertheless, the increased aggressive activity and reduced cooperation with adults frequently seen in day-care children might be due to an inhibitory effect of substitute care on general socialization. This might occur because the repeated separations from the primary caregiver necessitated by day care impair the mother-infant relationship and thereby hinder the socialization process.

The increased play activities and decreased exploration exhibited by day-care versus home-care children might be the result of the differences in architectural and social milieus between the home and the day-care facility (Cochran, 1977). The home, with its multilevel purposes of resting, entertaining, eating, and so forth, provides a rich environment conducive to exploration—especially in the presence of the mother, who, under normal conditions, provides a secure basis from which the child can set out to explore. The day-care setting, by contrast, is structured more rigidly to suit the purposes of limited child care. Thus, not only does this setting lack the security of the mother, which is conducive to exploration, there is in fact much less to explore.

Support for this interpretation comes from a study by Schindler and colleagues (1987), in which day care was seen to have beneficial effects. Children in three different day-care centers were studied. The centers varied widely in terms of location, program characteristics, and populations served. In this experiment, child age and sex were held constant in order to assess the relationship between time in care and social participation.

In general, the findings showed that extended day care had a positive impact on social interaction and development. With age and sex held constant in order to separate the effects of time in care from those of maturation, general experience, or gender-related role learning, increases in associative play activity and concomitant decreases in onlooker and unoccupied behaviors were observed as a function of increasing time in care. While these results are encouraging in terms of the growing trend toward placing children in day-care facilities, other studies have not substantiated these findings.

One of the few definitive findings regarding day care relates to its value in preserving or enhancing cognitive function in high-risk, economically disadvantaged children. Experience in a day-care facility appears to attenuate the declines in test scores that are typically associated with high-risk children after 18 months of age (Golden & Birns, 1976).

Belsky, Steinberg, and Walker (1982) and Belsky and Steinberg (1978), in their extensive and analytic reviews of the literature to date, pointed to several weaknesses in research methodologies that have led to the current lack of definitive information regarding the effects of day care on the preschool population. Unlike the study by Schindler and colleagues (1987), most studies have focused on high-quality, research-affiliated centers rather than sampling preschool facilities on a random basis. Furthermore, the great majority of studies have relied on standardized tests of intellectual and social development whose usefulness in comprehending development in real-life settings has frequently been called into question.

Belsky and co-workers also stressed the need to examine other, as yet neglected, features of the caregiving environment. They suggested that to obtain more useful and complete data it may prove useful to employ Bronfenbrenner's (1977, 1979) ecological approach to the study of day care. This approach, utilizing a concentric-circle model of the ecology of human development containing the micro-, meso-, exo-, and macro-systems, will permit coordinated inquiry at several levels of analysis. The microsystem is any immediate setting that contains the child. The mesosystem represents the interrelation of these settings. The exosystem is the formal and informal social structures that do not contain the child but impinge on the child's immediate surroundings. Finally, the macrosystem represents the overreaching patterns of ideology and organization that are characteristic of a particular culture or subculture.

According to Belsky and co-workers (Belsky et al., 1982; Belsky & Steinberg, 1978), until a substantial body of literature based on an ecological approach has been developed, definitive conclusions regarding the effects of day care will be difficult to come by. Based on their review of the literature, the only conclusions that appear justified at the present time apply largely to high-quality day-care centers. Thus far, care in these centers does not appear to help or hinder intellectual development, does not disrupt the child's emotional bond with the mother, and increases the degree to which the child interacts, both negatively and positively, with peers.

Separation from Peers

The generally poorly defined results of the many studies of child care illustrate the fact that the various factors contributing to the day-care experience have yet to be isolated and analyzed sufficiently. Outside the realm of mother-child interaction, even less is known about the effects of separation from peers.

However, observations of peer separations in both young primates and young children do suggest that loss or separation from peers is often stressful (Freud & Dann, 1951; Reite, Harbeck, & Hoffman, 1981; Suomi et al., 1976). In one attempt to resolve some of the issues of peer separation, Field and colleagues (1984) studied the play behaviors and sleep patterns of 12 infants who were 15 months old and 20 toddlers aged 24 months. The infants and toddlers were observed during the first and fourth weeks of the months preceding and following graduation to a new nursery class.

The changes in behavior noted in this study were similar to those cited in many studies for mother-child separations. There were increases in negative affect, activity level, physical aggression, and sleep disturbance, which were attributed to stress due to peer separation. As Field and colleagues pointed out, these reactions have also been noted in primates who are separated from their peers, but only after separation has occurred. In this study, however, the authors emphasized their observation that the toddlers manifested behavioral changes before separation, while the infants did not react until after separation.

Thus, it appears that "sometime late in infancy the necessary cognitive development has occurred for children to experience anticipatory reactions to separation stress" (Field et al., 1984, p. 283). The fact that toddlers feel sufficiently threatened by peer separation to develop anticipatory defenses and reactions argues in favor of considering this variable to be an important one in the day-care milieu.

The legitimacy of studying peer separations was demonstrated in another study by Field (1984). The behaviors of 28 preschool children who had been together for between 2 and 4 years were observed during the 2-week period prior to their transfer to a new school. These observations were compared to the behaviors they exhibited 3 months earlier and to the behaviors of children remaining in the school.

During the 2 weeks prior to leaving the school, teachers' questionnaires revealed an increase in the incidence of absenteeism, toileting accidents, failure to eat lunches, and difficulty sleeping during nap time. These observations were in general agreement with those of parents, who noted increases in illness, fussiness, eating changes, and disordered sleep and toileting.

An interesting finding in this study, and one that further emphasizes the stress inherent in peer separation, was that a greater number of children who remained at the school, according to parent reports, showed more unusual fussiness, sleep disturbances, and illness than those who had transferred to new schools. Field suggested that this increased agitation might represent a coping response to separation in an environment that is suffused with cues of the losses associated with separation. Thus, separation from peers appears to be a powerful factor operating to govern the behavior not only of those who are leaving but of those who must stay as well.

Ellen: Unhappy with School

Ellen is a $3\frac{1}{2}$-year-old girl who lives with her mother, her father, and her 6-week-old sister. Ellen was the product of her mother's second pregnancy; the first ended in miscarriage. Ellen was delivered by cesarian section at 40 weeks. Her parents describe her developmental milestones as within normal ranges. While Ellen's mother was in the 8th month of her pregnancy with her second child, Ellen's maternal grandfather was diagnosed with rectal cancer. Ellen's mother is currently pressed to return to work because the family is under financial strain; she has not worked since 5 months before Ellen's birth. Ellen's parents describe her as a cheerful child who began attending nursery school 1 month ago. At this time, they also initiated a search for day-care placement for their infant when Ellen's mother begins working. Ellen's behavior toward her baby sister is mixed. At times she is playful and gentle, but at other times she has picked up her sister and dropped her, and she has hit her several times. Her parents' reaction to Ellen's aggression toward her sister has been to restrict her access to the infant when possible and to teach her proper ways to interact with the baby.

In addition to her parents' nervousness about Ellen's handling of her sister, Ellen's teacher has indicated concern about her behavior in school. First, Ellen has tantrums when her parents drop her off at school, and these take anywhere from a few minutes to an hour to subside. Second, Ellen expresses much worry that something will happen to her parents and her sister while she is at school. She has behaved aggressively toward other children in class too, hitting them and taking toys from them. Her teacher says that Ellen clings to adults at the school and has trouble separating when assigned any activity. At home, Ellen sometimes has tantrums or complains of feeling sick when it is time to go to school. Lately, she has demanded that her mother stay in her room with her when it is time to go to sleep, and she awakens during the night from nightmares about her parents being killed in an accident.

At her teacher's suggestion and due to her parents' concerns, Ellen was referred for psychiatric evaluation. During the assessment interview, Ellen was slow to let her mother leave the room, and after finally allowing her to leave, she insisted on running to the waiting room several times during the interview to make sure she was okay. Ellen's motor behavior and speech were within the normal ranges, and she displayed a full range of affects. She demonstrated an intact sense of reality. All other elements of her mental status were also judged to be normal. She talked about her sister, indicating ambivalence toward her. Discussion with Ellen's mother revealed that both she and her husband are under much stress due to the responsibilities of a new baby, the recent diagnosis of Ellen's grandfather's cancer, and the financial strain pushing Ellen's mother back to work.

Ellen's symptoms indicate that she has separation anxiety disorder, which was precipitated by the stress of starting nursery school. The feelings of tension and anxiety in separating from her parents when left at school and from her teachers when in school, her refusal to go to sleep without an adult present, her physical complaints when it is time for school, and her excessive worry about something happening to her parents and sister while she is away are all common symptoms in separation anxiety disorder. It seems that Ellen reacts to the frustration of separation and the reduction in attention she receives at home due to her sister's birth through aggressive acts, although they are too restricted and isolated to be considered part of an additional diagnosis of conduct disorder. Her anxiety is restricted to her fear of separation and was therefore not judged to be part of overanxious disorder. Panic disorder with agoraphobia was also ruled out because Ellen does not experience panic attacks. Because she evidences no psychotic symptoms and her developmental level is age-appropriate, her maladaptive behavior was not assessed to be related either to pervasive developmental disorder or to schizophrenia. Major depression was also ruled out as a possible diagnosis because Ellen does not display characteristic symptoms of that disorder, such as disturbed appetite, self-doubt, and so forth.

Thus, a diagnosis of separation anxiety, related both to the stresses experienced at home and to starting school, has been assigned. Dyadic counseling of Ellen and her mother has been recommended, with emphasis on modeling limit-setting strategies and supportive techniques.

School Separation from Caregivers

Just as separation from peers at an early age can have a profoundly stressing influence, temporary daily separations from caregivers are also potentially stressing, and they can influence the child's affect and learning ability during the separation. This certainly seems to be a risk in Ellen's case, considering the intensity of her reaction. Field and co-workers (1984) observed the leave-taking and reunion behaviors of 56 infants, toddlers, preschoolers, and their parents as the children were dropped off and picked up before and after nursery school each day.

Toddlers displayed distress behaviors more frequently than any other group, and those who were dropped off by mothers rather than fathers showed more attention-getting behavior and crying. Furthermore, of significance to the upcoming discussion on loss through divorce, mothers engaged in more "distracting the child" behaviors and showed a longer latency in leaving the classroom.

This dynamic changed during the second semester, when parents and children spent less time relating to each other during leave taking. The children protested departures less frequently, and the parents left the classroom more quickly. While these phenomena did show some habituation in toddlers, *they never completely abated* despite experience with daily leave takings since infancy.

Distress behaviors also diminished significantly in infants, but they showed increasing amounts of clinging and hovering across the two semesters. Field and co-workers noted that these facts taken together suggest that "proximity-maintaining behaviors may be more influenced by developmental age than by amount of experience with leave-takings" (p. 634). Thus, in this study, leave-taking and reunion behaviors were segregated along with the variables of the child's age, sex, and duration of time in the school, as well as the sex of the parent.

In another study, Bloom-Feshbach and Blatt (1981) observed separation and adaptation to nursery school in 20 3-year-old children, emphasizing the need to view separation difficulties in terms of when they occur and how they are expressed. These investigators found that separation distress during the first 2 weeks correlates well with distress during the next 2 weeks. Thus, separation anxiety may easily last a month.

One element of the findings of this study may have relevance to the question of the relationship between separation stress during day care and later social outcome. Distress on entry in the early weeks was not seen to be related to stress during the second month. Therefore, the authors suggest, *separation distress manifested during the second month in school may be qualitatively different from that seen in the first month.* This may be especially true in light of the fact that distress at leave taking in the second month was associated with social-emotional problems of the "angry, defiant" type. Thus, there was a clear relationship between separation distress in the second month of school and later problematic social outcome. Furthermore, it might be inferred that children exhibiting distress in the second month were experiencing difficulty in their attachment bonds.

In assessing the contributions of stress resulting from separation from both peers and parents in nursery school, it appears at this time that peer separation may function generally as one of many normal environmental stressors. As long as other support is not unduly removed, the child should continue to function well. This appears to be true in the case of parental separation as well. However, because of the intense and intricate dynamics of the child-parent dyad, problems in separation/individuation occurring within the family outside the context of day care are likely to be exacerbated by the forced separation of school attendance.

SEPARATION DUE TO PARENTAL DIVORCE

Depression: A Possible Underlying Pathway to Pathology

As demonstrated in the study by Bloom-Feshbach and Blatt (1981), the relatively minor separations entailed in day-care attendance can prove problematic. Loss due to parental death or divorce or separation may have even more dire consequences. However, regardless of the relative severity of deviant social outcome, a study by Handford, Mattison, Humphrey, and McLaughlin (1986) has suggested that difficulties associated with separation may have a common pathway: depression due to the disruption of a highly valuable support system.

Handford and colleagues (1986) studied 105 boys and girls 8 to 16 years of age who had experienced the loss of one or both parents by death, divorce, or parental separation. The children were assessed for depressive syndrome, based on the Children's Depression Inventory (CDI), 9 months apart — first on admission to a private residential school and then at the end of the first school term. None of the children displayed any major medical, educational, or behavioral problems in their past histories.

Of the 105 children assessed, 31% were identified via the CDI as having a depressive syndrome 6 weeks after beginning their first year in a new residential school. At follow-up 9 months later, the depressed children had not adjusted as well as those in whom the CDI had not detected depression. Further, those who were depressed in the beginning of the year continued to have more self-rated depression and anxiety symptoms and more overall psychopathology.

Handford and co-workers observed that many of the children who were found to be depressed might have had a true primary depressive disorder or perhaps dysthymia. However, the CDI was not sensitive enough to differentiate these cases from those who might have had a depressive syndrome secondary to some other psychiatric disorder or from those who might have had an extended adjustment disorder resembling major depression.

Still, despite the nuances of etiology, the authors concluded that "children with similar life experiences who are entering a residential school such as the program in this study can be effectively screened with the

CDI to identify that group needing further evaluation and appropriate therapeutic intervention" (p. 413).

The detection of depression in 31% of the children studied by Handford and colleagues might provide a plausible explanation for the results obtained in a prospective study by Wallerstein and Kelly (1976), using an even younger population. These investigators followed 34 preschool children aged $2\frac{1}{2}$ to 6 years for 1 year following the divorce of their parents. At the time of the 1-year interview, 44% were found to be in significantly worsened psychological condition.

This sample was drawn from a normal family population (Marin County, California) with no previous psychiatric histories. Prior to the disruption of the family, all of the children were believed by their parents to be within the normal range of development. In addition to the finding that 15 (44%) of these children deteriorated noticeably following the divorce—a finding that may reflect the presence of depression in these children—there were certain patterns of response to divorce that were broadly age-specific and were also related to developmental and cognitive maturity.

In the youngest group ($2\frac{1}{2}$ to $3\frac{1}{2}$ years), the response to family disruption was characterized by regressions, fretfulness, cognitive bewilderment, heightened aggression, and neediness, the latter being the most enduring symptom. In the middle group ($3\frac{3}{4}$ to $4\frac{3}{4}$ years), reactions to divorce were apparently linked to superego development, demonstrating damage to the child's self-esteem and self-image. In the oldest group ($4\frac{3}{4}$ to 6 years), the divorce was handled with greater efficiency. Developmental stride was not broken and these children, for the most part, were able to generate some social distance between themselves and their parents. Significantly, for the most vulnerable children in all three groups (44% of the sample), poor outcome was associated with depressed state.

Social and Methodological Considerations

The existence of depression and related pathologies in children who endure parental divorce is of considerable social importance. It is estimated that 40 to 50% of children born in the 1970's will spend at least some time in a single-parent family (Hetherington, Cox, & Cox, 1979).

As is the case in nursery-school separations, reactions to loss due to divorce are highly dependent on developmental variables. In dealing with divorce situations, children must attempt to identify the motives of their parents and, in a sense, "divorce" themselves as being causative factors or from feelings of rejection. They must also experience some degree of control over the resolution of the situation if development is not to be seriously hampered.

In assessing the routes toward achieving these goals, Kurdek and Berg (1983) stressed the importance of understanding the divorce-related experiences of children within a hierarchically organized context of cultural, social, familial, and psychological variables. That is, assessments should focus on the following factors:

1. Cultural beliefs, values, and attitudes about family life.
2. The stability of the postdivorce environment and the social supports available to the restructured single-parent family.
3. The character of family interactions during the pre- and postseparation periods.
4. The individual competence of the child for dealing with stress.

In attempting to incorporate at least some elements of this hierarchical context, Wallerstein and Kelly (1980) performed a 5-year longitudinal study of 131 children from 60 divorcing families. They found that there is cause to question the assumption commonly held by many in the mental health and legal communities that the parent-child relationship that begins in a marriage is likely to endure past parental separation. In this study, men who had previously been very close to their children tended to visit sporadically after separation, while those who had previously responded to their children with indifference or annoyance began a surprising new level of interaction with them.

The dynamics behind this pattern were difficult to unravel. However, the changes were both age- and sex-related. Father-daughter relationships remained more stable over time, while father-son relationships were twice as likely to change over time. Further considerations were that the younger children experienced the disappearance of their father in "magical" terms, being happy to see, on visitation, that their fathers had refrigerators and television sets just like at home but fearing that the other parent might disappear at any moment as well.

Another methodological consideration emphasized by Wallerstein and Kelly was that paternal visitation patterns do not necessarily reflect the attitude of the father toward his child or children. Men who felt guilty about terminating their marriages had great difficulty in initiating and maintaining their visitations. This dynamic led to feelings of rejection on the part of the child.

Such dynamics in the complex milieu of a divorcing family can confound research results. This illustrates the necessity for both a hierarchical approach to research and scrupulous attention to the assumptions and needs of a child during the transition. Regarding the latter consideration, Kurdek and Berg (1983) reviewed the literature and identified several factors that alleviated adjustment problems within the contexts of social, emotional, and cognitive development: minimal depletion of financial resources, low levels of conflict and hostility between parents both before and after the divorce, cooperative parenting between former spouses, approval and love from both parents, authoritative discipline from the custodial parent, regular visitation by the noncustodial parent, and ample opportunity for the child to discuss and explore the reasons for and likely outcomes of the divorce.

SEPARATION DUE TO PARENTAL DEATH

Ian: Understandable Sadness

Ian is a 5-year-old boy who lives with his mother. A week ago, his father, a long-time heroin addict, died of an apparently accidental overdose. His parents had lived together until about a year ago, and Ian saw his father on weekends and on most holidays after the separation. Before the separation, the parents engaged in frequent verbal fights that Ian heard. Ian does not know that his father had a drug problem, and he interpreted his father's inconsistent behavior as a symptom of his having "a lot of problems." According to Ian and his mother, when Ian and his father were together, his father would cry and elicit emotional support from Ian. Ian said that he felt the need to ("I have to ...") help his father both to feel better emotionally and to improve his poor self-esteem. Since his father's death, Ian has behaved as before, except for occasionally reporting that he feels "sad." His kindergarten teacher has reported no overall change in Ian's school demeanor, although she did say that he told her about his father's death and said that it makes him feel sad sometimes. Ian's mother sought psychiatric assessment because she feared he might have difficulty coping with his father's death.

During assessment, Ian was alert and communicated remarkably clearly regarding his sad feelings about his father's death. He recounted events he participated in with his father prior to his death, such as going to a toy store and playing in a park. He told the clinician that it was his mother's wish for his parents to separate and that he suspected his mother was "hiding" something from him that was relevant to the circumstances surrounding his father's death. Ian stated that he would never see his father again, indicating his mature comprehension of one of the realities of death. Ian's attention and concentration were intact, and he exhibited no indications of either hallucinations or delusions. All other elements of the mental status examination were also judged to be within normal limits.

Ian's reaction to his father's death includes occasional and well-circumscribed sadness—which is a normal response to death of a loved one—without additional associated problems. Thus, from his present mental status, the clinician could infer that he is undergoing uncomplicated bereavement. Although his condition is not, at present, debilitating, the clinician recommended therapy sessions to monitor Ian. With uncomplicated bereavement, the concern is that Ian might begin to feel excessively guilty about or responsible for his father's death, especially because Ian expressed a responsibility for meeting his father's emotional needs. Other symptoms that might develop in Ian are insomnia, feelings of worthlessness, or wishes for his own death. These and other symptoms could develop unchecked, allowing the mourning process to become complicated and develop into, perhaps, a major depression. Therefore, while Ian currently exhibits what seems to be an appropriate adjustment to his father's death, it is imperative that he be observed and evaluated periodically for the next several months—the span of time within which uncomplicated bereavement most commonly is disturbed.

Reactive Mechanisms and the Variable of Age

Studies that have attempted to unravel the relationships between early loss and pathological outcome have yet to produce definitive results (Tennant, Bebbington, & Hurry, 1980). Nevertheless, a childhood history of the death or loss of a parent is common in adult psychiatric and social morbidity (Raphael, 1982), which leads to the speculation that relatively mild reactions like Ian's are in the minority. As discussed previously, depression in response to loss may be the substrate underlying development of other social pathologies (Birtchnell, 1972). Susceptibility to depression after losing someone whose existence is so closely tied to survival is certainly understandable.

However, the amount of time that may pass before all manifestations of loss are evident, the many hierarchical variables involved, and the numerous disruptions that occur with death in a family make it very difficult to assess the potential for later pathology. Nevertheless, it seems safe to say that while the child may well grieve in a manner similar to that of an adult (Bowlby, 1969; Elizur & Kaffman, 1982), he or she is not as well equipped intellectually and emotionally to handle the strong feelings involved. This inability is where the risk for future pathology resides.

Rather than engaging in repeated reality testing in order to disengage from an object that no longer exists, the child initially denies the loss and only gradually comes to resolution—a resolution that must march very much in step with the growth of the child's cognitive and emotional capacities (Miller, 1971). It is not difficult to see that there may be many traps along the way in which the child is at risk of becoming "stuck" or at the very least misguided, especially since the surviving parent may well be too consumed with his or her own grieving process to properly educate the child.

Thus, age, or at least the stage of development, may well be the primary factor influencing the child's adaption to loss of a parent (Trad, 1986). Unfortunately, the puzzle is so intricate that research is not consistent on this point either (Kurdek & Berg, 1983). However, the comprehensive study by Elizur and Kaffmann (1982) has served to illustrate the general dynamics of children's response to loss between the ages of 2 and 10 years.

Elizur and Kaffman observed the behavioral changes of 25 normal children, aged 2 to 10, living in a kibbutz over a period of $3\frac{1}{2}$ years following the deaths of their fathers in war. Data were drawn from interviews with the children's mothers and their teachers. Questions were asked to note any symptoms that were present before the bereavement in order to establish a pretraumatic baseline for each child.

A measure of pathological bereavement was used that applied to children who met the following criteria:

1. The presence of multiple, persistent clinical symptomatology severe enough to handicap the child in everyday life. The abnormal impairment must have persisted for at least 2 months following the loss.
2. The independent and concordant estimate by the mother and teacher on one side and the investigators on the other that the child needed psychological care.

Even within the social context of the supportive kibbutz environment, the experience of parental loss was profound. Mourning reactions observed in the children included sobbing and crying; expressions of sadness and longing; remembering the deceased father by recalling shared experiences, imitating him, talking to his photographs, and using his personal effects; denial of the fact of death; avoidance of the subject of death; or other coping reactions such as preoccupation with the theme of the nature of death or a search for a substitute father. These reactions are analogous to those noted in case studies by Barnes (1964) and Shambaugh (1961).

While the specific grief reactions decreased over time, there was a persistently high rate of behavior problems throughout the entire follow-up period. These problems included essentially every type of known childhood behavioral and emotional problem (overdependent behavior, night fears, withdrawal, rejection of strangers, "exemplary" behavior, enuresis, aggressive behavior, etc.).

More than 40% of the children showed clinical evidence of pathological bereavement, while less than a third were able to achieve adequate adjustment with regard to family and school. The two most common clusters of disorders were the overanxious-dependent type and the unsocial-aggressive type. The fact that there were no clear-cut boundaries between these clusters illustrates the fact that, as Elizur and Kaffman noted, "the bereavement reaction is not a set of symptoms which start after the loss and gradually fade away. Rather, it involves a succession of clinical pictures which blend into and replace one another" (1982, p. 477).

This study illustrates the fact that early loss of a parent is indeed a destabilizing event that could well place a child at risk for later behavioral pathology. The dynamics underlying the reactions of each child, however, are extremely difficult to detect and repair. At this point in time it seems advisable to concentrate on detecting abnormal levels of disturbance and supplying extra support to the child, both in the form of adult attachments and, if necessary, psychotherapy (Trad, 1987).

As Rutter (1980) pointed out, this approach is necessitated by the fact that it is still unknown whether the problems emanate from the disruption of bonds or the distortion of relationships. In this regard, Rutter noted that delinquency rates for boys with parents who had separated or divorced are much higher than for boys who lost a parent by death. Thus, it appears that discord within the family, rather than the family's dissolution, is the prime contributor to antisocial behavior, since delinquency is primarily associated with breaks that follow parental discord and not with the loss of a parent as such.

Block, Block, and Gjerde (1986) performed a prospective study that bears out the conclusions of Rutter. The personalities of children from 41 families who would later experience divorce or separation were assessed before and after family dissolution and compared at identical ages to the personalities of children from 60 families who remained intact. Comprehensive individual assessments were carried out at ages 3, 4, 5, 7, 11, and 14. Mothers and fathers were also included in the assessment.

Supporting the conclusions of Rutter (1980), Block and co-workers found that their descriptions of boys prior to parental divorce were very similar to those by others of children following divorce. In other words, the seeds for disordered behavior were present prior to the divorce and were generated by strained relationships within the family. Before divorce, the behavior of the boys was characterized by aggression, impulsivity, and an abundance of misguided energy.

As in nearly all other studies in this area, Block and co-workers noted far more disturbance in boys than in girls, both before and after family upheaval. The tendency of males to succumb more readily to psychological stress may be related, as Rutter (1980) has speculated, to the well-known fact that males are much more susceptible to biological stress. On the other hand, Block and colleagues (1986) have speculated that the basis for the sex difference may lie in the notion of differential parental salience. If, as Lamb (1981) stated, the bond between father and son is stronger than that between father and daughter, the lesser saliency of the father might attenuate the effects of parental disagreements for the girl. For sons, however, disagreements might be more anxiety inducing, since both parents are equally salient and arguments could thus generate conflicting loyalties.

While these explanations of the widely observed sexual difference in destabilization in boys versus girls might be plausible, Block and colleagues have generally agreed with Emery (1982) who stated, "Girls are likely to be just as troubled by marital turmoil as boys are, but they may demonstrate their feelings in a manner that is more appropriate to their sex role, namely, by becoming anxious, withdrawn, or perhaps very well-behaved" (p. 317).

Emery (1982) further summed up the argument in favor of the contention that parental conflict, and not separation from a parent, is the major contributor to negative outcome in children by citing the results of three groups of studies. First, as noted earlier by Rutter, more serious childhood problems exist in divorced families than in those experiencing a loss through death. A second group of studies showed that a child from a broken but conflict-free home is less likely to develop problems than a child from a family that is unbroken but full of strife. Finally, children of divorced parents who continue to fight after the divorce are observed to have more trouble than children from low-conflict divorces.

In light of these acknowledged trends, as well as the results of their own study, Block and colleagues stated that "the examination of families only after the divorce formally has occurred is a demonstrably insufficient means of fully comprehending the complex interpersonal processes influencing character development" (1986, p. 837).

CONCLUSION

As Freud (1915) pointed out, the loss of a parent or peer carries potentially more trouble than the simple loss of support. On the one hand, loved ones are "an inner possession, components of our own ego; but on the other hand they are partly strangers, even enemies. With the exception of only a very few situations, there adheres to the tenderest and most intimate of our love relations a small portion of hostility which can excite an unconscious death wish" (p. 298).

The potential for devastation following parental loss is even greater if the death occurs in synchrony with the normal child's sporadic impulse to wish a parent dead. Independent of this issue, however, Johnson and Rosenblatt (1981) have stressed the importance of differentiating between true cases of incomplete grief, which has continuity with the grieving state experienced immediately after the loss, and sporadic bouts with grief that arise later out of new experiences and thinking. It is important to realize that as the bereaved child matures he or she will discover previously unrecognized areas of loss and that this process is far from pathological.

In terms of the current understanding of the relationship between loss and disturbed behavior, perhaps Rutter (1980) has offered the best summation. Observing that while antisocial disorders seem largely related to family discord rather than divorce, separation, or death, Rutter pointed out that the psychological mechanisms mediating the interaction of family discord with the child's temperamental traits to produce the unproductive behavior are still unknown.

Rutter did suggest three possible mechanisms that need further exploration. First, data from retrospective and prospective studies alike indicate that the parents of delinquent boys employ a different approach to discipline and the supervision of their children than those of nondelinquent boys. Second, the well-known imitative capacities of young children make them very susceptible to learning aggressive behavior if an aggressive model operates in the home. The third possibility is that difficulties in interpersonal relationships may evolve in families with stressful intrafamilial interactions since the child's main avenue for learning social behavior is through a warm, stable relationship with parental figures.

Part V

Management

CHAPTER TWENTY-FOUR

Psychodynamic Interventions with Preschool Children

INTRODUCTION

Broadly speaking, the goal of individual psychotherapy is to allow pre-schoolers the opportunity for releasing, communicating, and coordinating their thoughts and feelings within a predictable and empathic environment. Over all, the child is helped to develop individuation, affective regulation, and impulse control and to separate fantasy from reality. Meeting these goals helps the child strengthen the internal structure of the sense of self. Because play provides children with a means through which they can represent fantasy and feelings, it is an important element in therapy. Pretend play episodes are one of the prime windows through which the therapist can perceive the child's inner panorama. Therapy helps the child regulate emotional distress, and it is also useful in promoting social, emotional, and cognitive development. Thus, the therapeutic situation gives the child the opportunity to practice and master skills in each of these areas.

Psychodynamic strategies focus primarily on supporting and/or interpreting the child's behaviors during treatment sessions. The goal is to help the child to gradually reveal subconscious feelings and thoughts. The therapeutic situation aims at supporting the child's affective states while enhancing cognitive skills. Labeling his or her feelings gives the child the opportunity to reason about them, thereby allowing an understanding of cause and effect. With continuous practice, the child learns to use cognitive skills to cope appropriately within the developmental context.

Interpretation of transference and countertransference phenomena is the major psychoanalytic instrument used to promote change. These phenomena are the unconscious recapitulation and projection of the thoughts and feelings of one party in the therapeutic context onto another party. Transference reactions give access to the foundations of conflict and provide the basis for interpretations. The therapist should be careful to forge the therapeutic alliance in such a way as to promote a positive transference and prevent the development of resistance on the part of the child. Elements such as accepting the child for who he or she is and allowing the child to take the lead in an uninhibited atmosphere can help in this respect.

STRUCTURING THE THERAPEUTIC ALLIANCE

Alliance means that the child and therapist are working together toward specific therapeutic goals. On the other hand, if the therapist and/or the child are opposed, or try to impose a personal agenda, then a misalliance will occur. During the course of therapy, confrontations and conflicts between patient and therapist will inevitably arise. The specific action the therapist takes during such situations will determine whether the patient and therapist can build an alliance or will become misallied.

Occasionally, the therapist is faced with a child who displays an affective demeanor that makes it difficult to communicate, whereas another child may comply with the therapy too adeptly. The therapist should be aware that the child who is too well behaved may be momentarily repressing symptoms in order to prevent therapeutic interventions (Gardner, 1979).

A strong therapeutic relationship between the child and therapist is a prerequisite for all subsequent work. In order for transference and countertransference to yield therapeutic profit, the therapist must plan and structure the relationship that is to exist with the child. Axline (1964a) argued that the success or failure of therapy depends to a large extent on the way in which the therapeutic alliance has been structured. An adequate structure provides the child with a means for understanding and defining the boundaries of his or her own personal needs. Otherwise, the lack of boundary distinctions and the interplay between past and present expectations, objective danger and neurotic anxiety, and wish and fantasy will overwhelm the child. If an alliance that promotes adaptation has not been created, the therapist may not be able to interpret the child's behaviors and communicate such interpretations to the child. In addition, a child who does not perceive the therapist as an ally may resist ventilating and expressing himself or herself in therapy. As Frankl and Hellman (1964) noted, the basis for therapy lies within the therapist's access to the child's subconscious transferences, so it is crucial that the therapist establish a positive therapeutic alliance that promotes such communication. Failure to do so dooms the therapeutic situation.

This section underscores the interactions that foster the therapeutic alliance. An examination of how resistances emerge and their effect on the formation of a therapeutic alliance will also be examined.

Principles

Axline (1964b) has defined the following principles for nondirective therapeutic alliances:

1. A benevolent relationship is established between the therapist and the child.
2. The therapist accepts the child for who he or she is.
3. The therapist creates an atmosphere in which the child is given the freedom to express himself or herself without inhibition.

4. The therapist is able to identify the child's feelings and counter-transfer them to the child, so that the child learns to identify his or her own feelings.

5. The therapist recognizes that, under certain circumstances, the child is able to solve his or her own conflicts and should be allowed to do so. The child, not the therapist, is responsible for introducing change.

6. The therapist follows the child's lead, making no attempt to direct and manipulate the child's behaviors.

7. The therapist realizes that therapy proceeds gradually. Therefore, the therapist does not hasten its end.

8. The therapist sets only those boundaries necessary to ground the therapy in reality and give the child an awareness of his or her responsibility to the therapeutic alliance.

Gardner (1979) has suggested five additional principles:

1. The therapist should be able to empathize with the child.

2. The therapist should be aware that if he or she misrepresents, the child may become aware of this eventually and lose trust and faith in the therapy.

3. If the situation arises, the therapist should be willing to confide in the child and validate the child's perceptions. The child, placed in such confidence by the therapist, will gain trust in the therapist and realize that the therapist is not a magician but an ordinary person with weaknesses.

4. If the therapist wants the child to express feelings and thoughts, then the therapist, too, must be willing to express himself or herself.

5. Given the fact that children would rather play than sit during therapy, the therapist should make the therapy an enjoyable and formative experience for the child.

Therapists should be aware that even though they follow the guidelines for the establishment of an alliance, it is still possible that a misalliance will occur.

The Role of Play in Individual Psychotherapy

During play, real-life conflicts and fears can be approached through symbolic representations that allow children to act them out without fear of repercussion (Harter, 1983b). In this fashion, play can aid the child by neutralizing the distress deriving from specific environmental circumstances (Barnett, 1984; Barnett & Storm, 1981; Erikson, 1940; A. Freud, 1946, 1962; Waelder, 1933; Winnicott, 1971). Barnett (1984) found that highly anxious children produced more fantasy and dramatic play than did the children with low anxiety, who tended to play at a more sensorimotor level. Thus, one of the primary values of play may be its capacity to alleviate emotional distress and consequently allow the child to master and achieve the skills needed to regulate distress in real life. Indeed, cognitive and emotional skills can be practiced and mastered during play situations, thus furthering the achievement of developmental skills.

Social, emotional, and cognitive play development must be carefully assessed before play therapy can be instituted. After mapping both the child's normal and pathological play behaviors, the therapist can continue to observe the individual deficits within the therapeutic setting and structure play situations to help resolve the child's internal conflicts. Once the therapeutic goals have been achieved, the modified behaviors and interests are transferred to the child's current and future environment and life experiences.

Amster (1964) posited that the purpose of play in therapy is distinct from that of the child's everyday play experiences. Regular play is a means through which the child expresses thoughts and feelings for private purposes. By contrast, in the therapeutic situation, play becomes a technique through which the therapist collaborates with the child to modify the child's behavior. Therapeutic play is an instrument to be manipulated by both therapist and child. It is also the means through which they interact and communicate with one another.

Play gives the therapist opportunities to establish contact with the child and obtain and interpret information. For a child who may be conscious of problems and yet unable to communicate them directly to the therapist, play can serve as a helpful mode of communication, enabling the child to ventilate his or her concerns through symbolic constructions. Initial observations and interviews portray for the therapist the various levels of emotional responses that the child may enact in different life situations.

Forging an Alliance

Given the importance of the therapeutic alliance, the therapist should be mindful of strategies that may be useful in promoting it. Gardner (1979) outlined five techniques that can help the therapist ally with the patient. These are the play interview, active play therapy, release therapy, relationship therapy, and nondirective therapy.

The Play Interview. The therapist should actively intervene, posing questions and structuring activities, in order to elicit specific responses from the child. The therapy centers around the child's past conflicts and the present circumstances that brought the child into therapy. The child gains an awareness of what he or she does to evoke the problems, and subsequent interventions help him or her modify these behaviors.

Active Play Therapy. Although the child's past does play an active role in the therapeutic process, present circumstances are also very important. The therapist can actively initiate play situations in order to provoke responses. Doll play is an example of a play situation from which the child can gain insight without becoming overly anxious or fearful.

Release Therapy. In release therapy, the therapist strategizes play activities to release strong, inhibited emotions from the child. Specific structuring of such play episodes forces the child to confront his or her conflicts. Here play serves as a catharsis for a traumatic event. However, therapists should be aware that such methods may force children into moments during which they have no means to cope with the anxiety and/or dysphoric reactions evoked. During these moments, children may experience powerful and frightening emotions without any resolution of the underlying conflict. Release therapy may thus serve only as temporary relief from the conflict, and given the possibility that the child may not be ready to deal with the emotions expressed, a therapist proposing such an approach in play should be aware of the possibility of negative repercussions.

Relationship and Nondirective Therapy. Allen (1942), Gardner (1979), and Axline (1964a,b) have expressed the belief that the therapeutic alliance determines the outcome in the therapeutic situation. If therapists create an environment in which children can freely express themselves, the children will likely gain insight into their conflicts. Since the affect of anxiety is an intrinsic element that gets woven into therapeutic situations, resistances commonly occur when a therapist attempts to direct a child into activities that produce anxiety.

During the play interview and active play therapy, the therapeutic alliance is directive in nature in that the therapist initiates play situations in order to evoke responses from the child. The child is placed in this structured environment so that he or she can deal with repressed conflicts. Nondirective therapy is a more mutually engaging situation in which the alliance is actively negotiated by the child and therapist. In this sense, the alliance is reciprocal. The child may take the lead by initiating and directing the therapy, while the therapist, through his or her responses, guidance, and interpretations of the child's behaviors, fosters such a situation. The therapist must accept the child and allow the child to act as he or she chooses, but the therapist must not remain passive, thereby making the situation less therapy and more play.

Close attention to the dynamics of the therapeutic relationship can clarify the strength of the alliance. An alliance can be directed and/or misdirected by both parties. Leland (1983) has suggested that directed interventions may be necessary when working with children who lack adequate coping skills. Depressed children, for example, may need more time to adjust to the therapy if they are to engage in communication with the therapist. Therefore, the therapist should be nondirective, providing the child with the necessary support that he or she needs to become comfortable with the therapeutic setting. Aggressive children may need additional interventions (e.g., limit setting) so as to prevent potentially destructive behaviors from occurring.

Limits must be established to teach the child not only the structure of the therapy but also his or her role in relation to the therapy. The therapeutic alliance, the play materials, and the time and place must have proscribed, defined limits. Once established, the limits serve to structure a safe therapeutic situation in order to prevent the child from acting out behaviors that may be damaging to others or the child. The limits defined with each particular child can be diagnostic of the nature of the alliance between the child and therapist.

The therapist must take the time to observe, analyze, and become comfortable with the child just as the child is keenly observing and adjusting his or her behavior to that of the therapist. An alliance founded upon mutual trust will provide the therapist with ample opportunities for therapeutic inquiry and will likely provide the therapist with cues as to how best to transmit such interpretations back to the child.

Play Materials as a Means of Enhancing the Therapeutic Alliance

Often, in order to prevent initial resistance, the therapist may introduce play materials into the therapeutic situation. These materials serve to take pressure off the child; they provide a means for strengthening the therapeutic alliance, as well as establishing a base from which to make future interpretations. Play materials that contribute the most are those that do not contain so-called *contaminants* (Gardner, 1979). Contaminants are play objects designed with specific, predetermined roles that are frequently fixed and inflexible. Their early presence in play therapy may only serve to "contaminate" the child's actions.

The therapist must present the child with play materials that increase the child's state of arousal. McDowell (1937) noted that children ages 2 to 4 years prefer to play with materials used for construction of other objects (e.g., wooden or plastic blocks). Toys employed for playing house, those involving small-muscle motor skills, creative materials, picture books, and toys involving a minimal amount of physical activity are respectively less popular. Thus, the therapist must be sure to usher into the therapeutic situation toys that arouse the child's interest in play.

The child who is given opportunities to play freely in therapy may relax and realize that therapy is not a punishment but an enjoyable experience. Employing artistic materials such as clay and paints, to which the child directly transfers thoughts and feelings, may reduce the child's anxiety and give the therapist opportunities to observe the child. Drawings, in general, can be employed throughout therapy as indicators of the child's progress as the therapy evolves. Ekstein (1983) has suggested that fairy tales and children's books may be useful for establishing an alliance. Reverie serves as a link between the child's and the therapist's minds, and therefore the stories may create a common foundation from which an alliance can be built. Gardner (1979) has found that Checkers and other board games may be of use with older children who are extremely resistant and who may be too inhibited to play with other materials. Also, with older children, structured board games reduce tension and allow the therapist opoportunities to gradually become less structured and more specifically addressed to the child's personal conflicts.

Acting Out, Play Acting, and Play Action

> *Whatever the patient produces . . . is to be understood within the framework of psychotherapy as the communication of the unconscious conflict that has driven the patient to seek the help of the psychotherapist.* (Ekstein & Friedman, 1957, p. 504)

Acting out, play acting, and play action are parameters through which the therapist can measure the therapeutic alliance (Ekstein & Freidman, 1957). The presence of such hallmarks indicates that the therapist is on the heels of meeting the needs of the child and is working with the child toward a mutual goal.

The enactment of spontaneous behavior on the part of the child will help the child eventually to master past conflicts. Although acting-out behavior does not provide the therapist with data to measure present object relationships or the child's reality-testing abilities, it is an indication of the child's attempt to recollect the past and represent it in play. Acting-out behaviors are rooted in preverbal forms of communication.

Since the child's language skills often are such that the child is unable to express conflicts, this preverbal mode of communication becomes the means through which the child adapts to his or her reality (Greenacre, 1952; Trad, 1988).

However, in addition to becoming a means of communicating unconscious conflicts, acting out may also serve as a means by which the child resists using language. This clouds the therapist's attempts to interpret the child's behaviors. While the child unconsciously defends against the therapist's proposed interpretations of current behavior, the operation of unconscious defenses can also be observed in the child's free play. Occasionally, when the child cannot play freely for a long period of time, play interactions are bound to modify themselves, and the child unconsciously defends against the anxiety induced during the therapy. Such resistance toward the therapist's interpretations may not indicate complete misalliance, but it does indicate the child's need for additional interpretations when faced with such conflicts. Unconscious thought processes, along with emotional endurance, may make the child resist going further without reassurance from the therapist that he or she will remain safe.

Acting out is a form of regression through which the child seeks to avoid anxiety. The child reverts back to earlier perceptual schemas and primitive thought processes as a method of coping, rather than relying on higher skills of ego organization. The ego is surreptitiously controlled and thus unable to organize adaptive behavioral responses. The mature ego coordinates hierarchically organized behaviors and allows the child to play-act the conflict. At the same time, it regulates the child's emotional reactivity so that the emergence of affective states can be used for the purposes of adaptation, thus leaving the child with an intact sense of self. Play action serves to coordinate the release of unconscious/repressed affective states into conscious affective states. Therefore, the child may choose to act out and regress in lieu of meeting the challenges (e.g., emotional dysregulation) posed by play action. The therapist must intervene so that the child can learn to progress toward assessment and mastery, rather than retreat into immature perceptual and thought schemas. The child's willingness to proceed and manifest the dysphoric feelings (e.g., anxieties produced by conflicts) relies to a large extent on how secure he or she feels in the therapeutic relationship.

Play action and play acting must be differentiated when assessing a child's behaviors in the therapeutic setting. During *play action*, children unconsciously attempt to master conflicts and inflexible states from the past. They unconsciously recollect the past and replay it through action until the past conflict has been mastered. In contrast, *play acting* refers to the future and serves as a means of adapting to current challenges.

In play acting, children do not wholly identify with the roles they act, but modify past identifications so that they can play act roles that they can identify with in the future. Play acting is based on imitation, whereas play action is grounded in identification. Play acting is a less developed activity than play action. While play action helps children master the past, play acting is indicative of their desire to move ahead.

In contrast to both play action and play acting, *acting out* is a means through which children resist the therapist's attempts to interpret play behaviors. Ekstein and Friedman (1957) posited that these three hall-marks are experimental versions of recollections represented by the ego as a means for reconstruction of the past. Their function is adaptive, not substitutive. These behaviors help the therapist to understand and interpret the child's conflicts if the therapeutic alliance has been struc-tured in such a way that it warrants such activities.

Whether a child chooses to communicate via play action, play acting, and/or acting out, the child must always feel that the therapist is capable of understanding meanings communicated through these channels. If the therapist supports the child, in time the child will imitate, identify with, and trust the therapist. Such an alliance serves as a buffer to offset the anxiety induced by unconscious conflicts.

PSYCHODYNAMIC INTERVENTIONS

Indications and Contraindications

Psychodynamic treatment strategies range from child analysis to sup-portive psychotherapy. The goal of insight-oriented psychotherapy is to help the child develop internal structure and to change the balance of ego, id, and superego. The child's inner conflicts are the central focus of the treatment, and transference reactions should be analyzed thor-oughly with reference to both the past and present. Child psychother-apy, on the other hand, seeks to resolve symptoms, eliminate develop-mental deficits, and promote behavioral adaptations. It is more structured and goal-oriented and relies less on insight and interpreta-tion than analysis.

Analysis is indicated whenever a child presents with a pervasive inter-nalized conflict. However, Mishne (1986) has suggested that in most cases involving children it is not the treatment of choice. He has noted that analysis is contraindicated for children who are weak intellectually or who have a poor understanding of their psychological processes. Other contraindications include psychosis, cognitive defects, weak ego- or self-boundaries, and particularly rigid defense systems. Successful treatment for these conditions requires a supportive environment both in the community and at home (Sours, 1978).

Mishne (1986) noted the indications for psychotherapy. Broadly speaking, psychotherapy is used for children with less severe neurotic conflicts, individuation-separation difficulties, structural ego defects, or preverbal disturbances.

There are no significant statistical data that compare the effectiveness of different analytic treatments. The therapist should, therefore, rely on a comprehensive assessment of the child to determine whether or not analysis is indicated. The assessment should consider biographical data, the nature and intensity of disturbances, the relationship between parent and child, and the prognosis of the disorder (Smirnoff, 1971).

Smirnoff (1971) suggested that, to determine whether child analysis is indicated, an assessment must focus on symptoms that indicate pathological structures of the ego and their defense mechanisms; libidinal developmental difficulties, emotional cathexes and their effect on object relations; intellectual and motor development; and pathological environmental effects that stimulate or hide a structural defect.

Once assessment is completed, a treatment plan is chosen. Individual plans range from those that are merely supportive in nature to those that are intensively insight-oriented. With psychotherapy, less restructuring is attempted and there is less emphasis on unconscious material. Its goals include conflict resolution, personality reintegration, maturation, and improvement in adaptation skills (Dewald, 1983). Unconscious motives, affective behavior, and defensive patterns are revealed and explored. In contrast to supportive treatment, the aim of insight-oriented therapy is to make a profound, lasting change that goes well beyond mere symptom reduction.

Freedheim and Russ (1983) classified individual child psychotherapy into the following three broad categories:

1. Insight-oriented therapy, the goals of which are conflict resolution and mastering of developmental crises. This form of therapy is indicated for children who have adequate overall ego development, are capable of tolerating anxiety, and are able to learn from their behavior.

2. Supportive psychotherapy, the goals of which are to help the child develop problem-resolving techniques and coping strategies. This therapy is indicated for children who have developmental deviations, a less-developed ego, and are not psychologically minded. The focus of such interventions is in the here and now, without uncovering anxiety-producing material.

3. The last form focuses on helping children develop an internal structure, which ultimately results in a better definition of self/

other boundaries and object relationships. This modality has ample applicability with children with borderline and narcissistic disorders.

Insight-oriented therapy should only be used with children who have strong enough egos to withstand the frustration and anxiety of grappling with conflict resolution. In addition, the patient must be motivated, trustful, and come from a supportive home. Individual outpatient therapy is contraindicated if the child's parents do not support such effort.

Within the bounds of improving the patient's perception of reality, supportive treatment, although it aims to relieve symptoms and effect overt behavioral change, leaves repression intact. Personality and unconscious conflicts are left unchanged, and only conscious material and the present are dealt with. Supportive treatment requires a more structured and less open-ended approach than insight-oriented therapy, with the therapist actively minimizing anxiety and reinforcing secondary ego processes (Marks, 1986). Dewald (1983) has suggested that supportive treatment is appropriate where the child is withdrawn and suspicious and has difficulties establishing object relationships. In addition, he has noted that it is suitable for those denying a physiological illness or for those pressured by family or community to attend treatment sessions.

Strategies and Techniques

Interpretations of the behaviors that take place during treatment sessions should serve the therapeutic aim of bringing subconscious feelings and thoughts into consciousness, thereby providing the child with the opportunity to recognize and label his or her own thoughts, feelings, and motivations (Harter, 1983a). The task of releasing, for other uses, the energy required to maintain the repression is made particularly difficult by this frequent misplacement of emerged emotions.

Fraiberg (1962) contended that intervention strategies should aim to interfere with the emotional and/or cognitive difficulties that have patterned. Since the ego operates to defend the child from subconscious impulses, Anna Freud (1966) posited that it is the child's ego that should be the object of the therapist's attention. The therapist interprets the child's defensive operations against the instincts, transformations undergone by the affects, and potential resistances in order to gradually bring subconscious residues into consciousness. Sharing information acts to further increase interactions between the therapist and the patient. Amster (1964) warned that not all children can tolerate the emergence of subconscious motives. Therefore, therapists must be careful when relaying interpretations to vulnerable children. Interpretations that fail to take into consideration a child's emotional make-up may perpetuate the child's condition. Furthermore, they may force the child to withdraw from the therapeutic orbit as a defensive move against the overwhelming anxiety experienced from such lack of empathy.

Play therapy is a mode of communication through which the child and therapist interact to reach a final therapeutic goal (Ekstein, 1983; Esman, 1983). Therapists should realize that their primary function is to interpret the child's behaviors and not to initiate and predetermine the child's play activities. Thus, the therapist should participate by following the child's lead. Once the child has begun the creation of a pretend episode, the therapist should carefully orchestrate a dialogue in order to gain as much knowledge about the child's emotional condition as possible. Harter (1983a) suggested that such therapeutic activity comes to life through the child's activities and not through the interjection of the therapist's own initiative. When given the necessary amount of time to adjust to and accept the therapeutic situation, the child will most likely initiate play activities that readily make themselves available for interpretation.

Therapeutic interventions are analogous to experimental independent variables in that they can be manipulated in order to test the validity of hypotheses regarding the origins of the child's behavior. Harter (1983a) stated that when testing hypothetical observations the therapist should give equal weight to what confirms and what disconfirms such conclusions. Harter also noted that, although the therapist may be able to gather the evidence necessary to support the interventions, he or she must be able to communicate such interpretations to the child. Communication must be carried out in the preschooler's language and at a level commensurate with the child's cognitive skills. Unless this accessibility is assured, the therapist's interpretations serve no purpose in the therapeutic process.

Clinicians should chart children's reactions to interpretations using three measures of confirmation: (1) The child accepts the therapist's intervention, (2) the child rejects or denies the therapist's intervention, or (3) the child meets such intervention by showing a change in the play sequence. Therapists should remember that when interpretations are met with no reaction from a child (that is, they arouse neither confirmation nor denial nor change in sequence), then the child's play situation may have to be considered invalid. In such cases, the therapist should actively consider new hypotheses.

Lewis (1974) contended that interventions should create an environment for the emergence and understanding of the transference and countertransference nuances between patient and therapist. This helps build trust between them and thus permits structural changes in the child. In Lewis's view, interpretation can be seen as a means through which many other communications can develop.

Types of Interventions

Lewis suggested that the interventions made by children's therapists can be broken down into the following six types, which are useful at different stages of therapy:

1. *Setting Statements.* The goal of these interventions is to create the necessary setting for the therapy to occur. The therapy begins by exploring and clarifying why the child is in therapy.
2. *Attention Statements.* Attention statements are made to call attention to particular behaviors of the child. These interventions provide factual information about either play behaviors that are evident or the absence of specific behaviors.
3. *Reductive Statements.* Reductive statements are aimed at reducing the child's disparate behaviors into comprehensive forms that define the origins of such behaviors.
4. *Situational Statements.* Situational statements follow the statements previously described. They draw attention to situations that trigger feelings (e.g., anger, aggression). They aim to show children the origins of their feelings and the ways in which they can repeat situations either outside or within the treatment.
5. *Transference Interpretation.* Once children have become accustomed to the therapeutic situation, accept its limit setting, and conceive of therapy as a means to help them understand their feelings and behaviors, then they begin to recognize that therapy is oriented toward a final goal. During play, children communicate revealing internal thoughts and feelings regarding objects, roles, actions, and dreams. They throw themselves into the present play situation with no thought of the past or future. As therapy progresses, a child will begin to transfer these emotions and actions onto the therapist. According to Lewis, the transference neurosis in the child is typically less stable than for adults. However, any degree of transference lends itself to interpretation by the therapist. Transference is most commonly seen when children attribute feelings and thoughts regarding their parents to the therapist.
6. *Etiological Statements.* Etiological statements derive from past events in the patient's life. They are recalled and reconstructed in order to associate them with the child's present behaviors.

The approach the therapist takes toward formulating an interpretation and proposing it to the child is extremely important. Interpretations of symbolic behaviors observed in play should be grounded in the child's personal experiences and not upon general models of definition (Fraiberg, 1962). Although excited about an interpretation, the therapist should remain attuned to the child's fundamental needs and not push the child into conclusions that may be beyond his or her comprehension. With this in mind, Loewenstein (1951) defined the following sequential steps toward making interpretations:

1. Make the child aware that events have certain common elements.
2. Point out to the child the behaviors that are similar in each of these situations.
3. Demonstrate to the child the circumstances that motivate such behaviors.
4. Point out that behaviors that are unconsciously motivated can be replaced by other kinds of behaviors.
5. Show how behaviors correlate with critical events of the patient's life.

Interpretations of play behaviors can be perceived as one mode through which the child's conflicts can be resolved. Conflicts can be worked through if the therapist repeatedly relates them to observed behaviors, feelings, and events during the child's play. By repeatedly working through the conflict, the conflict's structure can be broken down to its elements, thereby enabling the child to begin to understand and articulate the origins of such self-defeating behaviors.

During the course of development the child has a natural resistance to change, and this may challenge the therapeutic situation. Superego development, which intercedes by weakening defenses, facilitates behavior modifications (Lewis, 1974). Thus, in the young child, the less differentiated the superego, the more support and encouragement from the therapist may modify play behaviors. For the therapist, play's purpose is twofold: It serves as both a diagnostic and therapeutic tool for assessing and modifying psychopathology. The relationship between therapy and play and the way in which the two are interwoven help the child to benefit and grow from such a process.

Although the therapeutic situation can be a powerful force for change, the therapist should note that other factors outside of play therapy affect the child's ongoing life (e.g., parental psychopathology). Lewis (1974) cautioned that it may be difficult for a child to work through conflicts when they are specifically reinforced by the child's parents. Within the psychotherapeutic situation, regular, ongoing sessions with the child's parents help them recognize and modify these issues. The less the parents reinforce their child, the easier it is for maladaptive behavior modifications to be integrated into the child's personality. Therapists should split and contrast the behavioral activities in and outside the therapeutic situation, and, when it is therapeutically indicated, children should be made aware of such behaviors and relate them to their behaviors in their real environment. Without such awareness and without acquiring new strategies to replace those that are impaired, children are doomed to compulsively repeat behaviors that may not only serve to alienate them and their caregivers, but also prevent them from developing adaptively.

The Use of Imagery in Individual Psychotherapy

Imagery, the artificial imitation, metaphor, or mental representation of an external entity, is widely used for diagnosis, rapport building, and treatment of children with psychiatric disorders. This technique facilitates learning of visual materials and is especially useful in treatment of children who have poor verbal abilities. Piaget and Inhelder (1971) viewed assimilation as a function of imagery and considered this function to be the foundation of conceptual thinking.

Imagery can be measured using self-report, behavioral, physiological, and projective measures (Tower & Singer, 1981). These measures assess the child's imagery abilities and help distinguish whether the imagery is passive or active, its relationship to perception, its subjectivity versus objectivity, its consciousness, and the extent to which it can be differentiated stylistically from the imagery of others (Strosahl & Ascough, 1981). Differences along these dimensions are important in diagnosis and the choice of treatment strategies. Elliott and Ozolins (1983) noted that the ability to create subjective images is of particular concern for children who are frequently distressed by fear-provoking images, obsessive images, or images of unresolved conflict. Wilkins (1974) argued that an important function of imagery is to foster the affective elements of experience, especially where there are distortions of reality. This researcher suggested that when a child is helped to develop imagery skills, a desensitization effect occurs. In addition, Elliott and Ozolins (1983) noted that play therapy, which allows fantasies to be acted out, is probably more effective than purely covert strategies with young children. This is because only older children (7 or 8 years and up) are able to bring to mind and manipulate images as instructed (Levin, 1976).

Therapeutic techniques that make direct use of imagery include psychodrama and guided imagery. In psychodrama, group members play the roles in a drama designed to encourage the expression of feelings and the working through of conflicts. Members play roles and also offer feedback on what takes place. Psychodrama has been used to ascertain comprehension of responsibilities for maladaptive behaviors and, with children, to enhance decision-making skills (Elliott & Ozolins, 1983; Mathis, Fairchild, & Cannon, 1980). Guided imagery calls for the therapist to make suggestions to the child regarding imaginary situations. These suggestions are designed to elicit information in specific areas. Other, less-structured suggestions function like projective techniques for revealing subconscious material. Guided imagery has been used not only in diagnosis but also as a tool for teaching imagery skills.

Video Techniques in Psychotherapy

Videotape is frequently used in individual psychotherapy to seek clues and focus attention on especially important events during therapy sessions. While watching tapes of previous sessions, the therapist can offer interpretations of responses or behaviors and attempt to make the child explore conflicts and underlying motivations. Interpretations may be offered immediately or the therapist may aim for the emergence of spontaneous insight. The replayed visual recording makes it more difficult for the child to repress evidence of underlying conflicts, and it can help promote self-reflection and the formation of cause-effect hypotheses. Occasionally, voice-overs on tapes are used to promote this self-reflection and to incorporate the therapist's interpretations. The tapes may also be given to the child to take home, so that he or she can view them alone and respond in a way that is uninhibited by the presence of the therapist.

Videotape is generally used in the treatment of preschoolers with low self-esteem, poor body image, social withdrawal, and passivity, and it is particularly useful as an attraction with resistant children. It can also be used with children who have behavioral or skill deficits. On the other hand, its use is contraindicated in the treatment of psychotic, paranoid, or extremely depressed children (Heilveil, 1983).

Parents can be provided with a model tape of a typical therapy session so that their child can become sensitized to the new setting before treatment begins. Tapes can also be used to transfer information from one therapeutic context to another, as in cases where group or family therapy is used in combination with individual psychotherapy. Parents may be asked to allow family interactions to be taped so that patterns of interaction can be identified. This is particularly useful in helping family members realize their roles in the child's problems and in encouraging them to contribute to the treatment process.

The mutual storytelling technique is one of the many psychotherapeutic techniques that employ video. It is designed to overcome communication difficulties with children (Gardner, 1971). The child begins by telling a story and is followed by the therapist, who tells a similar story in the same language as the child. The video format is important because it encourages the child to tell a story. The key to the technique is that the therapist's story can explore the conflicts revealed in the child's story and suggest interpretations and solutions that are readily understandable by the child.

Other video techniques include freeze and half and half (Heilveil, 1983). In the freeze technique, freeze frames are used to highlight subtle nonverbal behavior and serve as the basis for a discussion of unconscious conflicts. In half-and-half techniques, only the sound or image is replayed, allowing the therapist and patient to focus attention on particular communication characteristics that might go unnoticed otherwise.

BUILDING AND UNDERSTANDING THE TRANSFERENCE RELATIONSHIP

As the skilled therapist creates an atmosphere of trust, the preschool child cooperates and eventually reveals to the therapist, either directly or through fantasy material, the nature of the conflict (Harley, 1971). The presence of the therapist during play situations allows the child opportunities to forge a transference relationship—a kind of relationship that was first alluded to by Freud (1905). A transference relationship occurs when the patient unconsciously recapitulates and projects onto the therapist thoughts and feelings about his or her caregivers and other important figures. In contrast, a "real relationship" (Greenson, 1971) refers to a new interaction that is not determined by the patient's past and that serves adaptive functions. In transference, children attribute to the therapist feelings and attitudes that originated from their caregivers (Fraiberg, 1962; Freud, 1905; Markowitz, 1959). Transference not only makes understanding, interpretation, and reconstruction possible but, as Ritvo (1978) has pointed out, it also "restores the feeling of immediacy, reality and conviction to psychological phenomena arising out of the past" (p. 299). Based on familiarity with the patient, the therapist has to distinguish transference reactions that have their root in memories, those that are extensions of current conflicts, and those that reflect a transference neurosis.

Anna Freud (1928) distinguished transference in children from that found in adults. Adult patients give up the objects on which they had been fixed and center their attention on the therapist. The child gradually replaces previous neurotic functioning with a "transference neurosis" in which the patient acts out neurotic reactions in relation to the therapist—the object of the transference. Tyson and Tyson (1986) have stated that transference neurosis is taking place when "those situations in which the child's feelings, attitudes and behavior originally expressed in interaction with important others are now expressed in a new form primarily in relation to the analyst and limited to the analytic situation, with a marked diminution in the expression of those feelings, attitudes and behaviors elsewhere" (p. 33).

In contrast to the objects of adult patients, the child's original objects (parents) presently exist as primary love objects, not merely in fantasy, as with the adult patients. The therapist enters the situation as a new person and shares with the parents the love or hate experienced by the child. In contrast to the original object (i.e., the parent), when this object is exchanged for a real person (i.e., the therapist), such a person does not offer all the advantages that the patient finds in his or her fantasy objects.

Although transference may consist of new or revived behaviors, these behaviors are limited to the relationship with the therapist. A third possibility involves a decrease in the expression of feelings and certain behaviors in their usual setting, with a concomitant increase in their expression in relation to the analyst. For example, the child may attempt to project images of important figures in his or her life onto the therapist. Such attempts to transform the analyst into someone else may lead to disappointment and frustration as the transference is continually interpreted. Transference behaviors not only will help to define the child's feelings toward caregivers, many of which the child cannot directly identify or verbalize, but also will help the child to overcome the ego's split that enables the child to maintain conflicting beliefs defensively.

Neubauer (1980) has pointed out, however, that transference reactions will not be evoked indiscriminately in all patients, primarily because this phenomenon is tied to the developmental status of the child. Certain developmental prerequisites must be achieved, including the ability to differentiate self-object representations and to maintain a stable representation of the object within the internal landscape. In other words, for transference to occur, the child must first develop object constancy (Kohrman, Fineberg, Gerlman, & Weiss, 1971; Neubauer, 1980), a concept that usually consolidates at around $3\frac{1}{2}$ years of age (Mahler et al., 1975). Prior to this development, the child focuses primarily on moving ahead and meeting the developmental challenges that prevail in his or her life and is without the capacity to edit past experiences. However, once the child acquires the ability to fully represent primary past relationships with growing degrees of stability and constancy, he or she can then transfer these representations onto the therapist during the current therapeutic situation. In young children, transference phenomena emerge as a consequence of both the child's effort to test reality perceptions against the coercive pull of primitive drives and the effort to differentiate new from primary objects. Seen in this light, transference reactions can be understood as a byproduct of the developmental pro-gression. Thus, even in young children, transference allows the repre-sentation in the present of events that the child experienced in the past (Neubauer, 1980). For this reason, the transference relationship can give even otherwise unimportant performances a definite symbolic signifi-cance (A. Freud, 1928).

Some of these repressed memories may contain deepseated conflicts that the patient, albeit unconsciously, will now attempt to master. The transference allows reenactment of these past conflicts. Its skillful han-dling will determine the actual contours of the therapist-patient rela-tionship and set the stage for behavioral change to take place.

Transference is more than just a reenactment of the past. It revives the feelings associated with those memories and gives them a convinc-ing immediacy (Ritvo, 1978). This reanimation of the past gives access to the foundations of conflict, thereby allowing direct exploration of these issues. The therapist makes interpretations about the conflicts that are being manifested via the transference, and these interpreta-tions, along with revealing the child's defensive mechanisms, are the major therapeutic instrument of change (A. Freud, 1927). Moreover, the transference restores the feelings of immediacy, reality, and the nature of psychological phenomena arising from the past (Ritvo, 1978).

The patient may have a compulsion to unconsciously repeat earlier experiences and relationships and may believe that these responses are entirely appropriate in the context of the present therapeutic situation (Sandler, Dare, & Holder, 1973). It is the extent of the distortion that makes these responses manifestations of the transference. Therapists should be careful to discriminate between nontransference and trans-ference elements. Furthermore, transference reactions may not be pro-jected solely onto the therapist, but may be projected onto the situation in its entirety.

Parallel to the transference relationship is the real relationship, which evolves from realistic perceptions of the therapist and interacts with the more purely transferential elements. Both are important to the child, serving adaptive, developmental, interpersonal, and emotional needs.

A further complication in the development of the transference is the child's limited ability to generalize, conceptualize, and coordinate ab-stract thoughts. This limits understanding of therapist's interpretations. Understanding of interpretations is essential if the child is to develop a realistic perception of his or her feelings and learn to distinguish between past and present-day real and fantasy influences. One tech-nique that is commonly used to overcome this problem is to tell a story about an animal or a child. One drawback is that stories are symbolic and therefore may not engage the child's ego, which is the focus of the intervention. When communicating interpretations, therapists should remember to avoid provoking anxiety, guilt, or loss of control.

MANAGING THE COUNTERTRANSFERENCE EFFECTIVELY

As the child transfers thoughts and feelings to the therapist, the therapist must, on the other hand, be capable of countertransferring effectively the feelings evoked within him by the child. Berlin (1987) noted that the therapist must keep in mind past relationships that were detrimental to the child, so as to avoid repeating any of these behaviors within the therapeutic milieu. The therapist must create a countertransference-free environment that is receptive to the child's transferences. Freud (1933), who introduced the concept, described countertransference as the numerous emotions triggered in the therapist as a consequence of the patient's influence on the therapist's unconscious feelings. The therapist's experience of the patient has diagnostic potential and therapeutic implications in that it can be used to understand and interpret the child's internal perceptions. As Winnicott (1949) put it, "However much he loves his patients he cannot avoid hating them, and fearing them, and the better he knows this the less will hate and fear be the motive determining what he does to his patients" (p. 6).

The key, then, is for the therapist to be aware of the compelling subjective element of his or her experience of the child and to use this information to discern what intervention will be appropriate for the management of the particular issue (Stein, 1985a,b,c). Depending on the nature of the countertransference, the therapist will be provided with a significant clue as to whether this particular patient responds in other relationships in a manner that thwarts interaction or fosters adaptive response. The more adept the therapist becomes at analyzing his or her countertransference reactions, the more equipped he or she will be in deciphering and delineating the internal experience of the child.

Countertransference responses are frequently evoked by acting-out behavior on the part of the patient. Acting out is the discharge of an impulse, emotion, fantasy, or memory in a spontaneous action devoid of conscious scrutiny. It may be provoked if the therapist uses free associations to stimulate memories and the feelings associated with them. The past and present may appear the same, and the child may project the reanimated feelings onto the readily available therapist. The patient may also be unconsciously testing the therapist by watching his or her reactions to provocations.

Esman (1983) stipulated that the therapist must keep an objective perspective of his or her role in the transference-countertransference interaction in order not to overidentify with, misinterpret, and/or become seduced by the child. In particular, the therapist should watch for warning signs such as overreluctance to see parents. In this regard, a question that might be usefully asked is whether the therapist views himself or herself as being a better father or mother to the child. Other warning signs include stereotypic behavior or an unusually high frequency of a particular behavior with a lack of explanation for it. Bick (1962) has pointed out that the child may induce feelings of anxiety and/or guilt in the therapist. If unaware of such feelings, the therapist may nurture the child to such an extent that the interactions are no longer therapeutic.

Esman contended that the therapist must feel relatively secure with regard to his or her own childhood conflicts in order to remain objective. Whereas an effective therapist is keenly aware of all the emotions that the patient's transference evokes in himself or herself, the child may be unaware of such feelings, and thus the child may actively pursue action-oriented responses from the therapist (Winnicott, 1949). The therapist, placed in this scenario by the child, should proceed carefully in order to respond optimally to the child's needs. Bick maintained that the child's dependence on and projections toward the therapist can evoke unconscious feelings that the therapist may not be able to suppress within himself or herself. Thus, the therapist must remain in a constant state of self-analysis. The hate the child thrusts on the therapist must be met objectively. The therapist should recognize any negative feelings toward the child and prevent these feelings from contaminating therapeutic strategies. The therapist must always interpret the child's transference reactions objectively rather than act out countertransference feelings (Kohrman et al., 1971) in the hopes of repairing the child's negative sense of self. Frequently, the very same needs and desires the child transfers to the therapist are the ones that the child puts forth when interacting with his or her parents (Rubenstein & Levitt, 1964). Inadequate handling of countertransference feelings elicited by the child's caregivers will most likely impair the therapy and prove counterproductive to the parent-child-therapist partnership.

Effective handling of countertransference feelings allows the therapist to objectively diagnose the child's progress regarding the transference. To maintain objectivity and enhance the potential usefulness of countertransference feelings, the therapist may use free-floating attention and response techniques—allowing thoughts, daydreams, and associations to freely emerge while listening to and observing the patient.

Bernstein and Glenn (1978) have cataloged the possible emotional responses of child therapists toward patients. These include identification, counteridentification, experiencing the patient as an extension of the self and, finally, responding to the patient as a real person. The therapist may perceive himself or herself to be a parent of the child or may view the child as a narcissistic extension of the self. If this response is not rectified, the therapist could fuse with the child and be hampered in dispensing therapeutic guidelines from an objective perspective. The final category involves responses to the child's transference reactions as a real person. These can be triggered by provocative behavior such as pushing away. Because these responses can be sudden and unexpected, the therapist may be caught off guard and respond in a manner designed to shield himself or herself from unpleasant assaults.

THE EMERGENCE OF RESISTANCE

Resistance refers to the behaviors the child may consciously or unconsciously employ in order to evade the therapist's interventions. Children may resist therapy, and subsequently the establishment of a therapeutic alliance, for various reasons. Being under the scrutiny of a stranger (the therapist) and encouraged to express unpleasant, dangerous emotions is a difficult experience. In addition, many children, unaccustomed to the therapeutic process, may thwart the therapist's efforts to establish an alliance because of the secondary gain that is derived from their ability to control an adult. In these instances, resistance serves to provide the child with a feeling of power over the environment. In other cases, such as abused children, children may initially resist therapy because they fear the therapist, like their parents, will randomly punish them for any behavior they may display.

When confronted with resistance that prevents the establishment of an alliance with the child, the therapist needs to actively intervene and direct the child's behaviors and/or thoughts from the outset. Indeed, resolution of the initial resistance between the child and the therapist may serve not only to alleviate the child's anxieties but also to induce a feeling of trust in the child. Thus, the child may begin to understand that the therapist exists not to dole out punishment for maladaptive behaviors but to relieve the dysphoric feelings borne from such behaviors.

Gardner (1979) posited that introducing therapy through the child's parents will serve to allay the child's initial fears about the therapist. Another means of allaying the child's anxieties may be to explore the child's feelings about being in therapy and explain the nuances of the therapeutic process. With some children, such as abused children, overcoming resistances may be the main goal of the therapy itself. Children who have learned to mistrust everyone they meet may be incapable of forming alliances since their relationships with their caregivers are of this nature. In this regard, the therapist who can bring the abused child to trust and ally with him or her has accomplished a goal that will leave the child feeling that new, trustworthy alliances can be formed.

Sigmund Freud (1926) defined the following three forms of ego resistance:

1. Repression resistance, born out of the need to maintain repressed id impulses.
2. Transference resistance, which evolves when the child repeats with the therapist past modes of reacting.
3. Secondary gain resistance, born out of the need to maintain a symptom because of the gains that derive from it.

Transference resistance and *secondary gain resistance* refer to the behaviors that may be acted out in the session in order to avoid therapeutic attempts at interpreting and/or modifying behavior. Gardner (1979) expressed the belief that the young child may engage in resistances as a defense against the development of specific object relationships in which the child fears the adult, who is a stranger and a representative of the parental role. One of the initial goals of therapy is to prevent or alleviate the anxieties that can cause such resistance. Over time, as fear and apprehension of the therapeutic situation diminish, so do these resistances, until eventually an adaptive alliance can be established that facilitates the establishment of therapeutic goals.

Repression resistance, on the other hand, is not a defense activated by the introduction of an external event into the therapy, but a defensive mechanism that the child carries from his or her real environment to the therapeutic relationship. This type of resistance may be resolved if the child experiences the therapist as being empathically interested and understanding of his or her condition. As the therapist verbalizes the child's feelings, the child's ego grows in the direction of self-assessment of personal thoughts and feelings (Frankl & Hellman, 1964). Gardner (1979) noted that the therapist must translate the observations he or she makes into words the child understands, so that the child, too, may draw conclusions from such statements. The therapist must keep abreast of any changes in attitude and realize that the child's mental capacities are developing at the same time as the therapeutic situation is progressing.

Frankl and Hellman warned that the therapist must be wary of making interpretations that bypass ego defenses and confront the child directly. The young child often makes his or her unconscious readily available for interpretations; however, the therapist must resist confronting the child in an abrupt fashion or be met with resistance. The therapist who directly transmits interpretations to the child's unconscious becomes less of a vehicle through which the child can gauge and differentiate between the reality-fantasy boundaries and more a person who has the power to read the child's secret, undisclosed thoughts. Direct confrontation of the child's unconscious may induce anxiety and counteract the therapeutic situation. Communication through the child's ego provides access to the derivatives of the unconscious and thus prevents anxiety from overwhelming the child. The therapist should establish a trusting alliance prior to making confrontational interventions.

OUTCOME PREDICTIONS

Cohen, Kolers, and Bradley (1987) studied treatment outcomes for preschool children who presented with emotional or behavioral problems and/or specific developmental delays. The children were of normal intelligence, and the setting was a multifocused therapeutic preschool program. The treatment was most successful when the child entered the program at a young age, had a relatively high developmental level, remained in the program for longer than 1 year, and had a family who were motivated. In some cases up to 2 years of treatment was required before progress was reasonable, although, in general, treatment duration was shorter and depended on the area of functioning being considered and the child's initial developmental level. The investigators also found that while parental involvement was generally important, it was not a determinant of change in receptive language or of reduction in withdrawal behavior. These were influenced by the age at which treatment began, the initial functioning level, and other environmental variables. Finally, biological risk factors were found to be useful predictors of outcome.

In a related study, Cohen, Bradley, and Kolers (1987) looked at a group of preschoolers with a broader range of intelligence. Again, the children were delayed or emotionally disturbed and the setting was a multifocused day-treatment program. They discovered that children with normal nonverbal intelligence benefitted most from treatment. Progress was slower, and the duration of required treatment longer, for those with below-average intelligence. In general, treatment was most successful with developmentally delayed children who were also withdrawn. Those treated primarily for behavioral problems showed the least progress. The best results, in terms of behavior, were found with children who had impulse-control difficulties. Family involvement was generally found to be very important, but not in terms of improving receptive language or reducing withdrawal behavior.

Heinicke and Ramsey-Klee (1986) studied the effect of session frequency on treatment outcome. They found that a frequency of more than once a week left children with more flexibility in their adaptations, a larger capacity for relationships, and less dependence on others for behavioral control. It was also discovered that children who had more sessions also had a better balance in their defensive organization, were able to regulate aggression as opposed to repressing it, and could elaborate an idea imaginatively. Greater session frequency was also associated with a greater improvement in reading, although arithmetic and spelling abilities were left unchanged.

The choice of a basic treatment approach is not influenced by social class. However, in the upper middle class, longer duration of treatment is associated with greater improvement (McDermott, Harrison, Schrager, Killins, & Dickerson, 1970). In addition, social class has not been found to be a determinant of the relative efficacy of "uncovering" versus "supportive" treatment.

FAMILY INTERVENTIONS

Clinicians who work with children in therapy must never forget that children are constantly affected by the behaviors of their families. Therefore, even if a child's behavior is modified, overall success cannot be assured unless the child's family supports and reinforces the modified behaviors and develops a clearer understanding of the child's problem. Additional family play therapy may be one means through which the child masters his or her difficulties. Mendell (1983) contended that therapeutic work with parents and other central figures in the child's life (e.g., foster parents) is crucial to the child's overall therapy. The child who perceives that his or her family supports the therapeutic process may enter into the therapy with a positive outlook. Families who participate in the child's therapy are more likely to empathize with their child and feel that growth is something they have supported. Greif (1983) and Ney and Mulvihill (1985) have agreed that family intervention should create for the parents and the child a comfortable environment that facilitates communication and understanding. Greif has suggested that family play therapy can be used as part of the therapeutic process with the child. Not surprisingly, this therapeutic approach is most successful when the therapist-caregiver relationship is a positive one in which all members are working toward a common goal.

Greif has noted that family play therapy may not be helpful when treating mentally retarded children. Unless the child's behavior has been previously modified, the goals of family therapy in these cases may prove difficult to meet, and therapy may serve only to frustrate the parents, the therapist, and the child.

Ney and Mulvihill have observed that parents like to attend family training sessions because they want to gain knowledge about their child. Through observations, the parents learn to become more objective when looking at their child and themselves, and they gain a better understanding of their relationship to the child. These researchers have posited that parents should learn to perceive and interpret their child's behaviors objectively and acquire and employ stronger communicative skills to further enhance their interactions with the child.

Greif has concurred, adding that family therapy gives the therapist an opportunity to act as a role model for the parents. For example, many parents who are abusers were abused themselves. Thus, family therapy may be one means of communication through which parents, who were taught bad parenting techniques by their parents, can learn positive parenting techniques from the therapist. As stated earlier in the section on transference and countertransference, the therapist must be aware of parental transferences during therapy. A parent may enter family therapy more to meet his or her own emotional needs and nurturance than to meet those of the child. Therefore, the therapist must remain aware, and make the parent aware, of the motivations behind both the therapist's and the parent's actions.

The therapist participates actively by becoming a guide, an organizer, and a role model in the therapeutic setting. Greif has stated that the therapist's role changes as the therapy evolves. Initially, the therapist chooses and guides activities for the family to follow. In later sessions, the therapist becomes the role model for the parents, demonstrating behaviors and skills for the parents to reenact with their child. In the final stages of treatment, the therapist steps back, supports the parents' interactions with their child, and encourages the parents to employ the new skills they have mastered.

Specific activities and games employed during the family play therapy sessions should be chosen in concert with the parents. Parents who accept the responsibility for organizing the session tend to adopt such skills to guide future real-life activities (Greif, 1983). Parents who are given control over the therapy feel the trust the therapist has placed in them and are more likely to open up during therapy sessions. The parents see the therapist not as a threat to their parenthood but as a support. Therapeutic techniques should be modified to meet the family's specific needs. Some parents might rather be told what to do initially, in fear of choosing the "wrong" game or activity. When these cases occur, the therapist can guide the therapeutic activity to master the parents' fears of the situation so that they will be better able to accept responsibility for structuring the therapeutic environment in later sessions.

However, as important as the parents' involvement in the family's therapeutic process is, in the psychodynamic framework the child remains the primary focus of the therapy. Ney and Mulvihill (1985) cited one problem that may possibly arise during family counseling: The child who has long been the force holding the family together may be unable to express himself or herself in therapy with the family present. The therapist must take the child's emotional state into account prior to introducing family therapy. The child should view therapy as an opportunity for self-expression to take place without repercussion. The therapist must make sure that family therapy retains a sense of comfort, primarily for the child. Family play therapy should be viewed as a cooperative medium of communication through which the parents, the child, and the therapist can interact in a relaxed and flexible environment. Family therapy that lacks such a cooperative atmosphere might generate counterproductive feelings that could only serve to betray the overall therapeutic goals.

CONCLUSION

Projection of the overtones of the unconscious relationship onto the therapist taxes both the child and the therapist. Within the therapeutic relationship the child reenacts the pain from the loss of the ideal parent. The therapist, on the other hand, has to interact with this transference component by continually reminding the child that he or she can interact in ways other than those introjected from interactions with caregivers. The process of treating a young child is an arduous one, since the child naturally tries to refocus into his or her fantasy each time the therapeutic relationship threatens the existence of this imaginary companion. A cure, in this sense, has been achieved when the child can share without fearing further losses.

By preschool age, children can differentiate good (nurturing) from bad (depriving) characteristics of their caregivers. They also have sufficient internal abilities to control and regulate their affective states. These skills allow preschoolers to test out their perceptions regarding caregivers' affective states and begin to experiment. That is, while controlling their affective states and remaining aware of these feelings, they can begin to contrast how their feelings evoke feelings in their caregivers. This process makes children aware that the way they feel does not necessarily represent the way their caregivers feel.

CHAPTER TWENTY-FIVE

Family, Behavioral, Cognitive, Group, and Pharmacotherapy Interventions

INTRODUCTION

Other strategies commonly used in the treatment of preschool children include family, behavioral-cognitive, and group therapies and pharmacotherapy. The more involved family therapies view the family system, rather than the child, as being disturbed, and the goal of treatment is to destabilize and replace existing family structures that are contributing to the child's symptoms. Knowledge of the type of family being dealt with is essential to determining whether family therapy is indicated and, if so, what modality should be followed. Less involved family treatment strategies, such as teaching family members behavioral-cognitive techniques, focus on the family contingencies surrounding the child's maladaptive behaviors and treat those behaviors directly. This training helps reinforce progress that has been made within the therapeutic context.

Behavioral therapies assume that behaviors are a function of their consequences and can be unlearned if responses to them are managed systematically. This approach is most successful when there is a predictable pattern of behavior, as in cases involving fears or obsessive-compulsive disorders. Cognitive therapies, on the other hand, focus on correcting maladaptive thoughts and feelings through various training methods. This is a prerequisite for successful psychotherapy that relies on well-developed cognitions to promote the process of learning.

Group therapy typically involves supervised activities such as sports, play, and teamwork, in which the social aspect of the group is considered therapeutic. Psychotherapy is also involved when the group activities include discussions of thoughts and feelings regarding psychological issues. Group therapies are usually used when the child's problem concerns conflicts in interpersonal relationships, and it can also be used to validate experiences and provide the mutual support necessary for working through problems. In the following sections, the role of each of these therapeutic modalities is discussed and the techniques employed are described.

FAMILY THERAPY

Engaging the family is virtually always a part of the treatment, although degrees of involvement vary. For example, the psychoeducational model combines individual therapy for the patient with extensive education and support for the family. In contrast, family therapy, in which the child's symptoms are perceived as part of the family system, requires even greater involvement since the family, and not the child alone, requires treatment.

The need for family therapy is particularly obvious when the child is a member of a "multiproblem family." These families are best distinguished from so-called normal families by the extensiveness of their contacts with professionals and agencies. Parents in these families frequently have a variety of interpersonal and emotional difficulties that place their children at risk for developing psychiatric disorders. In addition, the therapist commonly has to overcome the family's strong resistance to treatment.

Types of Family Functioning

Therapists should become adept at recognizing the three fundamental typologies of family functioning: optimal families, midrange families, and severely dysfunctional families (Beavers, 1982). The characteristics found in optimal families represent the highest level on a continuum of competence and they are used as a model of healthy interaction. These families have a capacity for and a continual striving toward intimacy. They demonstrate the skills that are crucial in dealing with the tensions between individual choices and group needs and between the need for individual freedom and the need for belonging. Within these families, the hierarchy of power is clearly delineated, with leadership firmly in the hands of the parents, who foster an egalitarian coalition.

Midrange families, on the other hand, seek control, and family members endlessly strive to obtain power via intimidation of other family members. A rigid and often harsh set of rules guides family interactions. According to Beavers, children in these families are likely to grow up with a coherent but limited sense of self and identity, which may manifest itself in neurosis and behavior disorders.

Severely dysfunctional families flounder in thwarted efforts at achieving coherence and genuine communication. They have poorly defined power structures; unclear, ineffective, and ungratifying communications; extreme problems in establishing interpersonal boundaries; and limited negotiation skills.

Knowledge of the type of family that is being dealt with should help the therapist determine whether family therapy is needed and, if so, what modality should be followed.

Liaisons with Other Agencies

Therapists should also broaden their perspective by forming liaisons with institutions other than the family. Although young children's lives are centered in the family, numerous health, educational, and social welfare agencies may be involved with families or with the children themselves. Therapists should be aware of the roles of these institutions and utilize the skills of co-professionals where appropriate.

The length of time and the variety of activities in which they have seen the child, as well as their relationship with the child's parents, make day-care and nursery-school teachers an invaluable source of information on a child's social, cognitive, and psychomotor functioning. The therapist can make recommendations to the teacher for dealing with the child, thus making the teacher a part of the treatment team.

Contacting the referral source can offer another perspective on the family structure. Often clinic or nursery referrals come from doctors whose knowledge of the family's patterns of compliance and noncompliance in health issues could influence the choice of therapeutic interventions.

If there is clinical evidence that suggests physical or sexual abuse or neglect of a child, practitioners are legally obligated to report it, to comply with relevant child protection laws and reporting procedures in their state.

Educating the Family

Regular contacts with parents are commonplace in individual child psychotherapy. Parents attempt to elicit a clear explanation of the etiology and treatment of the child's illness as well as its prognosis. Since treatment decisions are made in alliance with family members, it is essential to inform them of the precise diagnosis and the genetic and psychosocial risks of the disorder. It is critical for therapists to provide parents with a rationale for the chosen treatment. Possible side-effects from such interventions should be carefully spelled out. Informing parents of the basis for prognoses is also important because it allows them to have realistic expectations.

In addition to educating the family about the nature of the illness, the therapist should provide a "map" that includes practical information such as which local, state, and federal agencies provide funding for child patients. Local support groups can be mentioned, and community advocacy should also be suggested.

More complete family education may make family members less resistant to playing an active role in the treatment. In cognitive-behavioral therapy, this role involves the reinforcement of behavior modification outside the clinic setting. The psychoeducational model, used mostly in the treatment of autism and schizophrenia, provides multifamily support groups and instructions for managing with a recovering family member. Emphasis is placed on the family's maintenance of outside social ties and activities, reduction of guilt over the patient's illness, and limiting negative communications with the patient.

Treating the Family as the Patient

In contrast to these approaches, family therapy does not conceive of family work mainly as a helpful adjunct in treatment of the child patient. It perceives the whole family as the patient. The family as a unit, and not only the child, is disturbed. The child's symptoms are part of the family system and perform some function for the family (e.g., stopping parental fighting, increasing contact with a disengaged parent, expressing the suppressed feelings or wishes of another family member). The child's symptoms are important in the family, and changing them will modify the family's unhealthy balance. Family systems theory predicts that if only the child's symptoms are addressed in therapy and other crucial aspects of the family system are not explored, either the child will remain symptomatic ("the family will maintain the child's symptoms") or another symptom will arise in the family. For example, if a family's "difficult child" stops acting out, his younger sister might begin having problems in school or his parents might fight. Thus the balance of the system is maintained.

The treatment goals include not only symptomatic relief of the identified patient, but often change in family structure, that is, the pattern of coalitions and emotional distance among family members. Establishment of appropriate boundaries between generations is frequently important in the families of young patients. The theory behind this strategy is that children who become "triangulated" in the relationship with their parents, for example, are prevented from accomplishing age-appropriate developmental tasks. Therapeutic strengthening of the parental bond and the family hierarchy could leave the child free to grow up.

There are several schools of family therapy. They vary on questions of theory and technique such as how much to use individual psychodynamic material, insight, or members of the extended family. Examination of relationships within the family system and the significance of the child's symptom for each family member is their common theme. Family assessment resembles behavioral therapy in that it might start with similar questions regarding the frequency and context of a child's symptoms, but it diverges from the behavioral model in its style of family observation and its theory and practice of therapeutic intervention. Cognitive-behavioral observation is centered on the identified patient, focusing on the contingencies surrounding the child's maladaptive behaviors, and treats those behaviors directly. Family assessment widens its lens to take into consideration all family interactive patterns.

There is a widespread misconception that family members, particularly fathers and siblings, by nature tend to be uncooperative with family assessment. The perception is that they will be hostile or unable to reveal themselves and that their expectations and capacities will be incompatible with any sophisticated approach employed by the therapist. However, research has indicated that most parents are willing to participate in family assessment if they are invited to do so (Howells, 1980).

After the initial assessment, the therapist forms a hypothesis as to the nature of the family problem and then attempts to destabilize the current interactive patterns and establish new ones. This task is accomplished not only through behavioral contingencies but mostly through verbal therapeutic intervention (e.g., interpretation) that provides a new perspective on family assumptions. There is no limit to the additional techniques a creative therapist might conceive of.

Assessment and Treatment Techniques

Genograms, reframing, and unbalancing are three commonly used techniques for assessment and treatment. Genograms are family trees with representations of birth order, marriages, divorces, and personal characteristics of extended family members. They are used to inquire about established family patterns, roles, and myths. Reframing can then be employed by the therapist to offer family members a new way of thinking about a family assumption, rule, or interaction. If a more forceful intervention is required, the therapist uses unbalancing techniques to destabilize the existing hierarchical structure by allying himself or herself with certain members (Glick, Clarkin, & Kessler, 1987).

Another technique is sculpting or choreography. This technique involves having one family member briefly describe a setting, and, under guidance from the therapist, "sculpt" other members in physical positions representing their actions and emotions in the scene. This is a powerful technique for illustrating emotional closeness and distance and for communicating one member's feelings in a way others readily understand.

The therapist can also employ modeling and role playing in treatment. Modeling, often only an implicit component of family therapy, occurs when the therapist's behavior in treatment sessions exposes family members to a new repertoire of behaviors, emotions, and responses to situations such as challenge and misunderstanding. Sometimes modeling is also done explicitly to teach particular behaviors, as it is in behavioral therapy. In role-playing techniques, family members play themselves in a hypothetical situation or play other family members. The goal is to discover novel patterns of adaptation and develop empathy within the family (Glick, Clarkin, & Kessler, 1987).

Treatment can also involve homework and paradoxical techniques. With homework techniques, family members are assigned tasks—some of which might resemble behavioral techniques—whose goals are readily apparent (e.g., parents rewarding themselves after successfully responding to a child's acting out). Other tasks could be strategies intended to effect structural change, and their goals might not be evident to the family. Paradoxical techniques are used to push problem behaviors to their extremes in order to convince family members of their existence or enable the patient to realize that they are controllable.

Video can be used as an element of family therapy. It is particularly helpful in increasing awareness of family interaction patterns and in revealing conflicting parental messages. Video techniques include the serial argument and family role playing (Heilveil, 1983). In the serial argument technique, the therapist chooses a topic for the family to argue about. Each person is restricted to saying only a couple of sentences and speaking in turn. The argument is videotaped and replayed with stops for discussion after each person has said something. This process can be repeated several times to explore and reinforce what has been learned.

Family role playing also involves the repetition of family episodes. An event that is considered to be important is reenacted with family members playing themselves. A videotape recording is then played back to allow exploration of behaviors. The process is then repeated, with family members free to incorporate any insights they might have gained, and it is completed only when conflicts have been resolved.

Research findings in general have not shown pronounced differences in the effectiveness of the various treatment techniques. Therefore the choice of specific interventions is typically made on the basis of the particular circumstances of the case and the therapist's own predilection. However, the effectiveness of individual treatment techniques for some specific disorders has been supported by research. Gurman, Kniskern, and Pinsof (1986), for example, have stated that behavioral family therapy can be used effectively to treat schizophrenia, anxiety disorders, and conduct disorders, while structural family therapy can be used to treat psychosomatic disorders. Ziegler and Holden (1988) have suggested that family therapy can be used to improve the self-esteem, self-control, and frustration tolerance of children with learning disabilities or attention deficit disorders. The indications for and techniques of family intervention for disorders that involve a pattern of family interaction are discussed in the following chapter.

PARENT BEHAVIORAL TRAINING

Parent behavioral training attempts to employ parents, who are the child's most powerful behavior change agents, in extending the contingencies of the therapeutic environment beyond the clinic. This program focuses on teaching parents specific techniques designed to modify target behaviors of the child. In general, increased use of positive reinforcement is prescribed while coercive techniques are discouraged. The program also includes an education in the general principles of operant conditioning.

Parents become part of the treatment team, responsible for rewarding appropriate behavior. Parent competence may be augmented further through training in child management, household organization, and impulse control. Such formal inclusion of family members has other advantages, including actually changing the family system by drawing the parents together in a project; increasing positive interactions of the target child with parents and siblings; and allowing the family to feel themselves active and capable (Gordon & Davidson, 1981).

The efficacy of training parents in specific behavioral techniques has received considerable support from research (Trad, 1988). Research suggests that the following disorders can be treated successfully using parent training: encopresis (Edelman, 1971); nocturnal enuresis (Paschalis, Kimmel, & Kimmel, 1972); childhood obesity (Gillick, 1974; Grace, 1975); mental retardation (Mash & Terdal, 1973); pervasive developmental disorder (Graziano, 1974; Lovaas, Koegel, Simmons, & Long, 1973); attention deficit disorder (Johnson & Brown, 1969); severely aggressive boys (Patterson, Reid, Jones, & Conger, 1975); noncompliant children (Gardner et al., 1976); and elective mutism (Nolan & Pence, 1970).

Parents' characteristics are also important in deciding whether or not parent training in behavioral techniques is indicated. When marital difficulties exist, mothers are less successful at generalizing child management skills in the home (Reisinger, Frangia, & Hoffman, 1976). Also, while empirical research offers few guidelines, it is generally thought that the refusal of the father to participate in the training has a strong negative impact on the program's effectiveness.

Gordon and Davidson (1981) have described a typical parent training program. The program begins with a brief introduction to social learning theory. The parents are then taught to pinpoint behaviors objectively and define them in specific behavioral terms. If parents are to be fully informed and motivated partners in treatment, it is essential that behavioral terminology be either avoided or translated (Rinn, 1985). Next, parents learn how to analyze the effects of antecedents and consequences on those behaviors. By this stage, they are in a position to monitor their child's behavior purposefully and establish baseline data. Most training programs include lessons in the importance of consistent record keeping, although some practitioners report difficulties with noncompliance.

Actual behavioral intervention training begins with parents being shown how to identify and use potential reinforcers. The therapist should emphasize the importance of consistent rule enforcement. Reinforcement may simply involve using praise or giving attention to appropriate behavior. Parents are also taught how to evoke new behaviors using such techniques as shaping, modeling, and prompting.

Depending on the sophistication of the parents, training may include learning how to change antecedent events. For example, although the research evidence on the matter is ambiguous, some therapists train parents to make fewer commands in the hope that the child will become more compliant. Gordon and Davidson (1981) have suggested that it is appropriate to use fewer commands because this facilitates the use of reinforcement.

The program frequently includes some training in deceleration techniques, the most common of which is the time-out technique. This involves the removal of any opportunity the child might have for reinforcement of maladaptive behaviors. The child may be isolated from people who are reinforcing, materials stimulating maladaptive behaviors may be withdrawn, or the child may be ignored. Parents are taught the importance of both using contingent release from time out and forewarning children that time out will be used.

Other deceleration techniques taught to parents include negative attention, isolation, token systems, and ignoring (Gordon & Davidson, 1981). Negative attention typically involves the contingent use of verbal reprimands. With isolation, the parent takes the toys and leaves the room. In contrast, ignoring procedures call for the parent to stay in the room but withdraw all attention from the child. Token systems are a highly effective technique in which children are given rewards for appropriate behaviors. Punishment procedures may also be employed.

BEHAVIORAL AND COGNITIVE THERAPIES

Behavioral therapy derives from the work of B. F. Skinner and has been developed for work with children primarily by the social learning theorists. Operant conditioning procedures are used to increase the occurrence of targeted positive behaviors and to extinguish negative ones. Little or no attention is paid to etiology or internal dynamics; rather, current conditions under which a child behaves in a problematic way are assessed and new contingencies are assigned to those behaviors.

The assumption is that behavior is primarily learned and can therefore be unlearned. The operant model assumes that behavior is a function of its consequences, and therefore the child will respond to consistent negative and positive reinforcement and eventually alter behavior accordingly. The focus is on responses subsequent to maladaptive behaviors and on managing response contingencies.

This model is most effective in the treatment of fears and obsessive-compulsive disorders, particularly rituals. It is also indicated for social skills problems, disorders such as enuresis, control of aggression, and behavior disorders (Marks, 1986). Contraindications include severe depression, psychosis, or biological illness (Marks, 1986). In general, behavioral therapy is appropriate only when there is a predictable pattern of behavior. In addition, the therapist, parents, teachers, and patient must concur that a behavioral approach is correct and agree on clear behavioral goals. Finally, the application of behavioral techniques requires ongoing evaluation of their efficacy, which is best accomplished if there are no confounding treatments.

Cognitive techniques are frequently used along with strictly behavioral ones. Indeed, some behavioral techniques such as control of obsessions and covert desensitization make direct use of the child's cognitions. Cognitive work aims to identify and correct maladaptive thoughts and feelings through various training methods. Underlying the approach is an assumption that psychotherapy is a process of learning and that fully developed cognitive structures are necessary for the child to learn. For example, attempts to make children express themselves in make-believe play will not be successful if they have dysfunctional cognitions.

Another goal is to teach the child to correctly coordinate and integrate the need for a realistic perspective and the need to develop an internal fantasy world. The child learns both to explore his or her inner world and contrast it with reality and to experiment with and assimilate new experiences (Santostefano, 1985). These abilities are essential to normal personality development, learning, and proper adaptation.

Cognitive techniques are typically used when the child fails to respond to traditional play therapy and verbal psychotherapy. The techniques generally call for the child to master a succession of structured cognitive tasks that attempt to build or rehabilitate specific cognitive functions (Santostefano, 1985). They may be used to treat disorders such as short attention span, poor retention, and learning anxieties. In addition, they are frequently used to treat children who are withdrawn, have low self-esteem, or have aggressive outbursts (Santostefano, 1985).

Cognitive-behavioral techniques are most often used to develop a better self-image, overcome a fear, and develop an ability to recognize and express feelings. Cognitive-behavioral procedures used for adults are often based on verbal logic; with young children, a more didactic and experiential approach is called for.

Assessment

Both before and during treatment, behavioral assessments are made to determine the exact nature and dimensions of the problem behaviors. Assessment of preschool children typically involves several methodologies and instruments, the choice of which depends on the particular disorder. Observation techniques are useful in evaluation, diagnosis, and treatment planning. They are particularly useful in establishing baseline data on frequency of adaptive and maladaptive behaviors necessary for a systematic assessment.

Analog and naturalistic assessment methods are two of the more commonly used assessment techniques. The analog method, used in the clinic setting, involves asking the child to execute certain real-life tasks or participate in situations that might occur naturally (such as a parent asking the child to put away toys). This clinic analog to outside life allows the therapist to observe an approximation of the child's behavior patterns in the family.

Naturalistic assessment, in contrast, uses a natural setting in which to observe behaviors. One or two trained raters observe the child over several days, noting frequency of target behaviors and the behaviors' precedents and antecedents. This can also be done by parents or teachers, although reliability of reports on antecedents and precedents may be compromised. With independent raters, change in the child's behavior due to the presence of a stranger may also be a problem.

Other assessment methods include structured clinical interviews, self-report measures, and behavior ratings. Both the child and the child's parents are interviewed individually in structured clinical interviews. This provides information on observable symptoms and the context in which they occur. The interviews also serve to establish a rapport between the therapist and the family. Self-report measures call for the child to be taught to recognize target behaviors and report their occurrence. For preschool children the report method must be kept very simple (e.g., telling a parent or teacher or making a mark on a chart). An important consideration is that children tend to underreport negative characteristics.

Behavior ratings by parents and teachers can also be used in assessment. These rate the child's display of adaptive and maladaptive behaviors outside the clinic. Retrospective behavior ratings can be accomplished using adaptive behavior scales. These provide a comprehensive view of adaptive and maladaptive behavior in communication, daily living skills, social skills, and motor skills. In some cases assessment is required for possible contrast effects, where behavioral interventions in one setting are offset by negative effects in another.

Standardized intelligence and achievement tests are often used to measure academic skills and to map out the child's strengths and weaknesses. Physiological responses such as heart rate may also be measured while the child is in the presence of anxiety-provoking stimuli. Finally, the therapist is well advised to carry out a medical assessment in order to avoid making a behavioral diagnosis when a medical one is appropriate (Strayhorn, 1987).

Choice of a Treatment Protocol

Once an assessment of the child has been made, the therapist chooses from a variety of techniques to devise a treatment protocol. If the choice is uncertain, the therapist may use pertinent treatments on a trial basis to ascertain their suitability. Cognitive and behavioral techniques appropriate for the treatment of specific disorders of preschoolers are outlined later in the section on specific disorders. Some of the more commonly used techniques include operant strategies, shaping, systematic desensitization, and modeling.

Operant Strategies. Operant procedures such as positive reinforcement and extinction essentially use rewards to encourage desired behaviors and punishments to discourage inappropriate ones. Before operant procedures can be employed, a baseline frequency of target behaviors is established and goals and guidelines are explained to and negotiated with the child, parents, and teachers. To chart progress, observation of the child's behavior continues.

Positive reinforcement calls for the child to be rewarded for performance of desired behavior. The therapist must define target behaviors carefully, choose rewards that are meaningful to the child, and administer them swiftly and consistently. A variety of rewards have been used including praise, attention, and tokens. Tokens are explicit rewards that serve as "back-up reinforcers" that can be exchanged for certain privileges.

With negative reinforcement, the child is punished for the performance of an undesirable behavior, and choice and administration of punishment are necessary. Extinction procedures help identify and eliminate reinforcers of undesirable behaviors. This frequently takes the form of ignoring negative behaviors on the theory that attention of any sort, even punishment, is a reward. Finally, differential reinforcement techniques introduce and reinforce a desired behavior once an undesirable behavior has been extinguished.

Shaping. Shaping techniques reward the child for making steps toward a specific behavioral goal. As each level is mastered with a high

(70% to 80%) rate of adaptive behavior, the next step is proposed and encouraged. With young children, it is often important to provide training in compliance and delaying gratification and impulsive action. For delayed gratification and impulse control, children are rewarded for waiting increasingly longer periods of time before responding to provocation or having their parents answer their requests. Preschoolers can be taught to wait several minutes for their parents and to count up to 10 instead of acting impulsively. In compliance training, a hierarchy of requests is created and the child is rewarded for prompt response to increasingly harder parental requests.

Systematic Desensitization and Flooding. Systematic desensitization begins by establishing, with help from the child and parents, a hierarchy of anxiety-provoking situations. The child is exposed to relatively innocuous situations at first; as each step is mastered, the situations become increasingly more difficult. Relaxation training is often given concurrently to aid in quelling the anxiety. Covert modeling is a similar technique, except that the child's imagination is used rather than live or filmed models.

Another technique designed to develop anxiety-coping skills is flooding or implosion. In this technique, the child is exposed to the anxiety-provoking stimulus directly for a relatively long time. Since this technique can induce extremely high levels of anxiety that the child may not be able to control, it should be applied only after other methods have been exhausted. Flooding is contraindicated where ego strength is weak, as with a borderline or psychotic child.

Systematic desensitization, flooding, or implosion and relaxation training techniques make direct use of a child's ability to conjure up and manipulate images. Elliot and Ozolins (1983) noted that imagery is also an important mediator in operant techniques. The child receiving verbal reinforcement may be indirectly taught to form positive images, which promote the desired adaptive behaviors.

Modeling. With modeling, the desired behaviors are demonstrated to the child through film, video, role playing by the therapist or others, or real-life situations. This technique is most successful when the model is someone whom the child can identify with or would want to emulate. Modeling is an important method of teaching adaptive behaviors to children and parents, and it is often used in conjunction with many of the other techniques discussed here.

Other Techniques. There is an enormous variety of additional cognitive and behavioral techniques appropriate for use with preschoolers. Role playing teaches the child to take the perspective of others through play. Materials introduced in role playing provide clues to the child's home life and the contingencies expected for specific behaviors. The therapist can guide or ask questions.

Problem-solving therapy can also be used to train children in step-by-step techniques of asking themselves questions in order to master cognitive skills and devise effective solutions to problem situations. Another technique, self-regulation therapy, trains children to develop their skills at self-monitoring, standard setting, self-evaluation, and self-reinforcement. More generally, cognitive strategy training teaches children to become more conscious of their thought processes.

Other cognitive techniques include "Who is me?", "Where is me?", "Moving fast," "Moving slowly," "Follow me," "Which is big?", "Find the shapes," "Remember me," and "Where does it belong?". Among other things, these teach the child to experience and define the body, focus attention, be selectively attentive, construct images from memory, and categorize information.

Behavioral-cognitive programs may include such techniques as self-instruction training, stress inoculation techniques, correspondence training, and physical exercise. Self-instruction training calls for the child to be trained to follow the therapist's behavior in a specific task, repeating instructions out loud. As the child masters the behavior, the necessity for verbal repetitions of instructions diminishes. Stress inoculation techniques involve the child in using a combination of coping statements and positive self-statements following success.

To reinforce children for doing what they said they would do, correspondence training can be used. This involves using reinforcers in the hope of creating antecedent verbal control of motor behavior. Another technique is vigorous physical exercise, which can be used, on a contingent or noncontingent basis, to suppress unwanted behaviors.

Finally, social skills training, through modeling and rehearsal, teaches the child verbal and nonverbal communication skills such as eye contact, intonation, and turn taking. Teaching social cues also helps the child develop the ability to understand others. Such training enables the child to communicate more easily with others and make a more agreeable impression, leading to greater self-esteem and self-confidence.

Parent training in therapeutic techniques is an essential element in the treatment plan. Parents need to be taught the principles of modification of their child's behavior and given a specific therapeutic plan to follow. They are trained to deal effectively with their child's misbehavior by modifying it through reinforcement, modeling, and extinction during rehearsals of parent-child interactions with the therapist as "coach." Training in self-control helps parents implement a difficult home treatment plan. They may establish a list of activities they find pleasing and reward themselves with an activity from the list when a specific behavioral goal has been met in home therapy with the child.

APPLICATIONS OF VIDEO TECHNIQUES

Parents and other family members may also be called on to play a role in another increasingly important dimension of treatment: the video-tape recording. Family members may be asked to allow family interactions to be taped and segments replayed to demonstrate the existence of particular patterns. The video recording can also be used to enhance family members' understanding of each other's perspectives by placing the camera so that interaction is seen from the perspective of others.

In recent years, the widespread availability of videotape recording has given practitioners a new and powerful tool, especially but not exclusively as an attraction to otherwise resistant children. Although use of videotape is contraindicated with psychotic, paranoid, and extremely depressed patients, there are myriad other patients for whom incorporation of videotape recording into therapy can be beneficial. This is particularly true for children with low self-esteem, poor body image, social withdrawal, and passivity. In addition, behavioral problems and skill deficits are amenable to treatment with video techniques.

The first use of the videotape recording in a child's treatment may be to provide parents with a tape of a typical therapy session. The child can be shown the tape to reduce fears about the new setting. Therapeutic uses of videotape recording include taping and playing back positive, adaptive aspects of the child's behavior. This can help increase the child's self-esteem and reinforce the adaptive behavior. Taped segments of sessions or interactions can also be played back to allow the child to evaluate his or her actions, behavior, and social skills. The mere act of watching oneself promotes this self-reflection. Voice-overs can also be used to promote reflection and to incorporate the therapist's interpretations.

Tapes of other people are often used to model adaptive behaviors to be emulated by the child. These tapes have been shown to be successful in changing attitudes, fostering interpersonal skills, and teaching assertiveness (Heilveil, 1983). Self-modeling tapes can be used to increase the intensity of the identification. The desired behavior is taped under conditions especially conducive to it, and the goal is to transfer those behaviors to other conditions. With preschool children, for example, the tape may be shown directly prior to a play therapy session.

Tapes of other people can also be used to show people with different emotions and have the child identify them as part of learning about his or her own emotions and being trained in empathy and social skills. If the modeling is to be successful, it is important that the model be similar to the child (Kornhaber & Schroeder, 1975).

One of the most widely used applications of videotape recording is in systematic desensitization, with the child being shown tapes presenting a hierarchy of anxiety-provoking stimuli. The procedure can be almost completely automated, with the therapist merely providing a safe environment. Its advantage over live desensitization is that it is available on a continuous basis to the patient. Its disadvantage is that inadequate imagery can lead to failure. Another use of videotape recording is to allow a child a few minutes alone in front of the camera to tell any secret he or she has not been able to express to the therapist. Later, the child can give permission for the therapist to watch the tape.

Videotape also can be used in the mutual storytelling technique, which is designed to overcome difficulties in communicating with children (Gardner, 1971). In this technique, the child tells a story, which is followed by a story from the therapist told in the same language as the child. The therapist's story illustrates adaptive solutions to conflicts revealed in the child's story. Gardner has suggested that a videotape format can be used to encourage the child to tell a story. The child's production should be independent of therapist suggestions.

Heilveil (1983) discussed several uses of videotape in individual psychotherapy including freeze, half and half, and affect simulation. Freeze uses the freeze-frame capability of videotape replay to highlight subtle nonverbal behavior revealed in frozen images. These images form the basis for a discussion of unconscious conflicts. Half-and-half techniques involve replaying only the sound or image part of the recording. This allows the therapist and patient to focus attention on particular attributes of communication that might go unnoticed otherwise. Affect simulation uses videotapes of scenes to provoke affect. For example, a child might be asked to imagine that a character talking into the camera lens is talking to the child. If the child has difficulty coping with parental rejection, the videotape recording might convey this message so that the child can learn coping skills in the safe confines of the therapist's office. The child's reaction to the videotape recording may also be used as a basis for assessment and discussion.

Other uses of videotape include simultaneous feedback, serial viewing, "transfer, please," and video homework. Simultaneous feedback uses video monitors to allow children to view themselves as they are speaking. The therapist focuses the child on specific behaviors, especially responses to questions and interpretations. Unlike videotape replay, this technique is designed to promote spontaneous insight. Serial viewing involves showing a compendium of excerpts from tapings over the course of many sessions. The focus is on indicating change and discussing significant moments during treatment. "That's me, all right" is a self-modeling technique that also uses serial viewing. A tape is made of the child performing desired behaviors in order of successive difficulty. Repeated viewing and review of antecedents helps the child master the behaviors.

"Transfer, please" facilitates the transfer of information from one therapeutic context to another. For example, if the child's treatment strategy calls for group or family therapy, then videotapes of those sessions can be brought to therapy sessions. Videotapes can also be taken home so that the child can do "homework" specified by the therapist. This has the advantage of letting the child view the tapes alone and respond in a way that is uninhibited by the presence of the therapist.

PARENT BEHAVIORAL TRAINING IN GROUPS

Group behavioral training for parents is an important element in treatment of childhood disorders (Rinn, Vernon, & Wise, 1975; Rose, 1974). For example, it has been found to be more effective than so-called reflective parent group procedures with the parents of mentally retarded children (Tavormina, 1975). Moreover, Rinn (1985) has suggested that for mild childhood disorders it can be used as the only form of intervention.

Rinn (1985) described one such program, called the Positive Parent Training Class, which teaches parents the principles and techniques of social learning. In this program, parents pay an initial fee, a proportion of which is refunded depending on level of attendance, homework completion, and success in altering desired behaviors. Members are first taught to define, identify, and measure specific behaviors. Then they learn to choose appropriate reinforcers and to apply them swiftly and consistently.

GROUP THERAPY

There are two general types of group therapy for children. In the first, a therapeutic group is formed that involves the children in almost any supervised group activity such as sports, play, and teamwork. The social aspect of the activity itself is considered therapeutic, although psychologically oriented discussion is not undertaken. In contrast, the second type, group psychotherapy, involves discussion of thoughts and feelings relating to psychological issues. Both types purposefully shape the group situation to act in a predictable way.

Group therapy can be used in the treatment of preschool children to accomplish several goals. It can satisfy a need to interact with and be accepted by peers, and it is particularly recommended for children who need help in overcoming shyness, withdrawal, phobias, behavior disorders, or sexual abuse and for children experiencing separation and divorce (Kraft, 1985; Rossiter, 1988). Validation of experience and support for each other can be offered even by very young children, while working through is gently encouraged by the therapist. Normalization through socialization may also be helpful for young children with handicaps or medical conditions. Finally, behavioral group therapy can be used to provide a relaxed, playful context in which children can model and practice adaptive behaviors.

Who Can Benefit

Empirical research regarding when to recommend group treatment for preschool children has been limited and inconclusive. Greif (1978) studied families with young children experiencing behavior disorders and found that, while group treatment used a fraction of the time that individual treatment used, there were no significant differences in treatment outcomes. Johnson, Phillips, Glaswow, and Christenson (1980) studied individual and group behavioral treatment strategies for young problem children and also found no significant differences in treatment outcomes. In another study, Pevsner (1982) looked at children with problems such as noncompliance, tantrums, and fighting. He found that a group behavioral treatment program that included some education about behavioral principles was more successful than individual behavioral family therapy. Finally, Rutan and Alonso (1982) have suggested that individual treatment should be used in combination with group treatment for children who are afraid of the intimacy of individual therapy and the confrontation within groups.

In a review of the clinical and research literature, Toseland and Siporin (1986) discovered that, in 25% of the studies reviewed, group therapy was more effective than individual therapy. In the remaining 75%, the group approach was as effective. However, the authors argued that the results were not as impressive as they seemed, because no clear pattern emerged as to which disorders would benefit most from group treatment and some of the results were contradictory. They also noted that there were severe methodological shortcomings in many of the studies.

Clinical research gives less ambiguous answers. It suggests that group therapy is generally appropriate when the patient's problem concerns relationships with others, especially conflicts in interpersonal relationships (Francis, Clarkin, & Perry, 1984). The group setting allows patients to work through deficits and malformations in object relationships, experience separations and individuation, and improve psychosexual development (Soo, 1985). The therapist serves as a "new object," managing individual and group transferences and providing corrective emotional experiences.

The use of group therapy with ego-impaired children such as children with borderline, antisocial, or impulsive behaviors is problematic because group techniques generally assume that the child is capable of tolerating regression (Spinner & Pfeifer, 1986). To avoid creating a hostile therapeutic setting, therapists must contain the children's reenactment of destructive object relationships. The goal is to create an environment where emotional expression is encouraged while regression is limited through ego-development techniques. The group members are helped to develop organizing and stabilizing functions that, in turn, help them build and integrate the structures underlying internal organization.

When a treatment strategy combining group and individual psychotherapy is indicated, the patient's ego structure and adaptational skills are important considerations. Children with a well-developed ego structure are aware of the inevitable discontinuities between the two modalities and can integrate the split-off object representation, thereby strengthening the transference and the alliance between therapist and patient (Pfeifer & Spinner, 1985). In contrast, ego-impaired children, while they benefit from the group approach, tend to fuse the therapeutic contexts and thus experience unintegrated affects, which must be contained. The combination of approaches does, however, increase the potential effectiveness of transference as a therapeutic tool (Bromfield & Pfeifer, 1988).

Group therapy is particularly helpful with sexually abused preschool girls. The primary goal is to diffuse the sense of psychological isolation these girls generally experience. The group can also validate feelings and help prevent the development of potentially harmful counterphobic behaviors (Pescosolido & Petrella, 1986). Specific issues that may be addressed include issues of trust, guilty feelings, self-destructive ideation, and body image (Pescosolido & Petrella, 1986). Symbolic play materials and art activities can be used in exploring these issues.

Co-therapists are typically used in groups of sexually abused preschool girls. An abused child may perceive her mother as being weak and unable to protect her. The female co-therapist can, therefore, be used to present a model of maternal protectiveness. The male therapist presents a model of a caring, responsive, and respectful male. The sessions are usually highly structured and time limited in order to maintain the focus on sexual abuse. Subsequent to the group therapy, the girl may require prolonged individual therapy to address more individualized issues such as low self-esteem, separation and abandonment fears, and trust.

In previous sections, parent groups that teach behavioral-cognitive techniques and those used in family therapy were discussed. In general, parallel parent groups are used to help parents understand the nature of their child's illness and cope with guilt feelings. They are also used to provide mutual support and practical information about medical institutions. For example, in cases involving one-parent families, groups for mothers and sons may be used simultaneously. The children in these families are thought to be particularly vulnerable to emotional and behavioral disorders. The mothers' group serves to diminish the mothers' sense of isolation and give them an understanding of the problems inherent in their situation. They may also be taught intervention strategies for improving their children's behavior (Hoffman, Byrne, Belnap, & Steward, 1981).

Contraindications for Group Therapy

In general, group therapy is unlikely to be helpful in revealing an individual patient's intrapsychic conflicts, and individual therapy should be used with such patients. More specifically, group therapy is contraindicated for depressed patients with verbalization difficulties (Horowitz, 1976); patients with socially bizarre behaviors (Toseland & Rivas, 1984; Yalom, 1975); patients in crisis situations requiring immediate intervention (Horowitz, 1976); antagonistic and extremely competitive patients (Klein, 1972); patients with severe pathology and an inability to tolerate anxiety and frustration (Horowitz, 1976); and patients who fear self-disclosure in group situations (Toseland & Siporin, 1986).

Composition of Groups

Group composition is another important consideration in group therapy. In selecting group members, the therapist's main focus is on the overall group structure rather than on the characteristics of the individual patient. For example, if a group contains too many withdrawn children, member interaction is impeded and withdrawal patterns tend to be enhanced in all members. A group size of six is optimum, and both sexes may be included evenly (Kraft, 1985). Age distribution, racial balance, and the developmental stages of members are other important compositional considerations. Antisocial, homicidal, or overtly sexually deviant children are typically excluded. The importance of group composition depends on the types of disturbances to be addressed. Treatment of behavior extremes benefits from the presence of girls, who generally tend to be a moderating influence on the group.

Approaches to Group Therapy

Practical considerations are commonly thought to be important in deciding such issues as whether to use group or individual therapy, whether to use interviews or activity training, and whether a short- or long-term treatment should be undertaken. Scheidlinger (1984) argued that, quite apart from economic considerations, while short-term group psychotherapy is not indicated for problems such as character disorder and arrested development, it is the treatment of choice for problems such as reactive disorders.

The short-term approach has been used in many group therapy treatment strategies. Groups of children at risk, for example, are designed for family members of psychiatric patients. They are informational discussion groups that attempt to give children greater objectivity about their parents' or siblings' illness. Another short-term group is a crisis-intervention group, in which group members are all children in the midst of a similar crisis. The group attempts to prevent the development of psychopathology through the use of verbalization and shared information.

Therapeutic camping is often used by child guidance clinics or social service agencies as part of a broader treatment strategy. In this technique, cabin groupings and voluntary subgroupings are used for diagnosis and treatment using a variety of means including discussions of interpersonal issues, activities, and psychodrama.

Diagnostic groups are used for children about whom little is known. Dyadic child therapists also use them to answer specific diagnostic questions. The objective is to place the child in a revealing setting where detailed observation can be made. Churchhill (1972) noted that they are especially useful in revealing a child's ego functioning in regard to object constancy and relationships, impulse control, and adaptive patterns. Finally, there are sometimes therapeutic groups in pediatric hospital wards that commonly focus on mutual support, providing information to correct anxieties and distortions, and relieving fear through expression.

Group therapy with preschool children can include several elements. Most commonly it is structured around some sort of expressive activity such as artwork or puppetry. The expressive nature of play is particularly important in the treatment of children with poor verbal skills. The activities are designed to give an opportunity for expression of fantasies and impulses such as aggression in a safe and contained atmosphere. The therapist makes interpretations when appropriate. According to Ginott (1961), change in group therapy is accomplished through catharsis, insights, sublimation, reality testing, and relationships and identification with the therapist and other children.

Nondirective play therapy is particularly useful in encouraging expression and promoting a catalytic effect among members. Daniels (1964) argued that unobtrusive observation is an essential condition for spontaneity in play-group therapy. The therapist should leave the child free while playing and only participate in the play when asked.

In addition to expressive play, the therapy session may contain other elements. Education is often worthwhile for children with medical problems or behavioral deficits. Discussion allows children to focus on particular issues and emotions in a more concentrated way than is possible during less structured play. Use of a snack creates a nurturant atmosphere. Combining these elements in a systematic fashion and maintaining a standard procedure from session to session allow the children to feel the security of ritual, itself an important therapeutic experience.

The therapy room should be equipped with toys. The play can include imaginative play (pretend), art, water, paint, and skill games. It can also involve practice with rules.

Play has diagnostic, dynamic, and behavioral uses. In the play setting, children's choice of play articles, their use of them (appropriate/ inappropriate), and their ability to structure play fantasies may all reveal diagnostically relevant data. The therapist can also observe a child's level of psychosexual and social development and the child's ability to structure situations. The group provides a unique view of member interactions in a variety of situations. Areas of strength and weakness, danger points, positive and negative affect, and tolerance level can all be easily ascertained in a group play situation.

Dynamic uses include using play to decipher, interpret, and work through psychosexual issues. Leal (1966) reported that verbalization and understanding of emotional problems can be increased by therapist interpretations of play themes. Play is frequently used as a springboard for discussion, with the therapist giving the child instruction on feelings and situations. Other uses include using play to symbolically represent fears and to give structure where needed.

Hansen, Niland, and Zani (1969) stressed the importance of including appropriate role models in the group. If this is impractical, then a substitute such as videotaped models can be used. Cognitive games may also be chosen to enhance the child's self-image, lessen fears, and teach skills.

Family members can also be involved in play sessions. This gives the therapist the opportunity to observe interactions, assign role changes, form closeness, and show the family that being together can be an enjoyable experience. The play can also be used to model positive behavior or to bring out any untapped skills of the authoritarian parent. The treatment program may call for a progression from solitary play with others present to play as a group, with the focus on cooperation, teamwork, rules, and social skills. A parent can lead, follow, or just play along.

Videotaping is frequently used in group therapy. This record of interaction patterns serves to heighten self-awareness and encourage change. The way in which different members of a group react to seeing themselves allows direct intercomparisons, which are more revealing for understanding the nature of the behavior. Videotape can also be used as another toy in group play therapy.

Some of the group activities that use videotapes include "Working Together" and "I Am the Greatest" (talk show). "Working Together" involves replaying tapes of important team interactions and focusing on the degree of cohesiveness of the team. In "I Am the Greatest" activities, the therapist acts as the host of a talk show on which children play famous people who are interviewed. This helps reveal goals, build self-esteem, and provide a basis for subsequent group discussions.

ART THERAPY

Therapeutic media other than play include music therapy, art therapy, and movement/dance therapy. The goals of music therapy include providing an outlet for expression, increasing coordination, and allowing the child to perform well in a nonjudgmental area. The child's emotional reactions to different pieces of music can be used to explore and label feelings and emotions. Music can also be used in play, with the child drawing or dancing to the music. The family might be indirectly involved, with the therapist discussing what family members' tastes in music reveal about them and with the child making music for each of them.

Art therapy can be used in combination with play and music therapy. The child may be asked to draw feelings or draw family members during important family episodes. Having something concrete to bring home from each session promotes object constancy and security. In some cases, both art and music activities are used to illustrate the same issue. The hope is that presentation in different contexts will have a synergistic and reinforcing effect. Art and music are often used merely as activities designed to captivate the children, and not for any intrinsic therapeutic properties. Movement/dance therapy helps the child overcome shyness and improve his or her body image.

PHARMACOTHERAPY

Although pharmacotherapy is an infrequent treatment modality with preschool children, it can be used in combination with psychotherapy, and it may also be used as an adjunct to other treatment strategies. The therapist should know the precise developmental effect of the drugs, including the possible side effects to watch for, and should be aware of the drugs' comparative value relative to other treatment strategies.

Pharmacological treatment is indicated for disorders such as pervasive developmental disorders (Campbell, 1988; Fisher, Kerbeshian, & Burd, 1986; Rapoport & Kruesi, 1985); mental retardation (Rapoport & Kruesi, 1985); depression (McDaniel, 1983); attention deficit hyperactivity disorder (Rapoport & Kruesi, 1985; Speltz, Varley, Peterson, & Beilke 1988); enuresis (Fournier, Garfinkel, Bond, Beauchesne, & Shapiro, 1987; Rapoport & Kruesi, 1985), and school phobia and separation anxiety (Rapoport & Kruesi, 1985). The use of stimulants is contraindicated for psychotic children or children with thought disorders (Rapoport & Kruesi, 1985).

Gadow (1983) suggested several methods for improving compliance and thus the effectiveness of pharmacotherapy. He argued that the therapist should (1) open a channel of communication with the child's school; (2) use standardized procedures for ascertaining the effects of the medication; (3) discontinue medication now and then to determine its efficacy; and (4) find the appropriate dosage levels. The success of this form of treatment also depends on parental compliance with the medication schedules. The therapist should be careful to check whether the parents have prior experience with this drug and ascertain whether there are any negative attitudes toward it.

CONCLUSION

The therapist faces several challenges in choosing treatment strategies. The focus of treatment should be broad enough to involve family members and other institutions as partners in the treatment process. It is a misconception that they are generally unwilling to participate fully. The therapist must decide on the scope of treatment and whether to investigate the conflicts underlying particular symptoms or focus primarily on the contingencies surrounding a child's maladaptive behaviors. The therapist must also decide between short- and long-term interventions and between individual and group approaches. This chapter has provided information to guide therapists in making these decisions and forming successful treatment strategies.

CHAPTER TWENTY-SIX

Therapeutic Protocols for Disorders During the Preschool Years

INTRODUCTION

Once the therapist has evaluated the precise nature of the preschool child's disorder, he or she must determine the differential effectiveness of the techniques discussed in Chapter Twenty-Five for the particular disorder in hand. It is essential to consider the interrelatedness of the modalities and devise a protocol in which the individual elements complement, rather than counteract, each other. For example, Bromfield and Pfeifer (1988) have argued that whenever there is a weak alliance between child and therapist the alliance may be weakened further by the added psychological pressures of combining group therapy with individual therapy. The therapist should also be aware of the variations in a particular technique's implementation procedures as they relate to specific disorders.

In general, there is a place for family, behavioral, cognitive, group, and pharmacotherapy interventions in the treatment protocol chosen for any specific disorder. For example, whenever behavioral techniques are used, the simultaneous use of other modalities typically can enhance the effectiveness of those techniques. It is usually recommended that the family be trained in behavioral techniques so that they will become aware of the extent and nature of their influence on their child's behaviors and so that the treatment process will be generalized beyond the therapeutic context. A group setting can also be used to diagnose antecedents and precedents for maladaptive behaviors and to provide a relaxed, playful context in which the child can model and practice adaptive behaviors. Cognitive therapy might also be important if the child lacks the cognitive structures necessary for learning the new behaviors. Finally, pharmacotherapy can be used to facilitate the child's attempt to build a new repertoire of behaviors.

This chapter provides pointers as to which techniques might be included in the overall treatment package for a specific disorder. Each disorder's symptoms are specified, and the appropriate treatment techniques for ameliorating them are indicated.

SPECIFIC DISORDERS: TREATMENT AIMS AND GOALS

Pervasive Developmental Disorders

Symptoms of pervasive developmental disorders, particularly autism, may present in the form of social isolation, oppositional behavior, lack of environmental exploration, and communication difficulties. Treatment goals are focused on helping the child develop adaptive socialization, compliance, exploration, and communication skills. Therapeutic strategies also include methods that both relieve parents of feelings of blame for the child's maladaptive behaviors and train them to actively support the evolution of the child's therapy. Treatment methods include psychotherapy, behavioral strategies, pharmacotherapy, and family and psychoeducational interventions.

To improve the child's socialization skills the therapist begins by engaging the child in a therapeutic relationship. The therapist then promotes the child's sense of individuation by using photographs, mirrors, and video devices to enable the child to perceive and reflect about himself or herself as a separate individual from parents and others. Compliance skills are developed through modeling and role playing. Modeling, a technique in which adaptive behaviors are learned from observing and imitating models, is also used to help develop reciprocal communication skills, techniques such as appropriate use of eye contact, facial expression, and physical gesturing. Also, the therapist and child can mutually explore the environment until the child is ready to undertake his or her own explorations.

Behavioral strategies can be used to improve the child's social interests. For example, in order to encourage the frequency of adaptive behaviors, the therapist uses operant strategies such as reinforcement and behavior induction. Behavior reduction strategies, on the other hand, are employed to reduce maladaptive behaviors. Pharmacotherapy, such as the use of fenfluramine and haloperidol, can also be used to ameliorate the secondary symptoms of gross deficits in communication and social responsiveness (Campbell, 1988; Fisher et al., 1986; Rapoport & Kruesi, 1985). Rapoport & Kruesi (1985) have suggested that haloperidol is especially useful in treating children with Tourette syndrome, a disorder characterized by multiple skeletal and vocal tics.

Parallel group therapy can be used to increase an autistic child's social interactions and individuation. In the hope of interrupting autistic behavior, children are provided with toys that promote contact and sharing with each other. The therapist's interpretations should address such issues as withdrawal, rivalry, and the violation of property rights. Speers and Lansing (1982) found that after an initial period of panic reactions, interactions increased, individuation developed, and communicative speech became evident. Gratton and Rizzo (1969), on the other hand, used nonplay group therapy and found that progress was very slow, with the children remaining nonverbal.

Maintaining a flux in group composition benefits both newcomers and experienced group members. Group formation is promoted by the addition of new members, who, in turn, experience less anxiety due to the presence of more experienced children on whom they can model themselves.

Parent training in therapeutic techniques is an essential element in the treatment of children with pervasive developmental disorders. Parents can learn how to reinforce the behavior modification initiated by the therapist, and by engaging in this role they can relieve themselves of guilt feelings concerning their child. Parents' groups can also be formed to provide mutual support and enable parents to deal with conflicts of displacement and dependency.

Family and/or individual family member counseling can also be used to help family members adopt perspectives about the child's deficits and cope with their own relevant feelings and responsibilities. Two therapists might work together in the family home to allow sufficient time to be given to both child and parents. The aim is to promote a mutually satisfying relationship between parents and child and to focus the parents on the child's affective experience and needs while at the same time taking into account the parents' feelings. The parents are taught to empathize with the child and develop an adaptive relationship with him or her. They are also taught to explore their own feelings, especially as they relate to interacting with the child. However, one difficulty is that fathers are generally emotionally isolated and reluctant to participate fully in the treatment (Speers & Lansing, 1982).

Elective Mutism

Elective mutism usually results from struggles for autonomy between a child and his or her parents. The child usually perceives the parents as being overcontrolling and responds by punishing them via refusal to talk. The goal in treating the child with elective mutism is to help the parents and child cope with and resolve underlying dynamic issues. Psychotherapy, behavioral, and family intervention strategies are employed in treatment.

The therapist begins by providing a situation in which issues of parental control/child autonomy can be resolved with less intense conflicts. Conflict displacement techniques can be used to model appropriate behaviors during conflict situations. Conflict displacement is a learning process in which family members are helped to argue about issues that engender conflict.

Family counseling is aimed at helping family members understand and resolve issues that motivate overcontrol.

Mental Retardation

Children with mental retardation are unable to process environmental stimuli and respond appropriately; as a result they may be disruptive, ineffective at communicating, and unable to cope adaptively. The goals of treating a child with mental retardation are many, serving to help these children respond more adaptively to their environments and thus become more easily accepted by mainstream society. These treatment goals include the following:

- To develop coping skills to a level that enables the child to interact with the family and handle any social situations.
- To increase the child's ability to differentiate between real-life and pretend situations.
- To help the child develop a positive self-concept.
- To decrease self-stimulation and egocentric behaviors.
- To improve the child's impulse control.

These aims are accomplished via psychotherapy, behavioral strategies, pharmacotherapy, and family interventions.

To help a child with mental retardation achieve his or her full potential, the practitioner's first step is to become familiar with the child's strengths and deficits through naturalistic observations and analog assessments. The presence and frequency of particular behaviors can be rated by parents, teachers, or, depending on capability, the child. When coping skills and levels of motor, cognitive, emotional, and social adjustment have been evaluated, a treatment plan can be devised.

The self-stimulating, egocentric behaviors of retarded children are discouraged through behavior-reduction procedures such as extinction. Adaptive behaviors are encouraged through modeling, shaping, and reinforcement. Modeling is a technique in which adaptive behaviors are learned from models; shaping techniques reward the child for progress toward a specific behavioral goal; and reinforcement is a technique in which a system of rewards and punishments is employed to encourage adaptive behaviors and discourage undesirable ones. Through shaping and reinforcement, the child is taught to cope better and to help himself or herself. Bathing, dressing, and grooming can be taught, thereby allowing the child to be more self-reliant and less dependent on others for physical caretaking. Cognitive therapy is of use in at least two areas: training the child to improve concentration and attention spans, and practice in the recognition and expression of emotions. Skills such as interpreting feelings of others and engaging in reciprocal communication are developed through modeling and role playing.

Pharmacotherapy can also be used to diminish the self-stimulating and aggressive behaviors of mentally retarded children. Rapoport and Kruesi (1985) reported that haloperidol can be useful in this regard; however, they noted that the mere existence of mental retardation is not a sufficient indication for use of the drug.

Nondirective group play therapy can be used to help mentally retarded children become better adjusted emotionally and behaviorally.

The emphasis should be on nonverbal play and emotional, rather than intellectual, expression. The objective is to provide safe, stress-free settings in which supportive therapists can help these children release themselves from their inadequate level of functioning. Through repetitive experimentation, the mentally retarded child can develop and improve his or her self-image.

It is widely believed that mentally retarded children should be excluded from groups unless the group is specifically designed for such children. However, Scheidlinger, Eisenberg, King, and Ostrower (1962) reported a case in which a single mentally retarded child was included in an activity group. The treatment was surprisingly successful. The child developed a realistic view of his disabilities and improved his ability to interact with and identify with his peers in a positive way.

Mental retardation in many children results from interpersonal or familial deprivation. Even when its source is biological, family involvement may be necessary to overcome maladaptive reactions by family members. Parent training in behavioral techniques is essential. Supportive counseling and education regarding the nature of the child's disorder are also helpful. The therapist can provide practical help for the family in the form of referrals to appropriate schools, play groups, day-care facilities, and parent support associations.

Family therapy may be called for to explore parental and sibling feelings of ambivalence and guilt regarding the child. Therapists should be sensitive to family issues such as financial strain, sibling jealousy or parental overattention to the retarded child, and parental exhaustion. In a troubled family system, a retarded child may be prevented from attaining full potential due to ossification of family roles and the family's "need" for the retarded child's dependence.

Schizophrenia Spectrum

When working with schizophrenic children, the therapist serves as a liaison between the child's magical world and the real world. The goals of treating a child with schizophrenia are to develop the child's ego boundary awareness; to develop the child's cognitive skills; to help the child cope with emotional/cognitive discrepancies; and to promote adaptive behaviors. Play therapy can be used in conjunction with family therapy and other therapeutic strategies to modify the child's behavior.

When treating schizophrenic children, it is useful to work progressively, according to which of the three ego-boundary levels the child is acting at. At the first level, the therapist promotes the development of a realistic physical self-concept by using a mirror and by fixing ankle weights to the child in order to increase body boundary awareness. The child's sense of self-identity is further developed using autonomous ego skill developmental therapy.

At the second level, the therapist uses structured cognitive stimulation techniques and play therapy to promote the child's interest in environmental stimuli. Because of their difficulty in distinguishing between reality and their pervasive unreal perceptions, schizophrenic children may become anxious in play therapy; the similarity of toys and their referents may induce stress. Furthermore, they may be unenthusiastic about participating in play. Thus, the therapist who uses play therapy must act as an interpreter who aids the child in understanding distinctions between reality and play and aims to root the child in reality.

As the child moves to higher ego-boundary levels, techniques employed at earlier levels are continued to reinforce the development. However, the therapist can increase the complexity of treatment strategies as indicated by the child's progress.

Family counseling is useful in helping parents understand the level of ego boundaries the child has and to handle adaptively expressed emotions.

Affective Disorders

In affective disorders, the major symptom is a pervasive mood that colors the child's entire range of perceptions and behavior. In major depression, for example, the child's mental state can be influenced by feelings of helplessness and poor self-esteem. Treatment approaches for a child with major depression are designed to improve the child's self-esteem, help the child understand the relationship of his or her feelings to environmental changes, and promote competent and rewarding interactions with the environment. Psychotherapy, behavioral strategies, pharmacotherapy, and family interventions are employed to achieve these adjustments.

To assess the child's conceptualizations of his or her inner self and to monitor the changes in these conceptualizations over time, the therapist uses the "amorphous blob" technique at set intervals throughout the therapy. This technique involves having the child periodically draw a blob that reflects a description of his or her inner self. These drawings are used to explore and improve the child's self-image. A realistic self-concept can be developed using corrective feedback and self-esteem techniques to foster positive feelings and thoughts and help the child avoid being continually overwhelmed by negative feelings.

To help the child become more assertive and externalize aggression, assertiveness training and body painting techniques can be used. Body painting is a technique in which the child paints his or her own body, thereby making the child aware of the body's boundaries, parts, and properties. The child is also taught attribution retraining techniques to attribute negative outcomes to factors outside of himself or herself and develop realistic expectations of his or her ability to achieve positive outcomes. In addition, the therapist models and teaches the child social skills to increase effectiveness during and participation in social exchanges. Pharmacotherapy may involve the use of such tricyclic antidepressants as Imipramine and Nortriptyline (McDaniel, 1983).

Group activity therapy may be another element in the treatment strategy. The group provides a nonthreatening setting in which the child learns to express aggression through play. The child observes the other members and is eventually confident enough to experiment with establishing relationships. Another group technique for reducing social anxiety and shyness is assertiveness training. Leone and Gumar (1979) described a program in which behavioral contracts are used to promote assertive behaviors. When a child wants something from someone or wants to do something with someone, the child has to get the person to sign a contract. When the contract is completed, both children receive a reward. Group discussions, role playing, and modeling are also used to explore childrens' feelings about assertive behaviors.

Shy, withdrawn children are often treated using a group therapy program in which the therapist provides verbal or token reinforcement for selected behaviors. Clement and Milne (1967) found that using a tangible reward (token) as reinforcement was more effective than verbal reinforcement in improving social approach behaviors. As the treatment progresses, the child must make a more complete social approach to receive reinforcement. A variable-interval reinforcement schedule is used.

It is essential for the depressed child to experience a supportive family environment. The aim of family members is to learn models for interacting adaptively and positively with the child. Family members should not be critical of the depressed child or further the child's misconceptions about himself or herself. Recognition and individual treatment of any other member of the household who might be depressed are also very important.

Anxiety Disorders

In anxiety disorders, symptoms (e.g., separation anxiety) are usually accompanied by avoidance of the anxiety-evoking stimulus. Treatment goals include the development of coping mechanisms to be employed when confronted with the object of anxiety, as well as the eventual dissolution of the anxiety response to the object. The goals of treatment can be met through psychotherapy, behavioral strategies, pharmacotherapy, and family interventions.

To improve the child's coping skills, the therapist uses a combination of cognitive procedures, structured play therapy, and systematic desensitization techniques. The therapist models coping behaviors and teaches the child how to engage in other behaviors during an anxiety-provoking situation. Object-constancy reinforcement techniques and cognitive procedures are used to guide the child in discovering and verbalizing feelings. Pharmacotherapy, in the form of the tricyclic antidepressant Imipramine, can also be helpful, especially in the treatment of school-phobic children.

Desensitization during group therapy may also be used in treatment. Procedures are similar to those used in individual desensitization. The therapist counterconditions a hierarchy of anxiety-provoking events by repeatedly making the children relax and then asking them to imagine those events. To build self-confidence, group discussions are also employed. The use of a group is advantageous because it provides a setting for testing newfound social skills and the reinforcement of adaptive behaviors is immediate. The group also provides an environment for mutual support, and members can identify with each other.

Anxiety disorders are commonly treated with both individual and family therapy. A case in point is when a mother and her child have difficulty separating. Family therapy is called for because marital difficulties often exist in these cases. Family members are taught how to respond adaptively to the anxious child, and behaviors that act to extinguish maladaptive behaviors and encourage adaptive behaviors are modeled. Attachment figures should be encouraged to explore and deal adaptively with the ambivalent feelings of the child.

Montenegro (1968) reported that parents can be used in reciprocal inhibition, a behavioral technique, to successfully treat severe separation anxiety. Reciprocal inhibition is a desensitization technique that uses feeding responses to counteract anxiety. The child is gradually exposed to a hierarchy of anxiety-provoking events and is fed at the same time. With repetition, the effect becomes conditioned. The technique works best after the child has been fed poorly for a period of time.

Disruptive Behavior Disorders

Children who cannot control their impulses are at risk for harming themselves and others by acting out destructive impulses. In fire setting, for example, the child cannot resist urges to set fires because of the associated feelings of arousal and power. In treating such a child, the goal is to abolish the child's fascination with setting and watching fires.

This is accomplished through psychotherapy, cognitive therapy, and family therapy.

To inhibit the child, the therapist helps the child develop a comprehensive conceptualization of the consequences of his or her impulses. The therapist interprets the child's behaviors and shows the child, through pictures or visits, the real results of those behaviors. For example, a child who cannot resist setting fires could be shown a film that depicts the effects of fire on wildlife, could be taken to speak with firemen, and could be shown the effects of fire on property and life.

Family counseling should be used to help the parents observe the child closely and to help the child develop alternate ways of behaving.

Attention Deficit Disorder with Hyperactivity

Children with attention deficit disorder with hyperactivity usually have symptoms of inattention, an inability to control impulses, and a high level of motor activity. They may also have poor self-esteem and difficulty tolerating frustration. These behavioral elements typically interfere with the child's ability to learn. The desired goals of treatment of a child with attention deficit disorder with hyperactivity are to enable the child to control impulses, increase attention span, and provide a foundation for learning. Psychotherapy, pharmacotherapy, behavioral therapy, and family strategies are useful in achieving these goals.

The therapist helps the child learn how to control and regulate impulses using delayed impulse response techniques, operant techniques such as reinforcement, and behavior induction and reduction procedures. These techniques systematically manage behavior contingencies using rewards and punishments. The child is also encouraged to adhere to restrictions and external controls by using a set of behavioral guidelines provided by contingency management techniques. The therapist can use behavioral ratings as a basis for rewarding the decrease in maladaptive behaviors and as a means of monitoring progress. Pharmacotherapy may take the form of giving the child stimulants such as dextroamphetamine or methylphenidate. This can help change work behaviors and aggressiveness and reduce the frequency of tantrums (Barkley, 1988; Speltz, Varley, Peterson, & Beilke, 1987). Rapoport and Kruesi (1985) noted that such stimulants are contraindicated for thought disorders and psychosis.

Family intervention in the form of psychoeducation about the disorder is also advisable. In particular, the therapist should point out the physiological basis of the disorder and its implications for interaction with the child. Behavioral interventions among household members should also reduce the symptoms. Parents are given training in therapeutic techniques to enable them to reinforce progress made within the therapeutic setting.

Oppositional Defiant Disorder

Children with oppositional defiant disorder are noncompliant and resistant to adult requests. Often, oppositional behavior is unintentionally encouraged by parents who do not insist on the child's compliance; in this sense, the parents comply with the child's noncompliance. Thus, the goals of treating a child with oppositional disorder are to modify both the parents' and the child's behavior. The desired results of treatment are modification of oppositional tendencies and development of an emotionally secure and supportive family environment. Psychotherapy, behavioral strategies, and family interventions are used to achieve these goals.

Operant techniques such as reinforcement, behavior induction, and reduction techniques are used to encourage adaptive behaviors and discourage maladaptive behaviors. These can be taught to groups of parents via lectures, videotape presentations, modeling, and role playing.

Parent training is another essential element in the treatment program. Parents are trained in techniques to reinforce progress achieved within the therapeutic milieu. Parents are trained in social learning procedures to give them the tools needed to establish effective communication and a positive relationship with their child. They are taught to reward themselves for successful therapeutic interventions by allowing themselves to enjoy an activity they find pleasurable after the child has made progress. Family therapy can help parents cope with their feelings regarding distressing aspects of their involvement with the child.

Lavigne and Reisinger (1984) described two parent training programs, the University of Georgia Program, and the Regional Intervention Program. The University of Georgia Program calls for teaching parents behavioral management techniques and allowing them to practice these techniques under the supervision of the therapist in the clinic. Social reinforcement, contingent attention, contingent rewards, timeout techniques, modeling, and role playing are all elements of the program. Parents are also taught to eliminate vague or unsatisfactory commands. The Regional Intervention Program teaches parents similar techniques, but once they have mastered them, they go on to teach these skills to other parents, thus reinforcing their own progress. The program also uses reversal techniques, which call for the parent to only attend to the child when he or she is noncompliant. This serves to underscore in the parents' minds the role that their attention plays in the child's behavior.

Conduct Disorders

In treating children with conduct disorders, one goal is to decrease the incidence of their socially unacceptable behaviors (for example, disobedience or physical aggression toward others). To accomplish the reduction and eventual disappearance of such activities, children and parents must participate together in therapy. While the child is encouraged to cease unacceptable behaviors, the child's parents are trained in how to respond to the child's bad and/or adaptive behaviors. Another goal of therapy with conduct-disordered children is to improve parent-child relationships. Psychotherapy, behavioral strategies, and family interventions are used in treatment.

To motivate the child to recognize people's feelings, the therapist uses empathy training, which, in part, teaches the child to interpret facial expressions and other nonverbal communications. Operant techniques such as behavior induction and reduction techniques are also used to encourage adaptive behaviors and discourage maladaptive behaviors. These techniques systematically manage behavior contingencies using rewards and punishments for targeted behaviors. Adaptive behaviors are further promoted with contingency contracting, which furnishes the child with a set of rules to guide his or her behavior toward greater adaptability. The child enters into a contract to behave in a prescribed manner and is rewarded for meeting these obligations.

Group programs combining counseling and behavioral principles can be used to help undisciplined children adopt more appropriate patterns of thinking and behaving. This kind of program begins with group discussions that are nonjudgmental and focus on realistic assessments of situations and on problem solving. The therapist guides the discussions and reinforces appropriate behaviors. Later in the program, behavioral rules that stress discipline during discussions are adopted and a reward system can be instituted.

In the case of excessively aggressive behaviors, a combination of activity group therapy, verbal therapy, and behavior therapy can be used in treatment (Marks & Keller, 1977). The activities used include individual and group games, with the therapist using rewards to reinforce certain explicitly defined target behaviors. Half the time is devoted to discussions that focus on problem behaviors and exploring feelings. Parallel parent groups may also be formed so that treatment goals can be explained and the parents can be taught the behavioral skills necessary for the generalization of behavior modifications.

When delinquency is caused by acting out feelings, rather than verbalizing them, a group therapy program that uses token reinforcement is indicated. The rewards are given initially for simply speaking and later only for personal statements. In the final phase, only verbalizations of feelings and personal problems are rewarded. Throughout treatment, the children are also given verbal reinforcement by the therapist.

Children showing episodic dyscontrol tend to have an extremely strong emotional bonding with one parent and a weak one with the other (Howells, 1980). Parental inconsistency in reaction to aggression is also common. Family psychotherapy initially involves forcing the family to adopt a clear set of systematic steps to be taken when a violent episode occurs. Later, the therapist can work on the causes underlying overly close alliances.

Conduct disorders often reflect the unconscious needs of the parents, whose limits on the child's behavior are either extreme or inconsistent. Such familial motivations need to be ascertained in family therapy. Contingency contracting is also used to provide parents with appropriate responses to incidents of maladaptive behaviors.

Parent training in therapeutic techniques enables parents to reinforce modifications that were accomplished within the therapeutic milieu. Parent training in social learning principles gives them the necessary tools to develop effective communication and a more rewarding relationship with their child. In addition to training parents in how to reinforce therapeutic gains, family and/or individual family member therapy provides family members with the opportunity to develop skills for coping with their own feelings about the child's problematic behavior and its impact on them.

Functional Encopresis

Functional encopresis is commonly accompanied by a stressed parent-child relationship, anxiety and guilt feelings in the encopretic child, and the child's inability to modulate emotional conflicts and body functions. The goal of therapy when treating an encopretic child is to encourage the development of an emotionally secure family environment wherein the child is able to feel supported and subsequently gain control over emotional conflicts and body functions. Psychotherapy and family intervention techniques are used to reach that goal.

Self-esteem techniques are used to improve the child's self-concept. These techniques involve the use of modeling, monitoring, and goal setting to improve the child's self-perception. Improved self-esteem, in turn, helps to alleviate feelings of guilt and anxiety related to the encopresis. The child is educated about the emotional underpinnings, and self-control techniques are used to teach the child how to express emotions appropriately and manage emotional conflicts.

Family counseling is given to capitalize on the family's existing support structure and adaptive dynamics to encourage eradication of the child's stress and encopresis. Conflict displacement teaches families with an encopretic child to model behavior for confronting the child's encopresis appropriately. Family therapy is important in order to ensure family compliance to treatment therapies and provide opportunity for members to discuss and understand the implications of their personal involvement in the child's care.

Functional Enuresis

Functional enuresis is often associated with strained parent-child relationships and with the enuretic child's victimization by peers who tease. As a result, enuretic children are likely to develop a deficient self-concept. Treatment of an enuretic child is aimed at improving the parent-child relationship and helping the child understand and act on his or her personal rights. Psychotherapeutic behavioral strategies, pharmacotherapy, and family interventions are used in the treatment.

The child should be helped to learn how to assert himself or herself appropriately and interact more adaptively with others, especially with peers. Assertiveness training can be used to teach enuretic children to understand that they are entitled to personal rights and respect. This training involves self-affirming statements, modeling of assertive responses, and teaching the child to empathize and interpret social situations correctly. Pharmacotherapy, in the form of giving the child such tricyclic antidepressants as Imipramine, can also be used to control enuretic symptoms (Rapoport & Kruesi, 1985).

Conflict displacement is used with the intention of teaching families with enuretic children to model behaviors that serve as a guide for confronting the enuresis appropriately. Conflict displacement is a process of learning and practice whereby family members are helped to argue about issues underlying conflicts. Families of enuretic children can be trained to use supportive strategies, which involve charting progress while supplying praise to the child in response to successes. A second aspect of family participation in the enuretic child's treatment is observing and reporting on the child's progress along with use of reinforcers prescribed by the therapist.

Sleep Disorders

In treating children with sleep disorders, the goal is to help them develop an improved sleep pattern. For example, the desired outcome of treatment of a child with insomnia is the child's improved rate of initiating and maintaining sleep. Psychotherapeutic, behavioral, and family interventions are used in achieving this goal.

To encourage continued improvements in sleep patterns, the thera-pist uses a combination of positive reinforcement and shaping tech-niques. Shaping rewards the child for making incremental advances toward achieving the desired adaptive behavior; it is used to gradually acclimate the child to falling asleep at an earlier time. A clear distinc-tion should be made between day and night, and a bedroom ritual should be developed. The child may also be taught to get up each morn-ing at the same time and associate the bed and bedroom solely with sleep (Norton & Deluca, 1979).

Positive reinforcers for negative behaviors, such as parental attention given to the child when he or she is awake at bedtime, are discouraged by using extinction techniques. Richman, Douglas, Hunt, Lansdown, and Levere (1985) have suggested that such parental responses are ex-tremely important and have provided evidence that their elimination is particularly efficacious. It is useful to involve parents and the child in defining treatment goals while developing an individualized treatment program. This can help reduce guilt feelings when a parent has to be strict with the child. Parents are also taught how to record the child's progress.

Eating Disorders

Obesity. Obese children are likely to suffer also from poor self-esteem and high sensitivity to others' criticisms and have a distorted image of their bodies. Usually these personality traits are accompanied by a pattern of family relationships that precipitates negative feelings in the child, and the child may subsequently use overeating as a substi-tute for these unsatisfactory relationships. In treating an obese child, the therapist's goal is to improve the child's self-image and ability to interact with others effectively. It is also important that the child be helped to forge an accurate self-concept. Psychotherapy, behavioral therapy, and family interventions are useful in treating the obese child.

The therapist uses such techniques as body impulse directing with limit challenge, conflict displacement, and "listen to your body" to teach the obese child how to accurately conceptualize his or her body and how to control both the urge to eat and inappropriate outbursts related to conflicts over weight. Body impulse directing teaches the child to manage behavior using detailed observation and recordkeep-ing. Incentives may be an element in this procedure. Conflict displace-ment uses modeling and practice to teach the child to be responsive, in a controlled manner, to legitimate concerns. "Listen to your body" teaches the child to be sensitive to inner sensations. The child is also taught, using increased body awareness techniques, to develop a realis-tic perception of his or her body.

The treatment should also include assertiveness training, which helps obese children express themselves effectively and therefore increases their self-respect. Behavior in social situations can be further improved by using social skills training, which focuses on enabling obese children to interact effectively with others, especially with peers who tend to reject or victimize them.

Family members are taught how to promote the obese child's development of an accurate self-concept and improved self-esteem.

Refusal to Eat. Children who refuse to eat sufficient food may be using this refusal as a means to escape their parents' demands to eat (Hilton, 1987). These children may also present a variety of behaviors such as intentional vomiting, physical aggression, and self-mutilation. The goal of therapy is to reduce these behaviors and teach caregivers the mechanics of an effective feeding program. Psychotherapy, behavioral therapy, and family interventions are employed in treatment.

Hilton (1987) has suggested three behaviorally oriented interventions suitable for reducing escape-oriented behavior: shaping, fun and distraction, and continued demand. Shaping uses a system of rewards and punishments to promote adaptive behaviors and discourage maladaptive ones. The reward, in this case, may be to give the child high-preference foods whenever he or she eats some of the prescribed diet. Fun and entertainment accompanying feeding may be used to reduce the negative feelings the child has about feeding times. On the other hand, Handen, Mandell, and Russo (1986) have argued the importance of feeding the child in isolated areas so as to eliminate distractions. Finally, continued demand is a technique in which the therapist or parent demands that the child consume a predetermined amount of food regardless of the child's actions. Positive verbal feedback may be included.

In order to avoid making the feeding process aversive for the child, parents should be taught these behavioral techniques carefully. They should also be taught feeding techniques that promote the establishment of an appropriate diet. Stroh, Robinson, and Stroh (1986) have suggested that these children should be offered only simple foods in small amounts, and that food should be offered only after some sign that the child desires it. They have also emphasized the importance of the relationship between the feeder and the child. Finally, Handen, Mandell, and Russo (1986) have argued that it is best to provide many meals, each of short duration.

Pica. Aside from medical causes, children with pica often have concomitant behavioral and emotional problems that contribute to their condition. For example, pica may be considered as an infantile hand-to-mouth behavioral response to such family stresses as child abuse, parental neglect, or separation (Sayetta, 1986). The goal of treatment is to assess the impact of dietary factors, decrease mouthing and ingestion behaviors, and evaluate emotional conflicts that might underlie the disorder. Psychotherapy and medical, behavioral, and family interventions are used in treatment.

The therapist should complete a medical assessment that focuses on dietary irregularities—especially in regard to iron and calcium deficiencies—and on cultural food preferences, especially for children from underdeveloped regions. Groups with high nutritional demands, such as infants, are also at high risk. If a medical cause is determined, a new dietary regime can be established, packed red blood transfusions can be given, and the child's environment can be investigated for sources of minerals contributing to the disorder, such as lead in paint.

Treatment might also involve the use of behavioral techniques such as reinforcement, discrimination training, and enrichment of the environment by increasing the level of interaction with adults and making more varied toys available. Physical restraint of the child's arms for a brief period has been noted to be particularly useful in suppressing pica.

Family counseling and psychotherapy are also used to investigate any contributing emotional conflicts and to educate family members regarding their role in treatment.

Rumination. Symptoms of rumination may be caused by organic, behavioral, or psychodynamic problems. Herbst, Friedland, and Zboraliski (1971) suggested that rumination might be an attempt to empty refluxed gastric contents from the esophagus or a reflex response to retrograde esophageal dilation. Rumination might also reflect an inadequate caregiver-infant relationship and the child's retreat from the environment. Such children are often either overstimulated or understimulated, and they may use rumination to relieve tension. Their mothers tend to have personality problems, and marital conflicts are often present (Richmond, Eddy, & Green, 1958). Finally, rumination may be a learned behavior, and it might be negatively reinforced if it results in consequences that are less averse than those avoided by ruminating. Treatment methods include psychotherapy and medical, behavioral, and family interventions.

Medical treatment of the child might involve giving small, frequent meals and thickened foods and teaching the child to have an upright posture (Chatoor, Dickson, & Einhorn, 1984). Medications such as metaclopromide or the opiate agonist paregoric may be prescribed, and, in extreme cases, surgery may be indicated. Negative conditioning in the form of unpleasant taste stimuli can also be used.

Psychodynamic treatment methods can be used to help these children gratify themselves with external objects. This might involve using a surrogate mother to regulate stimulation and provide the child with nurturing. Families can be taught to understand the disorder, and puppet play can be used to help them deal with the child's anger and change family interactions.

Somatoform Disorders

Children with somatoform disorders are usually unable to recognize emotions that act to precipitate various physical symptoms for which no medical cause can be found. In treating children with this type of disorder, the therapist's goal is to teach the child how to identify and experience feelings affectively instead of manifesting them via physical symptoms. Individual and group psychotherapy and behavioral and family interventions are useful in achieving this goal.

To help the child learn about his or her emotional life, feeling rehearsal techniques can be used. These involve the use of pictures to teach the child to recognize particular emotions. The child is also taught to portray emotions effectively using mirrors. This knowledge, in turn, helps the child recognize feelings that usually result in the production of physical symptoms so that he or she can learn how to express these feelings in appropriate and effective ways.

A strong relationship between child and therapist is essential for success. The therapist can offer emotional support and subtly convey recognition of the feelings of hurt, lack of affection, and need for help that the child is unable to communicate except through physical symptoms. With encouragement and support from the therapist, the child can be taught a more direct expression of these emotions and needs. The ease of changing the child's behavior depends, in part, on the extent to which the child actually prefers the consequences of being ill (Ford, 1983).

Group psychotherapy can also be used to help the child communicate and improve his or her sense of belonging. Concomitant symptoms of depression can be treated with pharmacological agents or by using psychotherapy if the depression reaches psychotic proportions.

Parents are taught how to promote the child's affective and emotional expression. Family involvement is particularly important in cases of hysteria (Briquet's syndrome), because these children frequently have chaotic family circumstances.

Gender Identity Disorder of Childhood

Children with gender identity disorder are often victimized and rejected by peers because of their gender-inappropriate behaviors. Treatment of gender identity disorder is directed toward preventing the child's social ostracism; this is accomplished through modification of the child's gender-referenced behaviors to socially acceptable patterns. The nature of the treatment approach is to encourage increases in gender-appropriate behaviors rather than actively discouraging inappropriate behaviors (Bates, Skilbeck, Smith, & Bentler, 1975). Psychotherapy and behavioral, group, and family interventions are used to achieve this goal.

The child is taught to use self-assessment to recognize aspects of his or her behavioral patterns and to self-monitor and adapt inappropriate behaviors on a continuing basis. This self-assessment of cross-gender mannerisms is made through play sessions purposefully designed to decrease the occurrence of such mannerisms and increase the child's awareness of his or her behaviors. Play sessions are also used to model gender-appropriate behavior, and sex-related sport skills are taught to enable the child to behave adaptively in social situations.

Using self-control behavioral modification techniques, the child is taught when to monitor his or her feelings. These techniques are also useful in encouraging the child to make accurate assessments in order to exhibit gender-appropriate behaviors. Finally, reinforcement techniques are used to encourage the consistent use of socially accepted adaptive behaviors such as the appropriate sex-typed speech.

Sports groups in a parallel group therapy context are sometimes used in the treatment of feminine boys and their parents. Appropriate behaviors are verbally reinforced while the boys are participating in sports. Criticism of each other's inappropriate behaviors is encouraged, consequently teaching members to identify such behavior in themselves. The therapist serves as a role model, and in many cases is the first male authority figure in the boy's life.

Parent groups are used to explore the parents' role in promoting the feminine behaviors. In addition, the parents are taught how to maintain in the home setting the behavior modifications accomplished in treatment sessions. Parents are encouraged to devise methods for promoting preferred behaviors at home and are taught how to reinforce such actions. Parent groups are useful for helping parents learn how to modify their children's behaviors at home and for providing an opportunity to share successes and difficulties. Father-child/mother-child activities can be useful in improving the dynamics of those relationships, and family counseling may be beneficial to all members of a family with a child who has gender-identity disorder.

Boderline Psychopathology

Often children with borderline personality organization experience feelings of aloneness (Adler & Guie, 1979). They are also likely to be enmeshed with their caregivers, a contributing factor in the development of the disorder. Thus, the goals of therapy are to assist such children in recognizing and coping with the feelings that precipitate such overwhelming feelings of aloneness and to aid them in the individuation process. Psychotherapy, behavioral strategies, and family interventions can be used.

To help children understand their emotional lives and keep track of their feelings, therapists use a combination of feelings reversal techniques and self-control techniques. Children are taught to modulate and control their responses and develop adaptive methods of expression and social interaction.

Individuation techniques are used to separate not only children from parents but also parents from their children. These techniques involve getting children to describe themselves and their parents while the therapist provides corrective feedback. Children are also taught to assert themselves verbally with their parents. Therapists can use attribution retraining techniques to teach these children how to modify perceptions both of environmental control over them and of their capacities. Parents should be taught how to provide a more structured environment in which the exhibitions of symptomatic behaviors can decrease.

It is important for parents to be trained in how to behave with consistency in interactions with their children because borderline children will experience the greatest improvements within a consistent and controlled environment.

Developmental Learning Disorders

Learning disorders are often accompanied by poor self-esteem and hindered social relationships. The learning disordered child suffers difficulties in executing everyday activities as a result of the particular learning deficits and their resulting effects on the child's emotional well-being. The child may also have difficulties with self-control and tolerance of frustration. In treating a child with a learning disorder such as developmental reading disorder, for example, the therapist's goal is to facilitate the educational process that is aimed at helping the child remediate and become a better reader, which can improve the child's self-esteem and motivation to learn. These goals are accomplished through remediation, psychotherapy, and behavioral and family interventions.

The therapist uses contingency contracting techniques to provide guidelines for the child, thus helping the child identify and set attainable learning goals. The child enters a contract to behave in a specified manner and be provided with rewards for meeting those obligations. Reinforcement techniques are then employed to reward progress toward goals.

Group therapy, in combination with individual therapy, can be used to help underachievers reduce academic anxiety that is hindering the development of their learning abilities. The treatment focuses on discussions designed to help the children identify with their peers and separate from their families. To stimulate discussion, the children might also be asked to perform academic tasks before the group. This helps other members recognize their own difficulties. Behavioral problems and interpersonal problems are also discussed. As a basis for discussion, the children might be asked to use puppets to act out the roles of teachers and parents. The therapist also discusses behaviors evident in the group sessions that he or she believes relate to the members' difficulties in school.

Parents can help improve the child's reading, writing, and arithmetic skills by following the child's academic tasks at home. This motivates improvement by demonstrating that the parents value and are interested in the child's betterment. The child's self-esteem may also be improved if parents avoid grieving over their child's condition and attempt to communicate respect for the child. Family therapy is also important in improving the child's self-control and ability to tolerate frustration. The family's role is to provide a structure that supports the behavior management required to shape skills. They should develop realistic expectations regarding performance and learn to tolerate the child's failures.

Suicide

While known suicides and suicidal behavior are relatively rare in preschool children, evidence indicates that neither is negligible. A variety of factors may underlie the young child's suicidal ideation and/or attempts. The child might be trying to control, via suicide, an otherwise unmanageable situation, or the child might be struggling unsuccessfully to develop an autonomous sense of self. The goals of therapy when treating a suicidal child are as follows:

- To stimulate the child to cognitively grasp the dimension of irreversibility of the concept of death.
- To help the child develop alternatives to self-destructive behavior.
- To aid the child in his or her individuation process.
- To help the child and his or her parents cope adaptively with intrafamilial conflicts.

Treatment methods include psychotherapy and cognitive and family interventions.

The therapist uses both psychotherapy and cognitive strategies to promote the use of adaptive behaviors as substitutes for self-destructive behavior. Cognitive strategies are also used to stimulate the child to understand the many aspects of his or her environment. Finally, in order to teach the child how to express himself or herself more effectively and to be more independent of parents, the therapist can employ assertiveness training.

Family counseling is useful in helping to reduce parent-child conflicts. Family therapy may also serve to guide family members in making appropriate responses to the suicidal child. Strategies for promoting the child's successful adaptation are designed according to the family dynamics and social supports available.

Divorce

Children of divorced parents are at risk for arrested development in response to the stress of parental separation. An individual child's vulnerability to such setbacks depends on a variety of factors. For example, a child's developmental level, parental attitudes, characteristics of the home environment, and available support systems all must be considered in the development of the child's treatment plan. The goal of the treatment is to help the child cope effectively with stress in a manner that promotes normal development. Psychotherapeutic, behavioral, group, and family intervention techniques are used in reaching such goals.

The therapist focuses on promoting understanding of divorce issues through an education program concerning divorce. This education should also be directed at acknowledging the child's suffering and relieving feelings of self-blame (Rossiter, 1988).

Group treatment programs for children of divorce are generally designed to teach coping skills and prevent disruption of development. Coping skills are learned through group discussions in which members share information on issues such as having to choose between parents, visitation problems, separation problems, and difficulties with stepparents. These group discussions also serve as an emotional outlet for feelings that, if not worked through, might disrupt development. The therapist can use films, drawings, problem lists, and role playing to draw out the children's feelings. Children are taught to recognize their feelings and view their family situations realistically.

Schaefer, Johnson, and Wherry (1982) have pointed out that many parents are so preoccupied by their own problems and so emotionally drained that their children are neglected. Outsiders such as schools or day-care centers must therefore prompt parents to provide treatment for their children. Cantor (1977) argued that these institutions are the logical place to provide group therapy because they have trained staff, are well placed for recognizing problems, and are, after families, the most important institutions in a child's life. Such groups also help prevent stigmatization of the child as having a problem.

Parental guidance that focuses on the parent/child relationship and working with the parent helps to alleviate the distress of divorce for the child. Family therapy can help improve the home environment and provide support for other family members, who are also experiencing reactions to the divorce.

Abuse and Neglect

Children who have been abused or neglected by their parents are predisposed to many psychopathologies and deficits that can result in life-long impairment. Thus it is imperative that the depression, panic states, posttraumatic stress, self-destructive tendencies, school problems, and other presenting symptoms of abuse be recognized and addressed. Since the child's affective response might serve to encourage continued abusiveness by caretakers, the goals of therapy are directed toward both the parents and the child. These goals include the following:

- To reform the parent-child bond.
- To teach effective communication skills to family members.
- To work through traumas experienced by the child and help the child learn how not to provoke further abuse.
- To establish an environment in which parents can focus on parenting and improving their relationships.
- To teach family members methods of controlling violent impulses.

Psychotherapeutic and behavioral family strategies are used to achieve these goals.

A natural starting point for the treatment program is to use abreaction techniques, which attempt to diffuse emotional responses through reviewing the trauma that caused the distress and are employed to reduce the negative effects of the past. Individuation techniques are employed to help in separating parent and child, and adjunctive skills training is used to provide parents with other outlets for stress that might be precipitating their abuse of the child.

The child is taught to cope better by using a variety of techniques including compliance training, social skills training, and training to tolerate dependency and depression. Compliance training uses natural reinforcers to promote compliance. Social skills training uses discussions, modeling, and practice to improve the child's ability to interact. These techniques help the child tolerate his or her ambivalence toward parents and thus maximize opportunities for developing a sense of consistency of the child's caregivers. Delayed gratification techniques are also used to teach the child how to be patient in having needs attended to. Finally, the child can be given an understanding of the concepts associated with privacy and security of ownership of self and objects by employing locked-box techniques.

Both social skills training and adjunctive skills training call for parent involvement. Family counseling is used to derive ways in which existing family dynamics and support systems can be incorporated into treatment. Teaching parents how to interpret their child's behaviors enables them to interact more effectively with the child, thus preventing further abuse. Working through the trauma with the child is helpful in discouraging the child from repeating behaviors that trigger abuse. Training in child management is useful for helping parents learn how to solve problems effectively when the child misbehaves, rather than abusing the child. Parent training in social principles is useful in establishing a foundation for the development of effective communication and more rewarding relationships between parents and child.

CONCLUSION

The range of therapeutic techniques suggested for inclusion in each disorder's treatment package reflects the breadth of the origins of each disorder and the variety of influences impinging on them. With each modality the disorder is viewed from a particular perspective, and rarely does just one perspective suffice. The therapist should give due consideration to the other perspectives and adopt broad-based therapeutic strategies that include elements of the various family, behavioral, cognitive, group, and pharmacotherapy interventions discussed in this chapter.

References

Aarkrog, T. (1981). The borderline concept in childhood, adolescence and adulthood. *Acta Psychiatrica Scandinavica, 293* (Suppl.).

Aber, J. L., & Zigler, E. (1981). Developmental considerations in the definition of child maltreatment. *New Directions for Child Development, 11,* 1–29.

Abraham, K. (1927). Notes on the psychoanalytic investigation and treatment of manic depressive insanity and allied conditions. In *Selected papers.* London: Hogarth Press.

Ackerly, W. C. (1967). Latency-age children who threaten or attempt to kill themselves. *Journal of the American Academy of Child Psychiatry, 6,* 242–261.

Adam, K. S. (1982). Loss, suicide, and attachment. In C. M. Parkes & J. Stevenson-Hinde (Eds.), *The place of attachment in human behavior* (pp. 269–294). New York: Basic Books.

Adler, G., & Guie, D. H. Jr. (1979). Aloneness and borderline psychopathology: The possible relevance of child development issues. *International Journal of Psycho-Analysis, 60,* 83–96.

Agren, H. (1983). Life at risk: Markers of suicidiality in depression. *Psychiatric Developments, 1,* 87–104.

Agren, H., Terenius, L., & Wahlstrom, A. (1982). Depressive phenomenology and levels of cerebrospinal fluid endorphins. *Annals New York Academy of Sciences,* 388–398.

Ainsworth, M. D. S., Blehar, M., Waters, E., & Wall, S. (1978). *Patterns of attachment.* Hillsdale, New Jersey: Erlbaum.

Ainsworth, M. D. S., & Wittig, B. A. (1969). Attachment and exploration behavior of one-year-olds in a strange situation. In B. M. Foss (Ed.), *Determinants of infant behavior, 4,* (pp. 113–136). London: Methuen.

Akiskal, H. S. (1986). A developmental perspective on recurrent mood disorders: A review of studies in man. *Psychopharmacology Bulletin, 22,* 579–586.

Akiskal, H. S., & McKinney, W. T. (1975). Overview of recent research in depression: Integration of ten conceptual models into a comprehensive clinical frame. *Archives of General Psychiatry, 32,* 285–303.

Allen, F. H. (1942). *Psychotherapy with children.* New York: Norton.

American Humane Association, (AHA). (1985). *Highlights of official child neglect and abuse reporting.* (Annual Report). Denver: American Humane Association.

American Psychiatric Association, (APA). (1980). *Diagnostic and statistical manual of mental disorders* (3rd ed.). (DSM-III). Washington, DC: American Psychiatric Association.

American Psychiatric Association, (APA). (1987). *Diagnostic and statistical manual of mental disorders (3rd ed., rev.), (DSM-III-R).* Washington, DC: American Psychiatric Association.

Amster, F. (1964). Differential uses of play in treatment of young children. In M. R. Haworth, (Ed.), *Child psychotherapy: Practice and theory.* New York: Basic Books.

Anders, T., & Guilleminault, C. (1976). The pathophysiology of sleep disorders in pediatrics. I. Sleep in infancy. *Advances in Pediatrics, 22,* 151–174.

Anders, T. F., Sachar, E. J., Kream, J., Roffwarg, H., & Hellman, L. (1970). Behavioral state and plasma cortisol response in the human newborn. *Pediatrics, 46,* 532–537.

Anders, T. F., & Weinstein, P. (1972). Sleep and its disorders in infants and children: A review. *Pediatrics, 50,* 312–324.

Anderson, L. T., Campbell, M., Grega, D. M., Perry, R., Small, A. M., & Green, W. H. (1984). Haloperidol in the treatment of infantile autism: Effects on learning and behavioral symptoms. *American Journal of Psychiatry, 141,* 1195–1202.

Andreasen, N. C., Rice, J., Endicott, J., Coryell, W., Grove, W. M., & Reich, T. (1987). Familial rates of affective disorder. *Archives of General Psychiatry, 44,* 461–468.

Andrulonis, P. A., Glueck, B. C., Stroebel, C. F., & Vogel, N. G. (1982). Borderline personality subcategories. *Journal of Nervous and Mental Disease, 170,* 670–679.

Andrulonis, P. A., & Vogel, N. G. (1984). Comparison of borderline personality subcategories to schizophrenic and affective disorders. *British Journal of Psychiatry, 144,* 358–363.

Anthony, E. J. (1986). Terrorizing attacks on children by psychotic parents. *Journal of the American Academy of Child Psychiatry, 25,* 326–335.

Arai, K., Yanaihara, T., & Okinaga, S. (1976). Adrenocorticotropic hormone in human fetal blood at delivery. *American Journal of Obstetrics and Gynecology, 125,* 1136.

Archer, J. (1984). Gender roles as developmental pathways. *British Journal of Social Psychology, 23,* 245–256.

Arend, R., Gove, F., & Sroufe, L. A. (1979). Continuity of individual adaptation from infancy to kindergarten: A reductive study of ego resilience and curiosity in pre-schoolers. *Child Development, 50,* 950–959.

Armelius, B., Kullgren, G., & Renberg, E. (1985). Borderline diagnosis from hospital records: Reliability and validity of Gunderson's Diagnostic Interview for Borderlines (DIB). *Journal of Nervous and Mental Disorders, 173,* 132–134.

Asaad, G., & Shapiro, B. (1986). Hallucinations: Theoretical and clinical overview. *American Journal of Psychiatry, 143,* 1088–1097.

Asarnow, R., Sherman, T., & Strandburg, R. (1986). The search for the psychobiological substrate of childhood onset schizophrenia. *Journal of the American Academy of Child Psychiatry, 25,* 601–604.

Asberg, M., Bertilsson, L., & Martensson, B. (1984). CSF monoamine metabolites, depression and suicide. In E. Usdin (Ed.), *Frontiers in biochemical and pharmacological research in depression* (pp. 87–97). New York: Raven Press.

Asberg, M., & Traskman, L. (1981). Studies of CSF 5–HIAA in depression and suicidal behavior. *Advances in Experimental Medicine and Biology, 133,* 739–752.

Asberg, M., Traskman, L., & Thoren, P. (1976). 5HIAA in the cerebrospinal fluid—A biochemical suicide predictor? *Archives of General Psychiatry, 33,* 1193.

Asberg, M., Varpila-Hansson, R., Tomba, P., Aminoff, A. K., Martensson, B., Thoren, P., Traskman-Bendz, L., Encroth, P., & Astrom, G. (1981). Suicidal behavior and the dexamethasone suppression test. *American Journal of Psychiatry, 33,* 1193–1197.

Aserinsky, E., & Kleitman, N. (1953). Regularly occurring periods of eye motility and concomitant phenomena during sleep. *Science, 118,* 243–274.

Asnis, G. C., Sacher, E. J., Halbreich, U., Nathan, S. R., Novacenko, H., & Ostrow, L. (1981). Cortisol secretion in relation to age in major depression. *Psychosomatic Medicine, 43,* 235–242.

August, G. J., Raz, N., & Baird, T. D. (1987). Fenfluramine response in high and low functioning autistic children. *Journal of the American Academy of Child and Adolescent Psychiatry, 26,* 342–346.

August, G. J., Raz, N., Papanicolaou, A. C., Baird, T. D., Hirsh, S. L., & Hsu, L. L. (1984). Fenfluramine treatment in infantile autism. *Journal of Nervous and Mental Disease, 172,* 604–612.

August, G. J., & Stewart, M. A. (1983). Familial subtypes of childhood hyperactivity. *The Journal of Nervous and Mental Disease, 171,* 362–368.

Avant R. (1984). Anxiety and depression: Determining the predominant disorder. *Family Practice Recertification, 6,* 19–26.

Axline, V. M. (1964a). *Dibs: In search of self.* New York: Ballantine.

Axline, V. M. (1964b). The eight basic principles. In M. R. Haworth (Ed.), *Child psychotherapy: Practice and theory* (pp. 93–94). New York: Basic Books.

Azrin, N. H., & Nunn, R. G. (1977). *Habit control in a day.* New York: Simon & Schuster.

Bach-Y-Rita, G., Lion, J. R., Clement, C. E., & Ervin, F. R. (1971). Episodic dyscontrol: A study of 130 violent patients. *American Journal of Psychiatry, 127,* 49–54.

Bakan, D. (1971). *Slaughter of the innocents: Study of the battered child phenomenon.* San Francisco: Jossey-Bass.

Baker, H. L., & Leland, B. (1967). *Detroit Test of Learning Aptitude.* Indianapolis: Bobbs-Merrill.

Baker, L., & Cantwell, D. P. (1987a). A prospective psychiatric follow-up of children with speech/language disorders. *Journal of the American Academy of Child and Adolescent Psychiatry, 26,* 546–553.

Baker, L., & Cantwell, D. P. (1987b). Comparison of well, emotionally disordered, and behaviorally disordered children with linguistic problems. *Journal of the American Academy of Child and Adolescent Psychiatry, 26,* 193–196.

Bakwin, H. (1968). Deviant gender-role behavior in children: Relation to homosexuality. *Pediatrics, 41,* 620–629.

Bakwin, H. (1973). The genetics of bed wetting. In I. Kolvin, R. MacKeith, & R. S. Meadow (Eds.), *Bladder control and enuresis* (pp. 73–77). *(Clinics in Developmental Medicine, Nos. 48/49.)*

Baldessarini, R. J. (1983). *Biomedical aspects of depression and its treatment.* Washington, DC: American Psychiatric Press.

Baldwin, J. M. (1911). *Thought and things: Interest and art, or genetic epistemology (Vol. 3).* New York: Macmillan.

Ball, R. S., Merrifield, P., & Stott, L. H. (1978). *Extended Merrill-Palmer scale.* Chicago: Stoeling.

Banki, C. M. (1983). Evidence of disturbance of monoamines in depression. *Advances in Biological Psychiatry, 10,* 176–199.

Banki, C. M. (1985). Biochemical markers for suicidal behavior. *American Journal of Psychiatry, 142,* 147–148.

Banki, C. M., & Arato, M. (1983a). Amine metabolites, neuroendocrine findings, and personality dimensions as correlates of suicidal behavior. *Psychiatry Research, 10,* 253–261.

Banki, C. M., & Arato, M. (1983b). Amine metabolites and neuroendocrine responses related to depression and suicide. *Journal of Affective Disorders, 5,* 223–232.

Banki, C. M., Arato, M., Papp, Z., & Kurcz, M. (1984). Biochemical markers in suicidal patients: Investigations with cerebrospinal fluid amine metabolites and neuroendocrine tests. *Journal of Affective Disorders, 6,* 341–350.

Barasch, A., Frances, A., Hurt, S., Clarkin, J., & Cohen, S. (1985). Stability and distinctness of borderline personality disorder. *American Journal of Psychiatry, 142,* 1484–1486.

Barkley, R. A. (1988). The effects of methylphenidate on the interactions of preschool ADHD children with their mothers. *Journal of the American Academy of Child and Adolescent Psychiatry, 27,* 336–341.

Barnes, D. M. (1987). Biological issues in schizophrenia. *Science, 235,* 430–433.

Barnes, M. J. (1964). Reactions to the death of a mother. *Psychoanalytic Study of the Child, 19,* 334–357.

Barnett, L. (1984). Research note: Young children's resolution of distress through play. *Journal of Child Psychology and Psychiatry, 25,* 477–483.

Barnett, L. A., & Storm, B. (1981). Play, pleasure and pain: The reduction of anxiety through play. *Leisure Science, 4,* 161–175.

Baron, M., Gruen, R., Asnis, L., & Lord, S. (1985). Familial transmission of schizotypal and borderline personality disorders. *American Journal of Psychiatry, 142,* 927–934.

Baron-Cohen, S., Leslie, A. M., & Frith, U. (1985). Does the autistic child have a "theory of mind"? *Cognition, 21,* 37–46.

Barry, H., & Lindemann, E. (1960). Critical ages for maternal bereavement in psychoneuroses. *Psychosomatic Medicine, 22,* 166–181.

Bartak, L. (1978). Educational approaches. In M. Rutter & E. Schopler (Eds.), *Autism: A reappraisal of concepts and treatment* (pp. 423–438). New York: Plenum.

Bartak, L., & Rutter, M. (1976). Differences between mentally retarded and normally intelligent autistic children. *Journal of Autism and Childhood Schizophrenia, 6,* 109–120.

Bartak, L., Rutter, M., & Cox, A. (1975). A comparative study of infantile autism and specific developmental receptive language disorder. I: The children. *British Journal of Psychiatry, 126,* 127–145.

Barter, J., Swaback, D., & Todd, D. (1968). Adolescent suicide attempts: A follow-up study of hospitalized patients. *Archives of General Psychiatry, 19,* 523–527.

Bates, E., Camaioni, L., & Volterra, V. (1975). The acquisition of performatives prior to speech. *Merrill Palmer Quarterly, 21,* 205–226.

Bates, J. E., Skilbeck, W. M., Smith, K. V. R., & Bentler, R. (1975). Intervention with families of gender-disturbed boys. *American Journal of Orthopsychiatry, 45*(1), 150–157.

Bateson, G. (1955). A theory of play and fantasy. *Psychiatric Research Reports, 2,* 39–51.

Bateson, G. (1956). The message "This is play." In B. Schanner (Ed.), *Group processes.* New York: Macy Foundation.

Bauer, D. H. (1976). An exploratory study of developmental changes in children's fears. *Journal of Child Psychology and Psychiatry, 17,* 69–74.

Beavers, W. R. (1982). Indications and contradictions for couples therapy. *Psychiatric Clinics of North America, 5,* 469–478.

Beck, A., Steer, R., Kovacs, M., & Garrison, B. (1985). Hopelessness and eventual suicide: A ten-year prospective study of patients hospitalized with suicidal ideation. *American Journal of Psychiatry, 142,* 559–563.

Behar, D. & Rapoport, J. L. (1983). Play observation and psychiatric diagnosis. In C. E. Schaefer & K. J. O'Connor (Eds.), *Handbook of play therapy* (pp. 193–199). New York: Wiley.

Behrman, J. (1970). Neurophysiological studies on patients with hysterical disturbances of vision. *Journal of Psychosomatic Research, 14,* 187–194.

Beitchman, J. H. (1985). Childhood schizophrenia: A review and comparison with adult-onset schizophrenia. *Psychiatric Clinics of North America, 8,* 793–814.

Beitchman, J. H., Nair, R., Clegg, M., Ferguson, B., & Patel, P. G. (1986). Prevalence of psychiatric disorders in children with speech and language disorders. *Journal of the American Academy of Child Psychiatry, 25,* 528–535.

Bell, R. Q., & Costello, N. S. (1964). Three tests for sex differences in tactile sensibility in the new-born. *Biology of the Neonate, 7,* 335.

Bellman, M. (1966). Studies on encopresis. *Acta Paediatrica Scandinavica, 170* (Suppl.): 1.

Belsky, J. (1980). Child maltreatment: An ecological integration. *American Journal of Psychology, 35,* 320–335.

Belsky, J., & Steinberg, L. D. (1978). The effects of day care: A critical review. *Child Development, 49,* 929–949.

Belsky, J., Steinberg, L. D., & Walker, A. (1982). The ecology of day care. In M. E. Lamb (Ed.), *Nontraditional families: Parenting and child development* (pp. 71–116). Hillsdale, NJ: Erlbaum.

Bemporad, J. R., Ratey, J. J., & O'Driscoll, G. (1987). Autism and emotion: An ethological theory. *American Journal of Orthopsychiatry, 57,* 477–484.

Bender, L. (1938). A visual motor Gestalt Test and its clinical use. *Research Monographs of the American Orthopsychiatric Association, 3,* 2–7.

Bender, L., & Faretra, G. (1972). The relationship between childhood and adult schizophrenia. In A. R. Kaplan (Ed.), *Genetic factors in schizophrenia* (pp. 28–64). Springfield, IL: Charles C Thomas.

Benjamin, J. D. (1963). Further comments on some developmental aspects of anxiety. In H. S. Gaskill (Ed.), *Counterpoint: Libidinal object and subject* (pp. 121–153). New York: International Universities Press.

Bennie, E., & Sclare, A. (1969). The battered child syndrome. *American Journal of Psychiatry, 125,* 975–979.

Bentovim, A., & Boston, M. (1973). A day-centre for disturbed young children and their parents. *Journal of Child Psychotherapy, 3,* 46–60.

Berg, C. J., Zahn, T. P., Behar, D., & Rapoport, J. L. (1986). Childhood obsessive-compulsive disorder: An anxiety disorder? In R. Gittelman (Ed.), *Anxiety disorders of childhood* (pp. 126–135). New York: Guilford.

Berg, I., Butler, I., & Pritchard, J. (1974). Psychiatric illness in the mothers of school-phobic adolescents. *British Journal of Psychiatry, 125,* 466–467.

Berger, P. A., & Barchas, J. D. (1983). Pharmacologic studies of betaendorphin in psychopathology. *Psychiatric Clinics of North America, 6,* 377–391.

Berlin, I. N. (1987). Some transference and countertransference issues in the playroom. *Journal of the American Academy of Child and Adolescent Psychiatry, 26,* 101–107.

Berman, A., & Siegal, A. (1976). A neuropsychological approach to the etiology, prevention, and treatment of juvenile delinquency. In A. Davids (Ed.), *Child personality and psychopathology: Current topics* (Vol. 3, pp. 259–294). New York: Wiley.

Berman, S. (1964). Techniques of treatment of a form of juvenile delinquency, the antisocial character disorder. *Journal of the American Academy of Child Psychiatry, 2,* 24–52.

Bernstein, G. A., & Garfinkel, B. D. (1986). School phobia: The overlap of affective and anxiety disorders. *Journal of the American Academy of Child Psychiatry, 25,* 235–241.

Bernstein, I., & Glenn, J. (1978). The child analyst's emotional reactions to his patients. In J. Glenn & M. A. Scharfman (Eds.), *Child analysis and therapy.* New York: Jason Aronson.

Bick, E. (1962). Symposium on child analysis: I. Child analysis today. *International Journal of Psychoanalysis, XLIII,* 328–332.

Bidder, R. T., Gray, O. P., Howells, P. M., & Eaton, M. P. (1986). Sleep problems in preschool children: Community clinics. *Child-care, Health and Development, 12,* 325–337.

Biederman, J., Munir, K., & Knee, D. (1987). Conduct and oppositional disorder in clinically referred children with attention deficit disorder: A controlled family study. *Journal of the American Academy of Child and Adolescent Psychiatry, 26,* 724–727.

Biederman, J., Munir, K., Knee, D., Armentano, M., Autor, S., Waternaux, C., & Tsuang, M. (1987). High rate of affective disorders in probands with attention deficit disorder and in their relatives: A controlled family study. *American Journal of Psychiatry, 144,* 330–333.

Birtchnell, J. (1972). Early parent death and psychiatric diagnosis. *Social Psychiatry, 7,* 202–210.

Bithoney, W. G., Snyder, J., & Michalek, J. (1985). Childhood ingestions as symptoms of family distress. *American Journal of Diseases of Children, 139,* 456–459.

Bixler, E., Kaies, A., & Soldatos, C. (1979). Sleep disorders encountered in medical practice: A national survey of physicians. *Behavioral Medicine, 1,* 1–6.

Bland, R., & Orn, H. (1986). Family violence and psychiatric disorder. *Canadian Journal of Psychiatry, 31,* 129–137.

Blehar, M. C. (1974). Anxious attachment and defensive reactions associated with day care. *Child Development, 45,* 683–692.

Block, J. H., & Block, J. (1980). The role of ego-control and ego-resiliency in the organization of behavior. In W. A. Collins (Ed.), *Minnesota symposium on child psychology* (Vol. 13, pp. 39–101). New Jersey: Erlbaum.

Block, J. H., Block, J., & Gjerde, P. F. (1986). The personality of children prior to divorce: A prospective study. *Child Development, 57,* 827–840.

Block, J. H., Block, J., & Morrison, A. (1981). Parental agreement-disagreement on child-rearing orientations and gender-related personality correlates in children. *Child Development, 52,* 965–974.

Blomberg, P. A., Koplin, I. J., Gordon, E. K., Markey, S. P., & Ebert, M. H. (1980). Conversion of MHPG to vanillymandelic acid. *Archives of General Psychiatry, 37,* 1095–1098.

Bloom-Feschbach, S., & Blatt, S. J. (1981). Separation response and nursery school adaptation. *Journal of the American Academy of Child Psychiatry, 21,* 58–64.

Blurton-Jones, N. G. (1972). Categories of child-child interaction. In N. G. Blurton-Jones (Ed.), *Ethological studies of child behavior.* Cambridge, MA: Harvard University Press.

Boll, T. J. (1983). Neuropsychological assessment of the child: Myths, current status, and future prospects. In S. B. Filskov & T. J. Boll (Eds.), *Handbook of clinical child psychology* (pp. 186–208). New York: Wiley.

Bousha, D. M., & Twentyman, C. T. (1984). Mother-child interactional style in abuse, neglect, and control groups: Naturalistic observations in the home. *Journal of Abnormal Psychology, 93,* 106–114.

Bowers, M. B., Goodman, E., & Sim, V. M. (1964). Some behavioral changes in man following anticholinesterase administration. *Journal of Nervous and Mental Disease, 138,* 383–389.

Bowlby, J. (1944). Forty-four juvenile thieves: Their characters and home life. *International Journal of Psychoanalysis, 25,* 163–171.

Bowlby, J. (1951). Maternal care and mental health. *Bulletin of the World Health Organization, 3,* 355–533.

Bowlby, J. (1960). Grief and mourning in infancy and early childhood. *Psychoanalytic Study of the Child, 15,* 9–52.

Bowlby, J. (1963). Pathological mourning and childhood mourning. *Journal of the American Psychoanalytic Association, 11,* 500–541.

Bowlby, J. (1969). *Attachment and loss: Vol. 1. Attachment.* London, Hogarth.

Bowlby, J. (1973). *Attachment and loss: Vol. 2. Separation.* New York: Basic Books.

Bowlby, J. (1982). Attachment and loss: Retrospect and prospect. *American Journal of Orthopsychiatry, 52,* 664–678.

Brady, C. P., Bray, J. H., & Zeeb, L. (1986). Behavior problems of clinic children: Relation to parental marital status, age and sex of child. *American Journal of Orthopsychiatry, 56,* 399–412.

Brambilla, F., Genazzani, A., & Facchinetti, F. (1984). Endogenous opioid peptides in schizophrenia and affective disorders. In N. S. Shah & A. G. Donald (Eds.), *Psychoneuroendocrine dysfunction* (pp. 309–329). New York: Plenum.

Branyon, D. W. (1983). Dexamethason suppression test in children (Letter to the editor). *American Journal of Psychiatry, 140,* 1385.

Braverman, E. R., & Pfeiffer, C. C. (1985). Suicide and biochemistry. *Biological Psychiatry, 20,* 123–124.

Brazelton, T. B. (1962). A child-oriented approach to toilet training. *Pediatrics, 29,* 121.

Brehm, J. W. (1966). *A theory of psychological reactance.* New York: Academic.

Breier, A., Charney, D. S., & Heninger, G. R. (1985). The diagnostic validity of anxiety disorders and their relationship to depressive illness. *American Journal of Psychiatry, 142,* 787–797.

Brent, D. A. (1987). Correlates of the medical lethality of suicide attempts in children and adolescents. *Journal of the American Academy of Child and Adolescent Psychiatry, 26,* 87–91.

Broadwin, I. T. (1932). A contribution to the study of truancy. *American Journal of Orthopsychiatry, 2,* 253–259.

Bromfield, R., & Pfeifer, G. (1988). Combining group and individual psychotherapy: Impact on the individual treatment experience. *Journal of the American Academy of Child and Adolescent Psychiatry, 27,* 220–225.

Bronfenbrenner, U. (1977). Toward an experimental ecology of human development. *American Journal of Psychology, 32,* 513–529.

Bronfenbrenner, U. (1979). *The ecology of human development: Experiments by nature and design.* Cambridge, MA: Harvard University Press.

Bronson, G. W. (1972). Infants' reactions to unfamiliar persons and novel objects. *Monographs of the Society for Research in Child Development, 37* (3, Serial No. 148).

Broughton, R. (1968). Biorhythmic variations in consciousness and psychological functions. *Canadian Psychology Review, 16,* 217–239.

Brown, F., & Epps, P. (1966). Childhood bereavement and subsequent crime. *British Journal of Psychiatry, 112,* 1043–1048.

Brown, G. W., Briley, J. L. T., & Wing, J. F. (1972). Influences of family life on the course of schizophrenic disorders: A replication. *British Journal of Psychiatry, 121,* 241–258.

Brown, G. L., & Goodwin, F. K. (1986). Human aggression and suicide. *Suicide and Life-Threatening Behavior, 16,* 223–243.

Brown, G. W., & Harris, T. (1978). *Social origins of depression: A study of psychiatric disorder in women.* London: Tavistock.

Brown, J. L. (1963). Follow-up of children with atypical development (infantile psychosis). *American Journal of Orthopsychiatry, 38,* 846–857.

Brown, J. L. (1969). Adolescent development of children with infantile psychosis. *Seminars in Psychiatry, 1,* 79–89.

Brown, R. (1973). *A first language: The early stages.* Cambridge, MA: Harvard University Press.

Bruch, H. (1973). *Eating disorders: Obesity, anorexia nervosa, and the person within.* New York: Basic Books.

Bruch, H. (1981). Developmental considerations of anorexia nervosa and obesity. *Canadian Journal of Psychiatry, 26,* 212–216.

Bruette, V. (1984). Food tolerance and food aversion. A joint report of the Royal College of Physicians and the British Nutrition Foundation. *Journal of the Royal College of Physicians of London, 18,* 83–123.

Bruner, J. S. (1972). Nature and uses of immaturity. *American Psychologist, 27,* 687–708.

Buchsbaum, B. C. (1987). Remembering a parent who has died: A developmental perspective. In *The Annual of Psychoanalysis* (Vol. 15). Madison, CT: International Universities Press.

Buck, R. (1984). *The communication of emotion.* New York: Guilford Press.

Bunch, J., & Barraclough, B. (1971). The influence of parental death anniversaries upon suicide dates. *British Journal of Psychiatry, 118,* 621–626.

Bunney, W. E., Jr., & Davis, J. M. (1965). Norepinephrine in depressive reactions. *Archives of General Psychiatry, 13,* 483–494.

Burchfield, S. R., Elich, M. S., & Noods, S. C. (1977). Geophagia in response to stress and arthritis. *Physiology and Behaviour, 19,* 265–267.

Burd, L., Fisher, W., & Kerbeshian, J. (1987). A prevalence study of pervasive developmental disorders in North Dakota. *Journal of the American Academy of Child and Adolescent Psychiatry, 26,* 700–703.

Burd, L., & Kerbeshian, J. (1987). A North Dakota prevalence study of schizophrenia presenting in childhood. *Journal of the American Academy of Child and Adolescent Psychiatry 26,* 347–350.

Burd, L., Kerbeshian, J., Wikenheiser, M., & Fisher, W. (1986). A prevalence study of Gilles de la Tourette syndrome in North Dakota school-age children. *Journal of the American Academy of Child Psychiatry, 25,* 552–553.

Byrd, D. E. (1979). *Intersexual assault: A review of empirical findings.* Paper presented at the annual meeting of the Eastern Sociological Society, New York.

Caine, E. (1985). Personal communication on unpublished raw data.

Caldwell, B. M. (1968). The usefulness of the critical period hypothesis in the study of filiative behavior. In N. S. Endler, L. R. Boutler, & H. Ossef (Eds.), *Contemporary issues in developmental psychology* (pp. 213–223). New York: Holt, Rinehart & Winston.

Cameron, J. M., Johnson, H. R. M., & Campos, R. E. (1966). The battered child syndrome. *Medicine, Science, and the Law, 6,* 2–21.

Campbell, M. (1988). Annotation: Fenfluramine treatment of autism. *Journal of Child Psychiatry, 29,* 1–10.

Campbell, S. B. (1986). Developmental issues in childhood anxiety. In R. Gittelman (Ed.), *Anxiety disorders of childhood* (pp. 24–57). New York: Guilford.

Campbell, S. B., Breaux, A. M., Ewing, L. J., & Szumowski, E. K. (1984). A one-year follow-up study of parent-referred hyperactive preschool children. *Journal of the American Academy of Child Psychiatry, 23,* 243–249.

Campbell, S. B., Breaux, A. M., Ewing, L. J., & Szumowski, E. K. (1986). Correlates and predictors of hyperactivity and aggression: A longitudinal study of parent-referred problem preschoolers. *Journal of Abnormal Child Psychology, 14,* 217–234.

Campbell, S. B., Endman, M. W., & Bernfield, G. (1977). A three-year follow-up of hyperactive preschoolers into elementary school. *Journal of Child Psychology and Psychiatry, 18,* 239–250.

Campbell, S. B. & Werry, J. S. (1986). Attention deficit disorder (hyperactivity). In H. C. Quay & J. S. Werry (Eds.), *Psychopathological disorders of childhood* (3rd ed. pp. 111–155). New York: Wiley.

Campbell, S. B., et al. (1986). Parent-referred problem three-year-olds: Follow-up at school entry. *Journal of Child Psychiatry, 27,* 473–488.

Cantor, D. W. (1977). School-based groups for children of divorce. *Journal of Divorce, 1,* 183–185.

Cantor, S., Evans, J., Pearce, J., & Pezzet-Pearce, T. (1982). Childhood schizophrenia: Present but not accounted for. *American Journal of Psychiatry, 139,* 758–762.

Cantor, S., & Kestenbaum, C. (1986). Psychotherapy with schizophrenic children. *Journal of the American Academy of Child Psychiatry, 25,* 623–630.

Cantwell, D. (1983a). Assessment of childhood depression: An overview. In D. P. Cantwell & G. A. Carlson (Eds.), *Affective disorders in childhood and adolescence: An update* (pp. 3–18). New York: SP Medical and Scientific Books.

Cantwell, D. (1983b). Overview of etiologic factors. In D. P. Cantwell & G. A. Carlson (Eds.), *Affective disorders in childhood and adolescence: An update* (pp. 206–219). New York: SP Medical and Scientific Books.

Cantwell, D., & Baker, L. (1980). Psychiatric and behavioral characteristics of children with communication disorders. *Journal of Pediatric Psychology, 5,* 161–178.

Cantwell, D., Baker, L., & Rutter, M. (In press). A comparative follow-up study of infantile autism and developmental receptive dysphasia.

Cantwell, D., Rutter, M., & Baker, L. (1978). Family factors. In M. Rutter & E. Schopler (Eds.), *Autism: A reappraisal of concepts and treatment* (pp. 269–296). New York: Plenum.

Caplan, P. J., & Dinardo, L. (1986). Is there a relationship between child abuse and learning disability? *Canadian Journal of Behavioral Science/Review Canadiennese Science Comparative, 18,* 367–380.

Capute, A. J., Palmer, F. B., Shapiro, B. K., Wachtel, R. C., & Accardo, P. J. (1981). Early language development: Clinical application of the language and auditory milestone scale. In R. E. Stark (Ed.), *Language behavior in infancy and early childhood* (pp. 429–436). New York: Elsevier North Holland.

Carey, W. B., & McDevitt, S. C. (1978). Stability and change in individual temperament diagnoses from infancy to early childhood. *Journal of the American Academy of Child Psychiatry, 17,* 331–337.

Carey, W. B., & McDevitt, S. C. (1985). Use of the infant temperament questionnaire. *Journal of the American Academy of Child Psychiatry, 24,* 502–503.

Carlson, G. A. (1984). A comparison of early and late onset adolescent affective disorder. *Journal of Operational Psychiatry, 15,* 46–50.

Carlson, G. A., Asarnow, J. R., & Orbach, Israel. (1987). Developmental aspects of suicidal behavior in children: I. *Journal of the American Academy of Child and Adolescent Psychiatry, 26,* 186–192.

Carlson, G. A., & Cantwell, D. P. (1980). A survey of depressive symptoms, syndrome, and disorder in a child psychiatric population. *Journal of Child Psychology and Psychiatry and Allied Disciplines, 21,* 19–25.

Carlsson, A., Lindvist, M., & Magnusson, T. (1957). 3,4-Dihydroxyphenylalanine and 5-hydroxytryptophan as reserpine antagonists. *Nature, 180,* 1200.

Carroll, B. J. (1972). The hypothalamic-pituitary-adrenal axis in depression. In B. Davies, B. J. Carroll, & R. Mowbray (Eds.), *Depressive illness: Some research studies.* Springfield, IL: Charles C Thomas.

Carroll, B. J. (1984). Dexamethasone suppression test for depression. In E. Usdin (Ed.), *Frontiers in biochemical and pharmacological research in depression.* New York: Raven Press.

Carroll, B. J., Greden, & Feinberg, M. (1981). Suicide, neuroendocrine dysfunction and CSF 5-HIAA concentrations in depression. In B. Angrist, G. C. Burrows, M. Lader, O. Lindjaerde, G. Sedvall, & D. Wheatley (Eds.), *Recent advances in neuropsychopharmacology* (pp. 307-313). Oxford: Pergamon.

Casby, M. W., & Della Corte, M. (1986). Symbolic play performance and early language development. *Journal of Psycholinguistic Research, 16,* 31–42.

Cavanaugh, R. M. (1983). Encopresis in children and adolescents. *American Family Physician, 27,* 107–109.

Chabrol, H., Claverie, J., & Moron, P. (1983). TI DST, TRH test, and adolescent suicide attempts. *American Journal of Psychiatry, 140,* 265.

Chandler, M. J. (1978). Role taking, referential communication, and egocentric intrusions in mother-child interactions of children vulnerable to risk of parental psychosis. In E. J. Anthony, C. Koupernik, C. Chiland, A. Freud, & M. Mahler (Eds.), *The child in his family: Vol. 4, Vulnerable children* (pp. 347–357). New York: Wiley.

Charney, D. S., & Heninger, G. R. (1986a). Abnormal regulation of noradrenergic function in panic disorders: Effect of clonidine in healthy subjects and patients with agoraphobia and panic disorder. *Archives of General Psychiatry, 43,* 1042–1054.

Charney, D. S., & Heninger, G. R. (1986b). Serotonin function in panic disorders: The effect of intravenous tryptophan in healthy subjects and patients with panic disorder before and during alprazolam treatment. *Archives of General Psychiatry, 43,* 1059–1065.

Chatoor, I., Dickson, L., & Einhorn, A. (1984). Rumination: Etiology and treatment. *Pediatric Annals, 13,* 924–929.

Chazan, M., & Threlfall, S. (1978). Behavior problems in infant school children in deprived areas. In E. J. Anthony, C. Koupernik, C. Chiland A. Freud, & M. Mahler (Eds.), *The child in his family: Vol. 4. Vulnerable children* (pp. 383–399). New York: Wiley.

Chen, X., Yin, T., He, J., Ma, Q., Han, Z., & Li, L. (1985). Low levels of zinc in hair and blood, pica, anorexia, and poor growth in Chinese preschool children. *American Journal of Clinical Nutrition, 42,* 694–700.

Chess, S. (1970). Temperament and children at risk. In E. J. Anthony & C. Koupernik (Eds.), *The child and his family* (Vol. 1, pp. 121–130). New York: Wiley.

Chess, S., & Thomas, A. (1984). *Origins and evolution of behavior disorders: From infancy to early adult life.* New York: Brunner/Mazel.

Chess, S., & Thomas, A. (1985). Temperamental differences: A critical concept in child health care. *Pediatric Nursing, 11,* 167–171.

Chess, S., Thomas, A., & Hassibi, M. (1983). Depression in childhood and adolescence: A study of six cases. *The Journal of Nervous and Mental Disease, 171,* 411–420.

Chethik, M. (1986). Levels of borderline functioning in children: Etiological and treatment considerations. *American Journal of Orthopsychiatry, 56*(1), 109–119.

Chiles, J. A., Miller, M. L., & Cox, G. B. (1980). Depression in an adolescent delinquent population. *Archives of General Psychiatry, 37,* 1179–1184.

Christian, W. P. (1982). Childhood autism. In M. D. Levine, W. B. Carey., A. C. Crocker, & R. T. Gross (Eds.), *Developmental-behavioral pediatrics* (pp. 722–739). Philadelphia: Saunders.

Churchill, D. W. (1972). The relation of infantile autism and early childhood schizophrenia to developmental language disorders of childhood. *Journal of Autism in Childhood Schizophrenia, 2,* 182–197.

Ciaranello, R. D. (1982). Hyperserotonemia and early infantile autism. *New England Journal of Medicine, 307,* 181–183.

Cicchetti, D., & Rizley, R. (1981). Developmental perspectives on the etiology, intergenerational transmission, and sequelae of child maltreatment. *New Directions for Child Development, 11,* 31–55.

Clarke, A. M., & Clarke, A. D. B. (1978). Priorities for vulnerable children: The mentally retarded. In E. J. Anthony, C. Koupernik, C. Chiland A. Freud, & M. Mahler (Eds.), *The child and his family: Vol. 4. Vulnerable children* (pp. 89–97). New York: Wiley.

Clarke-Stewart, A. (1984). Day care: A new context for research and development. In M. Perlmutter (Ed.), *The Minnesota symposia on child psychology: Vol. 17. Parent-child interaction and parent-child relations in child development* (pp. 61–100). Hillsdale, NJ: Erlbaum.

Clarkson, S., Williams, S., & Silva, P. A. (1986). Sleep in middle childhood—A longitudinal study of sleep problems in a large sample of Dunedin children aged 5–9 years. *Australian Pediatric Journal, 22,* 31–35.

Clement, P. W., & Milne, D. C. (1967). Group play therapy and tangible reinforcers used to modify the behavior of 8-year-old boys. *Behavior Research and Therapy, 5,* 301–312.

Cochran, M. M. (1977). A comparison of group care and family child-rearing patterns in Sweden. *Child Development, 48,* 702–707.

Coddington, R. D. (1972). The significance of life events as etiologic factors in the diseases of children. II: A study of a normal population. *Journal of Psychosomatic Research, 16,* 205–213.

Cohen, D. J., Detlor, J., Young, J. G., & Shaywitz, B. A. (1980). Clonidine ameliorates Gilles de la Tourette's syndrome. *Archives of General Psychiatry, 37,* 1350–1357.

Cohen, D. J., Marans, S., Dahl, K., Marans, W., & Lewis, M. (1987a). Analytic discussions with Oedipal children. In P. B. Neubauer & A. J. Solnit (Eds.), *The psychoanalytic study of the child* (Vol. 42, pp. 59–83). New Haven: Yale University Press.

Cohen, D. J., Paul, R., & Volkmar, F. R. (1986). Issues in the classification of pervasive and other developmental disorders: Toward DSM-IV. *Journal of the American Academy of Child Psychiatry, 25,* 213–220.

Cohen, D. J., Riddle, M. A., & Leckman, J. F. (1987b). Tourette syndrome: Clinical features, etiology, and pathogenesis. In J. D. Noshpitz (Ed.), *Basic handbook of child psychiatry: Vol. 5. Advances and new directions.* New York: Basic Books.

Cohen, N. J., Bradley, S., & Kolers, N. (1987). Outcome evaluation of a therapeutic day treatment program for delayed and disturbed preschoolers. *Journal of the American Academy of Child and Adolescent Psychiatry, 26,* 687–693.

Cohen, N. J., Kolers, N., & Bradley, S. (1987). Predictors of the outcome of treatment in a therapeutic preschool. *Journal of the American Academy of Child and Adolescent Psychiatry, 26,* 829–833.

Cohen, N. J., Sullivan, J., Minde, K., Novak, C., & Keens, S. (1983). Mother-child interaction in hyperactive and normal kindergarten-aged children and the effect of treatment. *Child Psychiatry and Human Development, 13,* 213–224.

Cohen-Sandler, R., Berman, A. L., & King, R. A. (1982). Life stress and symptomatology: Determinants of suicidal behavior in children. *Journal of the American Academy of Child Psychiatry, 21,* 178–186.

Cole, D., & LaVoie, J. C. (1985). Fantasy play and related cognitive development in 2- to 6-year-olds. *Developmental Psychology, 21,* 233–240.

Coleman, L., Wolkind, S., & Ashley, L. (1977). Symptoms of behaviour disturbance and adjustment to school. *Journal of Child Psychology and Psychiatry, 18,* 201–209.

Connell, H. M., & Sturgess, J. L. (1987). Sleep phobia in middle childhood—A review of six cases. *Journal of the American Academy of Child and Adolescent Psychiatry, 26,* 449–452.

Conners, C. K. (1969). A teacher rating scale for use in drug studies with children. *American Journal of Psychiatry, 126,* 884–888.

Cooper, M. G. (1966). School refusal. *Educational Research, 8,* 115–127.

Corbett, J. A., Matthews, A. M., Connell, P. H., & Shapiro, D. A. (1969). Tics and

Gilles de la Tourette's syndrome: A follow-up study and critical reviews. *British Journal of Psychiatry, 115,* 1229-1241.

Corsaro, W. (1979). Young children's conception of status and role. *Sociology of Education, 52,* 46-59.

Coryell, W., & Schlesser, M. A. (1981). Suicide and the dexamethasone suppression test in unipolar depression. *American Journal of Psychiatry, 138,* 1120-1121.

Coryell, W., & Winokur, G. (1984). Depression spectrum disorders: Clinical diagnosis and biological implications. In R. M. Post & J. C. Ballenger (Eds.), *Neurobiology of mood disorders.* Baltimore: Williams and Wilkins.

Cottrell, L. S. (1969). Interpersonal interaction and the development of self. In D. Goslin (Ed.), *Handbook of socialization theory and research.* Chicago: Rand McNally.

Cox, A., & Rutter, M. (1985). Diagnostic appraisal and interviewing. In M. Rutter & L. Hersov (Eds.), *Child and adolescent psychiatry: Modern approaches* (pp. 233-248). Boston: Blackwell Scientific.

Cox, A., Rutter, M., Newman, S., & Bartak, L. (1975). A comparative study of infantile autism and specific developmental receptive language disorder: II. Parental characteristics. *British Journal of Psychiatry, 126,* 146-159.

Crittenden, P. M. (1985). Social networks, quality of child rearing, and child development. *Child Development, 56,* 1299-1313.

Crowell, J. A., Feldman, S. S., & Ginsberg, N. (1988). Assessment of mother-child interaction in preschoolers with behavior problems. *Journal of the American Academy of Child and Adolescent Psychiatry, 27,* 303-311.

Culbertson, J. L., & Ferry, P. C. (1982). Learning disabilities. *Pediatric Clinics of North America, 29,* 121-136.

Curtis, G. (1963). Violence breeds violence. *American Journal of Psychiatry, 120,* 386-387.

Cytryn, L., McKnew, D. H., & Levy, E. Z. (1972). Proposed classification of childhood depression. *American Journal of Psychiatry, 129,* 149-155.

Dahl, M., Eklund, G., & Sundelin, C. (1986). Early feeding problems in an affluent society. II. Determinants. *Acta Paediatrica Scandinavica, 75,* 380-387.

Dahl, M., & Sundelin, C. (1986). Early feeding problems in an affluent society. I. Categories and clinical signs. *Acta Paediatrica Scandinavica, 75,* 370-379.

Dahl, V. (1976). A follow-up study of a child psychiatric clientele with special regard to the diagnosis of psychosis. *Acta Psychiatrica Scandinavica, 54,* 106-112.

Dalton, J. E., Pederson, S. L., & McEntyre, W. L. (1987). A comparison of the Shipley vs. Wais-R subtests in predicting Wais-R full scale IQ. *Journal of Clinical Psychology, 43,* 278-280.

Daniels, C. R. (1964). Play group therapy with children. *Acta Psychotherapeutica, 12,* 45-52.

Dare, C. (1985). Psychoanalytic theories of development. In M. Rutter & L. Hersov (Eds.), *Child and adolescent psychiatry: Modern approaches* (2nd ed., pp. 204-215). Oxford: Blackwell Scientific.

Davidson, J. R. T., Miller, R. D., Turnbull, C. D., & Sullivan, J. L. (1982). Atypical depression. *Archives of General Psychiatry, 39,* 527–534.

Davis, G. C., Buchsbaum, W. E., Jr., DeFraites, E. G., Kleinman, J. E., van Kammen, D. P., Post, R. M., & Wyatt, R. J. (1977). Intravenous naloxone administration in schizophrenia and affective illness. *Science, 197,* 74.

Dehorn, A., & Klinge, V. (1978). Correlations and factor analysis of the WISC-R and the Peabody Picture Vocabulary Test for an adolescent psychiatric sample. *Journal of Consulting and Clinical Psychology, 46,* 1160–1161.

Dejonge, G. A. (1973). Epidemiology of enuresis: A survey of the literature. *Clinical Developments in Medicine, 48/49,* 39.

Deleon-Jones, F., Maas, J. W., Dekirmenjian, H., & Sanchez, J. (1975). Diagnostic subgroups of affective disorders and their urinary excretion of catecholamine metabolites. *American Journal of Psychiatry, 132,* 1141–1148.

Delgado, J. M. R. (1969). Offensive-defensive behavior in free monkeys and chimpanzees induced by radio stimulation of the brain. I. Aggressive behavior. In S. Garattini & E. B. Sigg (Eds.), *Proceedings of the international symposium of the biology of aggressive behavior* (pp. 109–119). Amsterdam: Excerpta Medical.

Dement, W., & Kleitman, N. (1957). Cyclic variations in EEG during sleep and their relationships to eye movements, body motility, and dreaming. *Electroencephalography and Clinical Neurophysiology, 9,* 673–679.

DeMyer, M. K., Hingtgen, J. N., & Jackson, R. K. (1981). Infantile autism reviewed: A decade of research. *Schizophrenia Bulletin, 7,* 388–451.

Denzin, N. (1977). *Childhood socialization.* San Francisco: Jossey-Bass.

Deren, S. (1986). Children of substance abusers: A review of the literature. *Journal of Substance Abuse Treatment, 3,* 77–94.

Derryberry, D., & Rothbart, M. K. (1984). Emotion, attention, and temperament. In C. E. Izard, J. Kagan, & R. B. Zajonc (Eds.), *Emotions, cognition and behavior* (pp. 132–166). Cambridge, England: Cambridge University Press.

Despert, J. L. (1961). Some considerations relating to the genesis of autistic behavior in children. *American Journal of Orthopsychiatry, 21,* 335–350.

Deutsch, H. (1965). In *Neuroses and character types.* New York: International Universities Press. (Original work published 1937).

Dewald, P. A. (1964). *Psychotherapy: A dynamic approach.* New York: Basic Books.

Dewald, P. A. (1983). Elements of change and cure in psychoanalysis. *Archives of General Psychology, 40,* 89–95.

Dewey, J. (1938). *Experience and education.* New York: Kappa Delta Pi.

Diamond, M. (1965). A critical evaluation of the ontogeny of human sexual behavior. *Quarterly Review of Biology, 40,* 147.

Dipietro, J. (1981). Rough and tumble play: A function of gender. *Developmental Psychology, 17,* 50–58.

Doleys, D. M. (1977). Behavioral treatments for nocturnal enuresis in children: A review of the recent literature. *Psychology Bulletin, 84,* 30–54.

Douglas, V. I., & Peters, K. G. (1979). Toward a clearer definition of the attentional deficit of hyperactive children. In G. A. Hale & M. Lewis (Eds.), *Attention and the development of cognitive skills* (pp. 173–247). New York: Plenum.

Dunn, L. M., & Dunn, L. M. (1981). *Peabody Picture Vocabulary Test-Revised.* Minnesota: American Guidance Service.

Earls, E., & Cook, S. (1983). Play observations of three-year-old children and their relationship to parental reports of behavior problems and temperament characteristics. *Child Psychiatry and Human Development, 13,* 225–232.

Earls, F. (1982). Epidemiology and child psychiatry: Future prospects. *Comprehensive Psychiatry, 23,* 75–84.

Earls, F. (1987). On the familial transmission of child psychiatric disorder. *Journal of Child Psychology and Psychiatry, 28,* 791–802.

Edelman, R. I. (1971). Operant conditioning treatment of encopresis. *Journal of Behavior Therapy and Experimental Psychiatry, 2,* 71–73.

Edgil, A. E., Wood, K. R., & Smith, D. P. (1985). Sleep problems of older infants and preschool children. *Pediatric Nursing, 11*(2), 87–89.

Edmonson, B., Leland, H., de Jung, J. E., & Leach, E. M. (1967). Increasing social cue interpretations (visual decoding) by retarded adolescents through training. *American Journal of Mental Deficiency, 71,* 1017–1024.

Edmonson, B., Leland, H., & Leach, E. M. (1970). Social inference training of retarded adolescents. *Education and Training of the Mentally Retarded, 5* (4), 169–176.

Egeland, B., Breitenbucher, M., & Rosenberg, D. (1980). Prospective study of the significance of life stress in the etiology of child abuse. *Journal of Consulting and Clinical Psychology, 48,* 195–205.

Eisenberg, L. (1958). Emotional determinants of mental deficiency. *American Medical Association Archives of Neurological Psychiatry, 80,* 114–121.

Eisenberg, L. (1971). Chairman's closing remarks. In M. Rutter (Ed.), *Infantile autism: Concepts, characteristics and treatment* (pp. 313–315). New York: Churchill Livingstone.

Ekstein, R. (1980). Borderline states and ego disturbances. In R. M. Benson & J. Barton (Eds.), *Emotional disorders in children and adolescents: Medical and psychological approaches to treatment* (pp. 403–413). New York: Spectrum.

Ekstein, R. (1983). Play therapy for borderline children. In C. E. Schaefer & K. J. O'Connor (Eds.), *Handbook of play therapy* (pp. 412–418). New York: Wiley.

Ekstein, R., & Friedman, S. W. (1957). The function of acting out, play action and play acting in the psychotherapeutic process. *Journal of the American Psychoanalytic Association, 5,* 581–629.

Ekstein, R., & Wallerstein, J. (1954). Observations on the psychology of borderline and psychotic children. *Psychoanalytic Study of the Child, 9,* 344–369.

Elizur, E., & Kaffman, M. (1982). Children's bereavement reactions following death of the father: II. *Journal of the American Academy of Child Psychiatry, 21,* 474–480.

Elkind, D. (1976). Cognitive development and psychopathology: Observation on egocentrism and ego defense. In R. Schopler (Ed.), *Psychopathology and child development* (pp. 167–183). New York: Plenum.

Elkind, D. (1978). *The Child's reality: Three developmental themes.* New Jersey: Erlbaum.

Elkind, D. (1979). The figurative and the operative in Piagetian psychology. In M. H. Bornstein & W. Kessen (Eds.), *Psychological development from infancy* (pp. 225–247). New York: LEA Associates.

Elkind, D. (1982). Piagetian psychology and the practice of child psychiatry. *Journal of the American Academy of Child Psychiatry, 21,* 435–445.

Elliott, C., & Ozolins, M. (1983). Use of imagery and imagination in treatment of children. In C. E. Walker & M. C. Roberts (Eds.), *Handbook of clinical psychology* (pp. 1026–1049). New York: Wiley.

Elmer, E., & Gregg, C. S. (1967). Developmental characteristics of abused children. *Pediatrics, 40,* 596–602.

Emery, R. E. (1982). Interparental conflict and the children of discord and divorce. *Psychological Bulletin, 2,* 1097–1126.

Emmerich, W. (1959). Young children's discriminations of parent and child roles. *Child Development, 30,* 403–419.

Emmerich, W. (1961). Family role concepts of children age six to ten. *Child Development, 32,* 609–624.

Emrich, H. M. (1982). A possible role of opioid substances in depression. In E. Costa & G. Racagni (Eds.), *Typical and atypical antidepressants: Clinical practice* (pp. 77–84). New York: Raven Press.

Erikson, E. H. (1940). Studies in the interpretation of play. *Genetic Psychology Monographs, 22,* 557–671.

Erikson, E. H. (1951). Sex differences in the play configurations of American pre-adolescents. *American Journal of Orthopsychiatry, 21,* 667–692.

Erikson, E. H. (1977). *Toys and reasons.* New York: Norton.

Esman, A. (1983). Psychoanalytic play therapy. In C. Schaefer & K. O'Connor (Eds.), *Handbook of play therapy* (pp. 11–20). New York: Wiley.

Essen, J., & Peckman, C. (1976). Nocturnal enuresis in childhood. *Developmental Medicine and Child Neurology, 18,* 577–589.

Fagot, B. I., & Leinbach, M. D. (1985). Gender identity: Some thoughts on an old concept. *Journal of the American Academy of Child Psychiatry, 24,* 684–688.

Fang, V. S., Tricou, B. J., Robertson, A., & Meltzer, H. Y. (1981). Plasma ACTH and cortisol levels in depressed patients: Relation to dexamethasone suppression test. *Life Sciences, 29,* 931–938.

Fein, G. (1979a). Echoes from the nursery: Piaget, Vygotsky, and the relationship between language and play. *New Directions for Child Development, 6,* 1–14.

Fein, G. (1979b). Play and the acquisition of symbols. In L. E. Katz (Ed.), *Current topics in early childhood education.* Baltimore, MD: University Park Press.

Fein, G. (1981). Pretend play in childhood: An integrative review. *Child Development, 52,* 1095–1118.

Fein, G. A. (1975). A transformational analysis of pretending. *Developmental Psychology, 11,* 291–296.

Fein, G. G., & Apfel, N. (1979a). The development of play: Style, structure and situation. *Genetic Psychology Monographs, 99,* 231–250.

Fenson, L., & Ramsay, D. S. (1980). Decentration and integration of the child's play in the second year. *Child Development, 51,* 171–178.

Ferber, R. (1985). Sleep, sleeplessness, and sleep disruptions in infants and young children. *Annals of Clinical Research, 17,* 227–234.

Ferguson, B. E. (1979). Preparing young children for hospitalization: A comparison of two methods. *Pediatrics, 64,* 656–664.

Fergusson, D. M., Horwood, L. J., & Shannon, F. T. (1984). Relationship of family life events, maternal depression, and child-rearing problems. *Pediatrics, 73,* 773–776.

Feshbach, N. D., & Feshbach, S. (1969). The relationship between empathy and aggression in two age groups. *Developmental Psychology, 1,* 102–107.

Field, T. (1984). Separation stress of young children transferring to new schools. *Developmental Psychology, 20,* 786–792.

Field, T. (1986). Affective responses to separation. In T. B. Brazelton & M. W. Yogman (Eds.), *Affective development in infancy* (pp. 125–143). Norwood, NJ: Ablex.

Field, T., De Stefano, L., & Koewler, J. H., III. (1982). Fantasy play of toddlers and pre-schoolers. *Developmental Psychology, 18,* 503–508.

Field, T., Gewirtz, J. L., Cohen, D., Garcia, R., Greenberg, R., & Collins, K. (1984). Leave-takings and reunions of infants, toddlers, preschoolers, and their parents. *Child Development, 55,* 628–635.

Field, T., Vega-Lahr, N., & Jagadish, S. (1984). Separation stress of nursery school infants and toddlers graduating to new classes. *Infant Behavior and Development, 7,* 277–284.

Fisch, G. S., Cohen, I. L., Wolf, E. G., Brown, W. T., Jenkins, E. C., & Gross, A. (1986). Autism and the fragile X syndrome. *American Journal of Psychiatry, 143,* 71–73.

Fischer, M., Rolf, J. E., Hasazi, J. E., & Cummings, L. (1984). Follow-up of a preschool epidemiological sample—Cross-age continuities and predictions of later adjustment with internalizing and externalizing dimensions of behavior. *Child Development, 55,* 137–150.

Fish, B. (1986). Antecedents of an acute schizophrenic break. *Journal of the American Academy of Child Psychiatry, 25,* 595–600.

Fish, B. (1987). Infant predictors of the longitudinal course of schizophrenic development. *Schizophrenia Bulletin, 13,* 395–409.

Fish, B., Shapiro, T., & Campbell, M. (1968). A classification of schizophrenic children under 5 years. *American Journal of Psychiatry, 124,* 109–117.

Fisher, S. H. (1958). Skeletal manifestations of parent-induced trauma in infants and children. *Southern Medical Journal, 51,* 956–960.

Fisher, W., Kerbeshian, J., & Burd, L. (1986). A treatable language: Pharmacological treatment of pervasive developmental disorder. *Developmental and Behavioral Pediatrics, 7,* 73–76.

Fisk, J. L., & Rourke, B. P. (1979). Identification of subtypes of learning-disabled children at three age levels: A neuropsychological, multivariate approach. *Journal of Clinical Neuropsychology, 1,* 289–310.

Flament, M. F., Rapoport, J. L., Murphy, D. L., Berg, C. J., & Lake, R. (1987). Biochemical changes during clomipramine treatment of childhood obsessive-compulsive disorder. *Archives of General Psychiatry, 44,* 219–225.

Flavell, J. H. (1986). The development of children's knowledge about the appearance-reality distinction. *American Psychologist, 41,* 418–425.

Flavell, J. H., Flavell, E. R., Green, F. L., & Wilcox, S. A. (1981). The development of three spatial perspective-taking rules. *Child Development, 52,* 356–358.

Flavell, J. H., Green, F. L., & Flavell, E. R. (1986). Development of knowledge about the appearance-reality distinction. *Monographs of the Society for Research in Child Development, 51*(1, Serial No. 212).

Fontana, V. J. (1985). Child abuse, past, present, and future. *Human Ecology Forum,* 5–7.

Ford, C. V. (1983). *The somatizing disorders: Illness as a way of life.* New York: Elsevier Biochemical.

Fournier, J. P., Garfinkel, B. D., Bond, A., Beauchesne, R. N., & Shapiro, S. K. (1987). Pharmacological and behavioral management of enuresis. *Journal of the American Academy of Child and Adolescent Psychiatry, 26,* 849–853.

Fraiberg, S. (1962). Technical aspects of the analysis of a child with a severe behavior disorder. *Journal of the American Psychoanalytic Association, 10,* 338–367.

Francis, A., Clarkin, J., & Perry, S. (1984). *Differential therapeutics in psychiatry.* New York: Bruner/Mazel.

Frankl, L. (1963). Self-preservation and the development of accident proneness in children and adolescents. *Psychoanalytic Study of the Child, 18,* 464–483.

Frankl, L., & Hellman, I. (1964). The ego's participation in the therapeutic alliance. In M. R. Haworth (Ed.), *Child psychotherapy: Practice and theory* (pp. 229–235). New York: Basic Books.

Freedheim, D. K., & Russ, S. R. (1983). Psychotherapy with children. In C. E. Walker & M. C. Roberts (Eds.), *Handbook of clinical child psychology* (pp. 978–994). New York: Wiley.

Freedman, J. L., Carlsmith, J. M., & Sears, D. O. (1974). *Social psychology.* Englewood Cliffs, NJ: Prentice-Hall.

Freedman, R., Adler, L. E., Waldo, M. C., Pachtman, E., & Franks, R. D. (1983). Neurophysical evidence for a defect in inhibitory pathways in schizophrenia: Comparison of medicated and drug-free patients. *Biological Psychiatry, 18,* 537–551.

Freidlander, B., Wetstone, H., & McPeek, D. (1974). Systematic assessment of selective language listening defect in emotionally disturbed preschool children. *Journal of Child Psychology and Psychiatry, 15,* 1–12.

Freis, E. D. (1954). Mental depression in hypertensive patients treated for long periods with large doses of reserpine. *New England Journal of Medicine, 251,* 1006–1008.

Freud, A. (1928). Introduction to the technique of child analysis. *Nervous and Mental Disease Monograph Series, 48,* 30–41.

Freud, A. (1946). *Psychoanalytic treatment of children.* London: Imago.

Freud, A. (1962). Assessment of childhood disturbances. *Psychoanalytic Study of the Child, 17,* 149–158.

Freud, A. (1966). *The ego and the mechanisms of defense.* New York: International Universities Press.

Freud, A. (1974). Four lectures on child analysis. In *The writings of Anna Freud (Vol. 1).* New York: International Universities Press. (Original work published in 1927).

Freud, A., & Dann, S. (1951). An experiment in group living. In R. Eisler, A. Freud, H. Hartmann, & E. Kris (Eds.), *The psychoanalytic study of the child* (Vol. 6, pp 127–168). New York: International Universities Press.

Freud, S. (1886–1957). *The standard edition of the complete psychological works of Sigmund Freud.* (23 vols.) J. Strachney (Ed. and trans.). London: Hogarth.

Freud, S. (1905). Three essays on the theory of sexuality. *Standard edition* (Vol. 7). London: Hogarth.

Freud, S. (1922). *Beyond the pleasure principle.* London: Hogarth.

Freud, S. (1932). Analysis of a phobia in a five-year old boy. *Standard edition* (Vol. 10). London: Hogarth. (Original work published 1909).

Freud, S. (1933). New introductory lectures on psycho-analysis. *Standard edition* (Vol. 22, pp. 81–111). London: Hogarth. (Original work published 1910).

Freud, S. (1957a). Mourning and melancholia. *Standard edition* (Vol. 14, pp. 237–258). London: Hogarth. (Original work published 1917).

Freud, S. (1957b). Thoughts for the times on war and death. *Standard edition* (Vol. 14, pp. 275–300). London: Hogarth. (Original work published 1915).

Freud, S. (1959). Inhibitions, symptoms, and anxiety. *Standard edition* (Vol. 20, pp. 87–172). London: Hogarth. (Original work published 1926).

Friedman, R. C., & Corn, R. (1985). Follow-up five years after suicide at age 7. *American Journal of Psychotherapy, 34,* 108–113.

Fries, M. E. (1937). Play technique in the analysis of young children. *The Psychoanalytic Review, 24,* 233–245.

Gadow, K. D. (1983, January). Pharmacotherapy for behavioral disorders. *Clinical Pediatrics,* 48-53.

Galambos, N. L., & Dixon, R. A. (1984). Adolescent abuse and the development of personal sense of control. *Child Abuse and Neglect, 8,* 285–293.

Galejs, I., & Hegland, S. (1982). Locus of control and task persistence in preschool children. *Journal of Social Psychology, 117,* 227–231.

Gardner, H. L., Forehand, R., & Roberts, M. (1976). Timeout with children: Effects of an explanation and brief parent training on child and parent behaviors. *Journal of Abnormal Child Psychiatry, 4,* 277–288.

Gardner, R. (1971). *Therapeutic communication with children: The mutual story telling technique.* New York: Science House.

Gardner, R. (1976). *Psychotherapy with children of divorce.* New York: Jason Aronson.

Gardner, R. A. (1979). Helping children cooperate in therapy. In J. D. Noshpitz

& S. I. Harrison (Eds.), *Basic handbook of child psychiatry* (Vol. 3, pp. 414–432). New York: Basic Books.

Garfinkel, B. D. (1986). Major affective disorders in children and adolescents. In G. Winokur & P. Clayton (Eds.), *The medical basis of psychiatry* (pp. 308–330). Philadelphia: W. B. Saunders.

Garmezy, N., & Masten, A. S. (1986). Stress, competence, and resilience: Common frontiers for therapist and psychopathologist. *Behavior Therapy, 17,* 500–521.

Garrison, E. G. (1987). Psychological maltreatment of children: An emerging focus for inquiry and concern. *American Psychologist, 42,* 157–159.

Garrison, W., & Earls, F. (1983). Life events and social supports in families with a two-year-old: Methods and preliminary findings. *Comprehensive Psychiatry, 24,* 439–452.

Garrison, W., & Earls, F. (1986). Epidemiological perspectives on maternal depression and the young child. *New Directions for Child Development, 34,* 13–30.

Garvey, C. (1977). *Play.* Cambridge, MA: Harvard University Press.

Gatchel, R. J., & Baum, A. (1980). Cognitive determinants of reactance and helplessness in a dormitory environment. *Personality and Social Psychology Bulletin, 6,* 180.

Gearheart, B. R., & Weishahn, M. W. (1976). *The handicapped child in the regular classroom.* St. Louis: C. V. Mosby.

Geller, B., Cooper, T. B., Farooki, Z. Q., & Chestnut, E. C. (1985). Dose and plasma levels of nortriptyline and chlorpromazine in delusionally depressed adolescents and of nortriptyline in nondelusionally depressed adolescents. *American Journal of Psychiatry, 142,* 336–338.

Geller, B., Rogol, A. D., & Knitter, E. F. (1983). Preliminary data on the dexamethasone suppression test in children with major depressive disorder. *American Journal of Psychiatry, 140,* 620–622.

Gelles, R. J. (1973). Child abuse as psychopathology: A sociological critique and reformulation. *American Journal of Orthopsychiatry, 43,* 611–621.

Gelles, R. J., & Straus, M. A. (1979). Determinants of violence in the family: Toward a theoretical integration. In W. R. Burr, R. Hill, & F. I. Nye (Eds.), *Contemporary theories about the family* (Vol. 1, pp. 549–581). New York: Free Press.

George, C., & Main, M. (1979). Social interactions of young abused children: Approach, avoidance and aggression. *Child Development, 50,* 306–318.

Gershen, S., & Shaw, F. H. (1961). Psychiatric sequelae of chronic exposure to organophosphorous insecticides. *Lancet, 1,* 1371–1384.

Gesell, A., & Amatruda, A. (1974a). The development of behavior. In A. Gesell & A. Amatruda (Eds.), *Developmental diagnosis: The evaluation and management of normal and abnormal neuropsychologic development in infancy and early childhood* (pp. 3–15). New York: Harper and Row.

Gesell, A., & Amatruda, A. (1974b). The developmental assessment of behavior. In A. Gesell, & A. Amatruda (Eds.), *Developmental diagnosis: The evaluation and management of normal and abnormal neuropsychologic development in infancy and early childhood* (pp. 16-24). New York: Harper and Row.

Gesell, A., Ilg, F. L., & Ames, L. B. (1974). *Infant and child in the culture of today* (rev. ed). New York: Harper and Row.

Gil, D. (1971). Violence against children. *Journal of Marriage and Family, 33,* 637-657.

Gillberg, C., Terenius, L., & Lonnerholm, G. (1985). Endorphin activity in childhood psychosis: Spinal fluid levels in 24 cases. *Archives of General Psychiatry, 42,* 780-783.

Gillick, S. (1974). *Training mothers as therapists in treatment of childhood obesity.* Unpublished doctoral dissertation, State University of New York at Buffalo.

Gilmore, J. B. (1966). The role of anxiety and cognitive factors in children's play behavior. *Child Development, 37,* 397-416.

Ginott, H. G. (1961). *Group psychotherapy with children.* New York: McGraw-Hill.

Gitlan, M., & Rosenblatt, M. (1978). Possible withdrawal from endogenous opiates in schizophrenics. *American Journal of Psychiatry, 135,* 377.

Gleser, G. C., Grenn, B. L., & Winget, C. (1981). *Prolonged psychosocial effects of disaster. A study of Buffalo Creek.* New York: Academic Press.

Glick, I. D., Clarkin, J. F., & Kessler, D. R. (1987). *Marital and family therapy.* New York: Harcourt Brace Jovanovich.

Goel, K. M., Thomson, R. B., Gibb, E. M., & McAinsh, T. F. (1984). Evaluation of nine different types of enuresis alarms. *Archives of Disease in Childhood, 59,* 748-753.

Gold, D., & Berger, C. (1978). Problem-solving performance of young boys and girls as a function of task appropriateness and sex-identity. *Sex Roles, 4,* 183-193.

Goldberg, I. D., Regier, D. A., McInerny, T. K., Pless, I. B., & Roghmann, K. J. (1979). The role of the pediatrician in the delivery of mental health services to children. *Pediatrics, 63,* 898-909.

Goldberg, S., & Lewis, M. (1969). Play behavior in the year-old-infant: Early sex difference. *Child Development, 40,* 21-31.

Goldberg, T. E., Maltz, A., Bow, J. N., Karson, C. N., & Leleszi, J. P. (1987). Blink rate abnormalities in autistic and mentally retarded children: Relationship to dopaminergic activity. *Journal of the American Academy of Child and Adolescent Psychiatry, 26,* 336-338.

Golden, M., & Birns, B. (1976). Social class and infant intelligence. In M. Lewis (Ed.), *Origins of intelligence.* New York: Plenum.

Goldenson, R. M. (1970). *The encyclopedia of human behavior: Psychology, psychiatry and mental health* (Vol. 2). Garden City, NY: Doubleday.

Goldney, R. D. (1981). Parental loss and reported childhood stress in young women who attempt suicide. *Acta Psychiatrica Scandinavica, 64,* 34-59.

Goldstein, M. J., & Doane, J. A. (1982). Family factors in the onset, course, and treatment of schizophrenic spectrum disorders. *The Journal of Nervous and Mental Disease, 170,* 692-700.

Golomb, C., & Cornelius, C. B. (1977). Symbolic play and its cognitive significance. *Developmental Psychology, 13,* 246–252.

Goodman, C. S., & Gilman, A. (1970). *The pharmacological basis of therapeutics* (4th ed.). New York: Macmillan.

Goodwin, F. K. (1976). Discussion remarks. In E. Usdin, D. A. Hamburg, & Y. D. Barchas (Eds.), *Neuroregulators and psychiatric disorders* (p. 192). New York: Oxford University Press.

Gordon, S. B., & Davidson, N. (1981). Behavioral parent training. In A. S. Gurman & D. P. Kniskern (Eds.), *Handbook of family therapy* (pp. 517–555). New York: Bruner/Mazel.

Gottesman, L., & Shields, J. (1982). *Schizophrenia the epigenetic puzzle.* Cambridge, England: Cambridge University Press.

Gould, J. (1986). The Lowe and Costello symbolic play test in socially impaired children. *Journal of Autism and Developmental Disorders, 16,* 199–213.

Grace, D. (1975). *Self-monitoring in the modification of obesity in children.* Unpublished doctoral dissertation, State University of New York at Buffalo.

Grad, L. R., Pelcovitz, D., Olson, M., Matthews, M., & Grad, G. (1987). Obsessive-compulsive symptomatology in children with Tourette's syndrome. *Journal of the American Academy of Child and Adolescent Psychiatry, 26,* 69–73.

Graham, P. (1985). Psychosomatic relationships. In M. Rutter & L. Hersov (Eds.), *Adolescent psychiatry: Modern approaches* (2nd ed., pp. 599–613). Oxford: Blackwell Scientific.

Graham, P., & Rutter, M. (1973). Psychiatric disorder in the young adolescent: A follow-up study. *Proceedings of the Royal Society of Medicine, 66,* 1226–1229.

Granville-Grossman, K. L. (1966). The early environment in affective disorder. In A. Coppen & A. Walk (Eds.), *Recent developments in affective disorders* (pp. 65–80). London: General Registry Office.

Gratton, L., & Rizzo, A. E. (1969). Group therapy with young psychotic children. *International Journal of Group Psychotherapy, 19,* 62–71.

Graziano, A. M. (1974). *Child without tomorrow.* New York: Pergamon.

Green, A. H. (1983). Child abuse: Dimensions of psychological trauma in abused children. *Journal of the American Academy of Child Psychiatry, 22,* 231–237.

Green, R. (1974). *Sexual identity conflict in children and adults.* New York: Basic Books.

Green, R. (1980). Sexual identity: Research strategies. In S. I. Harrison & J. F. McDermott (Eds.), *New directions in childhood psychopathology: Vol. 1. Developmental considerations.* New York: International Universities Press.

Green, R. (1985a). Atypical psychosexual development. In M. Rutter & L. Hersov (Eds.), *Child and adolescent psychiatry* (2nd. ed., pp. 638–649). Oxford: Blackwell Scientific.

Green, R. (1985b). Gender identity in childhood and later sexual orientation: Follow-up of 78 males. *American Journal of Psychiatry, 142,* 339–341.

Green, R., Fuller, M., & Rutley, B. (1972). It-Scale for Children and Draw-a-Person

Test; 30 feminine versus 15 masculine boys. *Journal of Personality Assessment, 36,* 349–352.

Greenacre, P. (1952). *Trauma, growth, and personality.* New York: Norton.

Greenman, D. A., Gunderson, J. G., Cane, M., & Saltzman, P. R. (1986). An examination of the borderline diagnosis in children. *American Journal of Psychiatry, 143,* 998–1003.

Greenson, R. R. (1968). Dis-identifying from mother: Its special importance for the boy. *International Journal of Psychoanalysis, 49,* 370.

Greenson, R. R. (1971). The "real" relationship between the patient and the psychoanalyst. In M. Kanzer (Ed.), *The unconscious today: Essays in honor of Max Schur* (pp. 213–232). New York: International Universities Press.

Greif, E. B. (1979). Sex-role playing in preschool children. In J. S. Bruner, A. Jolly, & K. Sylva (Eds.), *Play* (pp. 385–391). New York: Basic Books.

Greif, E. F. (1978). A comparison of individual and group parent-child interaction training. *Dissertation Abstracts International, 39,* 1436A. (University Microfilms No. 78-14, 671).

Greif, M. D. (1983). Family play therapy. In C. E. Schaefer & K. J. O'Connor (Eds.), *Handbook of play therapy* (pp. 65–75). New York: Wiley.

Grinker., R. R., Werble, B., & Drye, R. C. (1968). *The borderline syndrome: A behavioral study of ego-function.* New York: Basic Books.

Guillemin, R., & Borgus, R. (1972). The hormones of the hypothalamus. *Scientific American, 227,* 24–33.

Gunnar, M. R. (1987). Psychobiological studies of stress and coping: An introduction. *Child Development, 58,* 1403–1407.

Gunnar, M. R., Fisch, R. O., & Malone, S. (1984). The effects of a pacifying stimulus on behavioral and adrenocortical responses to circumcision in the newborn. *Journal of the American Academy of Child Psychiatry, 23,* 34–38.

Gunnar, M. R., Malone, S., Vance, G., & Fische, R. O. (1985). Coping with aversive stimulation in the neonatal period: Quiet sleep and plasma cortisol levels during recovery from circumcision. *Child Development, 56,* 824–834.

Gurman, A. S., Kniskern, D. P., & Pinsof, W. M. (1986). Research on the process and outcome of marital and family therapy. In S. L. Garfield & A. E. Bergin (Eds.), *Handbook of psychotherapy and behavior change* (3rd ed., pp. 565–624). New York: Wiley.

Halbreich, M. D., Asnis, G. M., Schindledecker, R., Zumoff, B., & Nathan, S. (1985). Cortisol secretion in endogenous depression. *Archives of General Psychiatry, 42,* 904–908.

Hamilton, M. (1960). A rating scale for depression. *Journal of Neurology, Neurosurgery, and Psychiatry, 23,* 56–61.

Hampton, R. L., & Newberger, E. H. (1985). Child abuse incidence and reporting by hospitals: Significance of severity, class, and race. *American Journal of Public Health, 75,* 56–60.

Handen, B. L., Mandell, F., & Russo, D. C. (1986). Feeding induction in children who refuse to eat. *American Journal of Diseased Children, 140,* 52–54.

Handford, H. A., Mayes, S. D., Mattison, R. E., Humphrey, F. J., Bagnato, S., Bixler, E. O., & Kales, J. (1986). Child and parent reaction to the Three Mile Island nuclear accident. *Journal of the American Academy of Child Psychiatry, 25,* 346–356.

Handford, H. A., Mayes, S. D., Mattison, R. E., Humphrey, F. J., & McLaughlin, R. E. (1986). Depressive syndrome in children entering a residential school subsequent to parent death, divorce, or separation. *Journal of the American Academy of Child Psychiatry, 25,* 409–414.

Hansen, J. C., Niland, T. M., & Zani, L. P. (1969). Model reinforcement in group counseling with elementary school children. *Personnel and Guidance Journal, 47,* 741–744.

Harding, G. & Golinkoff, R. (1979). The origins of intentional vocalizations in prelinguistic infants. *Child Development, 50,* 33–40.

Hargreaves, D., Stoll, L., Farnworth, S., & Morgan, S. (1981). Psychological androgyny and ideational fluency. *British Journal of Social Psychology, 20,* 53–55.

Harley, M. (1971). The current status of the transference neurosis in children. *Journal of the American Psychoanalytic Association, 19,* 26–40.

Harris, G., & Levine, S. (1962). Sexual differentiation of the brain and its experimental control. *Journal of Physiology, 162,* 42P, 43P.

Harter, S. (1983a). Cognitive-developmental considerations in the conduct of play therapy. In C. Schaefer & K. O'Connor (Eds.), *Handbook of play therapy* (pp. 95–127). New York: Wiley.

Harter, S. (1983b). Developmental perspectives on the self-system. In E. M. Hetherington (Ed.), *Socialization, personality, and social development: Vol. 4. Handbook of child psychiatry* (4th ed., pp. 275–385). New York: Wiley.

Hartzell, H. E., & Compton, C. (1984). Learning disability: 10-year follow-up. *Pediatrics, 74,* 1058–1064.

Haskins, R. (1985). Public aggression among children with varying day care experience. *Child Development, 57,* 202–703.

Head, H. (1926). *Aphasia and kindred disorders of speech.* Cambridge, England: Cambridge University Press.

Hebben, N., Benjamin, D., & Milberg, W. P. (1981). The relationship among handedness, sighting dominance, and acuity dominance in elementary school children. *Cortex, 17,* 441–446.

Hechtman, L. (1985). Adolescent outcome of hyperactive children treated with stimulants in childhood: A review. *Psychopharmacology Bulletin, 2,* 178–191.

Hegland, S. M., & Galejs, I. (1983). Developmental aspects of locus of control in preschool children. *Journal of Genetic Psychology, 143,* 229–239.

Heilveil, I. (1983). *Video in mental health practice.* New York: Springer.

Heinicke, C. M., & Ramsey-Klee, D. M. (1986). Outcome of child psychotherapy as a function of frequency of session. *Journal of the American Academy of Child Psychiatry, 25,* 247–253.

Helfer, R. E., McKinney, J. P., & Kempe, R. (1976). Arresting or freezing the developmental process. In R. E. Helfer & C. H. Kempe (Eds.), *Child abuse and neglect: The family and the community* (pp. 55–73). Cambridge, MA: Ballinger.

Hellman, D. S., & Blackman, N. (1966). Enuresis, firesetting and cruelty to animals: A triad predictive of adult crime. *American Journal of Psychiatry, 122,* 1431–1435.

Helveston, E. M. (1986). Learning disabilities. *Transactions—New Orleans Academy of Ophthalmology,* 517–525.

Heninger, G. R., Charney, D. S., & Sternberg, D. E. (1984). Serotonergic function in depression: Prolactin response to intravenous tryptophan in depressed patients and healthy subjects. *Archives of General Psychiatry, 41,* 398–402.

Herbst, J., Friedland G. W., & Zboraliski, F. F. (1971). Hiatal hernia and rumination in infants and children. *Journal of Pediatrics, 78,* 924–929.

Herjanic, B., & Campbell, W. (1977). Differentiating psychiatrically disturbed children on the basis of a structured interview. *Journal of Abnormal Child Psychology, 5,* 127–134.

Herrenkohl, R. C., Herrenkohl, E. C., & Egolf, B. (1983a). Circumstances surrounding the occurrence of child maltreatment. *Journal of Consulting and Clinical Psychology, 51,* 424–431.

Herrenkohl, R. C., Herrenkohl, E. C., & Toedter, L. J. (1983b). Perspectives on the intergenerational transmission of abuse. In D. Finkelhor, R. J. Gelles, & G. T. Hotaling (Eds.), *The dark side of families* (pp. 305–316). Beverly Hills, CA: Sage.

Herrenkohl, E. C., Herrenkohl, R. C., Toedter, L., & Yanushefski, A. M. (1984). Parent-child interactions in abusive and nonabusive families. *Journal of the American Academy of Child Psychiatry, 23,* 641–648.

Hershberg, S. G., Carlson, G. A., Cantwell, D. P., & Strober, M. (1982). Anxiety and depressive disorders in psychiatrically disturbed children. *Journal of Clinical Psychiatry, 43,* 358–361.

Hersov, L. (1985a). Faecal soiling. In M. Rutter & L. Hersov (Eds.), *Child and adolescent psychiatry: Modern approaches* (pp. 482–489). Boston: Blackwell Scientific.

Hersov, L. (1985b). School refusal. In M. Rutter & L. Hersov (Eds.), *Child and adolescent Psychiatry* (pp. 382–399). Oxford: Blackwell Scientific.

Hertzig, M. E. (1982). Stability and change in nonfocal neurologic signs. *Journal of the American Academy of Child Psychiatry, 21,* 231–236.

Hetherington, E. M., Cox, M., & Cox, R. (1979). Play and social interaction in children following divorce. *Journal of Social Issues, 35,* 26–49.

Hewitt, L. E., & Jenkins, R. L. (1946). *Fundamental patterns of maladjustment, the dynamics of their origin: A statistical analysis based upon five hundred case records of children examined at the Michigan Child Guidance Institute.* Springfield: State of Illinois.

Hill, O. W. (1969). The association of childhood bereavement with suicidal attempt in depressive illness. *British Journal of Psychiatry, 115,* 301–304.

Hilton, A. (1987). Approaches for feeding the young child with anorexia. *Journal of Pediatric Nursing, 2,* 45–49.

Hindeman, M. (1977). Child abuse and neglect: The alcohol connection. *Alcohol, Health and Research World, 3,* 2–7.

Hirschfeld, R. M., Klerman, G. L., Andreasen, N. C., Clayton, P. J., & Keller, M. B. (1985). Situational major depressive disorder. *Archives of General Psychiatry, 42,* 1109–1114.

Hobson, R. P. (1984). Early childhood autism and the question of egocentrism. *Journal of Autism and Developmental Disorders, 14,* 85–104.

Hoffman, T. E., Byrne, K. M., Belnap, K. L., & Steward, M. S. (1981). Simultaneous semipermeable groups for mothers and their early latency-age boys. *International Journal of Group Psychotherapy, 31*(1), 83–98.

Hollingshead, A. B., & Redlich, F. C. (1957). *Social class and mental illness: A community study.* New York: Wiley.

Holman, S. L. (1985). A group program for borderline mothers and their toddlers. *International Journal of Group Psychotherapy, 35,* 79–93.

Holter, J. C., & Friedman, S. B. (1968). Principles of management in child abuse cases. *American Journal of Orthopsychiatry, 38,* 127–136.

Horn, W. F., O'Donnell, J. P., & Vitulano, L. A. (1983). Long-term follow-up studies of learning-disabled persons. *Journal of Learning Disabilities, 16*(9), 542–555.

Horowitz, L. (1976). Indications and contraindications for group psychotherapy. *Bulletin of Menninger Clinic, 40,* 505–507.

Howells, J. G. (1980). Family diagnosis. *Psychological Bulletin, 10*(7), 6–14.

Hughes, C. W., Preskorn, S. H., Adams, R. N., & Kent, T. A. (1986). Neurobiological etiology of schizophrenia and affective disorders. In J. O. Cavenar, Jr. (Ed.), *Psychiatry* (Vol. 1). Philadelphia: Lippincott.

Hughes, M. (1987). The relationship between symbolic and manipulative (object) play. In D. Gorlitz & J. F. Wohlwill (Eds.), *Curiosity, imagination, and play* (pp. 247–257). Hillsdale, NJ: Erlbaum.

Hulme, I. L., & Lunzer, K. A. (1966). Play, language and reasoning in subnormal children. *Journal of Child Psychology and Psychiatry, 7,* 107–123.

Husain, S. A., & Vandiver, T. (1984). *Suicide in children and adolescents.* New York: Spectrum.

Husaini, B. A., & Neff, J. A. (1981). Social-class and depressive symptomatology—The role of life change events and locus of control. *Journal of Nervous and Mental Disease, 169,* 638–647.

Huttunen, M. O., & Niskanen, P. (1978). Prenatal loss of father and psychiatric disorders. *Archives of General Psychiatry, 35,* 429–431.

Irwin, E. (1983). The diagnostic and therapeutic use of pretend play. In C. Schaefer & K. O'Connor (Eds.), *Handbook of play therapy* (pp. 148–173). New York: Wiley.

Irwin, M., Daniels, M., & Weiner, H. (1987). Immune and neuroendocrine changes during bereavement. *Psychiatric Clinics of North America, 10,* 449–465.

Iverson, L. L. (1982). Neurotransmitters and CNS Disease. *Lancet, 2,* 914–918.

Iwanaga, M. (1973). Development of interpersonal play structure in three-, four-

and five-year-old children. *Journal of Research and Development in Education, 6,* 71–82.

Jacklin, C. N., DiPietro, J. A., & Maccoby, E. E. (1984). Sex-typing behavior and sex-typing pressure in child/parent interaction. *Archives of Sexual Behavior, 13,* 413–425.

Jacobson, R. R. (1985). Child firesetters: A clinical investigation. *Journal of Child Psychology and Psychiatry, 26,* 759–768.

Jacobvitz, D., & Sroufe, L. A. (1987). The early caregiver-child relationship and attention-deficit disorder with hyperactivity in kindergarten: A prospective study. *Child Development, 58,* 1488–1495.

Janowsky, D. S., El-Yousef, M. K., & Davis, J. M. (1974). Acetylcholine and depression. *Psychosomatic Medicine, 36,* 248–257.

Janowsky, D. S., El-Yousef, M. K., Davis, J. M., et al. (1972). A cholinergic-adrenergic hypothesis of mania and depression. *Lancet, 1,* 632–635.

Janowsky, D. S., El-Yousef, M. K., Davis, J. M., et al. (1973). Parasympathetic suppression of mania by physostigmine. *Archives of General Psychiatry, 28,* 542–547.

Jaspers, K. (1963). *General psychopathology* (H. J. Hamilton, Trans.). Manchester: University Press.

Jenson, K. (1959). Depressions in patients treated with reserpine for arterial hypertension. *Acta Psychiatrica et Neurologica Scandinavica, 34,* 195–204.

Jersild, A. T., & Holmes, F. B. (1935). *Children's fears.* New York: Teachers College, Columbia University.

Jeste, D. V., Karson, C. N., & Wyatt, R. J. (1984). Movement disorders and psychopathology. In D. V. Jeste & R. J. Wyatt (Eds.), *Neuropsychiatric movement disorders.* Washington, DC: American Psychiatric Press.

Johns, C. (1985). Encopresis. *American Journal of Nursing, 85,* 153–156.

Johnson, D. J., & Myklebust, H. R. (1967). *Learning disabilities.* New York: Grune & Stratton.

Johnson, P. A., & Rosenblatt, P. C. (1981). Grief following childhood loss of parent. *American Journal of Psychotherapy, 35,* 419–425.

Johnson, S. M., & Brown, R. A. (1969). Producing behavior change in parents of disturbed children. *Journal of Child Psychology and Psychiatry, 10,* 107–121.

Johnson, S., Phillips, S., Glaswow, R., & Christenson, A. (1980). Cost-effectiveness in behavior family therapy. *Behavior Research and Therapy, 11,* 208–226.

Kaffman, M., & Elizur, E. (1977). Infants who become enuretics: A longitudinal study of 161 kibbutz children. *Monographs for the Society of Research in Child Development, 42,* 2.

Kagan, J. (1980). Family experience and the child's development. *Annual Progress in Child Psychology and Child Development,* 21–30.

Kagan, J. (1984). The emergence of self. *Annual Progress in Child Psychology and Child Development,* 5–28.

Kagan, J., Reznick, S., & Snidman, N. (1987). The physiology and psychology of behavioral inhibition in children. *Child Development, 58,* 1459–1473.

Kalin, N. H., & Carnes, M. (1984). Biological correlates of attachment and bond disruption in humans and nonhuman primates. *Progress in Neuro-Psychopharmacology and Biological Psychiatry, 8,* 459–469.

Kandel, D. B., & Davies, M. (1982). Epidemiology of depressive mood in adolescents: An empirical study. *Archives of General Psychiatry, 39,* 1205–1212.

Kanner, L. (1943). Autistic disturbances of affective contact. *Nervous Child, 2,* 217–250.

Kanner, L., & Eisenberg, L. (1956). Early infantile autism, 1943–1955. *American Journal of Orthopsychiatry, 26,* 556–566.

Kanner, L. (1973). *Childhood psychosis: Initial studies and new insights.* Washington: Winston.

Kaplan, S. J., Pelcovitz, D., Salzinger, S., & Ganeles, D. (1983). Psychopathology of parents of abused and neglected children and adolescents. *Journal of the American Academy of Child Psychiatry, 22,* 238–244.

Karush, R. K. (1979). Obsessive-compulsive syndromes. In M. M. Josephson & R. T. Potter (Eds.), *Clinician's handbook of childhood psychopathology* (pp. 87–100). New York: Jason Aronson.

Kashani, J. H., Barbero, G. J., & Bolander, F. (1981). Depression in hospitalized pediatric patients. *Journal of the American Academy of Child Psychiatry, 20,* 123–134.

Kashani, J. H., & Cantwell, D. P. (1983). Etiology and treatment of childhood depression: A biopsychological perspective. *Comprehensive Psychiatry, 24,* 476–486.

Kashani, J. H., & Carlson, G. A. (1985). Major depressive disorder in a preschooler. *Journal of the American Academy of Child Psychiatry, 24,* 490–494.

Kashani, J. H., & Carlson, G. A. (1987). Seriously depressed preschoolers. *American Journal of Psychiatry, 144,* 348–350.

Kashani, J. H., Carlson, G. A., Horwitz, E., & Reid, J. C. (1985). Dysphoric mood in young children referred to a child development unit. *Child Psychiatry and Human Development, 15,* 234–242.

Kashani, J. H., Holcomb, W. R., & Orvaschel, H. (1986). Depression and depressive symptoms in preschool children from the general population. *American Journal of Population, 143,* 1138–1143.

Kashani, J. H., Horwitz, E., Ray, J. S., & Reid, J. C. (1986). DSM-III diagnostic classification of 100 preschoolers in a child development unit. *Child Psychiatry and Human Development, 16,* 137–147.

Kashani, J. H., McGee, R. O., Clarkson, S. E., Anderson, J. C., Walton, L. A., Williams, S., Silva, A., Robins, A. J., Cytryn, L., McKnew, D. H. (1983). Depression in a sample of 9-year-old children: Prevalence and associated characteristics. *Archives of General Psychiatry, 40,* 1217–1223.

Kashani, J. H., & Priesmeyer, M. (1983). Differences in depressive symptoms and depression among college students. *American Journal of Psychiatry, 140,* 1081–1082.

Kashani, J. H., & Ray, J. S. (1987). Major depression with delusional features in a preschool-age child. *Journal of the American Academy of Child and Adolescent Psychiatry, 26,* 110–112.

Kashani, J. H., Ray, J. S., & Carlson, G. A. (1984). Depression and depressive-like states in preschool-age children in a child development unit. *American Journal of Psychiatry, 141,* 1397–1402.

Kashani, J. H., & Simonds, J. F. (1979). The incidence of depression in children. *American Journal of Psychiatry, 136,* 1203–1205.

Kataria, S., Swanson, M. S., & Trevathan, G. E. (1987). Persistence of sleep disturbances in preschool children. *Journal of Pediatrics, 110,* 642–646.

Katz, P. A. (1979). Development of female identity. In C. B. Kopp (Ed.), *Becoming female* (pp. 3–28). New York: Plenum.

Kaufman, D. M. (1985). *Clinical neurology for psychiatrists* (2nd ed.) Orlando: Grune & Stratton.

Kazdin, A. E., Moser, J., Colbus, D., & Bell, R. (1985). Depressive symptoms among physically abused and psychiatrically disturbed children. *Journal of Abnormal Psychology, 94,* 298–307.

Keller, M. B., & Lavori, P. W. (1984). Double depression, major depression, and dysthymia: Distinct entities or different phases of a single disorder? *Psychopharmacology Bulletin, 20,* 399–402.

Kellman, S. G., Branch, J. D., Agrawal, K. C., & Ensminger, M. E. (1975). *Mental health and going to school.* Chicago: University of Chicago Press.

Kelly, A. E., & Stinus, L. (1984). Neuroanatomical and neurochemical substrates of affective behavior. In N. A. Fox & R. J. Davidson (Eds.), *The psychobiology of affective development* (pp. 1–75). Hillsdale, NJ: Erlbaum.

Kelso, J., & Stewart, M. A. (1986). Factors which predict the persistence of aggressive conduct disorder. *Journal of Child Psychology and Psychiatry, 27,* 77–86.

Kempe, C. H., Silverman, F. N., & Steele, B. F. (1962). The battered child syndrome. *Journal of the American Medical Association, 181,* 17–240.

Kempe, R. S., & Kempe, C. H. (1978). *Child abuse.* Cambridge, MA: Harvard University Press.

Kendler, K. S., Tsuang, M. T., & Hays, P. (1987). Age at onset in schizophrenia. *Archives of General Psychiatry, 44,* 881–890.

Kenny, T. J., Bergey, S. F. A., & Young-Hyman, D. (1983). Psychosomatic problems of children. In C. E. Walker & M. C. Roberts (Eds.), *Handbook of clinical psychology* (pp. 437–452). New York: Wiley.

Kerkhofs, M., Hoffman, G., DeMartelaere, V., Linkowski, A., & Mendlewica, J. (1985). Sleep EEG recordings in depressive disorders. *Journal of Affective Disorders, 9,* 47–53.

Kernberg, O. (1975). *Borderline conditions and pathological narcissism.* New York: Jason Aronson.

Kestenbaum, C. J. (1982, May). *Children and adolescents at risk for manic-depressive illness: Introduction and overview.* Paper presented at 134th annual meeting of the American Psychiatric Association, New Orleans.

Kirman, B. H. (1985). Mental retardation: Medical aspects. In M. Rutter & L.

Hersov (Eds.), *Child and adolescent psychiatry: Modern approaches* (2nd ed., pp. 650–660). Oxford: Blackwell Scientific.

Klackenberg, G. (1982). Sleep behavior studied longitudinally. *Acta Paediatrica Scandinavica, 71,* 501–506.

Klee, S. F., & Garfinkel, B. D. (1984). Identification of depression in children and adolescents: The role of the dexamethasone suppression test. *Journal of the American Academy of Child Psychiatry, 23,* 410–415.

Klein, A. (1972). *Effective group work.* New York: Association Press.

Kline, N. S., Li, C. H., Lehmann, H. E., Lajtha, A., Laski, E., & Cooper, T. (1977). Beta-endorphin-induced changes in schizophrenic and depressed patients. *Archives of General Psychiatry, 34,* 1111.

Knapp, P. H. (1980). Free association as a biopsychological probe. *Psychosomatic Medicine, 42* (1 Suppl.), 197–219.

Knight, R. B., Atkins, A., Eagle, C. J., Evans, N., Finkelstein, J. W., Fukushima, D., Katz, J., & Weiner, H. (1979). Psychological stress, ego defenses, and cortisol production in children hospitalized for elective surgery. *Psychosomatic Medicine, 41,* 40–49.

Knight, R. P. (1953). Borderline states. *Bulletin of Menninger Clinic, 17,* 1–12.

Kohlberg, L. (1966). A cognitive-developmental analysis of children's sex-role concepts and attitudes. In E. E. Maccoby (Ed.), *The development of sex differences* (pp. 82–173). Stanford, CA: Stanford University Press.

Kohlberg, L., LaCrosse, J., & Ricks, D. (1972). The predictability of adult mental health from childhood behavior. In B. B. Wolman (Ed.), *Manual of child psychopathology* (pp. 1217–1284). New York: McGraw-Hill.

Kohn, M., & Rosman, B. L. (1972). Relationship of preschool social-emotional functioning to later intellectual achievement. *Developmental Psychology, 6,* 445–452.

Kohn, M. (1977). *Social competence, symptoms and underachievement in childhood: A longitudinal perspective.* Washington, DC: Winston.

Kohrman, R., Fineberg, H., Gerlman, R. L., & Weiss, S. (1971). Technique of child analysis: Problems of countertransference. *International Journal of Psycho-Analysis, 52,* 487–497.

Kolvin, I., Ounsted, C., Richardson, L. M., & Garside, R. F. (1971). Studies in childhood-III. The family and social background in childhood psychoses. *British Journal of Psychiatrics, 118,* 396–402.

Kopp, C. B. (1982). Antecedents of self-regulation: A developmental perspective. *Developmental Psychology, 18,* 199–214.

Kornhaber, R. C., & Schroeder, H. E. (1975). Importance of model similarity on extinction of avoidance behavior in children. *Journal of Consulting and Clinical Psychology, 43,* 601–607.

Kosky, R. (1983). Childhood suicidal behavior. *Journal of Child Psychology and Psychiatry, 24,* 457–468.

Kosterlitz, H. W., & Hughes, J. (1975). Some thoughts on the significance of enkephalin, the endogenous ligand. *Life Sciences, 17,* 91.

Kovacs, M., Feinberg, T. L., Crouse-Novak, M. A., Paulauskas, S. L., & Finkelstein, R. (1984a). Depressive disorders in childhood. I. A longitudinal prospective study of characteristics and recovery. *Archives of General Psychiatry, 41,* 229–237.

Kovacs, M., Feinberg, T. L., Crouse-Novak, M. A., Paulauskas, S. L., Pollock, M., & Finkelstein, R. (1984b). Depressive disorders in childhood. II. A longitudinal study of the risk for a subsequent major depression. *Archives of General Psychiatry, 41,* 643–649.

Kovacs, M., & Paulaukas, S. L. (1984c). Developmental stage and the expression of depressive disorders in children: An empirical analysis. *New Directions for Child Development, 26,* 59–80.

Kraft, I. A. (1985). Group therapy with children and adolescents. In H. I. Kaplan & B. J. Sadock (Eds.), *Comprehensive textbook of psychiatry/IV* (Vol. 2, 4th ed., pp. 1785–1793). Baltimore/London: Williams and Wilkins.

Kraner, R. E. (1976). *Kraner Preschool Math Inventory.* Austin: Learning Concepts.

Kroll, P. D., Stock, D. F., & James, M. E. (1985). The behavior of adult alcoholic men abused as children. *Journal of Nervous and Mental Disease, 173,* 689–693.

Kurdek, L. A., & Berg, B. (1983). Correlates of children's adjustment to their parents' divorces. In L. A. Kurdek (Ed.), *Children and divorce* (pp. 47–60). San Francisco: Jossey-Bass.

Kurland, A. A., McCabe, O. L., Hanlon, T. E., & Sullivan, D. (1977). The treatment of perceptual disturbances in schizophrenia with naloxone hydrochloride. *American Journal of Psychiatry, 134,* 1408.

Lahey, B. B., Piacentini, J. C., McBurnett, K., Stone, P., Hartdagen, S., & Hynd, G. (1988). Psychopathology in the parents of children with conduct disorder and hyperactivity. *Journal of the American Academy of Child and Adolescent Psychiatry, 27,* 163–170.

Lahey, B. B., Schaughency, E. A., Hynd, G. W., Carlson, C. L., & Nieves, N. (1987). Attention deficit disorder with and without hyperactivity: Comparison of behavioral characteristics of clinic-referred children. *Journal of the American Academy of Child and Adolescent Psychiatry, 26,* 718–723.

Lamb, M. (1981). The role of the father: An overview. In M. E. Lamb (Ed.), *The role of the father in child development* (2nd ed., pp. 1–70). New York: Wiley.

Lane, R. D., & Schwartz, G. E. (1987). Levels of emotional awareness: A cognitive-developmental theory and its application to psychopathology. *American Journal of Psychiatry, 144,* 133–143.

Langdell, T. (1978). Recognition of faces: an approach to the study of autism. *Journal of Child Psychology and Psychiatry, 19,* 255–268.

Langdell, T. (1980, September). *Pragmatic aspects of autism: Or, why is 'I' a normal word?* Paper presented at the annual conference of the Developmental Section of the British Psychological Society.

Last, C. G., Francis, G., Hersen, M., Kazdin, A. E., & Strauss, C. C. (1987). Separation anxiety and school phobia: A comparison using DSM-III criteria. *American Journal of Psychiatry, 144,* 653–657.

Laufer, B. (1930). *Geophagy.* Chicago: Field Museum.

Lavigne, J. V., & Reisinger, J. J. (1984). Behavioral interventions with noncompliant preschoolers. In W. J. Burns & J. V. Lavigne (Eds.), *Progress in pediatric psychology*, (pp. 241–276). New York: Grune & Stratton.

Lawson, J. S., & Inglis, J. (1985). Learning disabilities and intelligence test results: A model based on a principal components analysis of the WISC-R. *British Journal of Psychology*, 76, 35–48.

Leal, M. R. M. (1966). Group-analytic play therapy with preadolescent girls. *International Journal of Group Psychotherapy*, 16, 58–64.

Leckman, J. F., Detlor, J., & Cohen, D. J. (1983). Gilles de la Tourette syndrome: Emerging areas of clinical research. In S. B. Guze, F. J. Earls, & J. E. Barrett, (Eds.), *Childhood psychopathology and development* (pp. 211–229). New York: Raven.

Lee-Dukes, G. (1986). Infantile autism. *American Family Physician*, 33, 149–155.

Leese, S. M. (1969). Suicide behavior in twenty adolescents. *British Journal of Psychiatry*, 115, 479–480.

Leland, H. (1983). Play therapy for mentally retarded and developmentally disabled children. In C. Schaefer & K. O'Connor (Eds.), *Handbook of play therapy* (pp. 436–454). New York: Wiley.

Lempers, J. D., Flavell, E. R., & Flavell, J. H. (1977). The development in very young children of tacit knowledge concerning visual perception. *Genetic Psychology Monographs*, 95, 3–53.

Leonard, M. F., Rhymes, J. P., & Solnit, A. J. (1966). Failure to thrive in infants. *American Journal of Diseases in Children*, 111, 600–612.

Leone, S. D., & Gumar, J. (1979). Group assertiveness training of shy children. *School Counselor*, 27, 134–141.

Leopold, R. L., & Dillon, H. (1963). Psycho-anatomy of disaster. A long-term study of post-traumatic neurosis in survivors of a marine explosion. *American Journal of Psychiatry*, 119, 913–921.

Lerner, J. A., Inui, T. S., Trupin, E. W., & Douglas, E. (1985). Preschool behavior can predict future psychiatric disorders. *Journal of the American Academy of Child Psychiatry*, 24(1), 42–48.

Lester, D. (1986). Genetics, twin studies, and suicide. *Suicide and Life-Threatening Behavior*, 16, 274–285.

Lever, J. (1976). Sex differences in the games children play. *Social Problems*, 25, 55–62.

Levin, H., & Turgeon, V. (1957). The influence of the mother's presence on children's doll-play aggression. *Journal of Abnormal Social Psychology*, 55, 304–308.

Levin, J. R. (1976). What have we learned about minimizing what children learn? In J. R. Levin & V. L. Allen (Eds.), *Cognitive learning in children: Theories and strategies*. New York: Academic.

Levine, M. D. (1975). Children with encopresis: A descriptive analysis. *Pediatrics*, 56, 412.

Levine, M. D., Busch, B., & Aufseeser, C. (1982). The dimension of inattention among children with school problems. *Pediatrics, 70,* 387–395.

Levine, M. D., Carey, W. B., Crocker, A. C., & Gross, R. T. (1983). *Developmental-behavioral pediatrics.* Philadelphia: Saunders.

Levy, F., & Hobbes, G. (1982). A 30-month follow-up of hyperactive children. *Journal of the American Academy of Child Psychiatry, 21,* 243–246.

Lewis, H. (1954). *Deprived children: The Mersham experiment, a social and clinical study.* London: Oxford University Press.

Lewis, M. (1974). Interpretation in child analysis. *Journal of Child Psychiatry 13,* 32–53.

Lidov, H. G. W., & Molliver, M. E. (1982). An immunohistochemical study of serotonin neuron development in the rat: Ascending pathways and terminal fields. *Brain Research Bulletin, 8,* 389–430.

Lieberman, J. N. (1965). Playfulness and divergent thinking: An investigation of their relationship at the kindergarten level. *Journal of Genetic Psychology, 107,* 219–224.

Lindquist, G. T. (1982). Preschool screening as a means of predicting later reading achievement. *Journal of Learning Disabilities, 15,* 331–332.

Lingjaerde, O. (1983). The biochemistry of depression. *Acta Psychiatria Scandinavica Supplementum, 302,* 36–51.

Linkowski, P., Van Wettere, J. P., Kerkhofs, M., Gregoire, F., Brauman, H., & Mendlewicz, J. (1984). Violent suicide behavior and the thyrotropin-releasing hormone-thyroid-stimulating hormone test: A clinical outcome study. *Neuropsychobiology, 12,* 19–22.

Linnoila, M., Virkkunen, M., Scheinin, M., Nuutila, A., Rimon, R., & Goodwin, F. K. (1983). Low cerebrospinal fluid 5-hydroxyindoleacetic acid concentration differentiates impulsive from nonimpulsive violent behavior. *Life Sciences, 33,* 2609–2614.

Litin, E. M., Giffen, M. E., & Johnson, A. M. (1956). Parental influence in unusual sexual behavior in children. *Psychoanalytic Quarterly, 25,* 37–55.

Livingston, R., Taylor, J. L., & Crawford, S. L. (1988). A study of somatic complaints and psychiatric diagnosis in children. *Journal of the American Academy of Child and Adolescent Psychiatry, 27,* 185–187.

Long, M. E. (1987). What is this thing called sleep? *National Geographic, 172,* 787–821.

Loomis, A., Harvey, E., & Hobart, G. (1937). Cerebral states during sleep as studied by human brain potentials. *Journal of Experimental Psychology, 21,* 127–144.

Loosen, P. T., & Prange, A. J., Jr. (1982). Serum thyrotropin response to thyrotropin-releasing hormone in psychiatric patients: A review. *American Journal of Psychiatry, 139,* 405–416.

Lopez-Ibor, J. J., Jr., Saiz-Ruiz, J., & de los Cobos, J. C. P. (1985). Biological correlations of suicide and aggressivity in major depressions (with melancholia): 5-hydroxyindoleacetic acid and cortisol in cerebral spinal fluid, dexamethasone suppression test and therapeutic response to 5-hydroxytyptophan. *Neuropsychobiology, 14,* 67–74.

Lotstein, O. D. (1984). Early brain injury and lateral development. *DAI, 46,* 1357.

Lovaas, I. I., Koegel, R., Simmons, J. Q., & Long, J. S. (1973). Some generalizations and follow-up measures on autistic children in behavior therapy. *Journal of Applied Behavior Analysis, 6,* 131–166.

Lowe, M. (1975). Trends in the development of representational play in infants from one to three years: An observational study. *Journal of Child Psychology and Psychiatry, 16,* 33–47.

Lowe, T. L., Cohen, D. J., Detlor, J., Kremenitzer, M. W., & Shaywitz, B. A. (1982). Stimulant medications precipitate Tourette's syndrome. *Journal of the American Medical Association, 247,* 1729–1731.

Lowenstein, R. M. (1951). The problem of interpretation. *Psychoanalytic Quarterly, 20,* 1–14.

Maas, J. W., Derkirmanjian, H., & Fawcett, J. A. (1971). Catecholamine metabolism and stress. *Nature, 230,* 330–333.

Mabry, P. D., & Campbell, B. A. (1974). Ontogeny of serotonergic inhibition of behavioral arousal in the rat. *Journal of Comparative Physiological Psychology, 86,* 193–201.

Maccoby, E. E., & Jacklin, C. N. (1974). *The psychology of sex differences.* Stanford, CA: Stanford University Press.

Mahler, M. S., Pine, F., & Bergman, A. (1975). *The psychological birth of the human infant.* New York: Basic Books.

Main, M., & Goldwyn, R. (1984). Predicting rejection of her infant from mother's representation of her own experience: Implications for the abused-abusing intergenerational cycle. *Child Abuse and Neglect, 8,* 203–217.

Maizels, M., & Firlit, C. F. (1986). Guide to the history in enuretic children. *American Family Physician, 33,* 205–209.

Makita, K. (1966). The age of onset of childhood schizophrenia. *Folia Psychiatrica et Neurologica Japonica, 20,* 111–121.

Maletzky, B. M. (1973). The episodic dyscontrol syndrome. *Diseases of the Nervous System,* 178–185.

Markowitz, J. (1959). The nature of the child's initial resistances to psychotherapy. *Social Work, 4,* 40–52.

Marks, F., & Keller, N. (1977). A short-term goal-oriented latency boys' group at a child guidance center. *Group Process, 7,* 66–75.

Marks, I. M. (1986). *Behavioral psychotherapy: Maudsley pocket book of clinical Management.* Bristol, England: Wright.

Marriage, K., Fine, S., Moretti, M., & Haley, G. (1986). Relationship between depression and conduct disorder in children and adolescents. *Journal of the American Academy of Child Psychiatry, 25,* 687–691.

Marshall, H. R. (1961). Relations between home experiences and children's use of language in play interactions with peers. *Psychological Monographs: General and Applied, 75,* 1–75.

Martin, H. P., & Beezley, P. (1977). Behavioral observations of abused children. *Developmental Medicine and Child Neurology, 19,* 373–387.

Marx, J. L. (1983). The two sides of the brain. *Science, 220,* 488–490.

Mash, E. J., & Terdal, L. (1973). Modifications of mother-child interactions: Playing with children. *Mental Retardation, 11,* 44–49.

Mason, E. A. (1965). The hospitalized child—His emotional needs. *New England Journal of Medicine, 272,* 406–414.

Masters, J. C. (1972). Effects of success, failure, and reward outcome upon contingent self-reinforcement. *Developmental Psychology, 7,* 110–118.

Mathis, J., Fairchild, L., & Cannon, T. (1980). Psychodrama and sociodrama in primary and secondary education. *Psychology in the Schools, 17,* 96–101.

Matthews, L. H., Leibowitz, J. M., & Matthews, J. R. (1983). Tics, habits, and mannerisms. In C. E. Walker & M. C. Roberts (Eds.), *Handbook of clinical child psychology* (pp. 406–436). New York: Wiley.

Mattsson, A., Seese, L. R., & Hawkins, J. W. (1969). Suicidal behavior as child psychiatric emergency: Clinical characteristics and follow-up results. *Archives of General Psychiatry, 20,* 100–109.

McCarthy, D. (1972). *Manual for the McCarthy Scales of Children's Abilities.* New York: Psychological Test Corporation.

McCune-Nicolich, L. (1981). Toward symbolic functioning: Structure of early pretend games and potential parallels with language. *Child Development, 52,* 785–797.

McDaniel, K. D. (1983). Pharmocological treatment of psychiatry and neurodevelopmental disorders in children and adolescents (Part 3). *Clinical Pediatrics, 25,* 198–204.

McDermott, J. F., Harrison, S. I., Schrager, J., Killins, E. W., & Dickerson, B. (1970). Social class and child psychiatric practice: The clinician's evaluation of the outcome of therapy. *American Journal of Psychiatry, 126,* 75–80.

McDevitt, J. B. (1985). The emergence of hostile aggression and its defensive and adaptive modifications during the separation-individuation process. In H. P. Blum (Ed.), *Defense and resistance: Historical perspectives and current concepts* (pp. 273–298). New York: International Universities Press.

McDonald, D. I., & Blume, S. B. (1986). Children of alcoholics. *American Journal of Diseases of Children, 140,* 750–754.

McDowell, M. S. (1937). Frequency of choice of play materials by preschool children. *Child Development, 8,* 305–310.

McGuire, D. (1983). The problem of children's suicide: Ages 5–14. *International Journal of Offender Therapy and Comparative Criminology,* 10–17.

McGuire, E. J., & Savastano, J. A. (1984). Urodynamic studies in enuresis and the nonneurogenic bladder. *Journal of Urology, 132,* 299–302.

McIntire, M. S., Angle, C. R., & Schlicht, M. L. (1977). Suicide and self-poisoning in pediatrics. *Advances in Pediatrics, 24,* 291–309.

McLaughlin, I. J. (1987). The picas. *British Journal of Hospital Medicine, 37,* 286–290.

McLoyd, V. C. (1980). Verbally expressed modes of transformation in the fantasy play of black preschool children. *Child Development, 51,* 1133–1139.

Mead, G. H. (1934). *Mind, self, and society.* Chicago: University of Chicago Press.

Melnick, B., & Hurley, J. R. (1969). Distinctive personality attributes of child-abusing mothers. *Journal of Consulting and Clinical Psychology, 33,* 746–749.

Meltzer, H. Y., Peline, R., Tricou, B., Lowry, M., & Robertson, A. (1984a). Effect of 5–hydroxytryptophan on serum cortisol levels in major affective disorders: II. Relation to suicide, psychosis, and depressive symptoms. *Archives of General Psychiatry, 41,* 379–387.

Meltzer, H. Y., Peline, R., Tricou, B., Lowry, M., & Robertson, A. (1984b). Effect of 5–hydroxytryptophan on serum cortisol levels in major affective disorders: III. Effect of antidepressants and lithium carbonate. *Archives of General Psychiatry, 41,* 391–397.

Mendell, A. E. (1983). Play therapy with children of divorced parents. In C. Schaefer & K. O'Conner (Eds.), *Handbook of play therapy* (pp. 320–354). New York: Wiley.

Merrill, E. J. (1962). *Physical abuse of children—An agency study in protecting the battered child.* Denver, CO: Denver Children's Division, American Humane Association.

Meschia, G. (1978). Evolution of thinking in fetal respiratory physiology. *American Journal of Obstetrics and Gynecology,* 132–806.

Meyer-Bahlburg, H. F. L. (1977). Sex hormones and male homosexuality in comparative perspective. *Archives of Sexual Behavior, 6,* 297–325.

Mikkelsen, E. J. (1982). Efficacy of neuroleptic medication in pervasive developmental disorders of childhood. *Schizophrenia Bulletin, 8,* 321–332.

Mikkelsen, E. J., Brown, G. L., Minichiello, M. D., Millican, F. K., & Rapoport, J. L. (1982). Neurologic status in hyperactive, enuretic, encopretic, and normal boys. *Journal of the American Academy of Child Psychiatry, 21,* 75–81.

Mikkelsen, E. J., & Rapoport, J. L. (1980). Enuresis: Psychopathology, sleep stage, and drug response. *Urologic Clinics of North America, 7,* 361.

Miller, F. W., Dawson, R. O., Dix, E. D., & Parnas, R. I. (1976). *The juvenile justice process.* New York: Foundation Press.

Miller, J. B. M. (1971). Children's reactions to the death of a parent: A review of the psychoanalytic literature. *Journal of the American Psychoanalytic Association, 19,* 697–719.

Milos, M. E., & Reiss, S. (1982). Effects of three play conditions on separation anxiety in young children. *Journal of Consulting and Clinical Psychology, 50,* 389–395.

Minuchin, S., Rosman, B. L., & Baker, L. (1978). *Psychosomatic families: Anorexia nervosa in context.* Cambridge, MA: Harvard University.

Minuchin, S., Baker, L., Rosman, B. L., Liebman, R., Milman, L., & Todd, T. C. (1975). A conceptual model of psychosomatic illness in children. *Archives of General Psychiatry, 32,* 1031–1038.

Mishne, J. M. (1983). *Clinical work with children.* New York: Free Press.

Moffatt, M. E. K., Kato, C., & Pless, I. B. (1987). Improvements in self-concept after treatment of nocturnal enuresis: Randomized controlled trial. *Journal of Pediatrics, 110,* 647–652.

Molina, J. A. (1983). Understanding the psychosocial model. *International Journal of Psychiatry in Medicine, 13,* 29–36.

Monane, M., Liechter, D., & Lewis, D. O. (1984). Physical abuse in psychiatrically hospitalized children and adolescents. *Journal of the American Academy of Child Psychiatry, 23,* 653–658.

Money, J., Hampson, J. G., & Hampson, J. L. (1955). Hermaphroditism: Recommendations concerning assignment of sex, change of sex and psychological management. *Bulletin of Hopkins Hospital, 97,* 284.

Montenegro, H. (1968). Severe separation anxiety in two preschool children: Successfully treated by reciprocal inhibition. *Journal of Child Psychology and Psychiatry, 9,* 93–103.

Moore N. V., Evertson, C. M., & Brophy, J. E. (1974). Solitary play: Some functional considerations. *Developmental Psychology, 10,* 830–834.

Moore, T. (1964). Realism and fantasy in children's play. *Journal of Child Psychology and Psychiatry, 5,* 15–36.

Morison, R., & Gardner, H. (1978). Dragons and dinosaurs: The child's capacity to differentiate fantasy and reality. *Child Development, 49,* 642–648.

Morley, M. E. (1965). *The development and disorders of speech in childhood.* Edinburgh & London: Livingstone.

Morris, M. G., & Gould, R. W. (1963). Neglected children. Role reversal: A necessary concept in dealing with the "battered child syndrome." *American Journal of Orthopsychiatry, 33,* 298–299.

Morse, C. W., Sahler, O. J. Z., & Friedman, S. B. (1970). A three-year follow-up study of abused and neglected children. *American Journal of Diseases of Children, 120,* 439–446.

Munir, K., Biederman, J., & Knee, D. (1987). Psychiatric comorbidity in patients with attention deficit disorder: A controlled study. *Journal of the American Academy of Child and Adolescent Psychiatry, 26,* 844–848.

Musatti, T. (1983). Peer interaction in pretend play. In M. Stambak, M. Barriere, L. Bonica, R. Maisonnet, T. Musatti, S. Rayna, & M. Verba (Eds.), *Among babies* (pp. 93–134). Paris: Presses Universitaires de France.

Musatti, T. (1986). Early peer relations: The perspectives of Piaget and Vygotsky. In E. C. Mueller & C. R. Cooper (Eds.), *Process and outcome in peer relationships* (pp. 25–53). New York: Academic.

Nee, L. E., Cairie, E. D., Polinsky, R. J., Eldridge, R., & Ebert, M. H. (1980). Gilles de la Tourette syndrome: Clinical and family study of 50 cases. *Annual Neurology, 7,* 41–49.

Nelson, W. (1983). Psychiatric disorders. In R. E. Behran & V. C. Vaughan, III (Eds.), *Nelson textbook of pediatrics* (12th ed., pp. 76–98). Philadelphia: Saunders.

Neubauer, P. (1980). The life cycle as indicated by the nature of the transference in the psychoanalysis of children. *International Journal of Psycho-Analysis, 61,* 137–144

Newton, R. W., Stack, T., Blair, R. E., & Keel, J. C. (1981). Pets, pica, pathogens and pre-school children. *Journal of the Royal College of General Practitioners, 31,* 740–742.

Ney, P. G., & Mulvihill, D. L. (1985). *Child psychiatric treatment: A practical guide.* London: Croom Helm.

Nolan, D. J., & Pence, C. (1970). Operant conditioning principles in the treatment of a selectively mute child. *Journal of Consulting and Clinical Psychology, 35,* 265–268.

Norton, C. R., & DeLuca, R. (1979). The use of stimulus control procedures to eliminate nocturnal awakening. *Journal of Behavior Therapy and Experimental Psychiatry, 10,* 65–67.

Nunn, K. (1986a). Annotation on the episodic dyscontrol syndrome in childhood. *Journal of Child Psychology and Psychiatry, 27,* 439–446.

Nunn, K. (1986b). The episodic dyscontrol syndrome in childhood. *Journal of Child Psychology and Psychiatry, 27,* 439–446.

Nunn, K. (1986c). The periodic dyscontrol syndrome in childhood. *Journal of Child Psychology and Psychiatry and Allied Disciplines, 27,* 439–446.

O'Connell, J. C., & Farran, D. C. (1982). Effects of day-care experience on the use of intentional communicative behaviors in a sample of socioeconomically depressed infants. *Developmental Psychology, 18,* 22–29.

Ogdon, D. P. (1982). *Psychodiagnostics and personality assessment: A handbook.* Los Angeles: Western Psychological Services.

Olweus, D. (1979). Stability of aggressive reaction patterns in males: A review. *Psychological Bulletin, 86,* 852–875.

Olweus, D. (1980). Familial and temperamental determinants of aggressive behavior in adolescent boys: A causal analysis. *Developmental Psychology, 16,* 644–660.

Oppel, W. C., Harper, P. A., & Rider, R. V. (1968). Social, psychological and neurological factors associated with enuresis. *Pediatrics, 42,* 627–641.

Ornitz, E. M. (1978). Neurophysiologic studies. In M. Rutter & E. Schopler (Eds.), *Autism: A reappraisal of concepts and treatment* (pp. 117–139). New York: Plenum.

Orr, W. C. (1985). Utilization of polysomnography in the assessment of sleep disorders. *Medical Clinics of North America, 69,* 1153–1167.

Orris, J. B. (1969). Visual monitoring performance in three subgroups of male delinquents. *Journal of Abnormal Psychology, 74,* 227–229.

Orsini, D. L., Fletcher, J. M., & Satz P. (1984). Developmental context of performance deficits in disabled learners. In M. D. Levine & P. Satz (Eds.), *Middle childhood: Development and dysfunction* (pp. 63–86). Baltimore: University Park Press.

Orvaschel, H., Weissman, M. M., & Kidd, K. K. (1980). Children and depression—The children of depressed parents; the childhood of depressed patients; depression in children. *Journal of Affective Disorders, 2*(1), 1–16.

Ounsted, C. (1969). Aggression and epilepsy: Rage in children with temporal lobe epilepsy. *Journal of Psychosomatic Research, 13,* 237–242.

Overton, W. F., & Jackson, J. P. (1973). The representation of imagined objects in action sequences: A developmental study. *Child Development, 44,* 309–314.

Palfrey, J. S., Levine, M. D., Walker, D. K., & Sullivan, M. (1985). The emergence of attention deficits in early childhood: A prospective study. *Developmental and Behavioral Pediatrics, 6*(6), 339–348.

Panksepp, J. (1986). The neurochemistry of behavior. *American Review of Psychology, 37,* 77–107.

Pare, C. M. B., & Sandler, M. (1959). A clinical and biochemical study of a trial of iproniazid in the treatment of depression. *Journal of Neurology, Neurosurgery, and Psychiatry, 22,* 247–251.

Parens, H. (1979). Developmental considerations of ambivalence: Part 2 of an exploration of the relations of instinctual drives and the symbiosis-separation-individuation process. *Psychoanalytic Study of the Child, 34,* 385–420.

Parke, R. D., & Collmar, C. W. (1975). Child abuse: An interdisciplinary analysis. *Review of Child Development Research, 9,* 509–590.

Parke, R. D., & Slaby, R. G. (1983). The development of aggression. In P. H. Mussen (Ed.), *Handbook of child psychology: Vol. 3. Cognitive development* (4th ed., pp. 548–641). New York: Wiley.

Parkes, K. R. (1984). Locus of control, cognitive appraisal, and coping in stressful episodes. *Journal of Perspectives in Social Psychology, 46,* 655–658.

Parmelee, A., & Michaelis, R. (1971). Neurological examination of the newborn. In J. Hellmuth (Ed.), *Exceptional infant: Studies in abnormalities.* New York: Brunner/Mazel.

Parten, M. (1932). Social participation among preschool children. *Journal of Social Psychology, 27,* 243–270.

Parten, M., & Newhall, S. M. (1943). Social behavior of preschool children. In P. Barker (Ed.), *Child behavior and development* (pp. 15–26). New York: McGraw-Hill.

Paschalis, A. P., Kimmel, H. D., & Kimmel, E. (1972). Further study of diurnal instrumental conditioning in the treatment of enuresis nocturna. *Journal of Behavior Therapy and Experimental Psychiatry, 3,* 253–256.

Patterson, B. R., McNeal, S., & Hawkins, N. (1967). Reprogramming the social environment. *Journal of Child Psychology and Psychiatry and Allied Disciplines, 8*(3), 181–195.

Patterson, G. R., Reid, J. B,, Jones, R. R., & Conger, R. E. (1975). *A social learning approach to family intervention. Families with aggressive children.* Eugene, OR: Castalia.

Pauls, D. L., & Leckman, J. F. (1986). The inheritance of Gilles de la Tourette's syndrome and associated behaviors. *New England Journal of Medicine, 315,* 993–997.

Paulsen, M. J. (1974). The law and abused children. In R. E. Hilfer & C. E. Kemp (Eds.), *The battered child* (pp. 153–178). Chicago: University of Chicago Press.

Paulson, M. G., Schwemer, F. T., & Bendel, R. B. (1976). Clinical application of the Pd, Ma, and (OH) Experimental MMPI Scales to further understanding of abusive parents. *Journal of Clinical Psychology, 32,* 558–564.

Pearce, J. W., Akamine, H. S. T., Kapuniai, L. E., & Crowell, D. H. (1986). Insomnia: Rational diagnosis and treatment. *Postgraduate Medicine, 80*(4), 151–156.

Peck, R. (1966). The development of the concept of death in selected male children: An experimental investigation of the development of the concept of death in selected children from the point of no concept to the point where a fully developed concept is attained with an investigation of some factors which may affect the course of concept development. *Dissertation Abstracts International, 27,* 1294B.

Peller, L. (1952). Models of children's play. *Mental Hygiene, 36,* 66–83.

Peller, L. (1954). Libidinal phases, ego development, and play. *Psychoanalytic Study of the Child, 9,* 178–198.

Pennington, B. F., & Smith, S. D. (1983). Genetic influences on learning disabilities and speech and language disorders. *Child Development, 54,* 369–387.

Pescosolido, F., & Petrella, D. (1986). The development, process, and evaluation of group psychotherapy with sexually abused preschool girls. *International Journal of Group Psychotherapy, 36,* 447–469.

Petti, T. A., & Law, W. (1982). Borderline psychotic behavior in hospitalized children: Approaches to assessment and treatment. *Journal of the American Academy of Child Psychiatry, 21,* 197–202.

Petty, L. K., Asarnow, J. R., Carlson, G. A., & Lesser, L. (1985). The dexamethasone suppression test in depressed, dysthymic, and nondepressed children. *American Journal of Psychiatry, 142,* 631–633.

Pevsner, R. (1982). Group parent training versus individual family therapy: An outcome study. *Journal of Behavior Therapy and Experimental Psychiatry, 13/a,* 119–122.

Pfeffer, C. R. (1985a). Death preoccupations and suicidal behavior in children. *Issues in Comprehensive Pediatric Nursing, 8*(1–6), 261–278.

Pfeffer, C. R. (1985b). Suicidal fantasies in normal children. *Journal of Nervous and Mental diseases, 173*(2), 78–84.

Pfeffer, C. R. (1986a). Suicide prevention. Current efficacy and future promise. *Annual, New York Academy of Science, 487,* 341–350.

Pfeffer, C. R. (1986b). *The suicidal child.* New York: Guilford.

Pfeffer, C. R., Conte, H. R., & Plutchnik, R. (1980). Suicidal behavior in latency-age children: An outpatient population. *Journal of the American Academy of Child Psychiatry, 19,* 703–710.

Pfeffer, C. R., Conte, H. R., Plutchnik, R., & Jerrett, I. (1979). Suicidal behavior in latency-age children: An empirical study. *Journal of the American Academy of Child Psychiatry, 18,* 679–692.

Pfeffer, C. R., Plutchnik, R., & Mizruchi, M. S. (1983). Suicidal and assaultive behavior in children: Classification, measurement, and interrelations. *American Journal of Psychotherapy, 140,* 154–157.

Pfeffer, C. R., Solomon, G., Plutchnik, R., Mizruchi, M. S., & Weiner, A. (1982). Suicidal behavior in latency-age psychiatric inpatients: A replication and cross validation. *Journal of the American Academy of Child Psychiatry, 6,* 564–569.

Pfeffer, C. R., Zuckerman, S., Plutchnik, R., & Mizruchi, M. S. (1984). Suicidal behavior in normal school children: A comparison with child psychiatric inpatients. *Journal of the American Academy of Child Psychiatry, 23,* 416–423.

Pfeifer, G., & Spinner, D. (1985). Combined individual and group psychotherapy with children: An ego developmental perspective. *International Journal of Group Psychotherapy, 35*(1), 11–35.

Pfohl, B., Sherman, B., Schlechte, J., & Stone, R. (1985). Pituitary-adrenal axis rhythm disturbances in psychiatric depression. *Archives of General Psychiatry, 42*, 897–903.

Phillips, D., McCartney, K., & Scarr, S. (1987). Child-care quality and children's social development. *Developmental Psychology, 23*, 537–543.

Piaget, J. (1929). *The child's conception of the world.* New York: Harcourt Brace.

Piaget, J. (1948). *The moral judgment of the child.* Glencoe, IL.: Free Press.

Piaget, J. (1951). *Play, dreams and imitation in childhood.* London: Heinemann.

Piaget, J. (1962). *Play, dreams and imitation in childhood.* New York: Norton.

Piaget, J. (1965). *The moral judgment of the child.* New York: Free Press.

Piaget, J. (1967). *Play, dreams and imitation in childhood.* London: Routledge & Kegan Paul.

Piaget, J., & Inhelder, B. (1971). *Mental imagery in the child.* New York: Basic Books.

Pilowsky, I., Bassett., D. L., Begg, M. W., & Thomas, P. G. (1982). Childhood hospitalization and chronic intractable pain in adults: A controlled retrospective study. *International Journal of Psychiatry in Medicine, 12*, 75–84.

Pine, F. (1986). On the development of the "borderline-child-to-be." *American Journal of Orthopsychiatry, 56*, 450–457.

Pine, F. (1974). *Developmental theory and clinical process.* New Haven: Yale University Press.

Pine, F. (1982a). *Developmental theory and clinical process.* New Haven: Yale University Press.

Pine, F. (1982b). On the concept "borderline" in children: A clinical essay. In S. I. Harrison & J. F. McDermott (Eds.), *New directions in childhood psychopathology: Vol. 2. Deviations in development* (pp. 857–881). New York: International Universities Press.

Plenk, A. M., & Hinchey, F. S. (1985). Clinical assessment of maladjusted preschool children. *Child Welfare, 64*(2), 127–134.

Pliszka, S. R. (1987). Tricyclic antidepressants in the treatment of children with attention deficit disorder. *Journal of the American Academy of Child and Adolescent Psychiatry, 26*(2), 127–132.

Plomin, R. (1982). Childhood temperament. In B. Lahey & A. Kazdin (Eds.), *Advances in clinical child psychology* (Vol. 6, pp. 45–92). New York: Plenum.

Pollock, G. H. (1978). Process and affect: Mourning and grief. *International Journal of Psychoanalysis, 59*, 255–276.

Potter, W. Z. (1986). Introduction: Norepinephrine as an "umbrella" neuromodulator. *Psychosomatics, 27*(11) (Suppl.), 5–9.

Powell, G. F., Brasel, J. A., & Blizzard, R. M. (1967). Emotional deprivation and growth retardation simulating idiopathic hypopituitarism: I. Clinical evaluation of the syndrome. *New England Journal of Medicine, 276*, 1271–1278.

Poznanski, E. O., Carroll, B. J., Banegas, M. C., Cook, S. C., & Grossman, J. A.

(1982). The dexamethasone suppression test in prepubertal depressed children. *American Journal of Psychiatry, 139,* 321–324.

Pradhan, S. N., & Pradhan, S. (1980). Development of central neurotransmitter systems and ontogeny of behavior. In H. Parvez & S. Parvez (Eds.), *Biogenic amines in development* (pp. 641–662). New York: Elsevier North-Holland.

Preston, M. (1945). Late behavioral aspects found in cases of prenatal, natal and post-natal anoxia. *Journal of Pediatrics, 26,* 353.

Prior, M., & Sanson, A. (1986). Attention deficit disorder with hyperactivity: A critique. *Journal of Child Psychology and Psychiatry, 27,* 307–319.

Prior, M., & Werry, J. S. (1986). Autism, schizophrenia, and allied disorders. In H. C. Quay & J. S. Werry (Eds.), *Psychopathological disorders of childhood* (pp. 156–210). New York: Wiley.

Prior, M., Leonard, A., & Wood, G. (1983). A comparison study of preschool children diagnosed as hyperactive. *Journal of Pediatric Psychology, 8,* 191–207.

Prugh, D. G., Staub, E. M., Sands, H. H., Kirschbaum, R. M., & Lenihan, E. A. (1953). A study of the emotional reactions of children and families to hospitalization and illness. *American Journal of Orthopsychiatry, 23,* 70–106.

Prugh, D. G. (1983). *The psychosocial aspects of pediatrics.* Philadelphia: Lea & Febiger.

Puig-Antich, J. (1982). Major depression and conduct disorder in prepuberty. *Journal of the American Academy of Child Psychiatry, 21,* 118–128.

Puig-Antich, J. (1986). Psychobiological markers: Effects of age and puberty. In M. Rutter, C. E. Izard, & P. B. Read (Eds.), *Depression in young people: Developmental and clinical perspectives* (pp. 341–381). New York: Guilford.

Puig-Antich, J., Goetz, D., & Davies, M. (1983a). *A controlled family history study of adolescent major depressive disorder.* Paper presented at the meeting of the American Academy of Child Psychiatry.

Puig-Antich, J., Goetz, R., Hanlon, C., Tabrizi, M. A., Davies, M., & Weitzman, E. (1983b). Sleep architecture and REM sleep measures in prepubertal major depressives: Studies during recovery from a major depressive episode in a drug free state. *Archives of General Psychiatry, 40,* 187–192.

Puig-Antich, J., & Rabinovich, H. (1986). Relationship between affective and anxiety disorders in childhood. In R. Gittelman (Ed.), *Anxiety disorders of childhood* (pp. 136–156). New York: Guilford.

Pynoos, R. S., Frederick, C., Nadar, K., Arroyo, W., Steinberg, A., Eth, S., Nunez, F., & Fairbanks, L. (1987). Life threat and posttraumatic stress in school-age children. *Archives of General Psychiatry, 44,* 1057–1063.

Quay, H. C. (1979). Classification. In H. C. Quay & J. S. Werry (Eds.), *Psychopathological disorders of childhood* (2nd ed., pp. 1–34). New York: Wiley.

Quay, H. C. (1986). Conduct disorders. In H. C. Quay & J. S. Werry (Eds.), *Psychopathological disorders of childhood* (pp. 35–72). New York: Wiley.

Quay, H. C., & LaGreca, A. M. (1986). Disorders of anxiety, withdrawal, and dysphoria. In H. C. Quay & J. S. Werry (Eds.), *Psychopathological disorders of childhood* (3rd ed., pp. 73–109) New York: Wiley.

Ramey, C., Dorval, B., & Baker-Ward, L. (1981). Group day care and socially disadvantaged families: Effects on the child and the family. In S. Kilmer (Ed.), *Advances in early education and day care* (pp. 69–106). Greenwich, CT: JAI Press.

Ramey, C., MacPhee, D., & Yeates, K. (1982). Preventing developmental retardation: A general systems model. In L. Bond & J. Joffee (Eds.), *Facilitating infant and early childhood development: Vol. 6. Primary prevention of psychopathology* (pp. 343–401). Hanover, NH: University Press of New England.

Raphael, B. (1982). The young child and the death of a parent. In C. M. Parkes & J. Stevenson-Hinde (Eds.), *The place of attachment in human behavior* (pp. 131–150). New York: Basic Books.

Rapoport, J. L. (1986). Childhood obsessive compulsive disorder. *Journal of Child Psychology and Psychiatry, 27*(3), 289–295.

Rapoport, J. L., & Ismond, D. R. (1984). *DSM-III training guide for diagnosis of childhood disorders.* New York: Brunner/Mazel.

Rapoport, J. L. & Kruesi, J. P. (1985). Organic therapies. In H. I. Kaplan, & B. J. Sadock (Eds.), *Comprehensive textbook of psychiatry/IV*, (Vol. 2, pp. 1793–1798). Baltimore: Williams & Wilkins.

Rapoport, J. L., Mikkelsen, E. J., Zavardil, A., et al. (1980). Childhood enuresis II. Psychopathology, tricyclic concentration in plasma, and antineuritic effect. *Archives of General Psychology, 37,* 1146–1152.

Rappaport, L., Landman, G., Fenton, T., & Levine, M. D. (1986). Locus of control as predictor of compliance and outcome in treatment of encopresis. *Journal of Pediatrics, 109,* 1061–1064.

Raskin, L. A., Shaywitz, S. E., Shaywitz, B. A., Anderson, G. M., & Cohen, D. J. (1984). Neurochemical correlates of attention deficit disorder. *Pediatric Clinics of North America, 31,* 387–396.

Reichlin, S. (1985). Neuroendocrinology. In J. D. Wilson & D. W. Foster (Eds.), *Textbook of endocrinology*, (7th ed., pp. 492–567). Philadelphia: Saunders.

Reed, B. C., Jr. (1984). Pediatric neuropsychology. In W. J. Burns & J. V. Lavigne (Eds.), *Progress in pediatric psychology* (pp. 103–134). New York: Harcourt Brace Jovanovich.

Reeves, J. C., Werry, J. S., Elkind, G. S., & Zametkin, A. (1987). Attention deficit, conduct, oppositional, and anxiety disorders in children: II. Clinical characteristics. *Journal of the American Academy of Child and Adolescent Psychiatry, 26*(2), 144–155.

Reichelderfer, T. E., & Rockland, L. (1963). Maternal deprivation and the effect of loving care. *Clinical Pediatrics, 2,* 449–452.

Reiser, D. E., & Brown, J. L. (1964). Patterns of later development in children with infantile psychosis. *Journal of the American Academy of Child Psychiatry, 3,* 650–667.

Reisinger, J. J., Frangia, G. W., & Hoffman, E. H. (1976). Toddler management training: Generalization and marital status. *Journal of Behavior Therapy and Experimental Psychiatry, 7,* 335–340.

Reite, M., Harbeck, R., & Hoffman, A. (1981). Altered cellular immune response following peer separation. *Life Sciences, 29,* 1133–1136.

Rekers, G. A. (1979). Sex-role behavior change: Intrasubject studies of boyhood gender disturbance. *The Journal of Psychology, 103,* 255–269.

Rekers, G. A. (1981). Childhood sexual identity disorders. *Medical Aspects of Human Sexuality, 15*(3), 141–142.

Rekers, G. A., Amaro-Plotkin, H. D., & Low, B. P. (1977). Sex-typed mannerisms in normal boys and girls as a function of sex and age. *Child Development, 48,* 275–278.

Rekers, G. A., Crandall, B. F., Rosen, A. C., & Bentler, P. M. (1979). Genetic and physical studies of male children with psychological gender disturbances. *Psychological Medicine, 9,* 373–375.

Rekers, G. A., & Mead, S. L. (1979). Early intervention for female sexual identity disturbance: Self-monitoring of play behavior. *Journal of Abnormal Child Psychology, 7,* 405–423.

Rekers, G. A., Mead, S. L., Rosen, A. C., & Brigham, S. L. (1983). Family correlates of male childhood gender disturbance. *Journal of Genetic Psychology, 142,* 31–42.

Rekers, G. A., & Yates, C. E. (1976). Sex-typed play in feminoid boys versus normal boys and girls. *Journal of Abnormal Child Psychology, 4*(1), 1–8.

Rescorla, L. A. (1986). Preschool psychiatric disorders: Diagnostic classification and symptom patterns. *Journal of the American Academy of Child Psychiatry, 25,* 162–169.

Rice, J., Reich, T., Andreasen, N. C., Endicott, J., et al. (1987). The familial transmission of bipolar illness. *Archives of General Psychiatry, 44,* 441–447.

Rice, P. L. (1987). *Stress and health: Principles and practice for coping and wellness.* Monterey, CA: Brooks/Cole.

Richman et al. (1982). *Preschool to school: A behavioural study.* London: Academic Press.

Richman, N. (1977). Behaviour problems in pre-school children: Family and Social Factors. *British Journal of Psychiatry, 131,* 523–527.

Richman, N. (1985). Disorders in pre-school children. In M. Rutter & L. Hersov (Eds.), *Child and adolescent psychiatry: Modern approaches* (pp. 336–350). Boston: Blackwell Scientific.

Richman, N., Douglas, J., Hunt, H., Lansdown, R., & Levere, R. (1985). Behavioral methods in the treatment of sleep disorders—A pilot study. *Journal of Child Psychology and Psychiatry and Allied Disciplines, 26,* 581–590.

Richman, N., & Graham, P. J. (1971). A behavioral screening questionnaire for use with three-year-old children. Preliminary Findings. *Journal of Child Psychology and Psychiatry, 12,* 5–33.

Richman, N., Stevenson, J. E., & Graham, P. J. (1975). Prevalence of behaviour problems in 3-year-old children: An epidemiological study in a London borough. *Journal of Child Psychology and Psychiatry, 16,* 277–287.

Richman, N., Stevenson, J. E., & Graham, P. J. (1982). *Preschool to school: A behavioral study.* New York: Academic Press.

Richmond, J. B., Eddy, E., & Green, M. (1958). Rumination: Psychosomatic syndrome of infancy. *Pediatrics, 22,* 49.

Rinn, R. C. (1985). Children with behavior disorders. In M. Hersen & A. S. Bellack (Eds.), *Behavior therapy in the psychiatric setting* (pp. 365–395). Baltimore: Williams & Wilkins.

Rinn, R. C., Vernon, J. C., & Wise, M. J. (1975). Training parents of behavior-disordered children in groups: A three years' program evaluation. *Behavior Therapy, 6,* 378–387.

Ritvo, E. R., Freeman, B. J., Scheibel, A. B., Duong, T., Robinson, H., Guthrie, D., & Ritvo, A. (1986). Lower purkinje cell counts in the cerebella of four autistic subjects: Initial findings of the UCLA-NSAC autopsy research report. *American Journal of Psychiatry, 143,* 862–866.

Ritvo, E. R., Mason-Brothers, A., Jenson, W. P., Freeman, B. J., Mo, A., Pingree, C., Petersen, P. B., & McMahon, W. M. (1987). A report of one family with four autistic siblings and four families with three autistic siblings. *Journal of American Academy of Child and Adolescent Psychiatry, 26,* 339–341.

Ritvo, E. R., Ritvo, E. C., & Brothers, A. M. (1982). Genetic and immunohemato-logic factors in autism. *Journal of Autism and Developmental Disorders, 12,* 109–114.

Ritvo, E. R., Spence, M. A., Freeman, B. J., Mason-Brothers, A., Mo, A., & Marazita, M. L. (1985). Evidence for autosomal recessive inheritance in 46 families with multiple incidences of autism. *American Journal of Psychiatry, 142,* 187–192.

Ritvo, S. (1978). The psychoanalytic process in childhood. *Psychoanalytic Study of the Child 33,* 295–305. New Haven: Yale University Press.

Robbins, D. R., & Alessi, N. E. (1985). Suicide and the dexamethasone suppression test in adolescence. *Biological Psychiatry, 20,* 94–119.

Roffwarg, H. (1979). Diagnostic classification of sleep and arousal disorders. *Sleep, 2,* 1–137.

Rose, S. D. (1974). Training parents in groups as behavior modifiers of their mentally retarded children. *Journal of Behavior Therapy and Experimental Psychiatry, 5,* 135–140.

Rosenberg, B. G., & Sutton-Smith, B. (1960). A revised conception of masculine-feminine differences in play activities. *Journal of Genetic Psychology, 96,* 165–170.

Rosenblatt, D. (1977). Developmental trends in infant play. In B. Tizard & D. Harvey (Eds.), *Biology of play.* London: Heineman.

Rosenfeld, S., & Sprince, M. (1963). An attempt to formulate the meaning of the concept "borderline." *Psychoanalytic Study of the Child, 18,* 603–635.

Rosenthal, M. J. (1981). Sexual differences in the suicidal behavior of young people. *Adolescent Psychiatry, 9,* 422–442.

Rosenthal, N. E., Carpenter, C. J., James, S. P., Parry, B. L., Rogers, S. L. B., & Wehr, T. A. (1986). Seasonal affective disorder in children and adolescents. *American Journal of Psychiatry, 143,* 356–358.

Rosenthal, P. A., & Rosenthal, S. (1983). Suicide among preschoolers: Fact or fallacy? *Child Today, 12,* 21–25.

Rosenthal, P. A., & Rosenthal, S. (1984). Suicidal behavior by preschool children. *American Journal of Psychiatry, 141,* 520–525.

Rosenthal, R. H., & Allen, T. W. (1978). An examination of attention, arousal, and learning dysfunctions of hyperkinetic children. *Psychological Bulletin, 85,* 689–715.

Rossiter, A. B. (1988). A model for group intervention with preschool children experiencing separation and divorce. *American Journal of Orthopsychiatry, 58,* 387–396.

Roth, M., Mountjoy, C. Q., & Caetano, D. (1982). Further investigations into the relationship between depressive disorders and anxiety state. *Pharmacopsychiatria, 15*(4), 135–141.

Roth, S., & Kubal, L. (1975). Effects of noncontingent reinforcement on tasks of differing importance: Facilitation and learned helplessness. *Journal of Personality and Social Psychology, 32,* 680–691.

Rothbart, M. K. (1986). Longitudinal observation of infant temperament. *Developmental Psychology, 22,* 356–365.

Rothbart, M. K., & Derryberry, D. (1981). Development of individual differences in temperament. In M. E. Lamb & A. L. Brown (Eds.), *Advances in developmental psychology* (Vol. 1, pp. 17–86). Hillsdale, NJ: Erlbaum.

Rothbaum, F. (1980). Children's clinical syndromes and generalized expectations of control. In H. W. Reese & L. P. Lipsett (Eds.), *Advances in child development and behavior* (Vol. 15, pp. 207–247). New York: Academic Press.

Rourke, B. P. (1982). Central processing deficiencies in children: Toward a developmental neuropsychological model. *Journal of Clinical Neuropsychology, 4*(1), 1–18.

Roy, A. (1986). Depression, attempted suicide, and suicide in patients with chronic schizophrenia. *Psychiatric Clinics of North America, 9*(1), 193–206.

Rubenstein, B. O., & Levitt, M. (1964). Countertransference. In M. R. Haworth (Ed.), *Child psychotherapy* (pp. 256–258). New York: Basic Books.

Rubenstein, J. L., & Howes, C. (1979). Caregiving and infant behavior in day care and in homes. *Developmental Psychology, 15,* 1–24.

Rubenstein, J. L., Howes, C., & Boyle, P. (1981). A two-year follow-up of infants in community-based day care. *Journal of Child Psychology and Psychiatry, 22,* 209–218.

Rubin, K. H., Fein, G. G., & Vandenberg, B. (1983). Play. In E. M. Hetherington (Ed.), P. H. Mussen (Series Ed.), *Handbook of child psychology: Socialization personality and social development* (Vol. 4). New York: Wiley.

Rubin, K. H., Maioni, T. L., & Hornung, M. (1976). Free play behavior in middle- and lower-class preschoolers: Partgen and Piaget revisited. *Child Development, 47,* 414–419.

Rubin, K. H., Watson, K. S., & Jambor, T. W. (1978). Free-play behaviors in preschool and kindergarten children. *Child Development, 49,* 534–536.

Rudel, R. G., Teuber, H. L., & Twitchell, T. E. (1974). Levels of impairment of sensori-motor functions in children with early brain damage. *Neuropsychologia, 12,* 95–108.

Rumsey, J. M., & Rapoport, J. L. (1983, August). *Autistic children as adults: Mental and behavioral status.* Paper presented at the meeting of the American Psychological Association, Anaheim, CA.

Rutan, J. S., & Alonso, R. (1982). Group therapy, individual therapy or both? *International Journal of Group Psychotherapy, 32,* 267–282.

Rutter, M. (1977). Brain damage syndromes in childhood: Concepts and findings. *Journal of Child Psychology and Psychiatry, 18,* 1–21.

Rutter, M. (1979a). *Changing youth in a changing society: Patterns of adolescent development and disorder.* Nuffield Provincial Hospitals Trust, London. Cambridge, MA: Harvard University Press.

Rutter, M. (1979b). Maternal deprivation, 1972–1978: New findings, new concepts, new approaches. *Child Development, 50,* 283–305.

Rutter, M. (1980). Parent-child separation: Psychological effects on the children. In S. Harrison & J. E. McDermott (Eds.), *New directions in childhood psychology: Vol 1. Developmental consideration* (pp. 321–353). New York: International Universities Press.

Rutter, M. (1981). Psychological sequelae of brain damage in children. *American Journal of Psychiatry, 138,* 1533–1544.

Rutter, M. (1982). Concepts of autism: A review of research. In S. I. Harrison & J. F. McDermott, Jr. (Eds.), *New directions in childhood psychopathology: Vol. 2, Deviations in development* (pp. 979–1017). New York: International Universities Press.

Rutter, M. (1983). Cognitive deficits in the pathogenesis of autism. *Journal of Child Psychology and Psychiatry, 24,* 513–531.

Rutter, M. (1985). Psychopathology and development: Links between childhood and adult life. In M. Rutter & L. Hersov (Eds.), *Child and adolescent psychiatry: Modern approaches* (2nd ed., pp. 720–739). Oxford: Blackwell Scientific.

Rutter, M., Graham, P., & Yule, W. (1970). A neuropsychiatric study in childhood. *Clinics in Developmental Medicine* (Nos. 35 and 36). London: Simp/Seineman.

Rutter, M., & Shaffer, D. (1980). A step forward or back in terms of the classification of child psychiatric disorders? *Journal of the American Academy of Child Psychiatry, 19,* 371–394.

Rutter, M., Yule, W., & Graham, P. J. (1973). Enuresis and behavioural deviance: Some epidemiological considerations. In I. Kolvin, R. MacKeith, & S. R. Meadow (Eds.), *Bladder control and enuresis. (Clinics in Developmental Medicine,* Nos. 48/49, 137–147.)

Ryan, E. B., Ledger, G. W., & Weed, K. A. (1987). Acquisition and transfer of an integrative imagery strategy by young children. *Child Development, 58,* 443–452.

Salzarulo, P., & Chevalier, A. (1983). Sleep problems in children and their relationship with early disturbances of the waking-sleeping rhythms. *Sleep, 6*(1), 47–51.

Sameroff, A., Seifer, R., Zax, M., & Barocas, R. (1987). Early indicators of developmental risk: Rochester longitudinal study. *Schizophrenia Bulletin, 13,* 383–394.

Sandler, J., Dare, C., & Holder, A. (1973). *The patient and the analyst: The basis of the psychoanalytic process.* London: Allen & Unwin.

Santostefano, S. (1985). *Cognitive control therapy with children and adolescents.* New York: Pergamon.

Sanua, V. D. (1983). Infantile autism and childhood schizophrenia: Review of the issues from the sociocultural point of view. *Social Science and Medicine, 17,* 1633–1651.

Sargent, W., & Dally, P. J. (1962). Treatment of anxiety states by antidepressant drugs. *British Medical Journal, 1,* 6–9.

Satter, E. M. (1986). Childhood eating disorders. *Journal of the American Dietetic Association, 86,* 357–361.

Sattler, J. M. (1982). *Assessment of children's intelligence and special abilities* (2nd ed.). Boston: Allyn & Bacon.

Satz, P., & Fletcher, J. M. (1981). Emergent trends in neuropsychology: An overview. *Journal of Consulting and Clinical Psychology, 49,* 851–865.

Sayetta, R. B. (1986). Pica: An overview. *AFP, 33*(5), 181–185.

Scarlett, W. G., & Wolf, D. (1979). When it's only make-believe: The construction of a boundary between fantasy and reality storytelling. *New Directions for Child Development, 6,* 29–40.

Scarr, S., & Salapatek, P. (1970). Patterns of fear development during infancy. *Merrill-Palmer Quarterly, 16,* 53–90.

Schaefer, C. E., Johnson, L., & Wherry, J. N. (1982). *Group therapies for children and youth: Principles and practices of group treatment.* San Francisco: Jossey-Bass.

Schally, A. V., Arimura, A., & Kastin, A. J. (1973). Hypothalmic regulatory hormones. *Science, 179,* 241–350.

Schatzberg, A. F., Rosenbaum, A. H., Orsulak, P. J., Rohde, W. A., Maruta, T., Kruger, E. R., Cole, J. O., & Schildkraut, J. J. (1981). Toward a biochemical classification of depressive disorders. III. Pretreatment urinary MHPG levels as predictors of response to treatment with Maprotiline. *Psychopharmacology, 75,* 34–38.

Schecter, D. E. (1978). Early developmental roots of anxiety. In M. B. Cantor & M. L. Glucksman (Eds.), *Affect: Psychoanalytic theory and practice* (pp. 115–130). New York: Wiley.

Scheidlinger, S. (1984). Short-term group psychotherapy for children: An overview. *International Journal of Psychotherapy, 34,* 572–585.

Scheidlinger, S., Eisenberg, M. S., King, C. H., & Ostrower, R. (1962). Activity group therapy of a dull boy with severe body ego problems. *International Journal of Group Psychotherapy, 12,* 41–55.

Schildkraut, J. (1965). The catecholamine hypothesis of affective disorders: A review of supporting evidence. *American Journal of Psychiatry, 122,* 508–522.

Schindler, P. J., Moely, B. E., & Frank, A. L. (1987). Time in day care and social participation of young children. *Developmental Psychology, 23,* 225–261.

Schmale, A. H. (1972). Giving up as a final common pathway to changes in health. *Advances in Psychosomatic Medicine, 8,* 20–40.

Schmideberg, M. (1959). The borderline patient. In S. Arieti (Ed.), *American handbook of psychiatry* (Vol. 1, pp. 398–416). New York: Basic Books.

Schmidt, C. R. (1976). Understanding human action: Recognizing the plans and motives of other persons. In J. S. Carroll & J. W. Payne (Eds.), *Cognition and social behavior.* Hillsdale, NJ: Erlbaum.

Schneider-Rosen, K., & Cicchetti, D. (1984). The relationship between affect and cognition in maltreated infants: Quality of attachment and the development of visual self-recognition. *Child Development, 55,* 648–658.

Schneidman, E. S. (1976). An overview of suicide. *Psychiatric Annals, 6,* 13–47.

Schneidman, E. S. (Ed.) (1976). *Suicidology: Contemporary developments.* New York: Grune & Stratton.

Schuckit, M. A. (1985). Studies of populations at high risk for alcoholism. *Psychiatric Developments, 3,* 31–63.

Schwartz, E. K. (1964). A psychoanalytic study of the fairy tale. In M. R. Haworth (Ed.), *Child psychotherapy: Practice and theory* (pp. 383–395). New York: Basic Books.

Schwarz, J. C., Krolick, G., & Strickland, R. (1973). Effects of early day care experience on adjustment to a new environment. *American Journal of Orthopsychiatry, 43,* 340–346.

Schwarz, J. E., Strickland, R. G., & Krolick, G. (1974). Infant day care: Behavioral effects at preschool age. *Developmental Psychology, 10,* 502–506.

Seligman, M. E. P. (1975). *Helplessness: On depression, development and death.* San Francisco: Freeman.

Seligman, M. E. P., & Maier, S. F. (1967). Failure to escape traumatic shock. *Journal of Experimental Psychology, 74,* 1–9.

Shaffer, D. (1982). Diagnostic issues in child and adolescent suicide. *Journal of the American Academy of Child Psychiatry, 21,* 414–416.

Shaffer, D. (1985a). Enuresis. In M. Rutter & L. Hersov (Eds.), *Child and adolescent psychiatry: Modern approaches* (pp. 465–481). Boston: Blackwell Scientific Publications.

Shaffer, D. (1985b). Brain damage. In M. Rutter & L. Hersov (Eds.), *Child and adolescent psychiatry: Modern approaches* (pp. 129–151). Oxford: Blackwell Scientific.

Shaffer, D. (1986). Developmental factors in child and adolescent suicide. In M. Rutter, C. E. Izard, & P. B. Read (Eds.), *Depression in young people,* (pp. 383–396). New York: The Guilford Press.

Shaffer, D., & Fisher, P. (1981). The epidemiology of suicide in children and young adolescents. *Journal of the American Academy of Child Psychiatry, 21,* 545–565.

Shaffer, D., Gardner, A., & Hedge, B. (1984). Behavior and bladder disturbance in enuretics: The rational classification of a common disorder. *Developmental Medicine and Child Neurology, 26,* 781–792.

Shaffer, D., Schonfeld, I., O'Connor, P. A., Stokman, C., Trautman, P., Shafer, S., & Ng, S. (1985). Neurological soft signs. *Archives of General Psychiatry, 42,* 342–351.

Shafii, M. S., Carrigan, S., Whittinghill, J. R., & Derrick, A. (1985). Psychological autopsy of completed suicide in children and adolescents. *American Journal of Psychiatry, 142,* 1061–1064.

Shambaugh, B. (1961). A study of loss reactions in a seven-year-old. *Psychoanalytic Study of the Child, 16,* 510–522.

Shapiro, B. K., Palmer, F. B., Watchel, R. C., & Capute, A. J. (1983). Issues in the early identification of specific learning disability. *Developmental and Behavioral Pediatrics, 5*(1), 15–20.

Shapiro, S. K., & Garfinkel, B. D. (1986). The occurrence of behavior disorders in children: The interdependence of attention deficit disorder and conduct disorder. *Journal of the American Academy of Child Psychiatry, 25,* 809–819.

Shapiro, T. (1979). *Clinical psycholinguistics.* New York: Plenum.

Shapiro, T., Chiarandini, I., & Fish, B. (1974). Thirty severely disturbed children. *Archives of General Psychiatry, 30,* 819–825.

Shapiro, T., & Fish, B. (1969). A method to study language deviation as an aspect of ego organization in young schizophrenic children. *Journal of the Academy of Child Psychiatry, 8,* 36–56.

Shaw, D. S., & Emery, R. E. (1987). Parental conflict and other correlates of the adjustment of school-age children whose parents have separated. *Journal of Abnormal Child Psychology, 15,* 269–281.

Sheldon, R. E., Peeters, L. I. H., Jones, M. D., Makowski, E. L., & Meschia, J. (1979). Redistribution of the cardiac output and oxygen delivery in the hypoxemic fetal lamb. *American Journal of Obstetrics and Gynecology, 135,* 1075–1978.

Sherman, M., Shapiro, T., & Glassman, M. (1983). Play and language in developmentally disordered preschoolers: A new approach to classification. *Journal of the American Academy of Child Psychiatry, 22,* 511–524.

Shore, C., O'Connell, B., & Bates, E. (1984). First sentences in language and symbolic play. *Developmental Psychology, 20,* 872–880.

Shultz, T. R., & Cloghesy, K. (1981). Development of recursive awareness of intention. *Developmental Psychology, 17,* 465–471.

Shultz, T. R., Wells, D., & Sarda, M. (1980). Development of the ability to distinguish intended actions from mistakes, reflexes, and passive movements. *British Journal of Social and Clinical Psychology, 19,* 301–319.

Siever, L. J., & Davis, K. L. (1985). Overview: Toward a dysregulation hypothesis of depression. *American Journal of Psychiatry, 142,* 1017–1031.

Sigman, M., Mundy, P., Sherman, T., & Ungerer, J. (1986). Social interactions of autistic, mentally retarded and normal children and their caregivers. *Journal of Child Psychology and Psychiatry, 27,* 647–656.

Sigman, M., & Ungerer, J. A. (1984). Cognitive and language skills in autistic, mentally retarded and normal children. *Developmental Psychology, 20,* 293–308.

Silver, L. B. (1982). The playroom diagnostic evaluation of children with neurologically based learning disabilities. In S. I. Harrison & J. F. McDermott, Jr. (Eds.), *New directions in childhood psychopathology: Vol. 2. Deviations in development* (pp. 709–727). New York: International Universities Press.

Silverman, J. J. (1986). Post-traumatic stress disorder. *Advances in Psychosomatic Medicine, 16,* 115–140.

Simeon, J. G. (1987). Sleep in children: Recent advances. In J. D. Noshpitz (Ed.), *Basic handbook of child psychiatry* (Vol. 5, pp. 327–337). New York: Basic Books.

Simmons, J. Q., & Baltaxe, C. (1975). Language patterns of adolescent autistics. *Journal of Autism and Child Schizophrenia, 5,* 333–352.

Simonds, J. F., & Parraga, H. (1982). Prevalence of sleep disorders and sleep behaviors in children and adolescents. *Journal of the American Academy of Child Psychiatry, 21*(4), 383–388.

Simpson, K. (1967). The battered baby problem. *Royal Society of Health Journal, 87,* 168–170.

Simpson, K. (1968). The battered baby problem. *South African Medical Journal, 42,* 661–663.

Singer, D. G., & Rummo, J. (1973). Ideational creativity and behavioral style in kindergarten aged children. *Developmental Psychology, 8,* 154–161.

Singer, J. L. (1973). *The child's world of make believe.* New York: Academic.

Singer, J. L. (1979). Affect and imagination in play and fantasy. In C. Izard (Ed.), *Emotions in personality and psychopathology* (pp. 13–34). New York: Plenum.

Singer, J. L., & Singer, D. G. (1978, August). *Some correlates of imaginative play in preschoolers.* Paper presented at the meeting of the American Psychological Association, Toronto.

Singer, J. L., Singer, D. G., & Sherrod, L. R. (1980). A factor analytic study of preschoolers' play behavior. *American Psychology Bulletin, 2,* 143–156.

Singhi, S., & Singhi, P. (1982a). Pica: Not a solitary problem! *Indian Pediatrics, 19*(7), 615–618.

Singhi, P., & Singhi, S. (1982b). Pica type of "nonfood" articles eaten by Amjer children and their significance. *Indian Journal of Pediatrics, 49,* 681–684.

Singhi, P., & Singhi, S. (1983). Nutritional status and psycho-social stress in children with pica. *Indian Pediatrics, 20*(5), 345–349.

Singhi, S., Singhi, P., & Adwani, G. B. (1981). Role of psychological stress in the cause of pica. *Clinical Pediatrics, 20*(12), 783–785.

Sjobring, H. (1973). Personality structure and development: A model and its application. *Acta Psychiatrica Scandinavica,* Suppl. *244,* 1.

Skrzypek, G. J. (1969). Effect of perceptual isolation and arousal on anxiety, complexity preference, and novelty preference in psychopathic and neurotic delinquents. *Journal of Abnormal Psychology, 74,* 321–329.

Sleator, E. K., & Ullman, R. K. (1981). Can the physician diagnose hyperactivity in the office? *Pediatrics, 67*(1), 13–17.

Slosson, R. L. (1963). *Slosson Intelligence Test (SIT) for Children and Adults.* New York: Slosson Educational Publications.

Smilansky, S. (1968). *The effects of sociodramatic play on disadvantaged children: Preschool children.* New York: Wiley.

Smirnoff, V. (1971). *The scope of child analysis.* New York: International Universities Press.

Smith, P. K., & Connolly, K. (1972). Patterns of play and social interaction in preschool children. In N. Blurton-Jones (Ed.), *Ethological studies of child behavior* (pp. 30–46). London: Cambridge University Press.

Smith, S. M., Hanson, R., & Noble, S. (1973). Parents of battered babies: A controlled study. *British Medical Journal, 4,* 388–391.

Socarides, C. W. (1980). Homosexuality and the rapprochement subphase crisis. In R. F. Lax, S. Bach, & J. A. Burland (Eds.), *Rapprochement: The critical subphase of separation-individuation* (pp. 331–352). New York: Jason Aronson.

Sokol, M. S., Campbell, M., Goldstein, M., & Kreichman, A. M. (1987). Attention deficit disorder with hyperactivity and the dopamine hypothesis: Case presentations with theoretical background. *Journal of the American Academy of Child Psychiatry,* 428–433.

Soo, E. S. (1985). Applications of object relations concepts to children's group psychotherapy. *International Journal of Group Psychotherapy, 35*(1), 37–47.

Sorosky, A. D., Ornitz, E. M., Brown, M. B., & Ritvo, E. R. (1968). Systematic observations of autistic behavior. *Archives of General Psychiatry, 18,* 439–449.

Sours, J. A. (1978). The application of child analytic principles to forms of child psychotherapy. In J. Glenn (Ed.), *Child analysis and therapy* (pp. 615–648). New York: Jason Aronson.

Sours, J. A. (1980). Lines of maturation and development through the Phallic-Oedipal years of childhood. In J. R. Bemporad (Ed.), *Child development in normality and psychopathology* (pp. 121–155). New York: Brunner/Mazel.

Sparrow, S. S., Rescorla, L. A., Provence, S., Condon, S. O., Goudreau, D., & Cicchetti, D. V. (1986). Follow-up of "atypical children"—A brief report. *Journal of the American Academy of Child Psychiatry, 25,* 181–185.

Speers, R. W., & Lansing, C. (1982). Parallel groups for autistic children and their parents. In C. E. Schaefer, L. Johnson, & J. N. Wherry (Eds.), *Group therapies for children and youth.* San Francisco: Jossey-Bass.

Speltz, M. L., Varley, C. K., Peterson, K., & Beilke, R. L. (1987). Effects of dextroamphetamine and contingency management on a preschooler with ADHD and oppositional defiant disorder. *Journal of the American Academy of Child Psychiatry, 27,* 175–178.

Spinetta, J., & Rigler, D. (1972). The child-abusing parent: A psychological review. *Psychological Bulletin, 77,* 296–304.

Spinner, D., & Pfeifer, G. (1986). Group psychotherapy with ego impaired children: The significance of peer group culture in the evolution of a holding environment. *International Journal of Group Psychotherapy, 36,* 427–446.

Spitz, R. A., & Wolf, K. M. (1946). Autoerotism: Some empirical findings and hypotheses on three of its manifestations in the first year of life. *Psychoanalytic Study of the Child, 2,* 313–342.

Spitzer, R. L., Endicott, J., & Robins, E. (1978). Research diagnostic criteria: Rationale and reliability. *Archives of General Psychiatry, 35,* 773–782.

Spreen, O. (1981). The relationship between learning disability, neurological impairment, and delinquency. *Journal of Nervous and Mental Disorders, 169,* 791–799.

Stanley, E. J., & Barter, J. T. (1970). Adolescent suicidal behavior. *American Journal of Orthopsychiatry, 40,* 87–96.

Starfield, S. B. (1967). Functional bladder capacity in enuretic and non-enuretic children. *Journal of Pediatrics, 70,* 777–781.

Staub, E. (1971). The learning and unlearning of aggression. In J. L. Singer (Ed.), *The control of aggression and violence* (pp. 93–124). New York: Academic.

Stayton, J., Ainsworth, M. D. S., & Main, M. B. (1973). Development of separation behavior in the first year of life: Protest, following, and greeting. *Developmental Psychology, 9,* 213–225.

Steele, B. F. (1983). The effect of abuse and neglect on psychological development. In J. D. Call, E. Galenson, & R. L. Tyson (Eds.), *Frontiers of infant psychiatry* (pp. 103–147). Chicago: University of Chicago Press.

Stein, H. F. (1985a). The ebb and flow of the clinical relationship. In H. F. Stein & M. Apprey (Eds.), *Series in ethnicity, medicine, and psychoanalysis: Vol. I. Context and dynamics in clinical knowledge* (pp. 211–220). Charlottesville: University Press of Virginia.

Stein, H. F. (1985b). Physician self-insight as a tool of patient care: A case study of behavioral science supervision in family medicine. In H. F. Stein & M. Apprey (Eds.), *Series in ethnicity, medicine, and psychoanalysis: Vol. I. Context and dynamics in clinical knowledge* (pp. 56–77). Charlottesville: University Press of Virginia.

Stein, H. F. (1985c). Whatever happened to countertransference? The subjective in medicine. In H. F. Stein & M. Apprey (Eds.), *Series in ethnicity, medicine, and psychoanalysis: Vol. I. Context and dynamics in clinical knowledge* (pp. 1–55). Charlottesville: University Press of Virginia.

Stewart, M. A., DeBlois, C. S., & Cummings, C. (1980). Psychiatric disorder in the parents of hyperactive boys and those with conduct disorder. *Journal of Child Psychology and Psychiatry, 21*(4), 283–292.

Stone, G. (1965). The play of little children. *Quest, 4,* 23–31.

Straker, N. (1979b). Impulse and conduct disorders. In M. M. Joseph & R. T. Porter (Eds.), *Clinician's handbook of childhood psychopathology* (pp. 351–363). New York: Jason Aronson.

Straker, P. D. (1979a). Effects of assertion training and social skills training on self-esteem and self-assertion in educable and trainable non-institutionalized mentally retarded adults. *Dissertation Abstracts International, 39*(12–B), 6103.

Strayer, J. (1980). A naturalistic study of empathic behaviors and their relation to affective states and perspective-taking skills in preschool children. *Child Development, 51,* 815–822.

Strayhorn, J. M. (1987). Medical assessment of children with behavioral problems. In M. Hersen & V. B. Van Hasselt (Eds.), *Behavior therapy with children: A clinical approach* (pp. 50–74). New York: Wiley.

Stroh, K., Robinson, T., & Stroh, G. (1986). A therapeutic feeding programme. I: Theory and practice of feeding. *Developmental Medicine & Child Neurology, 28,* 3–10.

Strosahl, K. D., & Ascough, J. C. (1981). Clinical uses of mental imagery: Experimental foundations, theoretical misconceptions, and research issues. *Psychological Bulletin, 89,* 422–438.

Stutsman, R. (1931). *Mental measurement of preschool children.* New York: World Books.

Sullivan, H. S. (1953). *The interpersonal theory of psychiatry.* New York: Norton.

Suomi, S. J., Collins, H. L., & Harlow, H. F. (1976). Effects of maternal and peer separations on young monkeys. *Journal of Child Psychology and Psychiatry, 17,* 101–112.

Susman, R. N., Trickett, P. K., Iannotti, R. J., Hollenbeck, B. S., & Zahn-Waxler, C. (1985). Child-rearing patterns in depressed, abusive, and normal mothers. *American Journal of Orthopsychiatry, 55,* 237–251.

Suter, B. (1976). Suicide and women. In B. B. Wolman (Ed.), *Between survival and suicide.* New York: Gardner Press.

Sutton-Smith, B. (1979). The play of girls. In C. B. Kopp & M. Kirkpatrick (Eds.), *Becoming female: Perspectives on development.* New York: Plenum.

Taitz, L. S., Wales, J. K. H., Urwin, O. M., & Molnar, D. (1986). Factors associated with outcome in management of defecation disorders. *Archives of Disease in Childhood, 61,* 472–477.

Tamer, S. K., Warey, P., Swarnkar, J. S., & Tamer, U. (1986). Pica in children. *Indian Journal of Pediatrics, 53,* 821–823.

Tauber, M. A. (1979). Parental socialization techniques and sex differences in children's play. *Child Development, 50,* 225–234.

Tavormina, J. B. (1975). Relative effectiveness of behavioral and reflective group counseling with parents of mentally retarded children. *Journal of Consulting and Clinical Psychology, 43,* 22–31.

Taylor, R. L., & Warren, S. A. (1984). Educational and psychological assessment of children with learning disorders. *Pediatric Clinics of North America, 31,* 281–297.

Tennant, C., Bebbington, P., & Hurry, J. (1980). Parental death in childhood and risk of adult depressive disorders: A review. *Psychological Medicine, 10,* 289–299.

Tennen, H., & Eller, S. J. (1977). Attributional components of learned helplessness and facilitation. *Journal of Personality and Social Psychology, 35*(4), 265–271.

Tennes, K., & Carter, D. (1973). Plasma cortisol levels and behavioral states in early infancy. *Psychosomatic Medicine, 35*(2), 121–128.

Tennes, K., Downey, K., & Vernadakis, A. (1977). Urinary cortisol excretion rates and anxiety in normal 1-year-old infants. *Psychosomatic Medicine, 39*(3), 178–187.

Tennes, K., Kreye, M., Avitable, N., & Wells, R. (1986). Behavioral correlates of excreted catecholamines and cortisol in second-grade children. *Journal of the American Academy of Child Psychiatry, 25,* 764–770.

Tennes, K., & Lampl, E. E. (1969). Defensive reactions to infantile separation anxiety. *Journal of the American Psychoanalytic Association, 17,* 1142–1162.

Terr, L. C. (1979). Children of Chowchilla. *The Psychosomatic Study of the Child, 34,* 552–632.

Terr, L. C. (1981). Psychic trauma in children: Observations following the Chowchilla school-bus kidnapping. *American Journal of Psychiatry, 138*(1), 14–19.

Terr, L. C. (1983). Chowchilla revisited: The effects of psychic trauma four years after a school-bus kidnapping. *American Journal of Psychiatry, 140,* 1543–1550.

Thomas, A., & Chess, S. (1984). Genesis and evolution of behavior disorders: From infancy to early adult life. *American Journal of Psychiatry, 141,* 1–9.

Thomas, A., Chess, S., & Birch, H. G. (1968). *Temperament and behavior disorders.* New York: New York University Press.

Thomas, A., Chess, S., Birch, H. G., Hertzig, M. E., & Korn, S. (1963). *Behavioral individuality in early childhood.* New York: New York University Press.

Thoren, P., Asberg, M., Cronholm, B., Jornestedt, L., & Traskman, L. (1980). Clomipramine treatment of obsessive-compulsive disorder: I. A controlled clinical trial. *Archives of General Psychiatry, 37,* 1281–1285.

Tinbergen, E. A., & Tinbergen, N. (1972). Early childhood autism: An ethological approach. *Advances in Ethology (Journal of Comparative Ethology,* Suppl.), 1–53.

Tinbergen, N. A. (1974). Ethology and stress diseases. *Science, 185,* 20–28.

Toolan, J. M. (1962). Suicide and suicidal attempts in children and adolescents. *American Journal of Psychiatry, 118,* 719–724.

Torgensen, A. M. (1981). Genetic factors in temperamental individuality. *Journal of the American Academy of Child Psychiatry, 20*(1–4), 702–711.

Torgensen, A. M., & Kringlen, E. (1978). Genetic aspects of temperamental differences in infants. *Journal of the American Academy of Child Psychiatry, 17,* 433–444.

Torgeson, J. K. (1977). The role of nonspecific factors in the test performance of learning disabled children: A theoretical assessment. *Journal of Learning Disabilities, 10,* 33–40.

Toseland, R., & Rivas, R. (1984). *An introduction to group work practice.* New York: Macmillan.

Toseland, R. W., & Siporin, M. (1986). When to recommend group treatment: A review of the clinical and the research literature. *International Journal of Psychotherapy, 36*(2), 171–201.

Tower, R. B., & Singer, J. L. (1981). The measurement of imagery: How can it be clinically useful? In P. C. Kendall & S. Hollon (Eds.), *Assessment methods for cognitive-behavioral interventions* (pp. 265–281). New York: Academic.

Trad, P. (1986). *Infant depression: Paradigms and paradoxes.* New York: Springer-Verlag.

Trad, P. (1987). *Infant and childhood depression: Developmental factors.* New York: Wiley.

Trad, P. (1988). *Psychosocial scenarios for pediatrics.* New York: Springer-Verlag.

Traskman, L., Asberg, M., Bertilsson, L., & Sjostrand, L. (1981). Monamine metabolites in cerebrospinal fluid and suicidal behavior. *Archives of General Psychiatry, 38,* 631.

Troy, M., & Sroufe, L. A. (1987). Victimization among preschoolers: Role of attachment relationship history. *Child and Adolescent Psychiatry, 26,* 166–172.

Turner-Boutle, T. (1984). School phobia. *Nursing Times, 11,* 55–58.

Tyson, R. L., & Tyson, P. (1986). The concept of transference in child psychoanalysis. *Journal of the American Academy of Child Psychiatry, 25*(1), 30–39.

Ungerer, J. A., & Sigman, M. (1981). Symbolic play and language comprehension in autistic children. *Journal of the American Academy of Child Psychiatry, 20,* 318–337.

Ungerer, J. A., Zelazo, P. R., Kearsley, R. B., & O'Leary, K. (1981). Developmental changes in the representation of objects in symbolic play from 18 to 34 months of age. *Child Development, 52,* 186–195.

Urban Institute. (1980). *The subtle revolution: Women at work.* Washington, DC: Author.

Uzgiris, I. E., & Hunt, J. M. (1975). *Assessment in infancy: Ordinal scales of psychologic development.* Urbana: University of Illinois Press.

Valman, H. B. (1987). Sleep problems. *British Medical Journal, 294,* 828–830.

Van Praag, H. M. (1986). Biological suicide research: Outcome and limitations. *Biological Psychiatry, 21,* 1305–1323.

Van Praag, H. M., & de Haan, S. (1980). Depression vulnerability and 5-hydroxotryptophan prophylaxis. *Psychiatry Research, 3,* 75–83.

Vandenberg, B. (1978). Play and development from an ethological perspective. *American Psychologist, 33,* 724–738.

Varley, C. K. (1984). Attention deficit disorder (the hyperactivity syndrome): A review of selected issues. *Journal of Developmental and Behavioral Pediatrics, 5*(5), 254–258.

Vaughan, C. E., & Leff, J. P. (1976a). The influence of family and social factors on the course of psychiatric illness: A comparison of schizophrenic and depressed neurotic patients. *British Journal of Psychiatry, 129,* 125–137.

Vaughan, C. E., & Leff, J. P. (1976b). The measurement of expressed emotion in the families of psychiatric patients. *British Journal of Social Clinical Psychology, 15,* 157–165.

Vaughn, B. E., Kopp, C. B., & Krakow, J. B. (1984). The emergence and consolidation of self-control from eighteen to thirty months of age: Normative trends and individual differences. *Child Development, 55,* 990–1004.

Verhulst, F. C. (1984). Diagnosing borderline children. *Acta Paedopsychiatrica, 50,* 161–173.

Volavka, J., Mallya, A., Baig, S., & Perez-Cruet, J. (1977). Nalaxone in chronic schizophrenia. *Science, 196,* 1227.

Volkmar, F. R., & Cohen, D. J. (1986). Current concepts: Infantile autism and the pervasive developmental disorders. *Journal of Developmental and Behavioral Pediatrics, 7,* 324–329.

Volkmar, F. R., Stier, D. M., & Cohen, D. J. (1985). Age of recognition of pervasive developmental disorder. *American Journal of Psychiatry, 142,* 1450–1452.

Vygotsky, L. (1962). *Thought and language.* Cambridge, MA: MIT Press.

Vygotsky, L. (1966). Play and its role in the mental development of the child. *Voprosy psikhologii, 12*(6), 62–76.

Vygotsky, L. (1967). Play and its role in the mental development of the child. *Soviet Psychology, 5,* 6–18.

Waelder, R. (1933). The psychoanalytical theory of play. *Psychoanalytic Quarterly, 2,* 208–224.

Waldrop, M. F., Bell, R. D., McLaughlin, B., & Halverson, C. F. (1978). Newborn minor physical anomalies predict short attention-span, peer aggression and impulsivity at age 3. *Science, 199,* 563–565.

Waldrop, M. F., & Halverson, C. F. (1975). Intensive and extensive peer behavior: Longitudinal and cross-sectional analyses. *Child Development, 46,* 19–26.

Walker, E., & Emory, E. (1983). Infants at risk for psychopathology: Offspring of schizophrenic parents. *Child Development, 54,* 1269–1285.

Wallace, J. L. (1988). The relationship between attention problems in childhood and antisocial behavior eight years later. *Journal of Child Psychology and Psychiatry and Allied Disciplines, 29*(1), 53–61.

Wallace, J. R., Cunningham, T. F., & Del Monte, V. (1984). Changes in the relationship between self-esteem and locus of control. *Journal of Social Psychology, 124,* 261–262.

Wallace, J. R., & Fonte, M. E. (1984). Piagetian and information processing approaches to concepts of chance and probability: Relationships among methods, age, and locus of control. *Journal of Genetic Psychology, 144,* 185–194.

Wallander, J. L. (1988). The relationship between attention problems in childhood and antisocial behavior eight years later. *Journal of Child Psychology and Psychiatry and Allied Sciences, 29,* 53–61.

Wallerstein, J. S. (1984). Children of divorce: Preliminary report of a ten-year follow-up of young children. *American Journal of Orthopsychiatry, 54,* 444–458.

Wallerstein, J. S., & Kelly, J. B. (1976). The effects of parental divorce: Experiences of the child in later latency. *American Journal of Orthopsychiatry, 46,* 256–259.

Wallerstein, J. S., & Kelly, J. B. (1980). Effects of divorce on the visiting father-child relationship. *American Journal of Psychiatry, 137,* 1534–1538.

Walsh, J. K., Sugerman, J. L., & Chambers, G. W. (1986). Evaluation of insomnia. *American Family Physician, 33*(4), 185–194.

Wasserman, A. L., Whitington, P. F., & Rivara, F. P. (1988). Psychogenic basis for abdominal pain in children and adolescents. *Journal of the American Academy of Child and Adolescent Psychiatry, 27,* 179–184.

Watson, B. U., Watson, C. S., & Fredd, R. (1982). Follow-up studies of specific reading disability. *Journal of the American Academy of Child Psychiatry, 21*(4), 376–382.

Watson, D. C., Katz, K., & Shepherd, M. (1983). The natural history of schizophrenia: A 5-year prospective follow-up of a representative sample of schizophrenics by means of a standardized clinical and social assessment. *Psychological Medicine, 13,* 663–670.

Watson, M. W., & Fischer, K. W. (1977). A developmental sequence of agent use in late infancy. *Child Development, 48,* 828–836.

Watt, D. C., Katz, K., & Shepherd, M. (1983). The natural history of schizophrenia: A 5-year prospective follow-up of a representative sample of schizophrenics by means of a standardized clinical and social assessment. *Psychological Medicine, 13,* 663–670.

Wechsler, D. (1949). *Manual: Weschler Intelligence Scale for Children.* New York: Psychological Corporation.

Weil, A. A. (1956). Ictal depression and anxiety in temporal lobe disorders. *American Journal of Psychiatry, 113,* 149–157.

Weiner, H. (1977). *Psychobiology and human disease.* New York: Elsevier.

Weiner, H. (1985). Schizophrenia: Etiology. In H. I. Kaplan & B. J. Sadock (Eds.), *Comprehensive textbook of psychiatry* (Vol. 1, 4th ed., pp. 1121–1153). Baltimore: Williams & Wilkins.

Weintraub, M., & Lewis, M. (1977). The determinants of children's responses to separation. *Monographs of the Society for Research in Child Development, 42*(4, Serial No. 172).

Weiss, J. M., Glazer, H. I., Pohorecky, L. A., Bailey, W. H., & Schneider, L. H. (1979). Coping behavior and stress-induced behavioral depression: Studies of the role of brain catecholamines. In R. A. Depue (Ed.), *The psychobiology of the depressive disorders: Implications for the effects of stress* (pp. 125–160). New York: Academic.

Weissman, A., & Worden, W. (1972) Risk-rescue rating in suicide assessment. *Archives of General Psychiatry, 26,* 553–560.

Weissman, M. M., Merikangas, K. R., Wickramaratne, P., Kidd, K. K., Prusoff, B. A., Leckman, J. F., & Pauls, D. L. (1986). Understanding the clinical heterogeneity of major depression using family data. *Archives of General Psychiatry, 43*(5), 430–434.

Weller, E. B., Weller, R. A., Fristad, M. A., & Preskorn, S. H. (1984). The dexamethasone suppression test in hospitalized prepubertal depressed children. *American Journal of Psychiatry, 141,* 290–291.

Werner, H., & Kaplan, B. (1963). *Symbol formation.* New York: Wiley.

Werry, J. S. (1986). Diagnosis and assessment. In R. Gittelman (Ed.), *Anxiety disorders of childhood* (pp. 73–100). New York: Guilford.

Werry, J. S., Reeves, J. C., & Elkind, G. S. (1987). Attention deficit, conduct, oppositional, and anxiety disorders in children: I. A review of research on differentiating characteristics. *Journal of the American Academy of Child and Adolescent Psychiatry, 26,* 133–143.

Weschler, D. (1967). *Manual for the Weschler Preschool and Primary Scale of Intelligence.* New York: Psychological Corporation.

Weschler, D. (1974). *Manual for the Weschler Intelligence Scale for Children–Revised.* New York: Psychological Corporation.

West, E. D., & Dally, P. J. (1959). Effect of iproniazid in depressive syndromes. *British Medical Journal, 1,* 1491–1494.

Whitam, F. L. (1977). Childhood indicators of male homosexuality. *Archives of Sexual Behavior, 6*(2), 89–96.

White, S. H. (1965). Evidence for a hierarchical arrangement of learning processes. In L. P. Lipsitt & C. C. Cpiker (Eds.), *Advances in child development and behavior* (Vol. 2). New York: Academic.

Whitehill, M., DeMyer, G. S., & Scott, T. J. (1976). Stimulation seeking in antisocial preadolescent children. *Journal of Abnormal Psychology, 85*(1), 101–104.

Whiting, B., & Edwards, C. P. (1973). A cross-cultural analysis of sex differences in the behavior of children aged three through 11. *The Journal of Social Psychology, 91,* 171–188.

Wilk, S., & Watson, W. (1973). VMA in spinal fluid: Evaluation of the pathways of cerebral catecholamine metabolism in man. In E. Usdin & S. Snyder (Eds.), *Frontiers in catecholamine research* (pp. 1067–1069). New York: Plenum.

Wilkins, W. (1974). Parameters of therapeutic imagery: Directions from case studies. *Psychotherapy: Theory, Research, and Practice, 11*(2), 163–171.

Williams, C., Sale, I., & Wignall, A. (1977), Correlates of impulsive suicidal behaviors. *New Zealand Medical Journal, 85,* 323–325.

Williams, D. T., Pleak, R., & Hanesian, H. (1987). Neuropsychiatric disorders of childhood and adolescence. In R. E. Hales & S. C. Yudofsky (Eds.), *Textbook of neuropsychiatry.* Washington, DC: American Psychiatric Press.

Willock, B. (1983). Play therapy with the aggressive, acting-out child. In C. E. Schaefer and K. J. O'Connor (Eds.), *Handbook of play therapy* (pp. 386–411). New York: Wiley.

Windle, M., Hooker, K., Lenerz, K., East, P. L., Lerner, J. V., & Lerner, R. M. (1986). Temperament, perceived competence, and depression in early and late adolescents. *Developmental Psychology, 22,* 384–392.

Wing, L., & Gould, J. (1979). Severe impairments of social interaction and associated abnormalities in children: Epidemiology and classification. *Journal of Autism and Development Disorders, 9*(1), 11–29.

Wing, L., Gould, J., Yeates, S., & Brierley, L. (1977). Symbolic play in severely mentally retarded and in autistic children. *Journal of Child Psychology and Psychiatry, 18,* 167–178.

Winnicott, D. W. (1949). Hate in the counter-transference. *International Journal of Psycho-Analysis, 30,* 69–74.

Winnicott, D. W. (1965). *The maturational processes and the facilitating environment.* London: Hogarth.

Winnicott, D. W. (1971). *Playing and reality.* London: Tavistock.

Wolfenstein, M. (1966). How is mourning possible? *Psychoanalytic Study of the Child, 21,* 93–123.

Wolff, S. (1961). Social and family background of pre-school children with behaviour disorders attending a child guidance clinic. *Journal of Child Psychology and Psychiatry,* 260–268.

Wolfson, J., Fields, J. H., & Rose, S. A. (1987). Symptoms, temperament, resiliency, and control in anxiety-disordered preschool children. *Journal of the American Academy of Child and Adolescent Psychiatry, 26,* 16–22.

Woltmann, A. G. (1964). Concepts of play therapy techniques. In M. R. Haworth (Ed.), *Child psychotherapy* (pp. 35–51). New York: Basic Books.

Woodcock, R. W., & Johnson, L. (1977). *Woodcock-Johnson Psychoeducational Battery.* Boston: Teaching Resources.

Woodward, M., & Stern, D. (1963). Developmental patterns of severely subnormal children. *British Journal of Educational Psychology, 33,* 10–21.

Woolston, J. L. (1983). Eating disorders in infancy and early childhood. *Journal of the American Academy of Child Psychiatry, 22*(2), 114–121.

Wulff, S. B. (1985). The symbolic and object play of children with autism: A review. *Journal of Autism and Development Disorders, 15*(2), 139–148.

Wynne, L. C. (1978). Family interaction: An alternative starting point for evaluating risk of psychosis. In E. J. Anthony, C. Koupernik & C. Chiland (Eds.), *The child in his family* (pp. 293–302). New York: Wiley.

Yalom, I. (1975). *The theory and practice of group psychotherapy.* New York: Basic Books.

Yanaihara, T., & Arai, K. (1981). In vitro release of steroids from the fetal adrenal tissue. *Acta Obstetricia et Gynocologica Scandinavica, 60,* 225–228.

Yates, F. E., & Maran, J. D. (1974). Stimulation and inhibition of adrenocorticotropin release. In E. Knobil & W. Saywer (Eds.), *Handbook of physiology: Section 7, Endocrinology: Vol. 4. The pituitary gland, Part 2.* Washington, DC: American Physiological Society.

Young, D. E., & Young, R. R. (1985). Nocturnal enuresis: A review of treatment approaches. *American Family Physician, 31*(3), 141–144.

Young, M., Benjamin, B., & Wallis, C. Mortality of widowers. *Lancet, 2,* 454.

Zachry, W. (1978). Ordinality and interdependence of representation and language development in infancy. *Child Development, 49,* 681–687.

Zahn-Waxler, C., Cummings, E. M., McKnew, D. H., Jr., & Radke-Yarrow, M. (1984). Altruism, aggression, and social interactions in young children with a manic-depressive parent. *Child Development, 55,* 112–122.

Zahn-Waxler, C., & Radke-Yarrow, M. (1982). The development of altruism: Alternative research strategies. In N. Eisenberg-Berg (Ed.), *The development of prosocial behavior* (pp. 109–137). New York: Academic.

Zalba, S. (1971). Battered children. *Transaction, 8,* 68–61.

Zeligs, R. (1967). Children's attitudes toward death. *Mental-Hygiene, 51,* 393–396.

Ziegler, R., & Holden, L. (1988). Family therapy for learning disabled and attention-deficit disordered children. *American Journal of Orthopsychiatry, 58,* 196–210.

Zimrin, H. (1986). A profile of survival. *Child Abuse and Neglect, 10,* 339–349.

Zohar, J., Mueller, E. A., Insel, T. R., Zohar-Kadouch, R. C., & Murphy, D. L. (1987). Serotonergic responsivity in obsessive-compulsive disorder. *Archives of General Psychiatry, 44,* 946–951.

Author Index

282, 286, 312, 325, 363, 369, 377, 392, 394, 398, 399, 444, 445, 446, 447, 450, 452, 459, 461, 462, 467, 471, 481, 483, 497, 524, 621
Traskman, L., 142, 145, 150, 169, 567, 621
Traskman-Bendz, L., 173, 567
Trautman, P., 61, 615
Trevathan, G. E., 354, 355–356, 595
Trickett, P. K., 448, 620
Tricou, B., 145, 157, 158, 602
Tricou, B. J., 156, 582
Troy, M., 452, 622
Trupin, E. W., 45, 598
Tsuang, M., 321, 571
Tsuang, M. T., 199, 595
Turgeon, V., 21, 598
Turnbull, C. D., 263, 580
Turner-Boutle, T., 300, 622
Twentyman, C. T., 449, 572
Twitchell, T. E., 132, 612
Tyson, P., 506, 622
Tyson, R. L., 506, 622

Ullman, R. K., 326, 617
Ungerer, J., 206, 616
Ungerer, J. A., 22, 117, 193, 622
Urban Institute, 471, 622
Urwin, O. M., 340, 620
Uzgiris, I. E., 132, 622

Valman, H. B., 351, 622
Vance, G., 589
Vandenberg, B., 92, 104, 105, 121, 612, 622
Vandiver, T., 430, 433, 461, 592
Van Praag, H. M., 165, 173, 175, 622
Van Wettere, J. P., 168, 599
Varley, C. K., 311, 540, 550, 618, 622
Varpila-Hansson, R., 173, 567
Vaughan, C. E., 622
Vaughn, B. E., 51, 428, 622
Vega-Lahr, N., 583
Verhulst, F. C., 236, 249, 250, 251, 622
Vernadakis, A., 161, 620
Vernon, J. C., 533, 611
Virkkunen, M., 165, 170, 599
Vitulano, L. A., 214, 592
Vogel, N. G., 236, 242, 567
Volavka, J., 149, 622
Volkmar, F. R., 187, 200, 622
Volmar, F. R., 182, 578
Volterra, V., 67, 113, 114, 117, 569
Vygotsky, L., 93, 111, 120, 622, 623

Wachtel, R. C., 190, 575
Waelder, R., 92, 493, 623
Wahlstrom, A., 146, 566
Waldo, M. C., 148, 584
Waldrop, M. F., 66, 313, 623
Wales, J. K. H., 340, 620
Walker, A., 472, 570
Walker, D. K., 314, 322, 606
Walker, E., 49, 50, 623
Wall, S., 299, 566
Wallace, J. L., 623
Wallace, J. R., 275, 623

Wallander, J. L., 320, 623
Wallerstein, J., 249, 581
Wallerstein, J. S., 469, 470, 479, 623
Wallis, C., 146, 626
Walsh, J. K., 350, 623
Walton, L. A., 270, 594
Warey, P., 365, 620
Warren, S. A., 118, 620
Wasserman, A. L., 393–394, 623
Watchel, R. C., 213, 231, 616
Waternaux, C., 321, 571
Waters, E., 299, 566
Watson, B. U., 213, 214, 623
Watson, C. S., 213, 214, 623
Watson, D. C., 623
Watson, K. S., 93, 612
Watson, M. W., 106, 624
Watson, W., 165, 625
Watt, D. C., 267, 624
Wechsler, D., 131, 132, 624
Weed, K. A., 255, 269, 270, 613
Wehr, T. A., 262, 263, 611
Weil, A. A., 624
Weiner, A., 174, 447, 606
Weiner, H., 146, 148, 151, 159, 160, 397, 592, 596, 624
Weinstein, P., 348, 356, 567
Weintraub, M., 299, 624
Weishahn, M. W., 209, 586
Weiss, J. M., 147, 624
Weiss, S., 507, 510, 596
Weissman, A., 433, 624
Weissman, M. M., 43, 46, 604, 624
Weitzman, E., 164, 357, 608
Weller, E. B., 157, 624
Weller, R. A., 157, 624
Wells, D., 108, 616
Wells, R., 159, 620
Werble, B., 235, 589
Werner, H., 13, 114, 624
Werry, J. S., 151, 153, 281, 300, 301, 303, 309, 321, 326, 405, 575, 608, 609, 624
Weschler, D., 624
West, E. D., 263, 624
Wetstone, H., 191, 584
Wherry, J. N., 562, 614
Whitam, F. L., 417, 418, 625
White, S. H., 19, 625
Whitehill, M., 310, 625
Whiting, B., 62, 63, 64, 65, 625
Whitington, P. F., 393–394, 623
Whittinghill, J. R., 435, 436, 615
Wickramaratne, P., 43, 624
Wignall, A., 428, 625
Wikenheiser, M., 383, 385, 574
Wilcox, S. A., 112, 584
Wilk, S., 165, 625
Wilkins, W., 504, 625
Williams, C., 428, 625
Williams, D. T., 377, 378–379, 625
Williams, S., 270, 354, 355, 356, 358, 577, 594
Willock, B., 116, 119, 120, 625
Windle, M., 455, 625
Wing, J. F., 51, 573
Wing, L., 117, 185, 202, 625

Subject Index